Developmental Psychopathology

Jim Stevenson

Developmental Psychopathology

Concepts, Methods, and Findings

Springer

Jim Stevenson
University of Southampton
Southampton, UK

ISBN 978-3-031-45786-9 ISBN 978-3-031-45787-6 (eBook)
https://doi.org/10.1007/978-3-031-45787-6

This Springer imprint is published by the registered company Springer Nature Switzerland AG
The registered company address is: Gewerbestrasse 11, 6330 Cham, Switzerland

Jim Stevenson

Developmental Psychopathology

Concepts, Methods, and Findings

Springer

Jim Stevenson
University of Southampton
Southampton, UK

ISBN 978-3-031-45786-9 ISBN 978-3-031-45787-6 (eBook)
https://doi.org/10.1007/978-3-031-45787-6

This Springer imprint is published by the registered company Springer Nature Switzerland AG
The registered company address is: Gewerbestrasse 11, 6330 Cham, Switzerland

Paper in this product is recyclable.

I dedicate this book to Pam with love.

Preface

In 1977, Mike Rutter and Lionel Hersov edited the First Edition of what has become the definitive textbook in child psychiatry – *Child Psychiatry: Modern Approaches.* The latest Sixth Edition published in 2015 is titled *Rutter's Child and Adolescent Psychiatry.* A textbook published now in the 2020s and presenting "modern approaches" would have to cover a range of concepts and methods that would be radically different from those in 1977. These subsequent 50 odd years have seen the development of major advances in the conceptualisation of child psychological problems, in the multivariate analysis of data sets, in the study of the structure and function of the brain and in the investigation of genetic influences. In 1977, the majority readers of the Rutter and Hersov textbook would have been able to understand and appraise most of the methods and findings being referred to and published in journals such as the *Journal of Child Psychology and Psychiatry*. Today the picture has been totally transformed. Most of the readers of the Sixth Edition would struggle to critically evaluate the primary research material being presented in such journals. The present book has been written with the aim of providing a guide as to what issues such research studies are addressing and to the methods that are being applied.

The scientific approach adopted in the studies being covered here is that of developmental psychopathology. This attempts to explain the origin of behavioural differences in terms of the interplay between genetic factors and experiences. It is a feature of studies in developmental psychopathology that an understanding of the origins of behaviour is best considered as being on a continuum with variations in the normal range. The term psychopathology does not mean that the children being studied are seen as having disorders. The framework has a focus on individual differences in behaviour in the population. However, at the extreme these behaviours may cause problems for the child and/or the family and thereby warrant the attention of clinical psychologists and psychiatrists.

The motivation for writing this book on developmental psychopathology came from two main sources. The first is my interest in the question "Why are children in the same family so different from one another?". This is what fascinates parents – particularly parents with more than one child. Brothers and sisters share a lot of experiences in common but behave very differently. This question just so happens to be the title of a landmark paper by Robert Plomin and Denise Daniels which is discussed in Sect. 3.1. The origin of differences between children is to my mind just the most engaging scientific enquiry. The second motivation is that this area of science has made such major advances in the past few decades that this progress presents a challenge to the interested reader. In each case, the methods used in these field are of a sophistication and technical complexity that it is daunting for the non-specialist to feel competent to appraise the studies using these methods. This challenge is exacerbated by two further factors. First is the multidisciplinary nature of much of this research. This is exemplified by the move to combine an examination of molecular genetics with studies of brain imaging. Second is the development of international collaborations to provide very large data sets by pooling measures from different studies. This has raised the possibility of applying esoteric methods from machine learning, artificial intelligence, and deep learning to "mine" the data. My hope is that the book can provide a guide to these advances that include the fields of psychometrics, statistics, brain imaging, and genetics.

The above examples are of ways in which developments in the study of behavioural differences have been driven by technologies. But there have also been advances in conceptualisation and theory. These can best be illustrated by two examples: the first is the advance in analysis of data from epidemiological studies and the second is the development of dimensional frameworks for understanding psychological problems.

My involvement with studies on behaviour in the young child originated in an epidemiological study in collaboration with Naomi Richman and Philip Graham at the Great Ormond Street Hospital for Children, London. The culmination of this work was the publication of a monograph summarising one of the first studies to systematically survey problems of emotion and behaviour problems in a large sample of preschool children from the general population – the Waltham Forest Study. This is an example of an epidemiology study which was concerned to establish prevalence rates and risk factors from associations found in the general population – a descriptive study. The conceptual and data analysis tools available for epidemiology studies have subsequently changed beyond recognition. The core of these changes are developments in research design and data analysis to provide more adequate tests of causality. Epidemiology is largely constrained to be a non-experimental science (but see Sect. 4.2 on natural experiments). Consequently, it has to rely on associations measured by correlations or relative risks, which by themselves do not demonstrate causality. This becomes crucial if epidemiology is to be used to inform interventions on either social or health issues. If these interventions are not directed at a causal factor, they are likely to fail. The developments in epidemiology to attempt to establish causality are discussed in Chap. 4.

The second conceptual advance concerns dimensional frameworks for understanding psychological problems. These will have a profound impact on both the study of behavioural differences but also in the way in which extremes of behaviour should be understood. Historically these extremes of behaviour have been conceptualised as distinction diagnostic categories of psychiatric disorder. There has been a longstanding challenge to this view from those who see these dysfunctional behaviours as extremes of individual differences that extend across the normal range. This latter view, that psychiatric disorders are on a continuum of behavioural variation, has come to maturity since the millennium. In parallel, there has been a realisation that what have been seen as distinct diagnoses or dimensions actually have a lot in common. These continua of behavioural variation are strongly associated with one another. These conceptual developments have come to radically reframe the questions addressed in research and the way treatment and interventions are planned.

These issues are clearly laid out by Ben Lahey in his 2021 book *Dimensions of Psychological Problems*. He argues that behaviour varies by degree rather than in qualitative differences and that problems in psychological functioning should be considered as extensions of normal experiences, which are exacerbated to different degrees by the interplay between genetic and environmental influences. In the main, psychological problems lie on a continuum of severity that arise from individual differences in normal psychological processes rather than from psychiatric illnesses or diseases of the mind. He argues that the adoption of such an orientation should reduce the stigmatisation that so often accompanies psychological problems.

My hope is that by reviewing both the concepts and methods adopted to study behavioural differences in children and some of the main findings, I can provide a bridge for the reader to a more detailed reading of the literature on developmental psychopathology. In a wide-ranging book of this kind, there is no scope to provide more than a rudimentary coverage of these topics. Accordingly, my aim is to give an orientation to the concepts, methods, and findings in research studies and to guide the reader as to where more detailed coverage can be accessed. For this reason, the material presented is supported by extensive references to specific related studies.

Southampton, UK Jim Stevenson

Contents

About the Author

Jim Stevenson is Emeritus Professor of Developmental Psychopathology at the University of Southampton. He has published over 200 papers in peer reviewed journals. For a decade, he served as Editor and then Senior Editor of the *Journal of Child Psychology and Psychiatry*. He has undertaken a wide range of research studies on behaviour problems in young children, hyperactivity/ADHD, language and reading development, child sexual abuse, food additives, the psychological development of children with a permanent childhood hearing loss, and on children born prematurely. A number of these research studies used twins to identify the role of genetic and environmental influences on individual differences in development.

Abbreviations

AB or ASB	Antisocial Behaviour
ABCD	Adolescent Brain Cognitive Development (study)
ACC	Anterior Cingulate Cortex
ACE	Adverse Childhood Experiences – NB the same letters are also used to refer to modelling genetic (A), shared environment (C), and non-shared environment (E) effects
ADHD	Attention-Deficit Hyperactivity Disorder
ALSPAC	Avon Longitudinal Study of Parents and Children
AL	Adolescence-Limited (antisocial behaviour)
ALT	Autoregressive Latent Trajectory (model)
ASD	Autism Spectrum Disorder
ASQ	Autism Spectrum Quotient
AUC	Area Under Curve
BAP	Broader Autistic Phenotype
BBT	Brief Behaviour Therapy
BCAA	Branched-Chain Amino Acids
BI	Behavioural Individuality
BMI	Body Mass Index
BPT	Behavioural Parent Training
BRIEF	Behavior Rating Inventory of Executive Function
BSQ	Behavioural Screening Questionnaire
BWAS	Brain Wide Association Study
c^2	Effect of shared environment
CAST	Childhood Autism Screening Test
CBCL	Child Behavior Checklist
CBT	Cognitive Behaviour Therapy
CCFI	Comparison Curve Fit Index
CD	Conduct Disorder
CFA	Confirmatory Factor Analysis
CFI	Comparative Fit Index
$CI_{.95}$	95% Confidence Interval

CLPM	Cross-Lagged Panel Model
CNV	Copy-Number Variant
CNS	Central Nervous System
CoT	Children-of-Twins (model)
CU	Callous-Unemotional
d	Cohen's d (form of SMD)
DAG	Directed Acyclic Graphs
DDA	Direction Dependence Analysis
DF	DeFries and Fulker regression method to estimate group heritability
DISC	Diagnostic Schedule for Children
DMN	Default Mode Network
DNA	Deoxyribonucleic Acid
DSM-IV	Diagnostic and Statistical Manual of Mental Disorders – Fourth Edition
DSM-5	Diagnostic and Statistical Manual of Mental Disorders – Fifth Edition
DTI	Diffusion Tensor Imaging
DZ	Dizygotic (twins)
e^2	Effect of the non-shared environment
EA	Educational Attainment
EBD	Emotional and Behavioural Difficulties
EC	Effortful control
ECOT	Extended Children-of-Twins (model)
ECBI	Eyberg Child Behavior Inventory
EEA	Equal Environments Assumption (in the twin method)
EEG	Electroencephalogram
EF	Executive Function
EFA	Exploratory Factor Analysis
ENIGMA	Enhancing NeuroImaging Genetics through MetaAnalysis Consortium
ERA	English Romanian Adoptees (study)
ERP	Event-Related Potentials
fMRI	Functional Magnetic Resonance Imaging
FSSC-R	Fear Survey Schedule for Children – Revised
g	Hedge's g (form of SMD)
GABA	Gamma-Aminobutyric Acid
GAD	Generalised Anxiety Disorder
GMV	Gray Matter Volume
GPF	General Psychopathology Factor
GWAS	Genome-Wide Association Study
GxE	Gene-Environment Interaction
h^2	Heritability
h^2_g	Group Heritability
h^2_{SNP}	SNP Heritability
HiTOP	Hierarchical Taxonomy of Psychopathology
HR	Hazard Ratio

ICD	International Classification of Disease
ITSEA	Infant-Toddler Social and Emotional Assessment
LC	Language Comprehension
LCM-SR	Latent Curve Model with Structured Residual
LCP	Life-Course-Persistent (antisocial behaviour)
LEA	Labour Epidural Analgesic
MAOA	Monoamine Oxidase A
MCOTS	Multiple-Children-of-Twins-and-Siblings (model)
MDD	Major Depressive Disorder
MEG	Magnetoencephalography
mPFC	Medial Prefrontal Cortex
MR	Mendelian Randomisation
MRI	Magnetic Resonance Imaging
MRS	Magnetic Resonance Spectroscopy
MST	Multisystemic Therapy
MTA	Multimodal Treatment Study of Children with ADHD
MZ	Monozygotic (twins)
NAA	N-acetylaspartate
NAS	Neuroimaging Association Scores
NDBI	Naturalistic Developmental Behavioural Intervention
OCD	Obsessive Compulsive Disorder
ODD	Oppositional Defiant Disorder
OR	Odds Ratio
PAE	Prenatal Alcohol Exposure
PAPA	Preschool Age Psychiatric Assessment
PBCL	Preschool Behaviour Checklist
PCHL	Permanent Childhood Hearing Loss
PRS	Polygenic Risk Scores
RDR	Relatedness Disequilibrium Regression
ROI	Regions of Interest (in the brain)
RCI	Reliable Change Index
RCT	Randomised Controlled Trial
RDoC	Research Domain Criteria (of the National Institute of Mental Health)
R-fMRI	Resting-state Functional Magnetic Resonance Imaging
RI-CLPM	Random Intercepts Cross-Lagged Panel Model
r_{GE}	Gene-Environment Correlation
RIBA	Repetitive Interests, Behaviours, and Activities
RMSEA	Root Mean Square Error of Approximation
RT	Reaction Time
SCQ	Social Communication Questionnaire
SCT	Sluggish Cognitive Tempo
SDQ	Strengths and Difficulties Questionnaire
SEM	Structural Equation Modelling
SMD	Standardised Mean Difference (see d and g)
SMFQ	Short Mood and Feelings Questionnaire

sMRI	Structural Magnetic Resonance Imaging
SN	Salience Network
SNAP-IV	Swanson, Nolan, and Pelham Questionnaire Version 4 (for ADHD)
SNP	Single Nucleotide Polymorphism
SNV	Single Nucleotide Variant
SWAN	Strengths and Weaknesses of ADHD-symptoms and Normal-behavior Scale
TAU	Treatment As Usual
TD	Typically Developing
TDCG	Typically Developing Comparison Group
TEACCH	Treatment and Education of Autistic and Related Communication Handicapped Children
TEDS	Twins Early Development Study
ToM	Theory of Mind
YSR	Youth Self Report

Chapter 1
Introduction

1.1 Overview

Some children are quiet, others noisy. Some children are apprehensive about the new, others curious. Some children are always on the go, others content to stay put. Such behavioural differences are pervasive – children differ from one another; there is variability in behaviour. This variability between children in emotions and behaviour is the starting point for the questions to be addressed in this book. For some children their behaviour and emotional reactions can become a problem for the children themselves or for their families. These problems of emotion and behaviour will be viewed here as on a continuum with variation in behaviour in children in general.

Behavioural variation has been the subject of extensive investigation and is the most active research area in child development studies. Its study has undergone revolutionary changes in the first two decades of the twenty-first century. In part this is due to emerging technologies that can address its biological origins using genetics and neuroscience, for example. There have also been less widely recognised developments in the way social influences on behavioural differences are investigated. The field of epidemiology has developed a set of study designs and methods of data analysis that move on from identifying factors that are *associated* with behavioural variation to factors that can be plausibly identified as *causes* of behavioural differences.

Many of these changes emerged before 2000, but what has been revolutionary is the way these have now come together to radically alter the design and interpretation of studies. The changes include the way studies are conducted and administered. Often to address the questions of interest, there is a need to obtain very large samples. This need is driven in part by the need to be able to detect the modest effect sizes involved, for example, in the impact of genetic variants on behaviour. In part, large samples are also needed to help address the problems that arise from

J. Stevenson, *Developmental Psychopathology*,
https://doi.org/10.1007/978-3-031-45787-6_1

heterogeneity. It is now recognised, for example, that autism spectrum disorders can arise from a number of different causes. Consequently during the twenty-first century, there have been innovations in the organisation of science to facilitate cooperation in the sharing of data between large research groups to form consortia and thereby produce pooled samples running into hundreds of thousands and even millions.

These are some of the changes and developments in the design, conduct, and analysis of research studies that constitute the twenty-first-century revolution. These are radical changes but perhaps do not yet constitute a paradigm shift in the Kuhnian sense (Sonuga-Barke, 2020). Such a paradigm shift would require an agreed consensus on how to proceed. In the field of developmental psychopathology, there is no such consensus. This is, perhaps, most strikingly illustrated by the distinction between network and latent variable models of the structure of psychopathology. This issue is addressed in Sect. 2.6.

There are some broader changes to the social context in which studies of behavioural variation are conducted, which are beyond the scope of the book. For example, there is an increasing diversity in the constitution of families (Biblarz & Savci, 2010). However the evidence reviewed by Golombok (2020) suggests that:

> the quality of family relationships and the wider social environment matter more for children's psychological wellbeing than the number, gender, sexual orientation, or biological relatedness of their parents. (Golombok, 2020, p. 743)

There are critiques that have arisen recently from the neurodiversity movement (Runswick-Cole, 2014), which has been a particular focus of studies on autism (Kapp et al., 2013) and about which there is little consensus on the terminology that should be adopted (Kenny et al., 2016). The disparate views within the autism community reflected in the neurodiversity movement create challenges for research, which Happé and Frith (2020) have outlined.

However there are areas where a consensus is being reached. It is a feature of the developments in studies of developmental psychopathology that an understanding of its origins is best considered in terms of their being on a continuum with variations in the normal range. This means that there is a complementarity between studies of behavioural variation in the general population and studies of groups showing psychopathology. How can these behavioural differences be identified? How can they be classified? How do these differences arise? How stable are these differences as children get older?

To answer these questions, it is necessary to understand how the issues are conceptualised and how methods have been developed to test them. For these reasons the details of the design, analysis, and interpretation of studies and methods of investigation are covered in Chaps. 2, 3, 4 and 5. There is a consensus that any account of behavioural variation needs to consider its hierarchical organisation and this issue is discussed in Chap. 6. It has become recognised that a wide range of psychopathologies tend to co-occur. The evidence that there is a general factor influencing psychopathology that can be found in children is appraised in this chapter. For children there are two broad continua of behavioural variation – internalising and externalising – and studies on these dimensions are considered in Chaps. 7 and 8. There are two additional behavioural dimensions on which children vary. They are attention-deficit hyperactivity disorder (ADHD) and autism, which is now classified as autism spectrum disorder (ASD). The ASD designation reflects the reconceptualisation of these disorders as being on a continuum (spectrum) that merges with variation in the normal range and arises from underlying variations neurodevelopment. The studies on ADHD and ASD are reviewed in Chaps. 9 and 10, respectively.

The emphasis on problems of emotion and behaviour in child development studies arises in part as a recognition of the extent of distress that these behaviours can cause over prolonged periods of time. Some extremes of behavioural variation can come to have adverse effects on how the child functions in relation to others in the context of the family, the peer group, and the school setting. Psychopathology is the term that is used to refer to such dysfunctional behaviour. It is a general term that describes extreme behaviour and includes child psychiatric disorders. A report by Gore et al. (2011) puts the material being covered in this book into a sobering context; they showed that in a global survey of the impact of disease on young people (10- to 24-year-olds), neuropsychiatric disorders were the main cause of "years lost to disability" – an index of the impact on quality of life. The extremes of the range of behavioural variability represent a major drain on the quality of life for children and young people.

Confusion can arise with the term "psychopathology" as there is a specific condition referred to as "psychopathy". This is behavioural tendency to show a lack of empathy, guilt, and shallow emotions (callous-unemotional traits) and antisocial behaviour. Precursors of psychopathy can be identified in young children (Viding et al., 2005) and will be discussed in Sect. 8.1. To reiterate the term psychopathology does not mean psychopathy – it is an umbrella term that refers in a more general sense, to any behaviour or emotion, which causes impairment, distress, or disability. The approach taken in the studies being covered in this book is that of developmental psychopathology.

Landmark papers by Sroufe and Rutter (1984) and Rutter and Sroufe (2000) identified the scope of developmental psychopathology. They identified two central components to the approach as follows:

> First, it is concerned with development and is therefore closely wedded to the whole of developmental psychology. The methods, theories, and perspectives of developmental psychology are important tools of inquiry. Second, the focus is on pathology, that is, developmental deviations. Developmental psychopathology may be defined as the study of the origins and course of individual patterns of behavioral maladaptation, whatever the age of onset, whatever the causes, whatever the transformations in behavioral manifestation, and however complex the course of the developmental pattern may be. (Sroufe & Rutter, 1984, p. 18)

A developmental perspective remains important in the present era of research, which examines very large data sets and which incorporates genetic information with epidemiological indicators of environmental risk (Thapar & Riglin, 2020). For example, such studies have shown that both the environmental risk factors and genetics of depression are different in childhood, adolescence, and adult life. Consequently research studies need to consider age at onset and changes over time as well as different developmental periods.

There is a real concern when discussing behaviour in the young child that normal variation may be interpreted as pathological. This dilemma was well described by Banaschewski (2010) as follows:

> Owing to the high level of behavioural variation and the enormous changes in organisation of behaviour during early childhood, the diagnostic challenge to differentiate psychopathological forms of preschool disruptive behaviour from early child temperament features and the broad range of normative misbehaviours poses a particular problem for the current psychiatric classification systems. Clinically, the question of whether, and under what circumstances, it is appropriate to apply the diagnostic category of disruptive behaviour disorder in preschool children is a crucial one. The answer should balance between the risk of over- pathologising normal behaviour in young children that represents developmentally deviant but transient manifestations of dysfunction on the one hand and the risk of missed opportunities for early recognition of clinically significant indicators for the later onset of a full-blown disorder and appropriate early intervention on the other. (Banaschewski, 2010, p. 1)

For this reason the use of the term "normal" will not be used to refer to children who do not show atypical behaviour – as this implies that children showing atypical behaviour are abnormal. Instead the term "typically developing" (TD) will be adopted to refer children who are being used for comparison purposes. Also the term "controls" should not be used routinely for these comparison groups. The term controls is only strictly appropriate when there is an experimental design, such as a randomised controlled trial, where there is random allocation to treatment and control conditions. The term "comparison group" will be adopted instead. For a discussion of the issues relating to the use of language in studies of behaviour differences, see the editorial by Patalay and MacDonald (2022) on the change of title from the *Journal of Abnormal Psychology* to the *Journal of Psychopathology and Clinical Science*.

Throughout the book there is an attempt to cover the most recent advances in concepts, methods, and data analysis, many of which are complex and increasingly make heavy demands to understand their mathematical and statistical bases. These emerging methods and technologies are described in Chap. 2. However, in describing studies the emphasis will be on the what the results mean, not on the way they are derived or calculated. Many references are provided that can be used for more detailed information for those readers wanting a more in-depth understanding of specific techniques.

When attempting to summarise findings, the burgeoning number of studies presents a challenge. It also presents a complex picture as "conclusions" from different studies often differ quite markedly. This is reflected in the "reproducibility crisis" – something that is not confined to studies on child behaviour (see Sect. 2.9 for details). To address this disparity between studies, wherever possible, reference will be made to the findings from meta-analyses that attempt to provide a quantitative synthesis of findings based on a systematic review of the research literature (see Sect. 2.7).

1.2 The Study of Variability

It is 100 years since Ronald Fisher (1919) developed the way to quantify and conceptualise variability. He also systematised the way estimates of the magnitude of genetic causes of variation in human characteristics can be calculated from information on the resemblance between family members (Fisher, 1918). As he says, in this 1918 paper, by integrating data from biometry (the measure of quantitative characteristics) with Mendelian genetics:

> It is hoped that in this way it will be possible to make a more exact analysis of the causes of human variability. (Fisher, 1918, p. 399)

Fisher has been vilified for his endorsement of eugenics (Evans, 2020), but his place as a major figure in the twenty-first-century science is assured by the work on population genetics (Fisher, 1930), statistics (Fisher, 1925), and research design (Fisher, 1935). The complexity of his personality and antagonisms with other scientists has been well described by Bodmer (2003), and Rutherford (2020) has given a valuable account of how eugenicists, such as Fisher, should be viewed. He provides the following apt conclusion:

> We cannot and should not abandon nor trash the scientific works of Galton, Fisher, and others on whose shoulders we stand. Their techniques are in constant use, for the betterment of science and all humans, and these are formidable legacies. But we can choose not to honor their names. (Rutherford, 2020, p. 4)

Individual differences and variation are the core of natural selection and of theories of evolution; selection pressures act to make some differences more common in a population and other less common. By this means, over time, populations and species change, that is, they evolve. Although Darwin (1859) did not know of the work of Mendel on inheritance, he did foresee the importance to psychology of such small differences:

> In the distant future I see open fields for far more important researches. Psychology will be based on a new foundation, that of the necessary acquirement of each mental power and capacity by gradation. (Darwin, 1859, p. 488)

Barash (1997) identified the importance of considering individual differences from the perspective of studies of human evolution and social biology. In particular he emphasised the significance of looking at variation and not just commonalities in behavioural development.

> We need a general theory of individual differences. Perhaps this is an oxymoron, since to recognize individual differences is to celebrate particularity, whereas any general theory must, by definition, submerge the individual case in a wider sea of pattern. Indeed, attention to individual differences runs the risk of being itself 'unscientific', insofar as science aims at generalizing, at raising our heads above the individual trees to recognize (and generalize about) the forest. Yet the need persists. (Barash, 1997, p. 153)

This book is about trees rather than the forest. Perhaps more correctly, this book is about saplings! While there will be a focus on behavioural variation in the young child, there cannot be a strict limit on the ages covered as studies of middle childhood and adolescence need to be considered when development is being viewed in a longitudinal perspective. There are also important questions that have not been addressed in studies of children resulting in the need to refer to research on adults.

1.3 The Nature/Nurture Question

A central strand through this book is the examination of the interplay between genes and environmental risk factors in producing behavioural variation. This has been a focus of research on behavioural variation over the last 30 years and one that is becoming more and more dominant through continuing developments in molecular genetics. However there are residual confusions about the interpretations of genetically informative studies. In a review of the nature/nurture issue, Rutter (1991) draws attention to the following popular beliefs, each of which, he says, is *mistaken*:

> that strong [genetic] effects mean that environmental influences must be unimportant; that genes provide a limit to potential; that genetic strategies are of no value for studying environmental influences; that nature and nurture are separate; that genes for serious diseases are necessarily bad; that diseases have nothing to do with normal variation; that genetic findings will not help identify diseases; that genetic influences diminish with age; that disorders that run in families must be genetic; that disorders that seem not to run in families cannot be genetic; and that single major genes lead only to specific rare diseases that follow a Mendelian pattern. (Rutter, 1991, p. 125)

A starting point for investigating gene-environment interplay is often the calculation of heritability from measures taken on twins. This calculation will be described in more detail in Sect. 3.1. Heritability is a number between 0 and 1 that estimates the proportion of the variation in a characteristic that is attributed to genetic differences between people. Patrick Bateson and Paul Martin (1999) provided a view of the development of behaviour that was highly critical of the notion of estimating heritability. They made the analogy that behavioural development was like baking:

> The processes involved in behavioural and psychological development have certain metaphorical similarities to cooking. Both the raw ingredients and the manner in which they are combined are important. Timing also matters. In the cooking analogy, the raw ingredients represent the many genetic and environmental influences, while cooking represents the biological and psychological processes of development. Nobody expects to find all the separate ingredients represented as discrete, identifiable components in a soufflé. Similarly, nobody should expect to find a simple correspondence between a particular gene (or particular experience) and a particular aspect of an individual's behaviour or personality. (Bateson & Martin, 1999, p. 9)

This position could not be more radically different from that put forward by behaviour geneticists who have followed Fisher in the estimation of heritability. This is highlighted by the heading of a section of Chap. 4 in Bateson and Martin (1999) as "The Great Blueprint Fallacy" and the contrast with a book by the behaviour geneticist Robert Plomin (2018), which is entitled "Blueprint"! The blueprint referred to here is the code in deoxyribonucleic acid (DNA) that influences behaviour.

However these two positions are not as different as it would first seem. Bateson and Martin are primarily concerned with how behaviour develops. In this sense they want to establish the causal processes that underlie the usual behavioural changes that occur with age. Robert Plomin on the other hand is concerned with individual differences in behaviour. Both Patrick Bateson and Robert Plomin recognise the essential interactions between nature and nurture underlying behavioural development. However Plomin uses methods and an analytic framework that can portion out the variance in behaviour that is attributable to nature, to nurture, and their interplay. Using Bateson's cooking analogy, Plomin is looking at whether the variation in the quality of a soufflé is determined more by the type of flour, the freshness of the eggs, or the cooking temperature. These are all essential for the soufflé to be baked, but each makes a discernible difference to the variation in the quality of the end product.

There is an ironic historical footnote to this disagreement. Patrick Bateson's grandfather's cousin was the geneticist William Bateson whose most influential book published in 1894 was entitled "Materials for the study of variation treated with especial regard to discontinuity in the origin of species". His interest was precisely the variation that was of interest to Plomin as the following quotations illustrate:

> Difficulty has hitherto arisen from the fact that Variation is not studied for its own sake. (Bateson, 1894, p. vii)

> For though on the whole the offspring is like the parent or parents, its form is perhaps never identical with theirs, but generally differs from it perceptibly and sometimes materially. To this phenomenon, namely, the occurrence of differences between the structure, the instincts, or other elements, which compose the mechanism of the offspring, and those which were proper to the parent, the name Variation has been given. (Bateson, 1894, p. 3)

> Everyone is interested in the causes of Variation and the nature of 'Heredity', a subject of extreme and peculiar difficulty. (Bateson, 1894, p. ix)

William Bateson was correct – this is a subject that is of interest to everyone, but perhaps it is most pertinent to those who are parents and are perplexed about how their children can have turned out so differently! He is also correct that investigating the causes of variation can be complex and difficult; this book is aimed to provide a guide through this complexity.

References

Banaschewski, T. (2010). Editorial: Preschool behaviour problems – Over-pathologised or under-identified? A developmental psychopathology perspective is needed. *Journal of Child Psychology and Psychiatry, 51*(1), 1–2. https://doi.org/10.1111/j.1469-7610.2009.02206.x

Barash, D. P. (1997). In search of behavioral individuality. *Human Nature-an Interdisciplinary Biosocial Perspective, 8*(2), 153–169. https://doi.org/10.1007/s12110-997-1009-3

Bateson, P., & Martin, P. (1999). *Design for life: How behaviour develops*. Jonathan Cape.

Bateson, W. (1894). *Materials for the study of variation treated with especial regard to discontinuity in the origin of species*. Macmillan.

Biblarz, T. J., & Savci, E. (2010). Lesbian, gay, bisexual, and transgender families. *Journal of Marriage and Family, 72*(3), 480–497. https://doi.org/10.1111/j.1741-3737.2010.00714.x

Bodmer, W. (2003). RA Fisher, statistician and geneticist extraordinary: A personal view. *International Journal of Epidemiology, 32*(6), 938–942. https://doi.org/10.1093/ije/dyg289

Darwin, C. (1859). *On the origin of species by means of natural selection, or the preservation of favoured races in the struggle for life*. John Murray.

Evans, R. J. (2020). RA Fisher and the science of hatred. *New Statesman ((28 July))*.

Fisher, R. A. (1918). The correlation between relatives on the supposition of Mendelian inheritance. *Transactions of the Royal Society (Edinburgh), 52*, 399–433.

Fisher, R. A. (1919). The causes of human variability. *Eugenics Review, 10*, 213–220.

Fisher, R. A. (1925). *Statistical methods for research workers*. Oliver and Boyd.

Fisher, R. A. (1930). *The genetical theory of natural selection*. Clarendon Press.

Fisher, R. A. (1935). *The design of experiments*. Oliver and Boyd.

Golombok, S. (2020). The psychological wellbeing of ART children: What have we learned from 40 years of research? *Reproductive Biomedicine Online, 41*(4), 743–746. https://doi.org/10.1016/j.rbmo.2020.08.012

Gore, F. M., Bloem, P. J. N., Patton, G. C., Ferguson, J., Joseph, V., Coffey, C., …, & Mathers, C. D. (2011). Global burden of disease in young people aged 10–24 years: A systematic analysis. *Lancet, 377*(9783), 2093–2102. https://doi.org/10.1016/s0140-6736(11)60512-6

Happe, F., & Frith, U. (2020). Annual research review: Looking back to look forward – changes in the concept of autism and implications for future research. *Journal of Child Psychology and Psychiatry, 61*(3), 218–232. https://doi.org/10.1111/jcpp.13176

Kapp, S. K., Gillespie-Lynch, K., Sherman, L. E., & Hutman, T. (2013). Deficit, difference, or both? Autism and neurodiversity. *Developmental Psychology, 49*(1), 59–71. https://doi.org/10.1037/a0028353

Kenny, L., Hattersley, C., Molins, B., Buckley, C., Povey, C., & Pellicano, E. (2016). Which terms should be used to describe autism? Perspectives from the UK autism community. *Autism, 20*(4), 442–462. https://doi.org/10.1177/1362361315588200

Patalay, P., & MacDonald, A. W. (2022). New titles can give new perspectives: Reflections on language and equity in clinical science. *Journal of Psychopathology and Clinical Science, 131*(1), 1–3. https://doi.org/10.1037/abn0000739

Plomin, R. (2018). *Blueprint: How DNA makes us who we are*. Allen Lane.

Runswick-Cole, K. (2014). 'Us' and 'them': The limits and possibilities of a 'politics of neurodiversity' in neoliberal times. *Disability & Society, 29*(7), 1117–1129. https://doi.org/10.1080/09687599.2014.910107

Rutherford, A. (2020). Race, eugenics, and the canceling of great scientists. *American Journal of Physical Anthropology*. https://doi.org/10.1002/ajpa.24192

Rutter, M. (1991). Nature, nurture, and psychopathology: A new look at an old topic. *Development and Psychopathology, 3*, 125–136.

Rutter, M., & Sroufe, L. A. (2000). Developmental psychopathology: Concepts and challenges. *Development and Psychopathology, 12*(3), 265–296. https://doi.org/10.1017/s0954579400003023

Sonuga-Barke, E. J. S. (2020). Editorial: 'People get ready': Are mental disorder diagnostics ripe for a Kuhnian revolution? *Journal of Child Psychology and Psychiatry, 61*(1), 1–3. https://doi.org/10.1111/jcpp.13181

Sroufe, L. A., & Rutter, M. (1984). The domain of developmental psychopathology. *Child Development, 55*(1), 17–29. https://doi.org/10.2307/1129832

Thapar, A., & Riglin, L. (2020). The importance of a developmental perspective in psychiatry: What do recent genetic-epidemiological findings show? *Molecular Psychiatry, 25*(8), 1631–1639. https://doi.org/10.1038/s41380-020-0648-1

Viding, E., Blair, R. J. R., Moffitt, T. E., & Plomin, R. (2005). Evidence for substantial genetic risk for psychopathy in 7-year-olds. *Journal of Child Psychology and Psychiatry, 46*(6), 592–597. https://doi.org/10.1111/j.1469-7610.2004.00393

Chapter 2
Data Analysis Frameworks for Investigating Behavioural Differences

In order to understand the ways differences in behaviour are studied, it is necessary to understand the data analysis frameworks that are used. Some of the major frameworks will be discussed in this chapter. However it would be impractical to cover basic statistical methods here, so some familiarity with of elements of data analysis such as the comparison of means, correlation, multiple regression, and exploratory factor analysis is assumed.

2.1 Path Analysis

There are various types of variable that will be discussed in this book. Those that measure characteristics that might influence behaviour will be labelled "risk" factors. These may be concurrently measured associates of behaviour or antecedents, either of which may or may not be causally related to behaviour (see Fig. 2.1). The variables subsequently associated with behaviour will be labelled "outcome". Again there is no restriction as to what an outcome may be – it could be later behaviour, academic attainment, occupation, or mental health. Sometimes a risk factor may also influence an outcome independently of the behaviour measure (the dotted arrow in Fig. 2.1). Under these circumstances the risk variable may be a confound to the behaviour/outcome relationship, i.e. the effects of the risk on outcome need to be taken into account to evaluate the behaviour/outcome relationship.

Path analysis is a method to display and analyse the relationships between a set of measured variables that extends regression so that dependent variables can at the same time be independent variables that predict others. The method was developed in the context of the genetic analyses of patterns of inheritance by Sewall Wright (1920). For an account of the way Sewell Wright's methods have influenced research in psychology and the social sciences, see Wolfle (2003).

J. Stevenson, *Developmental Psychopathology*,
https://doi.org/10.1007/978-3-031-45787-6_2

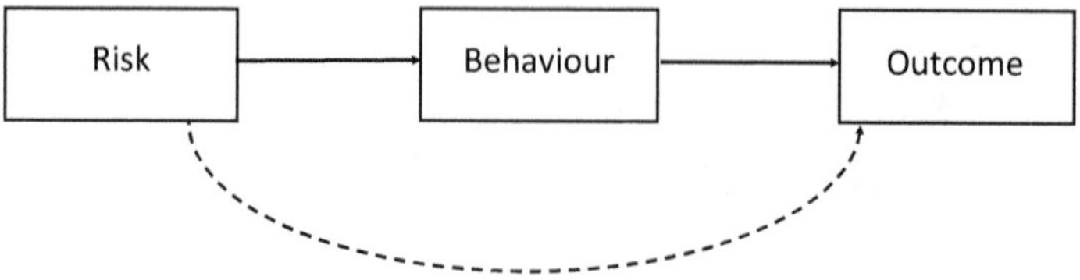

Fig. 2.1 Types of variable

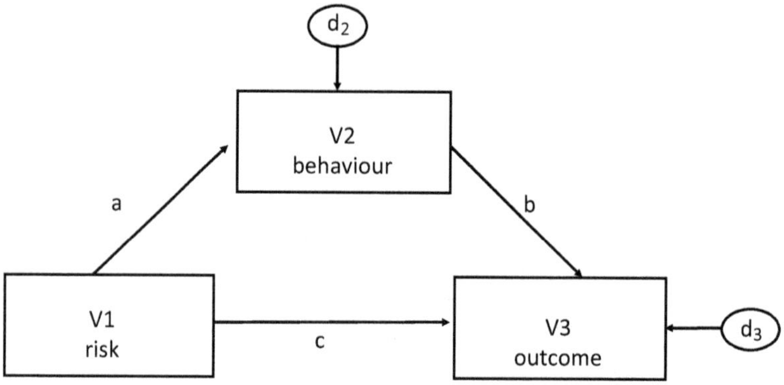

Fig. 2.2 Simple path diagram

A simple form of path analysis is shown in Fig. 2.2. Here the data on which the analysis is conducted are the correlations between three variables. Path analysis requires that a diagram (or model) be made representing the possible causal relationships between the variables that might produce these correlations. In this case the model proposes that *V*1 has an effect on (i.e. is a risk factor for) *V*2 and *V*3. *V*2 also has an effect on *V*3, which is an outcome variable. It must be emphasised that this is only one possible representation of the causal relationships that could be acting on these variables. For instance, the arrow between *V*2 and *V*1 might be reversed so that *V*2 influences *V*1 and *V*3. This is a real limitation on the extent to which path analysis can be thought to "prove" a set of causal relationships – there are always other models that could be considered and determining which is best is often uncertain. Consequently when the term "effect" is used here (as it commonly is in the description of the results of path analysis), it should not be interpreted to mean a causal effect.

The size of the effects of one variable on another is given by the path coefficient ("*a*", "*b*", "*c*" in Fig. 2.2). These are standardised partial regression coefficients, i.e. the number of standard deviation units a dependent variable would change in association with a one standard deviation change in the independent variable. These path coefficients can be multiplied and added together. A set of rules of path analysis can be applied to predict the influences of variables on each other – Wright's rules (Wright, 1934). For example, the total influence of *V*1 on *V*3 is $(c + a.b)$ ("*a.b*" stands for "*a*" times "*b*"), where "*c*" is the direct effect and "*a.b*" is the indirect effect. It is important to note that "*b*" is the effect of *V*2 on *V*3 with the effect of the confound (*V*1) taken into account.

The estimation of the values of the path coefficients is based on iterative methods. An initial solution is produced and then repeated iterations are applied to gradually improve the accuracy of the solution. Based on Wright's rules, estimates can be derived for expected correlations (variance/covariance) between the variables in the model. The accuracy (fit) of the solution is based on comparing the observed correlations and those expected under the model.

The measured variables in Fig. 2.2 are presented in the path diagram inside squares or rectangles. There are also two other variables, d_2 and d_3, which are presented inside circles or ovals. Variables presented in this way are not measured but are estimated within the model. These are latent variables. In this path diagram, the latent variables d_2 and d_3 are disturbance terms (or error variances). They represent all the other influences on *V*2 and *V*3 that are not explained by the variables in the model. These influences include both the measurement error for the variable and any other causal influences not included in the model. There is no disturbance term for *V*1 as this is not being predicted within the model.

An illustration of the use of path analysis is given in Fig. 2.3. This presents the prediction of child's sleep problems from measures of their caregiver's sleep problems and the quality of the relationship between the parents and the child's level of separation anxiety (Schlarb et al., 2016). The model postulates that the poor quality of the parents' relationship might influence the child's sleep problems via an increase in the child's separation anxiety. One feature of a path diagram that has been added in Fig. 2.3 is the double-headed curved arrow between "caregiver's

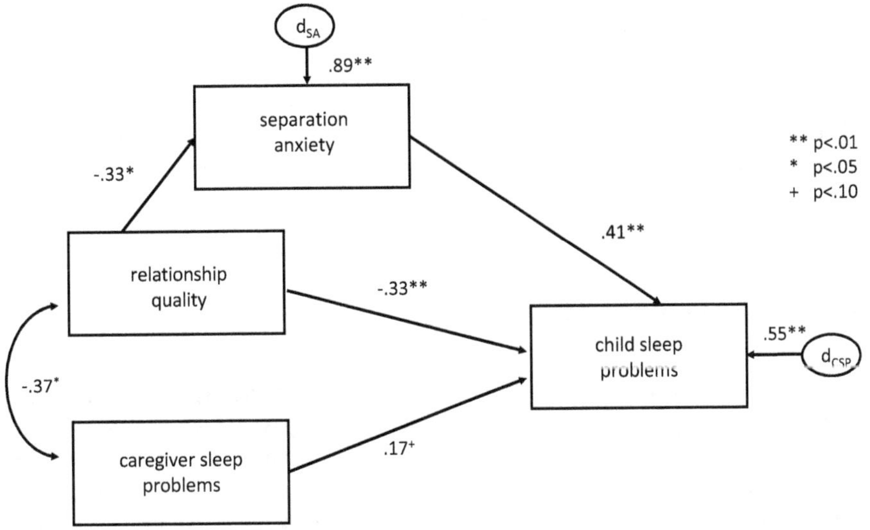

Fig. 2.3 Path model predicting child's sleep problems. (Adapted with the permission of Springer Nature BV from Fig. 1. Schlarb et al. (2016); permission conveyed through Copyright Clearance Center, Inc.)

sleep problems" and "relationship quality". This represents the correlation between these two variables but leaves open the question of direction of effect between the two. The results of the path analysis show that "child's sleep problems" are related to all these predictors with direct effects from "relationship quality" (−.33) and "separation anxiety" (.41) – indicating that the better the parental relationship, the fewer the child's sleep problems and the greater the child's separation anxiety, the more sleep problems shown by the child. There is also an indirect effect on "child's sleep problems" of "relationship quality" via "separation anxiety ($-.33 \times .41 = -.13$). These results suggest that whatever social and biological processes might lead a child with a parent with sleep problem to have poor sleep, the greater influence on the child's sleep problems stems from the quality of the parents' relationship ($-.33 + -.13 = -.46$). In this summary account, the paths linked by the correlation between "caregiver's sleep problems" and "relationship quality" have been ignored.

The final step in path analysis is to determine how well the model accounts for the observed correlations – more correctly the covariance and variances of the measured variables. This is the issue of model fit and will be discussed in more detail in the section on structural equation modelling (Sect. 2.5). In the Schlarb et al. (2016) example, the comparison between observed covariances and variances and those expected from the model was close, and the model fitted the data very well. As in the analysis of contingency tables, a χ^2 is calculated from the sum of the differences between the observed and expected values. For contingency tables, it is the observed and expected frequencies in the cells that are compared. In the modelling analyses, the chi-square compares the expected and observed correlations (variance and covariances). A non-significant chi-square indicates that the observed and expected correlations were similar. In the Schlarb et al. (2016) study, the model fit was good, i.e. $\chi^2 = 0.07$, $df = 1$, $p = 0.80$. The significance of individual paths can also be tested as being different from zero. In Fig. 2.3 there is one path that is not significant at the $p < .05$ level (from "caregiver's sleep problems" to "child's sleep problems").

An excellent introduction to path analysis is provided in Streiner (2005). Kline (2016) provides a more detailed text on the range of methods being discussed in the present chapter, i.e. path analysis, structural equation modelling, and causal analysis.

2.2 Mediation and Moderation

The distinction between mediation and moderation was made explicit by Baron and Kenny (1986) in one of the most highly cited papers in psychology. Up to that time, the terms were often used interchangeably. The terms are used to account for the role of a third variable in the relationship between an independent variable and a dependent variable. A moderator variable is one that changes the relationship between an independent variable and an outcome. A mediator variable is one that carries the effect of a risk on an outcome. Baron and Kenny (1986) provide data analysis methods for detecting moderation and mediation.

These methods vary depending on the nature of the measurement scale for the variables, but in the simplest case of a dichotomous risk variable, a dichotomous moderator, and a continuously measured outcome, a two-way analysis of variance can be applied. Moderation is detected by the presence of a significant interaction between the risk and moderator variables. In other cases, such as when the moderator variable and the outcome measures are on a continuous scale, regression is the recommended data analytic approach and again an interaction between the risk and potential moderator in predicting the outcome is used to detect moderation.

Baron and Kenny (1986) endorsed a regression-based method to detect mediation. This is illustrated in Fig. 2.4. For mediation to be present, the risk variable must be related to the mediator (path "*a*") and the mediator must predict the outcome (path "*b*"). If the risk variable no longer predicts outcome (i.e. path "*c*" is zero) when the mediator is added to the regression, then there is complete mediation. If "*c*" is reduced but remains significantly different from zero, then there is partial mediation. The value of path "*c*" is the measure of a direct effect of risk on outcome, and the product "*a.b*" indicates the strength of the mediated indirect effect. Baron and Kenny (1986) give a formula for the standard error of the indirect effect that can be used to test whether the "*a.b*" term is significantly different from zero.

There are a number of caveats concerning the interpretation of the results of mediation analyses based on the Baron and Kenny multiple regression approach (Lee et al., 2019; Zhao et al., 2010). These include the need to ensure that confounders have been controlled, that the potential effect of multiple mediators on each other has been taken into account (VanderWeele & Vansteelandt, 2014), and that possible reverse causation is excluded by the timing of the measurement of the mediator and outcome and by avoiding concurrent measurement. Kraemer et al. (2001) formulated a framework for a more extensive categorising of the way risk factors might act together to influence an outcome.

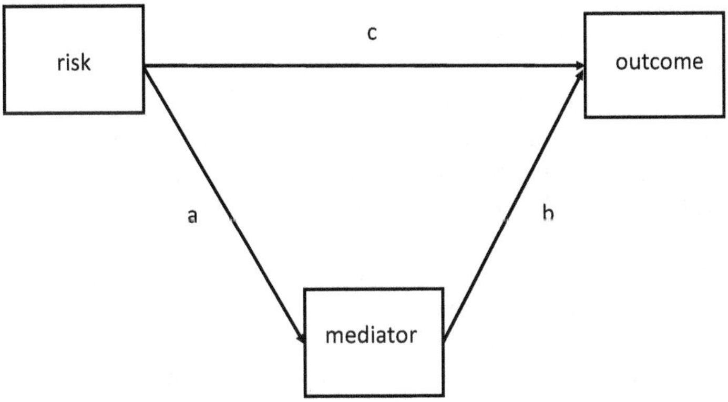

Fig. 2.4 Baron and Kenny (1986) mediation model

2.3 Cluster Analysis

Cluster analysis is a data analytic approach that identifies categories (Everitt et al., 2011). Based on a number of variables measured on a sample, it seeks to identify relatively homogeneous subgroups (clusters) within the sample, i.e. groups of individuals with a similar pattern of score on these measures. This is accomplished in a completely atheoretical and data-driven manner in that there is no a priori assumption about the number or nature of the clusters that will be identified. However considerations from theory are necessary to make an interpretation of the pattern of clusters identified.

A number of important decisions needed to be made before the cluster analysis can be conducted. The first decision is which method of clustering should be used. There are two broad classes of clustering: hierarchical agglomerative analysis and non-hierarchical analysis.

Hierarchical agglomerative analysis Hierarchical agglomerative cluster analysis starts with a set of individuals for whom there is a common set of measures. It then attempts to identify the two individuals with the most similar scores. At this first step in the analysis, these two individuals are merged to form a single cluster, which is treated as one individual at the next step in the analysis. This means that at the second step in the analysis, there is one less individual to be considered, and again the computer programme aims to identify the two individuals with the most similar scores. These two are then combined before entering the next step in the analysis. By this method the number of individuals decreases, and the number of clusters of individuals increases. Thus, increasingly groups of individuals (the clusters) are merged rather than just pairs of individuals at each step of the analysis. Eventually, the individuals are in just two clusters, which are then merged at the final step in the analysis. The clustering process can be summarised in a diagram called a dendrogram (Fig. 2.5).

The dendrogram shows which clusters have been joined at each stage of the analysis and the distance between clusters when they are being combined. A large increase in the distance between clusters being merged indicates that the clusters being merged are quite dissimilar from each other. In Fig. 2.5 this jump has been marked by a dotted vertical line. In this case it suggests that the most interpretable number of clusters is three. The dendrogram shows that Alan and Tom are quite distinct from the rest of the sample. Derek and Simone are also somewhat distinct from Alice, Deborah, and Tony. These three groups appear to be worth investigating further.

A decision needs to be made on the selection of a distance metric that will be used to measure how close individuals or clusters are to each other. This will depend on the nature of the scales for the variables, e.g. interval, ordinal, or binary. The most common choice for interval level measure is Euclidean distance; occasionally other metrics are used, such as City Block (sometimes referred to as Manhattan) metric. The difference between these two metrics is shown in Fig. 2.6. One advantage of using Euclidean distance is that it is commonly used in both hierarchical and

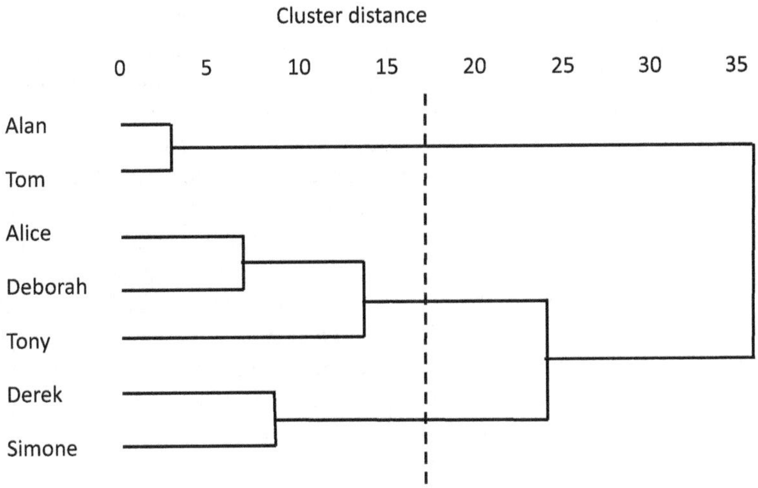

Fig. 2.5 A simplified example of a dendrogram

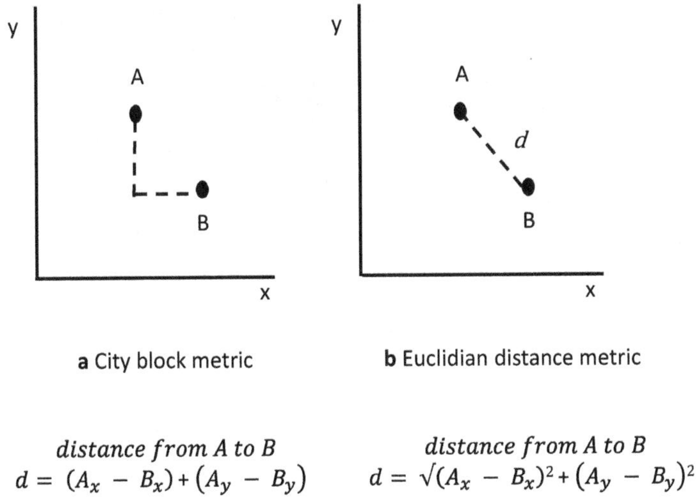

Fig. 2.6 Distance measures

k-means analyses (a non-hierarchical method – see below). This allows a more direct comparison between the results of these two methods. This comparison is a valuable test of the replicability of the cluster solution while also helping to identify whether the hierarchical agglomerative solution has been unduly influenced by outliers. This may arise when Ward's method (see below) has been adopted to select clusters for merging. It has become good practice to cluster analyse initially using Ward's method and then to apply k-means analysis to refine the cluster solutions.

This procedure was used, for example, in a study of teacher ratings of behaviour with a large sample of 6- to 11-year-old children from the general population. Kamphaus et al. (1997) and was also adopted in a study of children referred with pervasive developmental disorders (Lecavalier, 2006).

When using the hierarchical agglomerative approach, there are various options for the method to be adopted in deciding which clusters to combine. These methods differ in the way cluster distances are calculated. One such method is the average linkage method that is based on the average distance between all pairs of participants in the two clusters, and the pairs of clusters with the smallest average distance are then combined. Probably the most widely used approach is Ward's method, which combines all possible pairs of clusters and calculates the sum of the squared distances between the combined cluster members (error sum of squares). The two clusters with the smallest error sum of squares are then combined.

The large increase in the distance between clusters should not be treated in isolation as an indicator of the optimal number of clusters. It is here that expectations from prior studies and theory need to be considered to judge the interpretability of the cluster solution. Additionally it is valuable to investigate the extent to which the clusters differ on variables from outside the cluster analysis. Figure 2.7 presents the results of a cluster analysis of behaviour problems in preschool children (Wolkind & Everitt, 1974). The authors identified five cluster solutions based on the jump in the error sum of squares used in Ward's methods to indicate cluster similarity. This is marked by a dotted horizontal line in Fig. 2.7.

To obtain support for the five cluster solutions, the behaviours shown by the children in the clusters were inspected. Children in Cluster 1 showed problems related to developmental delays. Those in Cluster 2 showed problems with behavioural control. Those in Cluster 3 showed a typical pattern of behavioural development. Those in Cluster 4 showed a profile of social isolation and peer relationship difficulties. Those in Cluster 5 showed a high degree of anxiety and fearful behaviour. As a further test of the validity of these clusters, their mothers' mental health

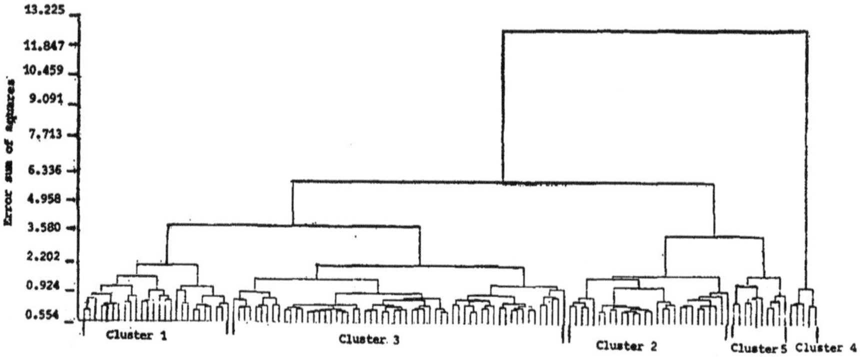

Fig. 2.7 Dendrogram of five cluster solutions on Ward's method. (Reproduced with the permission of Cambridge University Press from Wolkind and Everitt (1974); permission conveyed through Copyright Clearance Center, Inc.)

was measured 1 year later. Mothers of the children in the clusters indicating disturbed behaviour (Clusters 2, 4, and 5) reported significantly more mental health problems than the mothers of children in the other two clusters. By testing cluster differences on measures not used in the clustering, some independent support of the interpretability of the clusters is obtained.

Non-hierarchical analysis The most commonly used non-hierarchical cluster analysis is k-means. In this approach the number of clusters likely to be of interest is selected first, for example, four clusters. In this case a starting set of four-cluster seeds are selected as a guess as to where the cluster means might be. Each participant in the sample is then allocated to which of the four clusters it most resembles. The cluster means of the four clusters are then recalculated and the processes repeated again and again through a number of reiterations until eventually the cluster membership stabilises. A major problem with the k-means approach is that the initial cluster seeds can produce different results. This effect can be addressed by repeating the analysis a number of times using randomly selected alternative means for the initial clusters; the solution providing the best fit can then be selected. This is the solution with the lowest error sum of squares within the clusters. An additional uncertainty in the k-means method arises in the number of clusters that are expected to emerge. This uncertainty can in part be eased by reference to the results of previous studies or by theoretical considerations. However it is considered best practice to run the analyses repeatedly using varying number of initial clusters; the optimal solution can then be selected using a predefined criterion of adequacy of fit or with reference to external variables. For an account of these methods, see Jain (2010).

A study by Willems et al. (2016) illustrates the use of the k-means approach. They were investigating whether subgroups of children with reading disability could be identified based on their profiles of cognitive ability and whether family and environmental risk factors could distinguish the subgroups. They used a battery of reading-related measures (e.g. phonemics awareness and rapid naming) and found that there were homogenous sub-types of poor readers that could be identified based on their cognitive profiles. Moreover there were significant differences between these groupings in, for example, family history.

The k-means clustering approach has had a renascence (Jain, 2010) and has now become a major approach to data analysis used in studies of large and complex data sets such as arise in studies in genetics (McGuirl et al., 2020) and brain imaging (Aggarwal et al., 2021). Cluster analysis is also being applied to address the problem of heterogeneity in autism spectrum disorders (ASD) (see Sect. 10.8). For example, Lyons-Warren et al. (2022) used a k-means analysis to identify six clusters within a sample of people with ASD based on their sensory profile (e.g. tactile, auditory, and visual sensitivity). They then established that these six clusters had a distinctive pattern of gene variants.

2.4 Confirmatory Factor Analysis

When behavioural differences are measured, the question immediately arises as to the extent dimensions of behaviour are related to one another. Are they independent or do they tend to co-occur and, if so, do some groups of behavioural differences form more closely related subsets? The question of co-occurrence can be readily answered by calculating correlations between the measures. The question of identifying a more closely related subset of behaviours requires a more complex approach. The framework employed assumes that the relationship between subsets of variable comes about by the influence of underlying influences shared between them – these are called factors. These factors are unmeasured variables whose presence is inferred from the correlations that they produce; they are a form of latent variable. Identifying these factors has two particular benefits. One is to identify the possible common causes of different behaviours and thereby to gain some insight into the structure and organisation of behavioural differences. The second is to be able to use these factors to produce a smaller number of measures (factor scores) for data analysis. This helps to reduce the problem of multiple significance testing and can enhance the reliability of the variables in an analysis.

There are two broad categories of analyses that identify these subsets of variables with possible common causes. The first is exploratory factor analysis (EFA), which includes principal component analysis. The second is confirmatory factor analysis (CFA). The distinction here is that EFA is conducted without any specific hypotheses about the way the measures related to one another and what factors might be identified. The EFA simply extracts factors suggested by the pattern of intercorrelations between the measures (see Tabachnick & Fidell, 2013, for a good overview of EFA). By contrast in CFA a set of hypotheses (a model) is put forward, which should account for the way variables interrelate. This analysis produces a set of correlations that would be expected under the model and tests whether these hypotheses explain the observed correlations (see discussion of chi-square to test model fit in Sect. 2.1).

Scale development often starts with an EFA applied to a set of items that is then used to uncover the underlying structure for these sets of items. For example, the Strengths and Difficulties Questionnaire (SDQ, Goodman, 1997) was developed by revising and augmenting items from the Teacher and Parent Rutter Questionnaires (Rutter, 1967; Rutter et al., 1970) and the addition of items reflecting prosocial behaviour. These items were subsequently subject to EFA (Goodman, 2001). This analysis identified five factors responsible for the pattern of correlations observed between the scale items. These factors were labelled emotional symptoms, conduct problems, hyperactivity-inattention, peer problems, and prosocial behaviour. The implication of the analysis was that these five factors could be used to classify behavioural differences into groups of items with relatively higher correlations between items with a group and relatively lower correlations between groups of items.

Subsequent to this initial presentation of its psychometric properties, the SDQ has been subject to a number of CFAs. These analyses have been used to test whether

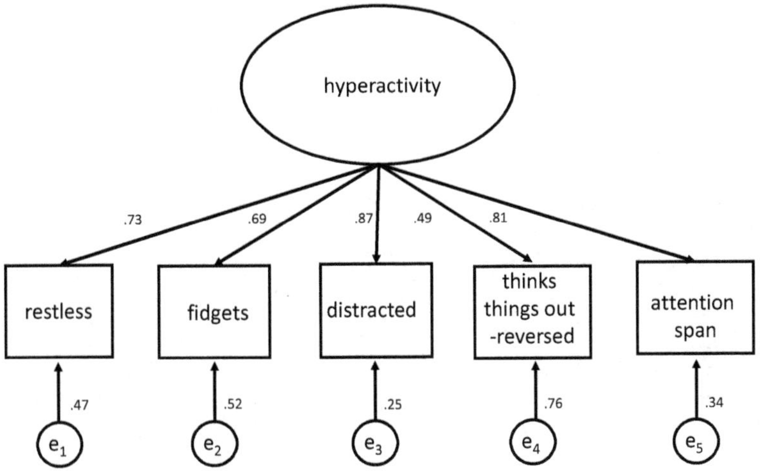

Fig. 2.8 Latent variable of hyperactivity for the SDQ in younger girls. (Adapted with the permission of Springer Nature BV from Fig. 1 in Niclasen et al. (2013); permission conveyed through Copyright Clearance Center, Inc.)

the five-factor model was robust and could be replicated, for example, in different age and gender groups. In a study of parent and teacher ratings of a sample of 60,000 children, Niclasen et al. (2013) applied CFA to SDQ ratings. Figure 2.8 shows the results of the CFA for just one factor (hyperactivity) and just one group (younger girls). There are both measures (in rectangles) and latent variable (in ovals). Figure 2.8 presents the latent variable "hyperactivity", which under the model accounts for the correlations between the five measure behaviour items. The unexplained variance in the items is shown by an error term (e.g. "e_1"). This is an example of another latent variable that is not observed but whose presence is inferred from the data. The values of the paths from the latent variable to each item indicate the strength of its effect on the items. The effect on "distracted" is greater (0.87) than that on "thinks things out" (0.49). The size of the unexplained variance for each item is the difference from 1 of the sum of squares of the path coefficients leading to it. For example, for "fidgets" the path from "hyperactivity" is 0.69 and the error variance is $1 - 0.69^2 = 1 - 0.48 = 0.52$.

The full model of the CFA for the SDQ from Niclasen et al. (2013) is shown in Fig. 2.9. The five latent variables representing the five SDQ factors each have five items loading on them; however the correlations between these four first-order latent variables are seen to be predicted by two further latent variables. These are second-order latent factors – "externalising" and "internalising". These second-order latent variables are themselves correlated (double-headed curved arrow). Since the latent variables "hyperactivity" and "conduct" are predicted by "externalising", they have an added error term and similarly for "emotional" and "peer problem". "Prosocial" is not predicted by another latent variable – it is just correlated with "externalising" and "internalising" and therefore does not have an error term.

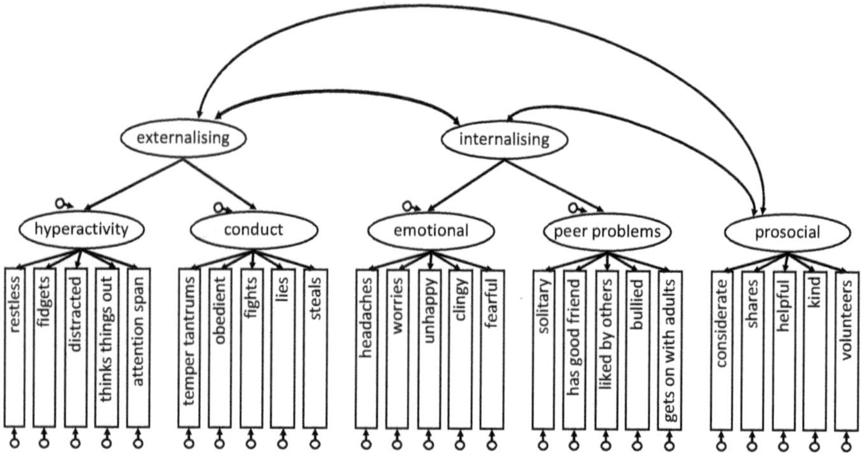

Fig. 2.9 Two second-order factors for the SDQ. (Adapted with the permission of Springer Nature BV from Fig. 1 in Niclasen et al. (2013); permission conveyed through Copyright Clearance Center, Inc.)

Having estimated the path values for the model (these are omitted from Fig. 2.9), the next step is to evaluate how well the model can reproduce the observed correlation matrix for the variables (again note for technical reasons this is done for the variance/covariance matrix). As for path analysis, a value of χ^2 provides an initial index of fit. If the fit is good, the χ^2 should not be significant – the observed and predicted correlations are close to one another. Good fit is not determined by χ^2 alone as χ^2 is influenced by the number of participants (N) in the study. As N increases so does χ^2 making it difficult for a study with a large number of participants to obtain a non-significant χ^2. Consequently a number of fit indices have been developed that are not sensitive to the effects of a large sample size. One of these is root mean square error of approximation (RMSEA). Values of RMSEA over 0.10 are considered to indicate poor fit, and those below 0.05 indicate good fit. There are a number of other indices of fit, e.g. comparative fit index (CFI). These should be greater than 0.90 to indicate reasonable fit. For these indicators of fit, there are no formal tests of statistical significance – the values suggested above are rules of thumb but very well-informed rules of thumb (Hu & Bentler, 1999). Kline (2016) provides a thorough account of CFA.

2.5 Structural Equation Modelling

Before considering the details of structural equation modelling (SEM), it is necessary to discuss the language that is used to describe the results of SEM. The American Medical Association has stipulated restrictions of the use of terms that indicate causation for studies other than randomised controlled trials (RCTs) (see Sect. 4.1) in papers in their journals:

> Causal language (including use of terms such as effect and efficacy) should be used only for randomized clinical trials. For all other study designs (including meta-analyses of randomized clinical trials), methods and results should be described in terms of association or correlation and should avoid cause-and-effect wording. (https://jamanetwork.com/journals/jama/pages/instructions-for-authors#SecUseOfCausalLanguage. Accessed 7 March 2021)

This creates a potential problem when reporting the results of structural equation modelling (SEM). The aim of SEM is to test the plausibility of a putative causal model – the results do not in and of themselves prove causality. However, SEM does aim to go beyond simply description of association, but it does not aim to establish causal relations from associations alone. This was expressed succinctly by Bollen and Pearl (2013) as follows:

> SEM is an inference engine that takes in two inputs, qualitative causal assumptions and empirical data, and derives two logical consequences of these inputs: quantitative causal conclusions and statistical measures of fit for the testable implications of the assumptions. Failure to fit the data casts doubt on the strong causal assumptions of zero coefficients or zero covariances and guides the researcher to diagnose, or repair the structural misspecifications. Fitting the data does not "prove" the causal assumptions, but it makes them tentatively more plausible. Any such positive results need to be replicated and to withstand the criticisms of researchers who suggest other models for the same data. (Bollen & Pearl, 2013, p. 310)

Lei and Wu (2007) provide an introduction to structural equation modelling (SEM). They conclude, echoing Bollen and Pearl (2013), that:

> A selected well-fitting model in SEM is like a retained null hypothesis in conventional hypothesis testing. It remains plausible among perhaps many other models that are not tested but may produce the same or better level of fit. SEM users are cautioned not to make unwarranted causal claims. Replications of findings with independent samples are essential especially if the models are obtained based on post hoc modifications. Moreover, if the models are intended to be used in predicting future behaviors, their utility should be evaluated in that context. (Lei & Wu, 2007, p. 40)

The Academy Medical Sciences (2007) gives a very helpful discussion of the limitations on SEM analyses but also identifies how SEM can provided a powerful addition to analyses where confounders need to be considered. This is particularly the case when longitudinal data are being analysed (VanderWeele, 2021).

There are a number of guidelines on the reporting of SEM (McDonald & Ho, 2002) and CFA (Jackson et al., 2009), but these do not deal with the question of the use of causal language when discussing the results of SEM. Here in this book the term "effect" will be used to label the unidirectional relations between one variable and other. This does not mean that a causal relationship has been identified. It simply means that within the context of the putative causal model being tested, one variable has dependent relationship on another of a certain magnitude. Double-headed arrows represent associations or correlation with no direction of effect assumed.

The role of CFA is to create a framework for understanding the influences underlying measures, i.e. providing a measurement model. These models identify the various theoretical constructs (latent variables) that can account for the relationships between the measures. SEM takes this formulation further by testing the proposed relationships between the latent variables. In the example of the CFA in Fig. 2.9, the second-order latent variables were correlated with each other and with the first-order latent variables. SEM extends such relationships to incorporate both prediction (single-headed arrows) and correlation (double-headed arrows). This process can be elaborated to create complex sets of latent variables correlated with and predicted by each other.

The input for SEM is the same as that for CFA – variance/covariance matrices for a set of variables. Like CFA the SEM model provides estimates of the strength of the relationships between the measures and latent variables and between the latent variables themselves. The process of estimating the model parameters is an iterative one. The computer programme has an initial set of start values for these parameters. The rules of reading path models (see above discussion of Fig. 2.3) are then used to calculate the predicted value of the covariances between the measured variables. These predicted values are subsequently compared with the observed covariances, and the path estimates are then revised to produce a closer agreement between the observed and predicted values. This is a process that is repeated over a large number of iterations until further improvements in agreement are minimal. At this final stage, the adequacy of the model is evaluated. The SEM models are appraised in the same way as the goodness of fit of the CFA measurement model by the use of χ^2, RMSEA, and the CFI. An unsurpassed introduction to SEM is provided by Kline (2016). The history of the development and application of SEM was reviewed by Bollen et al. (2022).

A study by Murray et al. (2010) on the long-term effects of maternal postnatal depression on the child's academic performance will be used to demonstrate the value of SEM. This was a longitudinal study of 50 children whose mothers were postnatally depressed and 39 children whose mothers were not depressed. For boys this exposure to postnatal depression had an adverse effect on cognitive development. Cognitive measures at 1.5, 5, and 8 years of age were used to identify a latent IQ variable. The child's academic performance was measured by GCSE results at age 16 years. The study also investigated the role of mother support for the cognitive development of the child at 5 and 8 years. These measures were obtained from videotaped sessions of mother-child interactions. The final element in the study was the role of the mother's IQ in influencing the child's development. The interplay between these factors was displayed in the path diagram shown in Fig. 2.10. The error variance for the dependent latent and measured variables are omitted from the diagram. The analysis indicated that postnatal depression has an effect on academic performance via two routes. One is via a negative impact on the boy's cognitive development in middle childhood. The other is by reducing the support given to cognitive development by the mother. The fit of this model was adequate ($\chi^2 = 48.28$, $d.f. = 39$, $p = .15$, CFI = .94, RMSEA = .07 ($CI_{.90}$ 0.00–0.13).

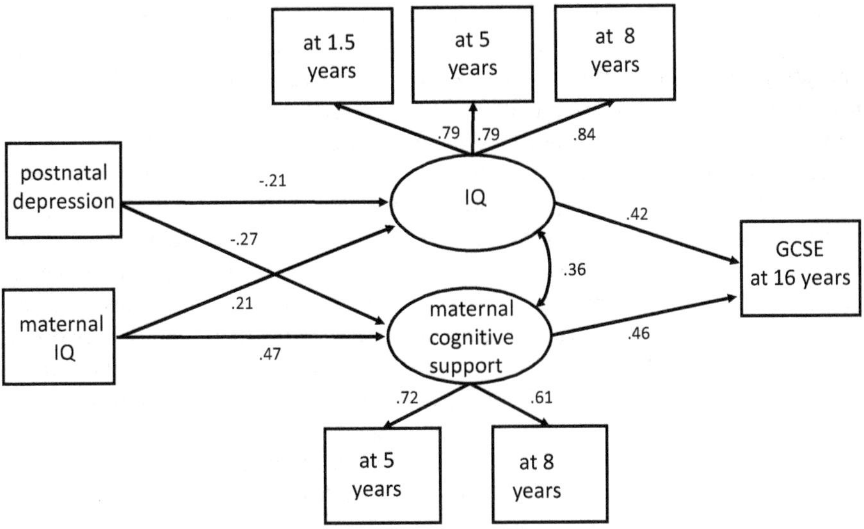

Fig. 2.10 Relationship between postnatal depression and academic attainment in boys. (Adapted with the permission of John Wiley & Sons from Fig. 2 in Murray et al. (2010); permission conveyed through Copyright Clearance Center, Inc.)

What is the value of SEM in this paper by Murray et al. (2010)? First, the path diagram provides a succinct and readily interpretable summary of a complex set of relationships. Second, the use of the latent variable for IQ and for mother's cognitive support reduces the number of variables whose relationship with academic performance has to be tested. Third, the latent variables are free from measurement error and therefore reflect the reliable association with academic performance.

What do latent variables mean? Latent variables are theoretical constructs that account for the correlation between behaviours, but the mechanisms producing these associations is an open question. For example, for the latent variable underlying a wide range measures of psychopathology – the *p*-factor or general psychopathology factor (GPF) – a number of mechanisms have been proposed that range from the genetic ("generalist genes") to features of brain structure and function and adverse experiences such as child maltreatment (see Sect. 6.7 for more details on the interpretation of this factor). By itself the SEM does not identify how the latent variable has an effect. This needs to be investigated by relating the latent variable to other measures.

Tackett et al. (2013) undertook such a study to test the hypothesis that the general factor (latent variable) influencing psychopathology was strongly related to negative emotionality. This is the temperamental disposition to experience negative effect and distress. They measured negative emotionality in a large twin sample aged 6–17 years as well as measures of psychopathology. Applying a bifactor model (see Sect. 6.2), they were able to obtain a latent variable that was a general factor of psychopathology. They showed that this latent variable was correlated (r = 0.58) with negative emotionality. As twin data was available, they were able to estimate the extent to which additive genetic influences were shared between the general psychopathology latent variable and negative emotionality. They found that on parent ratings this genetic correlation (see Sect. 3.1) was substantial ($r = 0.71$). The results of the study indicate that the latent variable underlying the correlation between measures of psychopathology in children and adolescents was closely related to negative emotionality both at the level of the phenotype (i.e. measured behaviour) and the genotype (i.e. shared genetic influences).

SEM is premised on the notion that there is a dimensional latent variable that produces the correlations between the measured variables. There are a number of related model fitting analyses that have different approaches. Latent class analysis is designed to place individuals into groups (classes) with others with similar values on a set of measured variables. SEM produces latent variables that account for the correlations between variables, i.e. its group variable. Latent class analysis groups individuals. This is achieved by identifying an underlying categorical latent variable that determines an individual's class membership. It should be noted that latent class analysis produces results that parallel those from cluster analysis (see Sect. 2.3). Nylund et al. (2007) used this approach to identify three classes of middle-school pupils based on the severity of peer victimisation they experienced – victimised, sometimes victimised, and not victimised. The predictive validity of this structure of classes was tested by examining the mean scores of the classes on an independent measure of depression, and the victimised group consistently had higher depression scores that the other two classes.

Latent class analysis addresses the question of heterogeneity within a population. There are a number of other related types of analyses doing a similar job (e.g. latent profile analysis, see Wade et al., 2021). Latent transition analysis defines classes at each time point and then groups individuals by how they change from class to class over time (for an example see Wiggins et al., 2021). There are methods for combining both a dimensional latent variable and a latent class approach. These factor mixture model approaches have applied to the heterogeneity in children with autism spectrum disorder (Eagle et al., 2010; Georgiades et al., 2013). Johnson (2021) provides an overview of the how to conduct, interpret, and report these factor mixture model analyses.

2.6 Network Analysis

A radical critique of the latent variable modelling approach has been made by those endorsing a network approach to psychopathology (Borsboom et al., 2019; Cramer et al., 2012; Fried & Cramer, 2017; Saxe et al., 2016). In a network model, the symptoms of disorders are not seen as arising from an underlying common cause identified by a latent variable. Instead the associations between the symptoms arise from their causal effects on each other. An example of this given by Fried and Cramer (2017) is that:

> from the network perspective, certain symptoms like insomnia, fatigue, and concentration problems in patients with Major Depression co-occur not because they result from an underlying brain disorder or neurochemical imbalance but because not sleeping well leads to being tired and having concentration problems. (Fried & Cramer, 2017, p. 999)

McNally (2016) provides an excellent introduction to network analysis outlining how its distinction from a latent variable formulation and how some of the analytic methods are used and interpreted. Epskamp et al. (2018) have provided a tutorial on the methods used to estimate the psychometric characteristics of networks. The network represents the pattern of putative causal relationships between the symptoms.

In a psychopathology network, the measures of symptoms are referred to as nodes, the links between nodes are referred to as edges, and if the strengths of the links are estimated, these are referred to as weighted edges. The importance of a node within a network is indicated by measures of centrality with those with high centrality being the most influential in terms of their impact on other symptoms. Centrality measures include degree (number of edges connected to a node) and strength (the sum of weighted of edges connected to a node).

The results of a network analysis are presented in Fig. 2.11, which is based on a small selection of behaviour items from the analysis by Hukkelberg (2019) of conduct problems in Norwegian children aged 3–12 years. The thickness of the edges (lines) in the network is an indication of their strength. It can be seen that there are strong connections between the conduct items (steal, lies, destroys toys) and between the inattention items (easily distracted, poor concentration, short attention span, fails to finish). There are a few and only weak connections between these two sets of behaviours.

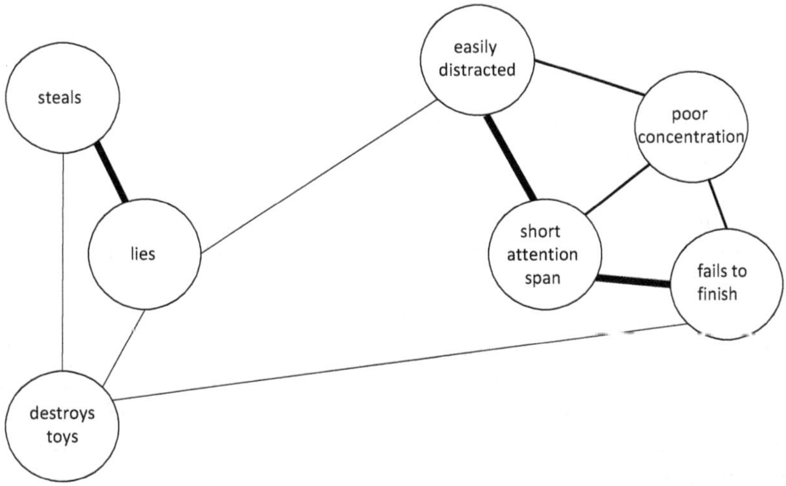

Fig. 2.11 Causal network model of selected conduct and inattention problems. (Adapted with the permission of Springer Nature BV from Fig. 2 in Hukkelberg (2019); permission conveyed through Copyright Clearance Center, Inc.)

The particular value of longitudinal data in examining networks was shown by Funkhouser et al. (2021) in an investigation of internalising, externalising, and attention symptoms in 4093 10- to 11-year-olds. This found that depressed mood, inattention, and worry were potent influences on other symptoms.

A meta-analysis of network analysis studies published between 2010 and 2017 found 65 such studies, of which just 8 investigated children or adolescents (Contreras et al., 2019). This meta-analysis concluded that the network approach can identify novel features of psychopathology symptomatology, such as the centrality of certain symptoms in a given disorder and the dynamic relationships among symptoms. There are a number of examples of the application of network analysis to the structure of problems of emotion and behaviour in children. For example, Rouquette et al. (2018) examined the relationship between disruptive and emotional symptom measures at ages 6, 8, and 10 years in a sample of 932 elementary school girls and anxiety disorders at 15 and 22 years. They found that the symptoms "irritable", "blames others", "not liked", "often cries", and "solitary" represented the most direct relationships between the disruptive and internalising grouping. These "bridge symptoms" could represent key targets for intervention. The network structure of symptoms was relatively stable during middle childhood. Using the prospective design of the study, they were able to show that the "not liked by other children", "disobedient", and "irritable" were predictive of later diagnoses of anxiety disorders.

A number of examples of the value of network analysis will now be discussed. An illustration of the combined use of network analysis and CFA with behaviour in young children is given by Bansal et al. (2020). They were interested in the structure of callous and unemotional traits (see Sect. 8.1) in the preschool child. As had been found previously in preschool children (Kimonis et al., 2016), the CFA identified two factors underlying these traits – callous and uncaring. The network analysis extended this by identifying items that were most central to the network, which were "Does not care who he/she hurts to get what they want", "Does not care if he/she is in trouble", and "Seems very cold and uncaring". These items may be particularly valuable in developing a screening measure for callous-unemotional traits in the preschool child. This would be valuable given the adverse long-term outcome of this trait (Frick et al., 2014).

Groen et al. (2019) used network analysis to address the question of how the nature of an underlying condition might change with increasing degrees of symptom severity. The study used measures of depressive symptoms, fatigue, fearfulness, medically unexplained pain, worrying, impulsivity, attention problems, hyperactivity/restlessness, emotional dysregulation, and substance use for a sample of 1933 adolescents in their late teens. They found no support for the hypothesis that the manifestation of psychopathology along the severity continuum changes from non-specific to specific. Across groups with increasing illness severity, there was a consistent pattern of symptom clustering and interrelationships. These results support the notion that psychopathology should be considered as a continuum as there is no evidence that there is substantial change in the relationships between symptoms as severity increases.

Boschloo et al. (2016) applied a network analysis to items from the Youth Self-Report (YSR) on a sample of 2175 10- to 12-year-olds. Broadly the results replicated the original principal component analysis of this measure (Achenbach & Rescorla, 2000). They found that problems within the same domain, in general, showed more and stronger connections than problems belonging to different domains, but some problems showed substantially more or stronger associations than others. They argue therefore that problems cannot be considered interchangeable indicators of their domain. However they conclude that the study does not detract from the use of scale scores derived from the YSR factor structure.

The symptoms of depression and obsessive-compulsive disorder (OCD) in adolescents were investigated using network analysis by Jones et al. (2018). They found that OCD and depression emerged as separate syndromes linked by bridge symptoms, i.e. obsessional problems in the OCD syndrome, and guilt, concentration problems, and sadness in the depression syndrome. They say that such findings from network analysis can inform improvements in the study and treatment of such conditions.

A particularly informative application of network analysis was that undertaken by Martel et al. (2016). They address the question of how the symptoms of attention-deficit hyperactivity disorder (ADHD) change with age and in particular which symptoms represent a core to the condition. They compared community samples across four age groups: preschool (aged 3–6 years), childhood (aged 6–12 years), adolescence (aged 13–17 years), and young adulthood (aged 18–36 years). Broadly the structure of ADHD symptoms became more differentiated in the older samples. However they found that "often easily distracted" and "difficulty sustaining attention" were central symptoms across age groups, as shown by the network analysis centrality indices of closeness and degree, and may therefore represent the core of ADHD, regardless of developmental period.

Network analysis was applied to measures of posttraumatic stress disorder obtained from samples of children (aged 8–13 years) and adolescents (aged 14–18 years) (Russell et al., 2017). The network analysis indicated that there were age-related changes in the pattern of symptoms. Some associations between symptoms appeared to be consistent across age groups, e.g. such as the link between avoiding activities and physiologic reactivity. Other symptom associations were particular to each age group. For example, a strong association between "numbness/sadness/anger" and "amnesia" was found among children but not adolescents. Russell et al. (2017) suggest that network analysis may have particular value in guiding clinical practice by guiding treatment to target symptoms for that have or are likely to have consequent effects on other symptoms, i.e. symptoms that have a high degree of centrality in the network.

The sharp distinction between network analysis and a common cause (latent variable based) approach made by advocates of a network has been criticised by Bringmann and Eronen (2018). They argue that there is much in common between the two approaches and indeed that networks can be analysed using a latent variable approach. Consequently they cannot identify a "clear border where network models end and latent variable or common cause models begin". There have been concerns about the extent to which the findings from network analysis are replicable (Forbes et al., 2017). Indeed Forbes et al. (2017) conclude that novel results originating from psychopathology networks need to be shown to be robust before they are disseminated or used in clinical practice.

There is a basic similarity between the approach to the analysis of structure of behaviour problems by latent variable and by network analyses. Both are based on data that represents the correlation (variance/covariance) between the measures of behaviour. Consequently, although representing the relationships between behaviour problems in radically different formats, correspondences should be found between the results of two analyses. This is well illustrated by the study reported by McElroy et al. (2018). They examined the network structure of Diagnostic and Statistical Manual of Mental Disorders – Fourth Edition (DSM-IV) disorders at ages 7.5, 10.5, and 14 years in 4405 children from the Avon Longitudinal Study of Parents and Children. Specifically they were interested in the relationship between internalising and externalising problems. They found a high degree of stability in the internalising and externalising clusters with generalised anxiety disorder (GAD) and oppositional defiant disorder (ODD) as the most central disorders in each. However in addition there were numerous associations between disorders across these two major clusters; that between depression and ODD was the most consistent across age groups. They conclude that these network findings are consistent with a p-factor model (see Sect. 6.2). Indeed the findings provide a possible mechanism underlying the *p*-factor. They suggest that the dimensions internalising and externalising are correlated by the *p*-factor as a result of local interactions and reinforcements between conditions that represent "bridges" between the broad dimensions.

Hallquist et al. (2019) have provided a clear account of the distinction between network and latent variable models of psychopathology symptoms. Do symptoms tend to co-occur because they are a product of an underlying comment cause, i.e. latent factor, or because they directly and causally influence one another, i.e. mutualism? They show that if network analyses ignore latent factors, spurious relationships may emerge from the analysis and indeed causally important influence may fail to be detected. They propose that:

> the classification of mental illness will be best advanced by examining parameters from formal models that are sensitive to latent structure and that instantiate specific hypotheses about the basis of symptom co-occurrence. (Hallquist et al., 2019, p. 22).

This is an approach to the analysis of patterns of symptom co-occurrence that incorporates both latent variables and symptom-to-symptom influences as per network analysis. In fact there is great degree of statistical equivalency between latent factor and network models (Christensen & Golino, 2020). Eadeh et al. (2021) provided an important test of the latent variable and network approaches by analysing the same data set of neurocognitive measures from a sample of 6- to 17-year-olds using both approaches. They found more agreement than disagreement between the results of the two sets of analyses. They conclude that latent variable and network analyses be considered valuable complementary tools for psychopathology research.

However there are concerns that many network studies are not designed to test adequately the causal relationships between symptoms that lie at the core of the network paradigm. For example, Huang et al. (2023) undertook a systematic review of network studies applied to depression that included some studies on children and adolescents. They concluded that few network studies tested key features to support causality, such as the absence of confounders between risk and outcome. Without such rigorous tests, network analyses are based on predictions rather than causation (see Sect. 4.13). Huang et al. (2023) suggest that:

> The lack of empirical evidence for symptom causal relationships is a critical threat to the paradigm and studies which adopt this paradigm. (Huang et al., 2023, p. 1666)

So how can the relative merits of network analysis and of latent factors be judged? The issue of adopting a latent factor or a network model is one of theoretical not statistical importance (Christensen et al., 2020). It is more a question of adopting the data analytic approach that best suits the needs of the user. It appears that clinicians find network models helpful in planning approaches to treatment. However there is a need for further investigations of the application of network analysis to understanding symptom development in individuals, and these need to apply an approach that utilises measurement of within-person changes over time (McNally, 2021). This form of network analysis could suggest symptoms that might provide an optimal focus for intervention. The latent factor models are valuable to guide the search for causes that are shared between symptoms. For this reason quantitative and molecular genetic studies have adopted the latent factor approach to the modelling of the structure of psychopathology.

2.7 Meta-analysis

Meta-analysis is a statistical approach that synthesises the results of a series of studies to provide an overall aggregate quantitative summary. This is optimally beneficial if the studies whose findings are being integrated have been identified comprehensively and in an unbiased way. For this reason meta-analyses are often based on systematic reviews of the literature, which have been conducted using a recommended set of procedures for identifying relevant studies and on reporting on the meta-analysis: the PRISMA statement (Moher et al., 2009). This systematic approach can be applied to any set of studies but has a particular value in identifying effect sizes from randomised controlled trials (see Sect. 4.1). There is also a set of recommended practices specific to the design of RCTs and how they should be reported: the CONSORT statement (Moher et al., 2010).

An excellent textbook on meta-analysis is that by Borenstein et al. (2009). The core component of a meta-analysis is an effect size calculation. The most commonly effect size used is based on the comparison of mean scores from a treatment and a control group, often on a continuous outcome measure. Different studies will use different outcome measures that require the difference between means converted to be on the same scale. This is achieved by calculating the standardised mean difference (SMD). Here for each study the difference between the means is divided by the pooled within group standard deviation for the treatment and control groups to give an effect size in standard deviation units. Consequently the SMD is calibrated on a scale that can be equated across very different measures. This SMD is then analysed across the studies in the meta-analysis to give an average effect size and indicators of the variation in effect sizes between the studies.

The test of the overall effect is whether the average SMD is significantly greater than zero. One commonly used SMD effect size is called Cohen's "*d*". A related effect size, Hedges's "*g*", corrects for a slight bias in "*d*" and is particularly valuable for small sample sizes. Meta-analysis can also be applied to studies that have estimated the relationship between continuous variables. Here the product moment correlation coefficient (*r*) is used to calculate an aggregated effect size. There are a range of other effect sizes given in Borenstein et al. (2009). A brief introduction to both systematic reviews and meta-analysis is provided by Siddaway et al. (2019). A more comprehensive overview has been produced by the Cochrane Collaboration (Higgins et al., 2019). For ease of comparison, throughout in this book, where possible, effect sizes have been converted to SMD using the methods given in Borenstein et al. (2009). These conversions assume equal sample size groups.

One of the most common uses of meta-analysis is to provide a quantitative assessment of the impact of treatments. This is of particular value in reporting the results of RCTs. There are however important provisos on the way effect sizes – especially standardised mean difference (SMD) – are reported (Cuijpers et al., 2017). It is essential that such reports do not rely on just calculating changes within a treated group. Such pre-post effect sizes are subject to a number of problems, the most important of which is that the effects of intervention cannot be distinguished from other concurrent changes, for example, those happening with age. For unbiased estimates to be obtained, it is necessary to compare the change in a treated group with concurrent changes in a comparison group – preferably one created by random allocation in an RCT.

An extension of meta-analysis is the network meta-analysis of treatment studies (Mavridis et al., 2015). Usually meta-analyses compare the results from a treatment and control groups from different studies. Meta-analyses are also conducted to compare two alternative treatments and effect sizes calculated to identify which is most efficacious (head-to-head studies). Network meta-analysis provides a way of estimating the relative merits of alternative treatments that have not necessarily be compared on a direct head-to-head basis. Cortese et al. (2019) introduce the calculations and methods in a network meta-analysis and provide a systematic review of such studies on mental health in children and adolescents.

A preferable option is to conduct a mega-analysis (Riley et al., 2010; Eisenhauer, 2021). A meta-analysis integrates the summary of often disparate statistics from different studies. A mega-analysis is based on raw data pooled across studies. Historically this was problematic as raw data was not readily available. However the large sample requirements of molecular genetic studies (e.g. Sullivan & Kendler, 2021) and brain imaging studies (e.g. Schilling et al., 2013) have led to many international cooperating consortia being established where data is obtained with common protocols and where raw data are pooled. Indeed there is a consortium that is pooling data on both molecular genetics and brain imaging (Thompson et al., 2014), thereby increasing both sample size and the range of data available for analysis.

There are distinct advantages to meta-analyses that are based on the pooling across studies of data on individuals, i.e. mega-analyses. For example, this allows the analysis of possible moderators of effects. One such "individual participant data" meta-analysis was reported by Gardner et al. (2019). They were interested in identifying whether interventions for child behaviour problems based on parenting programmes were more effective if applied at a younger age, i.e. is age a moderator of treatment efficacy? The age range in the studies was between 2 and 11 years. They conducted both an individual participant data mega-analysis and the more typical meta-analysis based on aggregated data. In both analyses they found no evidence that interventions at an earlier age were more effective.

There are great advantages to synthesising the results from disparate studies. The results from any one study are unlikely to be definitive as individual studies may be unrepresentative in the sample used and may be under-powered and the results possibly biased by the measures employed. Meta-analyses can help to minimise these potential problems. Network meta-analysis can extend the scope of the comparison between alternative treatments. There is a further stage that can be taken in the integration of findings across studies. This is called an umbrella review (Ioannidis, 2009). The umbrella review is a review of previously published systematic reviews, meta-analyses, and network meta-analyses. They attempt to repeat the meta-analyses following a standard protocol to achieve more accurate comparisons. A guide to the production of umbrella reviews has been produced by Fusar-Poli and Radua (2018). An example of the value of this approach is the umbrella review on child mental health by Correll et al. (2021). This provides evidence-based guidance to clinicians on the efficacy of pharmacological, psychosocial, and brain stimulation interventions.

2.8 Machine Learning and Big Data

Big Data is that derived from sources where there is a variety of measures available on very large samples. These data are often obtained with no specific research question in mind. An example of such a source relevant to behaviour is routinely obtained medical records. A pervasive problem with Big Data in studies of developmental psychopathology is that for reasons of economy, feasibility, and participant acceptability, there usually has to be reliance on measures of behaviour with tenuous validity. The measures have to be brief and superficial and have been labelled "shallow phenotypes". The importance of "deep phenotypes" has been argued by Phillips and Kendler (2021). They give the example of the study by Cai et al. (2020), which used both shallow and deep phenotype measures of depression in a genome-wide association study (GWAS) (see Sect. 3.2). This showed that shallow phenotypes provide lower estimates of heritability and were associated with genes with less specific links to depression. They conclude that shallow phenotypes may provide a biased picture of the genetic architecture of a condition and detract from the identification of specific pathways giving rise to a condition. It is therefore essential to consider the impact of the fidelity of the measures on the results from Big Data studies.

Machine learning is a group of mathematical techniques that exploit the power of the modern computer to identify patterns in large complex ill-defined data sets, such as Big Data, as well as in more structured large data sets. By learning about the relationship between measures in multidimensional data sets, the aim is then to make generalisable predictions about individuals. Usually such studies are in two phases. The first is a learning or training phase, which develops a model of the patterns in an initial data set. The second testing phase applies this model to a new data set. The key to evaluating the results of the machine learning process is in how accurately it predicts patterns in this second a data set. An important feature of the approach is the emphasis on identifying complex multidimensional patterns in the data. The patterns emerge from the data set usually without prior reference to theoretical expectations. There is an aspiration that machine learning can be effective in aiding the development of personalised treatments in the clinical setting, i.e. identifying what treatment works for whom and under what circumstances – sometimes referred to as precision medicine (Bzdok & Meyer-Lindenberg, 2018; Bzdok et al., 2021). The procedure for applying machine learning in the context of clinical psychology is clearly set out in Coutanche and Hallion (2020).

Machine learning has been used in a number of contexts: imaging genetics (Bogdan et al., 2017), the diagnosis of autism (Bone et al., 2016), genomics (Zou et al., 2019), in the analysis of brain imaging in children with ADHD (Johnston et al., 2014), applications in psychiatry (Huys et al., 2016; Iniesta et al., 2016), applications in clinical psychology (Dwyer et al., 2018), cognitive neuroscience (Wiecki et al., 2015), and to shift the focus of psychological research from explanation to prediction (Yarkoni & Westfall, 2017). An overview of the application of machine learning in child and adolescent psychiatry has been produced by Dwyer and Koutsouleris (2022). A meta-analysis of the performance of prediction models in child and adolescent mental health suggested that none of the models produced so far is of sufficient quality to be recommended for adoption in clinical practice (Senior et al., 2021).

A study by Miotto et al. (2016) will be used to illustrate an application of machine learning. The data were obtained from routinely collected health records such as clinical notes, diagnoses, medications, lab tests, and demographic features. Unsupervised machine learning then extracted representations of risks of future diagnoses for each patient. The training data were records on patients over a 34-year period. The testing data were diagnoses made in 1 subsequent year. The total number patients in the data set was about 1.2 million. The testing examined the accuracy with which machine learning predicted new diagnoses. The machine learning prediction was applied to 78 diverse conditions. For attention-deficit hyperactivity disorder, the area under curve (AUC) was 0.86. AUC represents how well a prediction is made by plotting true positives against false positives. If the prediction is only at chance level, the AUC will be 0.50. If the prediction is perfect, the AUC will be 1.00. In addition to ADHD, the method did well at predicting severe diabetes and schizophrenia but was not so successful in predicting new diagnoses of hypertension.

Miotto et al. (2016) provide an example of machine learning applied to Big Data – this is an imprecise term that refers not just to the number of units (individuals) being analysed, but often such data is also characterised by a loose if not unstructured format and by having many variables. Machine learning can be applied to more modest data sets. For example, Iniesta et al. (2018) examined whether patients' responses to antidepression medication could be predicted using a training sample of 280 people. They then tested the model derived on a new sample of 150 participants. The predictors were genetic polymorphisms and clinical variables. Separate models were derived for two antidepressants (escitalopram and nortriptyline) and achieved AUC of 0.77 in each case. They concluded that machine learning can be applied to achieve validated predictions about the likelihood of a positive response to treatment based on a relatively small set of genetic and clinical variables.

There are examples of machine learning being applied to data on children. Machine learning has shown its value in a study attempting to identify children who will show low language skills at age 11 years from measures readily obtainable under the age of 36 months (Gasparini et al., 2023). Such a prediction is crucial to the provision of timely support for those with continuing language difficulties, a group who are at risk of range of later problems (Yew & O'Kearney, 2013). The measures in this study were easily answered questions for parents and relate to aspects of children's language, play, and parent-child interactions. The sample was a longitudinally studied cohort from the general population. Using the measures obtained at 36 months, the machine learning algorithm was able to identify an aggregate of these measures that could predict low language skills at 11 years with a sensitivity of 0.75 and a specificity of 0.84. The real test of the importance of this results will be whether the predictions can be replicated in another general population sample. The authors have pre-registered their intention to conduct such a study (https://osf.io/jk32c/).

Machine learning has been used successfully to develop methods for diagnosis children with autism (Bone et al., 2015; Bone et al., 2016). It has also been shown that machine leaning can be trained to differentiate children with ADHD or bipolar disorders based on brain volume and thickness measures from structural magnetic resonance images (Gaus et al., 2023). However the prediction is too imprecise to allow the method to be applied as an aide to clinical diagnosis. Carpenter et al. (2016) used a machine learning approach to demonstrate the possibility of developing an efficient screening tool for anxiety disorders in preschool children. They suggest that the machine learning solution was a first step towards development and validation of a relatively short screening tool feasible for use in clinical settings.

A detailed guide to the analysis of Big Data has been provided by Chen and Wojcik (2016). The limitations on the value of the largely inductively derived findings from the analysis of Big Data and the importance of integrating such findings with those of more hypothesis driven studies have been highlighted by Sonuga-Barke (2023).

2.9 The Reproducibility Crisis

How much faith can you have in the studies that will be summarised in this book? Can the findings be replicated when attempts are made to repeat them? Surely they must be able to be reproduced – why else would they be of interest? These are issues that are confronting scientists in a number of fields – it is labelled the "reproducibility crisis". Addressing this crisis has important implications for the conduct of data analysis and how its results are reported. It is for this reason that the issues related to the "reproducibility crisis" will be discussed at length here in a chapter on data analysis.

The problems that arise from the analysis of data obtained from small samples (Button et al., 2013) are at the heart of the non-reproducibility crisis in psychology (Open Science Collaboration, 2015) (OSC-2015), but psychology is not alone with these difficulties. For example, see Begley and Ellis (2012) for related concerns in preclinical cancer research. The OSC-2015 undertook a replication of 100 experimental and correlational studies that had been published in 3 psychology journals. They concluded that:

> A large portion of replications produced weaker evidence for the original findings despite using materials provided by the original authors, review in advance for methodological fidelity, and high statistical power to detect the original effect sizes. (Open Science Collaboration, 2015, p. 943)

There is disagreement over how to interpret the findings of the OSC-2015. Gilbert et al. (2016) suggest that as a result of a number of statistical errors, OSC-2015 provides no support for the conclusion that reproducibility of psychology studies is very low. They argue that OSC-2015 used a benchmark that did not take into account the multiple sources of error in their data, used a relatively low-powered design that demonstrably underestimates the true rate of replication, and permitted considerable infidelities that almost certainly biased their replication studies towards failure. As a result, they concluded that OSC-2015 seriously underestimated the reproducibility of psychological science; Gilbert et al. (2016) suggest that to the contrary reproducibility is quite high. In response the authors of OSC-2015 step back a little and suggest that their results and its interpretation are somewhat equivocal (Anderson et al., 2016). They make the point that exact replication is a goal that it is impossible to achieve. They suggest that "both optimistic and pessimistic conclusions about reproducibility are possible and neither are yet warranted". Clearly the evaluation of reproducibly of findings is a complex issue.

One further reason for concern is that the suggestion that publications are not replicated is more likely to be cited than those that are replicated (Serra-Garcia & Gneezy, 2021). Why should that be? They suggest that results that are more "interesting" and are more likely to be published and subsequently cited. They are more "interesting" because they are unexpected. When submitted to journals, a less stringent review process is applied to such papers as they are attractive to journal editors. They are more attractive as they are thought to be likely to receive more citations and thereby boost a journal's impact factor.

There can be no doubt that scientists across the physical, biological, and social sciences are aware of a crisis related to reproducibility. Baker (2016) reports on a survey of over 1500 scientists, 52% of whom agreed that there is a significant "crisis". It has been suggested that studies in developmental psychology may be particularly prone to a lack of attention to the reproducibility of research and to a failure to test the robustness of findings within research reports (Duncan et al., 2014). They suggested that:

> leading journals in developmental psychology rarely include explicit replications of prior research conducted by different investigators, and few require authors to establish in their articles or online appendices that their key results are robust across estimation methods, data sets, and demographic subgroups. (Duncan et al., 2014, p. 2417)

Pre-registration Of the potential factors contributing non-reproducibility, the respondents in the Baker (2016) report identified selective reporting as the largest contribution. One major aspect of selective reporting is "p-hacking" where results are trawled to identify those that provide an *p* value below .05 (Nelson et al., 2018). One way to limit this practice is the pre-registration of studies. Nelson et al. (2018) identify two platforms for pre-registration – AsPredicted (http://AsPredicted.org) and the OSF (http://osf.io). An illustration of the way pre-registration is becoming standard good practice is the guidance from the Journal of Child Psychology and Psychiatry (a leading journal in the field of developmental psychology) that:

> Trials should be registered in one of the ICJME-recognised trial registries… Trial registration must include a pre-registered, date stamped, publicly available protocol setting out, at least, the research question, hypotheses, primary outcome and statistics plan.

This requirement is extended to other non-trial studies as follows:

> Pre-registration of studies with all other types of designs on publicly available platforms is encouraged. (https://acamh.onlinelibrary.wiley.com/hub/journal/14697610/forauthors.html#tr. Accessed 25 April 2023)

It may be thought that meta-analysis (see Sect. 2.7), by quantitatively synthesising the results from many studies, would address some of the problems of non-reproducibility and p-hacking. But, as Nelson et al. (2018) show, meta-analysis does not necessarily solve the problem. They suggest that:

> if one out of five studies is poorly done or obviously p-hacked, that study can be easily and safely ignored. However, if it is combined with the other studies into one analysis, it will taint them all (and that taint is likely to go unnoticed). (Nelson et al., 2018, p. 528)

Terminology What are the implications of these problems in the replicability and reliability of the studies in this field? There is a need to clarify the terminology being adopted in the discussion around reproducibility (Goodman et al., 2016). For example, some of the basic terms – reproducibility, replicability, reliability, robustness, and generalisability – are not standardised. This is an impediment to "understanding the relationships between reproducibility, cumulative evidence, and the truth of scientific claims". To address this inconsistency in the usage of terms, they proposed the following definitions:

Methods reproducibility – the ability to implement, as exactly as possible, the experimental and computational procedures, with the same data and tools, to obtain the same results
Results reproducibility (also replicability) – obtaining the same results from the conduct of an independent study whose procedures are as closely matched to the original experiment as possible
Robustness – the stability of experimental conclusions to variations in either baseline assumptions or experimental procedures
Generalisability – the persistence of an effect in settings different from and outside of an experimental framework [this is especially pertinent to randomised clinical trials – will the results generalise to delivery in everyday clinical practice]
Inferential reproducibility – the drawing of qualitatively similar conclusions from either an independent replication of a study or a reanalysis of the original study.

Goodman et al. (2016) suggest that

> Multiplicity, combined with incomplete reporting, might be the single largest contributor to the phenomenon of nonreproducibility, or falsity, of published claims. Multiplicity can arise in many ways, including testing many hypotheses in one experiment, testing one hypothesis many times or in multiple ways in one or more studies, and other manoeuvres that virtually guarantee a chance observation that will appear to strongly support some hypotheses. (Goodman et al., 2016, p. 4)

The manoeuvres they are referring to here include HARKing (i.e. Hypothesising After the Results are Known) and p-hacking (applying many analyses to seek out significant results in a manner that is not driven by theory and that is often unreported). The dangers arising from these manoeuvres in child studies were drawn out by Rutter and Pickles (2016) especially what they refer to as "unregulated flexibility" in data analysis.

One clear implication is that no reliance should be placed on isolated studies (Shrout & Rodgers, 2018). However, if replications are needed before confidence can be placed on findings, the OSC-2015 results need to be borne in mind. It is also important not to rely on replications from studies using a single methodology (Munafò & Davey Smith, 2018). Lawlor et al. (2016) make the case for triangulation, which is based on the principle that knowledge can best be advanced by integrating results from several different approaches, where each approach has different key sources of potential bias that are unrelated to each other.

The issues concerning how replications should be attempted were reviewed by Zwaan et al. (2018). One approach that may not be feasible for many studies is to conduct a multiverse reanalysis of the data (Steegen et al., 2016). This works on the basis that any data set provides the possibility of recoding the data values in multiple ways by collapsing values into categories, by combining variables, by transforming the scale, and by data exclusion. These processes can provide diverse data sets (what they call a multiverse of data sets), which can be analysed. The problem that they are seeking to address is the sensitivity of the results of studies to often arbitrary decisions that are made in data preparation and the possible lack of robustness of the findings that are claimed. Steegen et al. (2016) conclude that:

> Admittedly, performing a multiverse analysis will often be difficult, and to a large extent subjective, but that does not change the fact that it is a necessary step for increasing transparency. (Steegen et al., 2016, p. 710)

In part as a reaction to these reproducibility issues, the American Psychological Association produced revised guidelines on the reporting of the results of quantitative research in psychology (Appelbaum et al., 2018). This made a broad range of guidelines to improve the quality of reports of quantitative research to take into account such recent developments as the pre-registration of randomised controlled trials, the increasing frequency of data sharing, and secondary data analysis of very large data sets. Others have placed emphasis on making greater demands on the probability levels for identifying an effect as significantly different from zero (Benjamin et al., 2018). They argue that:

> The lack of reproducibility of scientific studies has caused growing concern over the credibility of claims of new discoveries based on 'statistically significant' findings. There has been much progress toward documenting and addressing several causes of this lack of reproducibility (e.g., multiple testing, P-hacking, publication bias, and under-powered studies). However, we believe that a leading cause of non-reproducibility has not yet been adequately addressed: Statistical standards of evidence for claiming new discoveries in many fields of science are simply too low. Associating 'statistically significant' findings with $P < 0.05$ results in a high rate of false positives *even in the absence of other experimental, procedural and reporting problems*. (Benjamin et al., 2018, p. 6)

Their solution is to require $p < .005$ as the threshold for claiming that new discoveries are significant. This they recognise is an arbitrary value but one that would address the problem of false positives. Of course it increases the likelihood of false negatives and would require much larger sample sizes to achieve the conventional 80% power requirement.

Power and *p* values The power of a study is defined as the probability of correctly rejecting the null hypothesis that there is no effect. The methods for the estimation of power of studies were laid out in classic text by Cohen (1988). A central aspect of these power calculations was the determination of effect sizes. There is an interplay between the desired significance level (i.e. the probability of falsely accepting the null hypothesis), sample size, effect size, and power. The larger the sample size, the greater the power. The smaller the effect size and the lower the desired significance level, the lower the power. It has become a convention that the required power of a study should be at least 80% (Cohen, 1992). Cohen has also provided guidelines on the judgement of the importance of different effect sizes (Cohen, 1992). For example, for the standardised mean difference (SMD), effect sizes of 0.20, 0.50, and 0.80 are deemed to be small, medium, and large, respectively. The equivalent sizes for correlation coefficients were 0.10, 0.30, and 0.50. It has been argued that these required values for correlations are too high and that more appropriate values are 0.10, 0.20, and 0.30 (Gignac & Szodorai, 2016).

Greenland et al. (2016) provide a cautionary account of the ways the misapplication and interpretation of tests of significance can lead to seriously incorrect conclusions. In particular they contend that the adoption of a cut-off p values into significant and non-significant (usually at the .05 level) is "an especially pernicious statistical practice". They provide guidelines on the way test of significance should be treated but suggest that:

> there are no interpretations of these concepts that are at once simple, intuitive, correct, and foolproof. (Greenland et al., 2016, p. 337)

The fundamental problems associated with the misinterpretation of p values have been laid out by Cohen (1994). His recommendations for dealing with the logical problems of inference from null hypothesis statistical testing are the adoption of effect size estimates and the reporting of confidence intervals. In this book, wherever possible, effect sizes and 95% confidence intervals ($CI_{.95}$) will be reported rather than p values. The final requirement for the generalisation of a finding must come from replication. A similar but wider-ranging critique was presented by Meehl (1990), who is the most engaging methodologist. It is sometimes challenging to go through the formal presentation of the logic of his arguments but worth the effort to enjoy the bravura of his writing!

Effect sizes When genetic studies are considered in Sect. 3.2, it will be seen that molecular genetic studies, in particular genome-wide association studies, have found that there are very few genes with large effects on behaviour. Instead behaviour is influenced by an aggregation of genes with small effect acting in concert. The same is true of most influences, both biological and experiential, on a wide range of behaviours (see Götz et al., 2022, for a review). They make a persuasive argument that the emphasis on large effects is misplaced and that by underplaying small effect sizes, reliable and reproducible findings are being ignored. Carey et al. (2023) have shown how small effect sizes in terms of changes in mean score can have a marked effect at the extremes of the population.

To put this into context, one of the largest effect sizes in relation to child behaviour is that of stimulant medication on ADHD. Meta-analyses have reported effect sizes of around SMD = 0.80 (see Sect. 9.6). More typical effect sizes for social influences on behaviour are those reported by Peverill et al. (2021) for the relationship between socioeconomic factors and child psychopathology: family income (SMD = 0.19), low parental education (SMD = 0.25), and poverty status (SMD = 0.25). Götz et al. (2022) conclude:

> It is only once psychological science accepts that small effects are to be expected—as the norm, rather than the exception—that we have any realistic hope of understanding causal processes in our field. Only then can we start building a cumulative psychological science— on the foundation of small effects. (Götz et al., 2022, p. 209)

Funder and Ozer (2019) provide guidance on how small effect sizes can be treated more appropriately in reports of psychological research. They have three recommendations on the interpretation of research findings. First, "Researchers should not automatically dismiss 'small' effect sizes". One reason for this is that small effect sizes can accumulate over time to produce greater benefits. For example, the Matthew effect arises from reciprocal (and possible modest) effects that amplify over time. This was illustrated by Stanovich (1986) in relation to the development of reading ability:

> The very children who are reading well and who have good vocabularies will read more, learn more word meanings, and hence read even better. Children with inadequate vocabularies— who read slowly and without enjoyment—read less, and as a result have slower development of vocabulary knowledge, which inhibits further growth in reading ability. (Stanovich, 1986, p. 37)

The second recommendation is that "Researchers should be more skeptical about 'large' effects". They point out that replications usually produce smaller effect sizes. For example, Camerer et al. (2018) found that in replications effect sizes were on average 50% of that originally reported. The third recommendation is that "Researchers should be more realistic about the aim of their programs of psychological research". The complexity of factors acting on behaviour makes it unlikely that any one causal factor is going to have more than a modest effect. When designing studies the sample size needs to be sufficiently large to detect what are likely to be small effect size. Accordingly power calculations need to incorporate the expectation of small effect sizes, and they recommend that a smaller number of studies with a larger N are to be preferred as a more appropriate use of resources.

A separate but related issue is the judgement as to whether a treatment intervention produces a change that is of "real-world" importance. This is the question of clinically significant change. Whatever the effect size produced, is it sufficiently large to make a difference to the quality of life of participants? The approaches to assessing clinically significant change are discussed in Sect. 9.6.

Moves to address reproducibility An important component of the approach to increase reproducibility is that of the use open-source software (Buck, 2015). This provides an account of the history of decisions that were made in the course of the analysis of data sets, and this history is open to inspection by others. The adoption of open data approach as a means to improve reproducibility has been endorsed by Lowndes et al. (2017) who illustrate the cost-effectiveness of use of free software tools (such as R Markdown and GitHub) in collaborative research.

One novel development in the UK has been the establishment of the UK Reproducibility Network, which has the following aims:

> The UK Reproducibility Network (UKRN) is a national peer-led consortium that aims to ensure the UK retains its place as a centre for world-leading research. We do this by investigating the factors that contribute to robust research, promoting training activities, and disseminating best practice. We also work collaboratively with various external stakeholders to ensure coordination of efforts across the sector.
>
> We seek to understand the factors that contribute to poor research reproducibility and replicability, and develop approaches to counter these, in order to improve the trustworthiness and quality of research. These issues affect all disciplines, so we aim for broad disciplinary representation. We believe that ongoing efforts to address these issues represent an opportunity to improve our research by reforming culture and practice. (Extract from https://www.ukrn.org. Accessed 25 April 2023)

The importance of these factors for the lack of reproducibility of studies was identified by Camerer et al. (2018) in a replication of 21 experimental studies in the social science published in Nature and Science between 2010 and 2015. They suggest that these systematic biases can be reduced by implementation of pre-registration of analysis plans. This will reduce the likelihood of false positives, and registration and reporting of all study results will reduce the effects of publication bias in inflating effect sizes. They are optimistic that such changes will gradually improve repeatability of studies in psychology. Others are even more sanguine about the health of science research. Fanelli (2018) argues that the ways in which science in general has developed in the recent past in terms of increased transparency and in the application of technologies have made science more accurate, powerful, open, democratic, transparent, and self-correcting than ever before.

2.10 Final Thoughts on Data Analysis

The approaches to data analysis in the study of developmental psychopathology outlined in this chapter have concentrated largely on those methods that have been adopted in the studies referred to in later chapters. They have by no means covered all the relevant data analysis techniques. In particular there are methods that have been developed for the analysis of intervention studies and repeated measures, such as linear mixed models (Gueorguieva & Krystal, 2004), that have not been addressed. Often the methods covered have been developed to take advantage of the opportunities that large sample sizes have provided. However there are disadvantages too that arise from large sample sizes, such as opportunity costs to undertake other studies (Finkel et al., 2017) and from studies with multiple measures, such as the need to adjust for multiple tests of significance (Bender & Lange, 2001). The critical issue in data analysis is not the rudimentary inspection of results for statistical significance but a more nuanced inspection of effect sizes with an appreciation that important effects will often be carried by variables producing modest or even small effect sizes.

References

Academy of Medical Sciences. (2007). *Identifying the environmental causes of disease: How should we decide what to believe and when to take action? An Academy of Medical Sciences working group report chaired by Michael Rutter*. Academy of Medical Sciences.

Achenbach, T. M., & Rescorla, L. A. (2000). *Manual for the ASEBA Preschool Forms & Profiles*. University of Vermont, Research Center for Children, Youth, and Families.

Aggarwal, N., Moody, J. F., Dean, D. C., Tromp, D. M., Kecskemeti, S. R., Oler, J. A., et al. (2021). Spatiotemporal dynamics of nonhuman primate white matter development during the first year of life. *NeuroImage, 231*. https://doi.org/10.1016/j.neuroimage.2021.117825

Anderson, C. J., Bahnik, S., Barnett-Cowan, M., Bosco, F. A., Chandler, J., Chartier, C. R., et al. (2016). Response to comment on "Estimating the reproducibility of psychological science". *Science, 351*(6277). https://doi.org/10.1126/science.aad9163

Appelbaum, M., Cooper, H., Kline, R. B., Mayo-Wilson, E., Nezu, A. M., & Rao, S. M. (2018). Journal article reporting standards for quantitative research in psychology: The APA Publications and Communications Board Task Force Report. *American Psychologist, 73*(1), 3–25. https://doi.org/10.1037/amp0000191

Baker, M. (2016). Is there a reproducibility crisis? *Nature, 533*(7604), 452–454. https://doi.org/10.1038/533452a

Bansal, P. S., Goh, P. K., Lee, C. T. A., & Martel, M. M. (2020). Conceptualizing callous-unemotional traits in preschool through confirmatory factor and network analysis. *Journal of Abnormal Child Psychology, 48*(4), 539–550. https://doi.org/10.1007/s10802-019-00611-9

Baron, R. M., & Kenny, D. A. (1986). The moderator mediator variable distinction in social psychological-research – Conceptual, strategic, and statistical considerations. *Journal of Personality and Social Psychology, 51*(6), 1173–1182. https://doi.org/10.1037/0022-3514.51.6.1173

Begley, C. G., & Ellis, L. M. (2012). Raise standards for preclinical cancer research. *Nature, 483*(7391), 531–533. https://doi.org/10.1038/483531a

Bender, R., & Lange, S. (2001). Adjusting for multiple testing – When and how? *Journal of Clinical Epidemiology, 54*(4), 343–349. https://doi.org/10.1016/s0895-4356(00)00314-0

Benjamin, D. J., Berger, J. O., Johannesson, M., Nosek, B. A., Wagenmakers, E. J., Berk, R., et al. (2018). Redefine statistical significance. *Nature Human Behaviour, 2*(1), 6–10. https://doi.org/10.1038/s41562-017-0189-z

Bogdan, R., Salmeron, B. J., Carey, C. E., Agrawal, A., Calhoun, V. D., Garavan, H., et al. (2017). Imaging genetics and genomics in psychiatry: A critical review of progress and potential. *Biological Psychiatry, 82*(3), 165–175. https://doi.org/10.1016/j.biopsych.2016.12.030

Bollen, K. A., & Pearl, J. (2013). Eight myths about causality and structural equation models. In S. L. Morgan (Ed.), *Handbook of causal analysis for social research* (pp. 301–328). Springer.

Bollen, K. A., Fisher, Z., Lilly, A., Brehm, C., Luo, L., Martinez, A., & Ye, A. (2022). Fifty years of structural equation modeling: A history of generalization, unification, and diffusion. *Social Science Research, 107*. https://doi.org/10.1016/j.ssresearch.2022.102769

Bone, D., Goodwin, M. S., Black, M. P., Lee, C. C., Audhkhasi, K., & Narayanan, S. (2015). Applying machine learning to facilitate autism diagnostics: Pitfalls and promises. *Journal of Autism and Developmental Disorders, 45*(5), 1121–1136. https://doi.org/10.1007/s10803-014-2268-6

Bone, D., Bishop, S. L., Black, M. P., Goodwin, M. S., Lord, C., & Narayanan, S. S. (2016). Use of machine learning to improve autism screening and diagnostic instruments: Effectiveness, efficiency, and multi-instrument fusion. *Journal of Child Psychology and Psychiatry, 57*(8), 927–937. https://doi.org/10.1111/jcpp.12559

Borenstein, M., Hedges, L., Higgins, J., & Rothstein, H. (2009). *Introduction to meta-analysis*. Wiley.

Borsboom, D., Cramer, A. O. J., & Kalis, A. (2019). Brain disorders? Not really: Why network structures block reductionism in psychopathology research. *Behavioral and Brain Sciences, 42*. https://doi.org/10.1017/s0140525x17002266

Boschloo, L., Schoevers, R. A., van Borkulo, C. D., Borsboom, D., & Oldehinkel, A. J. (2016). The network structure of psychopathology in a community sample of preadolescents. *Journal of Abnormal Psychology, 125*(4), 599–606. https://doi.org/10.1037/abn0000150

Bringmann, L. F., & Eronen, M. I. (2018). Don't blame the model: Reconsidering the network approach to psychopathology. *Psychological Review, 125*(4), 606–615. https://doi.org/10.1037/rev0000108

Buck, S. (2015). Solving reproducibility. *Science, 348*(6242), 1403–1403. https://doi.org/10.1126/science.aac8041

Button, K. S., Ioannidis, J. P. A., Mokrysz, C., Nosek, B. A., Flint, J., Robinson, E. S. J., & Munafo, M. R. (2013). Power failure: Why small sample size undermines the reliability of neuroscience. *Nature Reviews Neuroscience, 14*(5), 365–376. https://doi.org/10.1038/nrn3475

Bzdok, D., & Meyer-Lindenberg, A. (2018). Machine learning for precision psychiatry: Opportunities and challenges. *Biological Psychiatry-Cognitive Neuroscience and Neuroimaging, 3*(3), 223–230. https://doi.org/10.1016/j.bpsc.2017.11.007

Bzdok, D., Varoquaux, G., & Steyerberg, E. W. (2021). Prediction, not association, paves the road to precision medicine. *JAMA Psychiatry, 78*(2), 127–128. https://doi.org/10.1001/jamapsychiatry.2020.2549

Cai, N., Revez, J. A., Adams, M. J., Andlauer, T. F. M., Breen, G., Byrne, E. M., et al. (2020). Minimal phenotyping yields genome-wide association signals of low specificity for major depression. *Nature Genetics, 52*(4), 437-+. https://doi.org/10.1038/s41588-020-0594-5

Camerer, C. F., Dreber, A., Holzmeister, F., Ho, T. H., Huber, J., Johannesson, M., et al. (2018). Evaluating the replicability of social science experiments in Nature and Science between 2010 and 2015. *Nature Human Behaviour, 2*(9), 637–644. https://doi.org/10.1038/s41562-018-0399-z

Carey, E. G., Ridler, I., Ford, T. J., & Stringaris, A. (2023). Editorial perspective: When is a 'small effect' actually large and impactful? *Journal of Child Psychology and Psychiatry*. https://doi.org/10.1111/jcpp.13817

Carpenter, K. L. H., Sprechmann, P., Calderbank, R., Sapiro, G., & Egger, H. L. (2016). Quantifying risk for anxiety disorders in preschool children: A machine learning approach. *PLoS One, 11*(11). https://doi.org/10.1371/journal.pone.0165524

Chen, E. E., & Wojcik, S. P. (2016). A practical guide to Big Data research in psychology. *Psychological Methods, 21*(4), 458–474. https://doi.org/10.1037/met0000111

Christensen, A., & Golino, H. (2020). On the equivalency of factor and network loadings. *Behavior Research Methods, 53*, 1563–1580.

Christensen, A. P., Golino, H., & Silvia, P. J. (2020). A psychometric network perspective on the validity and validation of personality trait questionnaires. *European Journal of Personality, 34*(6), 1095–1108. https://doi.org/10.1002/per.2265

Cohen, J. (1988). *Statistical power analysis for the behavioral sciences* (2nd ed.). Erlbaum.

Cohen, J. (1992). A power primer. *Psychological Bulletin, 112*(1), 155–159. https://doi.org/10.1037/0033-2909.112.1.155

Cohen, J. (1994). The earth is round (p-less-than .05). *American Psychologist, 49*(12), 997–1003. https://doi.org/10.1037/0003-066x.49.12.997

Contreras, A., Nieto, I., Valiente, C., Espinosa, R., & Vazquez, C. (2019). The study of psychopathology from the network analysis perspective: A systematic review. *Psychotherapy and Psychosomatics, 88*(2), 71–83. https://doi.org/10.1159/000497425

Correll, C. U., Cortese, S., Croatto, G., Monaco, F., Krinitski, D., Arrondo, G., et al. (2021). Efficacy and acceptability of pharmacological, psychosocial, and brain stimulation interventions in children and adolescents with mental disorders: An umbrella review. *World Psychiatry, 20*(2), 244–275. https://doi.org/10.1002/wps.20881

Cortese, S., Tomlinson, A., & Cipriani, A. (2019). Meta-review: Network meta-analyses in child and adolescent psychiatry. *Journal of the American Academy of Child and Adolescent Psychiatry, 58*(2), 167–179. https://doi.org/10.1016/j.jaac.2018.07.891

Coutanche, M., & Hallion, L. (2020). Machine learning for clinical psychology and clinical neuroscience. In A. Wright & M. Hallquist (Eds.), *The Cambridge handbook of research methods in clinical psychology*. Cambridge University Press.

Cramer, A. O. J., Van der Sluis, S., Noordhof, A., Wichers, M., Geschwind, N., Aggen, S. H., et al. (2012). Dimensions of normal personality as networks in search of equilibrium: You can't like parties if you don't like people. *European Journal of Personality, 26*(4), 414–431. https://doi.org/10.1002/per.1866

Cuijpers, P., Weitz, E., Cristea, I. A., & Twisk, J. (2017). Pre-post effect sizes should be avoided in meta-analyses. *Epidemiology and Psychiatric Sciences, 26*(4), 364–368. https://doi.org/10.1017/s2045796016000809

Duncan, G. J., Engel, M., Claessens, A., & Dowsett, C. J. (2014). Replication and robustness in developmental research. *Developmental Psychology, 50*(11), 2417–2425. https://doi.org/10.1037/a0037996

Dwyer, D., & Koutsouleris, N. (2022). Annual Research Review: Translational machine learning for child and adolescent psychiatry. *Journal of Child Psychology and Psychiatry, 63*(4), 421–443. https://doi.org/10.1111/jcpp.13545

Dwyer, D. B., Falkai, P., & Koutsouleris, N. (2018). Machine learning approaches for clinical psychology and psychiatry. In T. Widiger & T. D. Cannon (Eds.), *Annual Review of Clinical Psychology, 14*, 91–118.

Eadeh, H.-M., Markon, K. E., Nigg, J. T., & Nikolas, M. A. (2021). Evaluating the viability of neurocognition as a transdiagnostic construct using both latent variable models and network analysis. *Research on Child and Adolescent Psychopathology, 49*(6), 697–710. https://doi.org/10.1007/s10802-021-00770-8

Eagle, R. F., Romanczyk, R. G., & Lenzenweger, M. F. (2010). Classification of children with autism spectrum disorders: A finite mixture modeling approach to heterogeneity. *Research in Autism Spectrum Disorders, 4*(4), 772–781. https://doi.org/10.1016/j.rasd.2010.02.001

Eisenhauer, J. G. (2021). Meta-analysis and mega-analysis: A simple introduction. *Teaching Statistics, 43*(1), 21–27. https://doi.org/10.1111/test.12242

Epskamp, S., Borsboom, D., & Fried, E. I. (2018). Estimating psychological networks and their accuracy: A tutorial paper. *Behavior Research Methods, 20*, 195–212.

Everitt, B. S., Landau, S., Leese, M., & Stahl, D. (2011). *Cluster analysis* (5th ed.). Wiley.

Fanelli, D. (2018). Is science really facing a reproducibility crisis, and do we need it to? *Proceedings of the National Academy of Sciences of the United States of America, 115*(11), 2628–2631. https://doi.org/10.1073/pnas.1708272114

Finkel, E. J., Eastwick, P. W., & Reis, H. T. (2017). Replicability and other features of a high-quality science: Toward a balanced and empirical approach. *Journal of Personality and Social Psychology, 113*(2), 244–253. https://doi.org/10.1037/pspi0000075

Forbes, M. K., Wright, A. G. C., Markon, K. E., & Krueger, R. F. (2017). Evidence that psychopathology symptom networks have limited replicability. *Journal of Abnormal Psychology, 126*(7), 969–988. https://doi.org/10.1037/abn0000276

Frick, P. J., Ray, J. V., Thornton, L. C., & Kahn, R. E. (2014). Can callous-unemotional traits enhance the understanding, diagnosis, and treatment of serious conduct problems in children and adolescents? A comprehensive review. *Psychological Bulletin, 140*(1), 1–57. https://doi.org/10.1037/a0033076

Fried, E. I., & Cramer, A. O. J. (2017). Moving forward: Challenges and directions for psychopathological network theory and methodology. *Perspectives on Psychological Science, 12*(6), 999–1020. https://doi.org/10.1177/1745691617705892

Funder, D. C., & Ozer, D. J. (2019). Evaluating effect size in psychological research: Sense and nonsense. *Advances in Methods and Practices in Psychological Science, 2*(2), 156–168. https://doi.org/10.1177/2515245919847202

Funkhouser, C. J., Chacko, A. A., Correa, K. A., Kaiser, A. J. E., & Shankman, S. A. (2021). Unique longitudinal relationships between symptoms of psychopathology in youth: A cross-lagged panel network analysis in the ABCD study. *Journal of Child Psychology and Psychiatry, 62*(2), 184–194. https://doi.org/10.1111/jcpp.13256

Fusar-Poli, P., & Radua, J. (2018). Ten simple rules for conducting umbrella reviews. *Evidence-Based Mental Health, 21*(3), 95–100. https://doi.org/10.1136/ebmental-2018-300014

Gardner, F., Leijten, P., Melendez-Torres, G. J., Landau, S., Harris, V., Mann, J., et al. (2019). The earlier the better? Individual participant data and traditional meta-analysis of age effects of parenting interventions. *Child Development, 90*(1), 7–19. https://doi.org/10.1111/cdev.13138

Gasparini, L., Shepherd, D. A., Bavin, E. L., Eadie, P., Reilly, S., Morgan, A. T., & Wake, M. (2023). Using machine-learning methods to identify early-life predictors of 11-year language outcome. *Journal of Child Psychology and Psychiatry*. https://doi.org/10.1111/jcpp.13733

Gaus, R., Pölsterl, S., Greimel, E., Schulte-Körne, G., & Wachinger, C. (2023). Can we diagnose mental disorders in children? A large-scale assessment of machine learning on structural neuroimaging of 6916 children in the adolescent brain cognitive development study. *JCPP Advances*, e12184. https://doi.org/10.1002/jcv2.12184

Georgiades, S., Szatmari, P., Boyle, M., Hanna, S., Duku, E., Zwaigenbaum, L., et al. (2013). Investigating phenotypic heterogeneity in children with autism spectrum disorder: A factor mixture modeling approach. *Journal of Child Psychology and Psychiatry, 54*(2), 206–215. https://doi.org/10.1111/j.1469-7610.2012.02588.x

Gignac, G. E., & Szodorai, E. T. (2016). Effect size guidelines for individual differences researchers. *Personality and Individual Differences, 102*, 74–78. https://doi.org/10.1016/j.paid.2016.06.069

Gilbert, D. T., King, G., Pettigrew, S., & Wilson, T. D. (2016). Comment on "Estimating the reproducibility of psychological science". *Science, 351*(6277). https://doi.org/10.1126/science.aad7243

Goodman, R. (1997). The Strengths and Difficulties Questionnaire: A research note. *Journal of Child Psychology and Psychiatry, 38*(5), 581–586. https://doi.org/10.1111/j.1469-7610.1997.tb01545.x

Goodman, R. (2001). Psychometric properties of the Strengths and Difficulties Questionnaire. *Journal of the American Academy of Child and Adolescent Psychiatry, 40*(11), 1337–1345. https://doi.org/10.1097/00004583-200111000-00015

Goodman, S. N., Fanelli, D., & Ioannidis, J. P. A. (2016). What does research reproducibility mean? *Science Translational Medicine, 8*(341). https://doi.org/10.1126/scitranslmed.aaf5027

Götz, F. M., Gosling, S. D., & Rentfrow, P. J. (2022). Small effects: The indispensable foundation for a cumulative psychological science. *Perspectives on Psychological Science, 17*(1), 205–215. https://doi.org/10.1177/1745691620984483

Greenland, S., Senn, S. J., Rothman, K. J., Carlin, J. B., Poole, C., Goodman, S. N., & Altman, D. G. (2016). Statistical tests, P values, confidence intervals, and power: A guide to misinterpretations. *European Journal of Epidemiology, 31*(4), 337–350. https://doi.org/10.1007/s10654-016-0149-3

Groen, R. N., Wichers, M., Wigman, J. T. W., & Hartman, C. A. (2019). Specificity of psychopathology across levels of severity: A transdiagnostic network analysis. *Scientific Reports, 9*. https://doi.org/10.1038/s41598-019-54801-y

Gueorguieva, R., & Krystal, J. H. (2004). Move over ANOVA – Progress in analyzing repeated-measures data and its reflection in papers published in the Archives of General Psychiatry. *Archives of General Psychiatry, 61*(3), 310–317. https://doi.org/10.1001/archpsyc.61.3.310

Hallquist, M. N., Wright, A. G. C., & Molenaar, P. C. M. (2019). Problems with centrality measures in psychopathology symptom networks: Why network psychometrics cannot escape psychometric theory. *Multivariate Behavioral Research*. https://doi.org/10.1080/00273171.2019.1640103

Higgins, J. P. T., Thomas, J., Chandler, J., Cumpston, M., Li, T. Y., Page, M. J., & Welch, V. A. (Eds.). (2019). *Cochrane handbook for systematic reviews of interventions* (2nd ed.). John Wiley & Sons.

Hu, L. T., & Bentler, P. M. (1999). Cutoff criteria for fit indexes in covariance structure analysis: Conventional criteria versus new alternatives. *Structural Equation Modeling-A Multidisciplinary Journal, 6*(1), 1–55. https://doi.org/10.1080/10705519909540118

Huang, D. B., Susser, E., Rudolph, K. E., & Keyes, K. M. (2023). Depression networks: A systematic review of the network paradigm causal assumptions. *Psychological Medicine, 53*(5), 1665–1680. https://doi.org/10.1017/s0033291723000132

Hukkelberg, S. (2019). The quintessence of child conduct problems: Identifying central behaviors through network analysis. *Journal of Psychopathology and Behavioral Assessment, 41*(2), 175–184. https://doi.org/10.1007/s10862-018-9713-3

Iniesta, R., Stahl, D., & McGuffin, P. (2016). Machine learning, statistical learning and the future of biological research in psychiatry. *Psychological Medicine, 46*(12), 2455–2465. https://doi.org/10.1017/s0033291716001367

Iniesta, R., Hodgson, K., Stahl, D., Malki, K., Maier, W., Rietschel, M., et al. (2018). Antidepressant drug-specific prediction of depression treatment outcomes from genetic and clinical variables. *Scientific Reports, 8*. https://doi.org/10.1038/s41598-018-23584-z

Ioannidis, J. P. A. (2009). Integration of evidence from multiple meta-analyses: A primer on umbrella reviews, treatment networks and multiple treatments meta-analyses. *Canadian Medical Association Journal, 181*(8), 488–493. https://doi.org/10.1503/cmaj.081086

Jackson, D. L., Gillaspy, J. A., & Purc-Stephenson, R. (2009). Reporting practices in confirmatory factor analysis: An overview and some recommendations. *Psychological Methods, 14*(1), 6–23. https://doi.org/10.1037/a0014694

Jain, A. K. (2010). Data clustering: 50 years beyond K-means. *Pattern Recognition Letters, 31*(8), 651–666. https://doi.org/10.1016/j.patrec.2009.09.011

Johnson, S. K. (2021). Latent profile transition analyses and growth mixture models: A very non-technical guide for researchers in child and adolescent development. *New Directions for Child and Adolescent Development.* https://doi.org/10.1002/cad.20398

Johnston, B. A., Mwangi, B., Matthews, K., Coghill, D., Konrad, K., & Steele, J. D. (2014). Brainstem abnormalities in Attention Deficit Hyperactivity Disorder support high accuracy individual diagnostic classification. *Human Brain Mapping, 35*(10), 5179–5189. https://doi.org/10.1002/hbm.22542

Jones, P. J., Mair, P., Riemann, B. C., Mugno, B. L., & McNally, R. J. (2018). A network perspective on comorbid depression in adolescents with obsessive-compulsive disorder. *Journal of Anxiety Disorders, 53,* 1–8. https://doi.org/10.1016/j.janxdis.2017.09.008

Kamphaus, R. W., Huberty, C. J., DiStefano, C., & Petoskey, M. D. (1997). A typology of teacher-rated child behavior for a national US sample. *Journal of Abnormal Child Psychology, 25*(6), 453–463. https://doi.org/10.1023/a:1022681630818

Kimonis, E. R., Fanti, K. A., Anastassiou-Hadjicharalambous, X., Mertan, B., Goulter, N., & Katsimicha, E. (2016). Can callous-unemotional traits be reliably measured in preschoolers? *Journal of Abnormal Child Psychology, 44*(4), 625–638. https://doi.org/10.1007/s10802-015-0075-y

Kline, R. (2016). *Principles and practice of structural equation modelling* (4th ed.). Guilford Press.

Kraemer, H. C., Stice, E., Kazdin, A., Offord, D., & Kupfer, D. (2001). How do risk factors work together? Mediators, moderators, and independent, overlapping, and proxy risk factors. *American Journal of Psychiatry, 158*(6), 848–856. https://doi.org/10.1176/appi.ajp.158.6.848

Lawlor, D. A., Tilling, K., & Smith, G. D. (2016). Triangulation in aetiological epidemiology. *International Journal of Epidemiology, 45*(6), 1866–1886. https://doi.org/10.1093/ije/dyw314

Lecavalier, L. (2006). Behavioral and emotional problems in young people with pervasive developmental disorders: Relative prevalence, effects of subject characteristics, and empirical classification. *Journal of Autism and Developmental Disorders, 36*(8), 1101–1114. https://doi.org/10.1007/s10803-006-0147-5

Lee, H., Herbert, R. D., & McAuley, J. H. (2019). Mediation analysis. *JAMA-Journal of the American Medical Association, 321*(7), 697–698. https://doi.org/10.1001/jama.2018.21973

Lei, P.-W., & Wu, Q. (2007). Introduction to structural equation modeling: Issues and practical considerations. https://onlinelibrary.wiley.com/doi/pdf/10.1111/j.1745-3992.2007.00099.x

Lowndes, J. S. S., Best, B. D., Scarborough, C., Afflerbach, J. C., Frazier, M. R., O'Hara, C. C., et al. (2017). Our path to better science in less time using open data science tools. *Nature Ecology & Evolution, 1*(6). https://doi.org/10.1038/s41559-017-0160

Lyons-Warren, A. M., Wangler, M. F., & Wan, Y. W. (2022). Cluster analysis of Short Sensory Profile data reveals sensory-based subgroups in Autism Spectrum Disorder. *International Journal of Molecular Sciences, 23*(21). https://doi.org/10.3390/ijms232113030

Martel, M. M., Levinson, C. A., Langer, J. K., & Nigg, J. T. (2016). A network analysis of developmental change in ADHD symptom structure from preschool to adulthood. *Clinical Psychological Science, 4*(6), 988–1001. https://doi.org/10.1177/2167702615618664

Mavridis, D., Giannatsi, M., Cipriani, A., & Salanti, G. (2015). A primer on network meta-analysis with emphasis on mental health. *Evidence-Based Mental Health, 18*(2), 40–46. https://doi.org/10.1136/eb-2015-102088

McDonald, R. P., & Ho, M. H. R. (2002). Principles and practice in reporting structural equation analyses. *Psychological Methods, 7*(1), 64–82. https://doi.org/10.1037//1082-989x.7.1.64

McElroy, E., Shevlin, M., Murphy, J., & McBride, O. (2018). Co-occurring internalizing and externalizing psychopathology in childhood and adolescence: A network approach. *European Child and Adolescent Psychiatry, 27*(11), 1449–1457. https://doi.org/10.1007/s00787-018-1128-x

McGuirl, M. R., Smith, S. P., Sandstede, B., & Ramachandran, S. (2020). Detecting shared genetic architecture among multiple phenotypes by hierarchical clustering of gene-level association statistics. *Genetics, 215*(2), 511–529. https://doi.org/10.1534/genetics.120.303096

McNally, R. J. (2016). Can network analysis transform psychopathology? *Behaviour Research and Therapy, 86*, 95–104. https://doi.org/10.1016/j.brat.2016.06.006

McNally, R. J. (2021). Network analysis of psychopathology: Controversies and challenges. In T. D. Cannon & T. Widiger (Eds.), *Annual Review of Clinical Psychology, 17*, 31–53. https://doi.org/10.1146/annurev-clinpsy-081219-092850

Meehl, P. E. (1990). Why summaries of research on psychological theories are often uninterpretable. *Psychological Reports, 66*(1), 195–244. https://doi.org/10.2466/pr0.66.1.195-244

Miotto, R., Li, L., Kidd, B. A., & Dudley, J. T. (2016). Deep patient: An unsupervised representation to predict the future of patients from the electronic health records. *Scientific Reports, 6*. https://doi.org/10.1038/srep26094

Moher, D., Liberati, A., Tetzlaff, J., Altman, D. G., & Grp, P. (2009). Preferred reporting items for systematic reviews and meta-analyses: The PRISMA statement. *BMJ-British Medical Journal, 339*. https://doi.org/10.1136/bmj.b2535

Moher, D., Hopewell, S., Schulz, K. F., Montori, V., Gotzsche, P. C., Devereaux, P. J., et al. (2010). CONSORT 2010 explanation and elaboration: Updated guidelines for reporting parallel group randomised trials. *BMJ-British Medical Journal, 340*. https://doi.org/10.1136/bmj.c869

Munafò, M., & Davey Smith, G. (2018). Repeating experiments is not enough. *Nature, 553*(7689), 399–401. https://doi.org/10.1038/d41586-018-01023-3

Murray, L., Arteche, A., Fearon, P., Halligan, S., Croudace, T., & Cooper, P. (2010). The effects of maternal postnatal depression and child sex on academic performance at age 16 years: A developmental approach. *Journal of Child Psychology and Psychiatry, 51*(10), 1150–1159. https://doi.org/10.1111/j.1469-7610.2010.02259.x

Nelson, L. D., Simmons, J., & Simonsohn, U. (2018). Psychology's renaissance. In S. T. Fiske (Ed.), *Annual Review of Psychology, 69*, 511–534.

Niclasen, J., Skovgaard, A. M., Andersen, A.-M. N., Somhovd, M. J., & Obel, C. (2013). A confirmatory approach to examining the factor structure of the Strengths and Difficulties Questionnaire (SDQ): A large scale cohort study. *Journal of Abnormal Child Psychology, 41*(3), 355–365. https://doi.org/10.1007/s10802-012-9683-y

Nylund, K., Nishina, A., Bellmore, A., & Graham, S. (2007). Subtypes, severity, and structural stability of peer victimization: What does latent class analysis say? *Child Develeopment, 78*(6), 1706–1722. https://doi.org/10.1111/j.1467-8624.2007.01097.x

Open Science Collaboration. (2015). Estimating the reproducibility of psychological science. *Science, 349*(6251). https://doi.org/10.1126/science.aac4716

Peverill, M., Dirks, M. A., Narvaja, T., Herts, K. L., Comer, J. S., & McLaughlin, K. A. (2021). Socioeconomic status and child psychopathology in the United States: A meta-analysis of population-based studies. *Clinical Psychology Review, 83*. https://doi.org/10.1016/j.cpr.2020.101933

Phillips, M. L., & Kendler, K. S. (2021). Three important considerations for studies examining pathophysiological pathways in psychiatric illness in-depth phenotyping, biological assessment, and causal inferences. *JAMA Psychiatry, 78*(7), 697–698. https://doi.org/10.1001/jamapsychiatry.2021.0022

Riley, R. D., Lambert, P. C., & Abo-Zaid, G. (2010). Meta-analysis of individual participant data: Rationale, conduct, and reporting. *BMJ-British Medical Journal, 340*. https://doi.org/10.1136/bmj.c221

Rouquette, A., Pingault, J. B., Fried, E. I., Orri, M., Falissard, B., Kossakowski, J. J., et al. (2018). Emotional and behavioral symptom network structure in elementary school girls and association with anxiety disorders and depression in adolescence and early adulthood A network analysis. *JAMA Psychiatry, 75*(11), 1173–1181. https://doi.org/10.1001/jamapsychiatry.2018.2119

Russell, J. D., Neill, E. L., Carrion, V. G., & Weems, C. F. (2017). The network structure of posttraumatic stress symptoms in children and adolescents exposed to disasters. *Journal of the American Academy of Child and Adolescent Psychiatry, 56*(8), 669–677. https://doi.org/10.1016/j.jaac.2017.05.021

Rutter, M. (1967). A children's behaviour questionnaire for completion by teachers: Preliminary findings. *Journal of Child Psychology and Psychiatry, 8*(1), 1–11. https://doi.org/10.1111/j.1469-7610.1967.tb02175.x

Rutter, M., & Pickles, A. (2016). Annual Research Review: Threats to the validity of child psychiatry and psychology. *Journal of Child Psychology and Psychiatry, 57*(3), 398–416. https://doi.org/10.1111/jcpp.12461

Rutter, M., Tizard, J., & Whitmore, K. (1970). *Education, health and behaviour*. Longmans.

Saxe, G. N., Statnikov, A., Fenyo, D., Ren, J. W., Li, Z. G., Prasad, M., et al. (2016). A complex systems approach to causal discovery in psychiatry. *PLoS One, 11*(3). https://doi.org/10.1371/journal.pone.0151174

Schilling, C., Kuhn, S., Paus, T., Romanowski, A., Banaschewski, T., Barbot, A., et al. (2013). Cortical thickness of superior frontal cortex predicts impulsiveness and perceptual reasoning in adolescence. *Molecular Psychiatry, 18*(5), 624–630. https://doi.org/10.1038/mp.2012.56

Schlarb, A. A., Jaeger, S., Schneider, S., In-Albon, T., & Hautzinger, M. (2016). Sleep problems and separation anxiety in preschool-aged children: A path analysis. *Journal of Child and Family Studies, 25*(3), 902–910. https://doi.org/10.1007/s10826-015-0262-z

Senior, M., Fanshawe, T., Fazel, M., & Fazel, S. (2021). Prediction models for child and adolescent mental health: A systematic review of methodology and reporting in recent research. *JCPP Advances, 1*(3), e12034. https://doi.org/10.1002/jcv2.12034

Serra-Garcia, M., & Gneezy, U. (2021). Nonreplicable publications are cited more than replicable ones. *Science Advances, 7*(21). https://doi.org/10.1126/sciadv.abd1705

Shrout, P. E., & Rodgers, J. L. (2018). Psychology, science, and knowledge construction: Broadening perspectives from the replication crisis. In S. T. Fiske (Ed.), *Annual Review of Psychology, 69,* 487–510.

Siddaway, A. P., Wood, A. M., & Hedges, L. V. (2019). How to do a systematic review: A best practice guide for conducting and reporting narrative reviews, meta-analyses, and meta-syntheses. *Annual Review of Psychology, 70,* 747–770. https://doi.org/10.1146/annurev-psych-010418-102803

Sonuga-Barke, E. J. S. (2023). Editorial: 'Safety in numbers?' Big data discovery strategies in neuro-developmental science – Contributions and caveats. *Journal of Child Psychology and Psychiatry, 64*(1), 1–3. https://doi.org/10.1111/jcpp.13723

Stanovich, K. E. (1986). Matthew effects in reading – Some consequences of individual differences in the acquisition of reading. *Reading Research Quarterly, 21*(4), 360–407. https://doi.org/10.1598/rrq.21.4.1

Steegen, S., Tuerlinckx, F., Gelman, A., & Vanpaemel, W. (2016). Increasing transparency through a multiverse analysis. *Perspectives on Psychological Science, 11*(5), 702–712. https://doi.org/10.1177/1745691616658637

Streiner, D. L. (2005). Finding our way: An introduction to path analysis. *Canadian Journal of Psychiatry-Revue Canadienne De Psychiatrie, 50*(2), 115–122.

Sullivan, P. F., & Kendler, K. S. (2021). The state of the science in psychiatric genomics. *Psychological Medicine*, 1–3. https://doi.org/10.1017/s0033291720004900

Tabachnick, B. G., & Fidell, L. S. (2013). *Using multivariate statistics* (6th ed.). Pearson.

Tackett, J. L., Lahey, B. B., van Hulle, C., Waldman, I., Krueger, R. F., & Rathouz, P. J. (2013). Common genetic influences on negative emotionality and a general psychopathology factor in childhood and adolescence. *Journal of Abnormal Psychology, 122*(4), 1142–1153. https://doi.org/10.1037/a0034151

Thompson, P. M., Stein, J. L., Medland, S. E., Hibar, D. P., Vasquez, A. A., Renteria, M. E., et al. (2014). The ENIGMA Consortium: Large-scale collaborative analyses of neuroimaging and genetic data. *Brain Imaging and Behavior, 8*(2), 153–182. https://doi.org/10.1007/s11682-013-9269-5

VanderWeele, T. J. (2021). Can sophisticated study designs with regression analyses of observational data provide causal inferences? *JAMA Psychiatry, 78*(3), 244–246. https://doi.org/10.1001/jamapsychiatry.2020.2588

VanderWeele, T. J., & Vansteelandt, S. (2014). Mediation analysis with multiple mediators. *Epidemiologic Methods, 2*(1), 95–115.

Wade, M., Carroll, D., Fox, N. A., Zeanah, C. H., & Nelson, C. A. (2021). Associations between early psychosocial deprivation, cognitive and psychiatric morbidity, and risk-taking behavior in adolescence. *Journal of Clinical Child and Adolescent Psychology*, 1–14. https://doi.org/10.1080/15374416.2020.1864737

Wiecki, T. V., Poland, J., & Frank, M. J. (2015). Model-based cognitive neuroscience approaches to computational psychiatry: Clustering and classification. *Clinical Psychological Science, 3*(3), 378–399. https://doi.org/10.1177/2167702614565359

Wiggins, J. L., Briggs-Gowan, M. J., Brotman, M. A., Leibenluft, E., & Wakschlag, L. S. (2021). Toward a developmental nosology for Disruptive Mood Dysregulation Disorder in early childhood. *Journal of the American Academy of Child and Adolescent Psychiatry, 60*(3), 388–397. https://doi.org/10.1016/j.jaac.2020.04.015

Willems, G., Jansma, B., Blomert, L., & Vaessen, A. (2016). Cognitive and familial risk evidence converged: A data-driven identification of distinct and homogeneous subtypes within the heterogeneous sample of reading disabled children. *Research in Developmental Disabilities, 53–54*, 213–231. https://doi.org/10.1016/j.ridd.2015.12.018

Wolfle, L. M. (2003). The introduction of path analysis to the social sciences, and some emergent themes: An annotated bibliography. *Structural Equation Modeling, 10*(1), 1–34. https://doi.org/10.1207/s15328007sem1001_1

Wolkind, S. N., & Everitt, B. (1974). Cluster-analysis of behavioral items in preschool-child. *Psychological Medicine, 4*(4), 422–427. https://doi.org/10.1017/s0033291700045876

Wright, S. (1920). The relative importance of heredity and environment in determining the piebald pattern of Guinea-pigs. *Proceedings of the National Academy of Sciences USA, 6*, 320–332. https://doi.org/10.1073/pnas.6.6.320

Wright, S. (1934). The method of path coefficients. *Annals of Mathematical Statistics, 5*, 161–215. https://doi.org/10.1214/aoms/1177732676

Yarkoni, T., & Westfall, J. (2017). Choosing prediction over explanation in psychology: Lessons from machine learning. *Perspectives on Psychological Science, 12*(6), 1100–1122. https://doi.org/10.1177/1745691617693393

Yew, S. G. K., & O'Kearney, R. (2013). Emotional and behavioural outcomes later in childhood and adolescence for children with specific language impairments: Meta-analyses of controlled prospective studies. *Journal of Child Psychology and Psychiatry, 54*(5), 516–524. https://doi.org/10.1111/jcpp.12009

Zhao, X. S., Lynch, J. G., & Chen, Q. M. (2010). Reconsidering Baron and Kenny: Myths and truths about mediation analysis. *Journal of Consumer Research, 37*(2), 197–206. https://doi.org/10.1086/651257

Zou, J., Huss, M., Abid, A., Mohammadi, P., Torkamani, A., & Telenti, A. (2019). A primer on deep learning in genomics. *Nature Genetics, 51*(1), 12–18. https://doi.org/10.1038/s41588-018-0295-5

Zwaan, R. A., Etz, A., Lucas, R. E., & Donnellan, M. B. (2018). Making replication mainstream. *Behavioral and Brain Sciences, 41*. https://doi.org/10.1017/s0140525x1700197

Chapter 3
Investigating the Biology of Behavioural Differences

Behaviour genetics studies have emerged as a central strand of research into the basis of behavioural differences. Such studies can be broadly classified into two groups. The first are based on the analysis of behavioural similarities between people with differing degrees of genetic relatedness. These are quantitative genetic studies. The second are molecular genetic studies in which there is an analysis of differences in the DNA and an examination of how these differences relate to behaviour.

Historically molecular genetics examined the association between known variants of a gene and phenotypic variation. For our purposes the phenotype refers to behavioural differences. One such approach are candidate gene association studies where genes are selected that are thought to be physiologically related to the behaviour. A second approach are linkage studies that examine the way DNA variants are inherited alongside behaviour variations in a family pedigree.

Molecular genetics is now dominated by genome-wide association studies (GWASs) that have superseded candidate gene association and linkage approaches. GWAS examines the association between thousands of DNA variations and behaviour. These variants are not necessarily known at the outset to be related to the behaviour of interest. It is important to note that GWAS does not identify an association with a gene but merely (but valuably) with a site on a chromosome with DNA variants that are associated with the behaviour. The actual gene involved may be nearby and this is likely to be only one of large number (thousands) of genes involved in the polygenic system influencing the behaviour. Sections 3.1, 3.2, and 3.4 will outline the application of quantitative and molecular genetics in the study of behavioural differences.

Section 3.3 deals with separate mechanisms whereby genetic effects are moderated by environmental influences. These are epigenetic influences on behaviour that can be transmitted across generations but that do not involve changes in the DNA base-pair sequence (the genetic code). Instead epigenetic mechanisms influence gene expression by, for example, methylation. This is a chemical change to the

J. Stevenson, *Developmental Psychopathology*,
https://doi.org/10.1007/978-3-031-45787-6_3

DNA that modifies the expression of a gene, i.e. how it influences cellular processes. This methylation can persist and the gene that includes this piece of DNA is said to be imprinted. This imprinting can be transmitted across generations. However there is as yet little evidence to support a major role for epigenetic changes in such transmissions of differences in behaviour.

The biological bases of behavioural differences have been the subject of extensive studies using various techniques to examine brain structure and brain function. These studies will be the subject of Sect. 3.6.

The material on genetic influences on behaviour covered in this chapter is the subject of an excellent textbook by Flint et al. (2020). This should be consulted for a more detailed coverage of the question of "how genes influence behaviour" – the title of their book! Flint et al. (2020) also provide an antidote to the notion that the study of behavioural differences has become "gene crazy". They point out that identifying a gene that makes a difference to behaviour is only a start.

> The real action begins when we try to understand how these genes act within cells, and within organisms who interact with an unpredictable environment that is at best indifferent to their existence and often openly hostile. It will not work, we believe, to assume that the little 'bits' of this puzzle all just add together. We know already that they don't. (Flint et al., 2020, p. 283)

This book will make extensive references to genetic influences on behaviour because they are pervasive. However these influences can only be understood if their joint actions and interactions with experiences (the environment) are incorporated into explanations of behavioural differences. This gene-environment interplay is discussed at the end of Sect. 3.1.

3.1 Quantitative Genetics

In order to identify the relative strength of genetic and environmental influences on behavioural differences, it is necessary to study the differential resemblance in behaviour between groups of people who vary in the degree of genetic relatedness. If the behaviour is more similar in individuals with more similar genetic make-ups, the more likely it is that genetic factors play a role influencing behaviour. Twins represent such a group of people with twin pairs varying in their degrees of genetic similarity – adopted children and their non-adopted siblings are another example. Twins are particularly valuable as members of a twin pair are of the same age and have many experiences in common, thereby controlling for a number of possible confounds.

Twin Studies The first person to suggest the potential of twins to identify the role of nature and nurture in influencing human characteristics was Frances Galton (1876). It seems he was surprised to find a predominance of nature in his study of twins:

> ...it seems contrary to all experience that nurture should go for so little. (Galton, 1876, p. 404)

Although often referred to as the origin of the twin method for estimating the strength of genetic and environmental influences, the Galton (1876) paper is based on the presentation of case study material; he was not able to differentiate the zygosity of the twins. Consequently there is no analysis of the differential similarity of monozygotic (MZ) or identical twins and dizygotic (DZ) or fraternal twins; this is the core of the twin method. So who did produce the first quantitative twin study comparing MZ and DZ twins?

Rende et al. (1990) reviewed this question and suggested that this was shared by two authors publishing in 1924. The first is Curtis Merriman who was an American Professor of Education. Merriman (1924) analysed the correlation in measures of intelligence in fraternal and duplicated (identical twins), but since he could not identify zygosity directly, he had to work indirectly through physical similarity. He was able to identify putative duplicated twins by the degree of physical similarity within the group of same-sex twins. He noted that this subset of physically similar twins had very high correlations for measures of intelligence, e.g. 0.986 for the Stanford-Binet test. The second author identified by Rende et al. (1990) was a German dermatologist named Siemens (1924). Mayo (2009) also examined the history of the twin method and identified yet another publication in 1924 that examined the difference in the correlation of characteristics in MZ and DZ twins (Bonnevie, 1924). Kristine Bonnevie was a Norwegian Professor of Biology; one of her students was the explorer Thor Heyerdahl whose Kon-Tiki expedition she helped to sponsor. She too had to rely on physical appearance to determine putative zygosity. She found that the correlation in fingerprint patterns in identical twins was 0.924 and in fraternal twins was 0.535.

So the answer to the question of who first applied the twin study method quantitatively is that we can't be sure, but whoever it was, it looks as if it was in the year 1924!

The formulation of heritability as the proportion of the variance in a characteristic that is attributable to genetic influences (h^2) was developed by Fisher (1918) and by Wright (1920). For Fisher this was part of broader ambition to account for variability in traits (Fisher, 1919) and to develop a theory of the genetic basis of evolution and natural selection (Fisher, 1930). Kohn (2004) gives an account of how Fisher was at the heart of a scientific development in England during the twentieth century to establish the biological basis of population genetics, natural selection, and evolution (the "modern synthesis"). The modern synthesis as an integrated account of the genetic basis of evolution has stood the test of time. However there have been recent attempts to revise this framework with an "extended evolutionary synthesis", which incorporates consideration of the role in evolution of developmental plasticity and other processes (Laland et al., 2015). Developmental plasticity refers to the capacity to modify characteristics in response to environmental changes. This extended evolutionary synthesis has created a vigorous debate in biology and is far from widely accepted (Futuyma, 2017).

Sewell Wright too made important contributions to population genetics and theories of evolution. His concept of genetic drift is an important adjunct to the modern synthesis. It refers to the influence of chance factors in evolution, especially in small populations, resulting in the disappearance of particular genes as individuals die or do not reproduce. (Wright, 1948). In addition, Wright's development of path analysis has had a major impact on the analysis of data in the social sciences and in causal modelling (see Pearl & Mackenzie, 2018).

The logic of the twin method to estimate heritability is based on assumptions about the origins of resemblances between the two types of twin. Monozygotic (MZ) twins resemble one another because they shared 100% of their genes and because they are reared in the same family. Dizygotic (DZ) twins are expected not to be as similar as MZ twins as, although they too share the experience of being raised in the same family, they have (on average) only 50% of their genes in common.

The variance in a behaviour can be divided into that arising from genetic differences (heritability) and designated *A* (this term has come to replace h^2 in publications in quantitative genetics). The shared environment (*C* or c^2) captures the effects of experiences that generate similarities between siblings. The non-shared environment (*E* or e^2) reflects the effects of experiences contributing to differences between siblings. The estimate of variance is also influenced by measurement error, which in the twin method is confounded within *E*.

Falconer (1960) showed that the size of the genetic influence (heritability) on the variance in a characteristic could be estimated based on the following equations:

$$\text{The total variance:} 1 = A + C + E$$

$$\text{The correlation between MZ twins:} r_{\text{mz}} = A + C$$

$$\text{The correlation between DZ twins:} r_{\text{dz}} = 0.5\,A + C$$

These simultaneous equations can be solved to produce the following estimates:

$$A = 2\left(r_{\text{mz}} - r_{\text{dz}}\right)$$

$$C = r_{\text{mz}} - A$$

$$E = 1 - r_{\text{mz}}$$

In this way the estimates of *A*, *C*, and *E* can be derived from the correlations between members of MZ and DZ twin pairs. This method for the analysis of twin data based on correlations has been superseded. The current approach is to use structural equation modelling (SEM) (see Sect. 2.5), and this has been applied to data from samples with a wide range of types of relative, for example, twins, parents, siblings, cousins, and those related via adoption. Specialist computer programmes have been produced for these SEM analyses such as Mx, developed by Michael Neale in the 1980s. This is now freely available as the OpenMx software package (Neale et al., 2016) from https://vipbg.vcu.edu/vipbg/OpenMx2/docs//OpenMx/latest/OpenMxUserGuide.pdf.

Pooling data from studies on 14,558,903 twin pairs (yes, 14 million!), the MaTCH website provides a unique opportunity to identify heritability and shared environment estimates. By accessing the website at http://match.ctglab.nl/#/home, estimates of A and C can be obtained for a wide range of biological and social traits. The effects of factors such as age and country on the estimates can be interrogated using the software provided. Results from this database have been summarised in Polderman et al. (2015). For psychiatric disorders A is 0.46 and C is 0.16. When the analysis for psychiatric disorders is separated by age, the following are obtained: age 0–11 years $A = 0.52$ and $C = 0.17$, 12–17 years $A = 0.46$ and $C = 0.21$, 18–65 years $A = 0.42$ and $C = 0.11$, and over 65 years $A = 0.43$ and $C = 0.16$. There is a consistent pattern of A being 0.50 or just under and of C being 0.20 or under for psychiatric disorders. Accordingly for psychiatric disorders E is approximately 0.30. Similar modest effects of the shared environment were obtained by Kendler et al. (2019) for psychiatric disorders from a Swedish general population register using data on the correlations between twins, step, and half siblings. Here the shared environment estimate across the pooled groups was 0.08 for anxiety and for depression and 0.17 for externalising disorders.

A recent innovation providing further opportunities to identify estimates of genetic and environmental effects comes from the ABCD study (https://abcdstudy.org/about/). This initiative is assembling a data set of brain imaging and cognitive and behavioural measures on 11,880 children ages 9–10 that will track their biological and behavioural development through adolescence into young adulthood. The ABCD is operating on an Open Science model that makes data sets available for analysis by the broader scientific community. The ABCD sample includes over 700 twin pairs. A means of accessing the results of analyses of this data set to obtain estimates of genetic and environmental effects on a wide range of behavioural and brain imaging is provided at https://abcdtwinhub.shinyapps.io/baselineTwinResults/#section-introduction.

Maes et al. (2023) provide an introduction to the use of this invaluable resource.

One of the main concerns with the twin method is whether the equal environment assumption (EEA) is valid. This is the assumption that in terms of experience, MZ and DZ twins are treated equally alike and have equally alike experiences. It may be thought the greater similarity in appearance and behaviour in MZ might have arisen because they have more similar experiences. If that were the case, then the twin method would overestimate the size of genetic effects. To test the validity of the EEA, Lytton (1977) used a variety of methods to examine the experiences of young twins. One method was to observe how parents interacted with the twins in the home environment. As a result of this work, Hugh Lytton concluded that:

> (a) parents do treat MZ twins more alike than DZ twins in some respects, but (b) they do not introduce systematically greater similarity of treatment for MZ twins in actions which they initiate themselves, and (c) the greater homogeneity of treatment of MZ twins, where it occurs, is in line with their actual, rather than their perceived, zygosity. In other words, parents respond to, rather than create, differences between the twins. (Lytton, 1977, p. 456)

The EEA may be violated, but this does not invalidate the twin method because the unequal shared environments are a *consequence* not a *cause* of the twins behaviour. In support of the validity of the twin method, it is also important to recognise the convergence in the estimates from the twin method and that derived from other designs such as adoption studies.

Quantitative Behaviour Genetic Estimation Methods The methods of analysing twin data and the wider range of genetically informative designs have developed radically since the work of Falconer. The extended analysis of genetic influences using twin and family data was established in the early 1970s. There were two particularly significant innovations in methodology and analysis. The first by Jinks and Fulker (1970) was based on the biometrical genetic approach of Fisher (1918, 1919). The second is by Morton (1974) and Rao et al. (1974) who applied the path analysis developed by Wright (1921). Historical accounts of some of the main subsequent methodological innovations in the biometrical genetic approach are given in Eaves (2020).

The path analysis approach informed the development of structural equation modelling (see Sect. 2.5), which has become the dominant method for analysis of quantitative behaviour genetic data. The basic structural equation model for twin data (ACE model) is represented in Fig. 3.1, which in graphical form represents the equations above from Falconer (1960). The analysis attempts to identify values for the unknown parameters (i.e. a, c, e) that will best reproduce the observed correlations between the twins' behaviour given the theoretically specified values for other paths, i.e. shared environment C is perfectly correlated for both types of twin, i.e. $r = 1.00$ (the EEA discussed above), and genes are perfectly correlated for MZ twins ($r = 1.00$) and correlate $r = 0.5$ for DZ pairs.

The model in Fig. 3.1 is for the quantitative genetic analysis of a single measure of behaviour. The ACE model has been elaborated to produce a variety of more complex analyses. For example, Maes et al. (2021) have shown that 25 different structural equation models can be tested to estimate the role of genetic and environmental factors in influencing just 2 measured variables in twins!

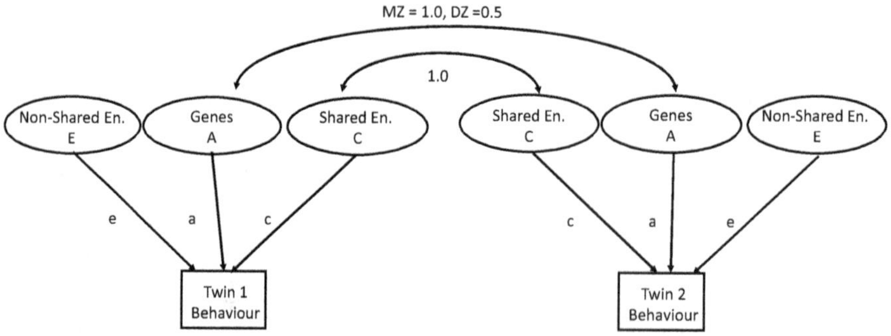

Fig. 3.1 ACE twin model

Often quantitative behaviour genetics is thought to be synonymous with twin studies, but there are a wide variety of research designs to which it can be employed, such as family and adoption studies. The association between characteristics in these various relationships can be measured, e.g. between biological parents and their children, adopted children and biological offspring, and adopted children and adopting parents. There will be different expectations for the correlations depending on the degree of their genetic relatedness and the extent of shared experiences. For example, biological parents and their biological children share some genes in common (on average 50%), and biological siblings share both some of their genes (on average 50%) and have common experiences in the shared environment. The adopted children and biological offspring in the same family will only have similarities that arise from the shared environment. Thereby expectations about the sources of resemblances between these family members can be generated. These can be tested against the observed correlations. In this way the size of genetic, shared, and non-shared environments can be estimated from a variety of family research designs.

There have been a very large number of studies applying quantitative genetic methods to behavioural differences. In relation to two dimensions of behaviour that will be discussed in more detail in Chaps. 7 and 8, a meta-analysis of twin and adoption studies by Burt (2009) produced an estimate of heritability for externalising behaviours of 0.59 and for internalising behaviours of 0.51.

Gene-Environment Interplay So far the effects of genes, the shared environment, and non-shared environment have been discussed as if they were independent and acted additively. However it is clear that behaviour is influenced by correlations between genes and the environment (r_{GE}) and by interactions between genes and the environment (G × E). These processes were delineated in a landmark paper by Plomin et al. (1977). These effects in aggregate have come to be termed "gene-environment interplay" (Rutter et al., 2006).

Plomin et al. (1977) argued that genes and the environment are not necessarily independent. Different genes can lead to changes in the types of environment the child will experience. These effects produce a correlation between genes and the environment. They identified three types of correlation between genes and the environment. The first is a *passive genotype-environment correlation* that will arise as parents pass on genes to the child and under the influence of their own genes may provide an environment that fosters a particular trait. For example, parents who are particularly verbally able will pass on genes for this ability and will provide an environment in the family particularly rich in opportunities to develop language. This type of correlation is labelled "passive r_{GE}" as it will arise independently of any behaviour by the child. The second is a *reactive genotype-environment correlation*, which arises from the impact of the child's genes (via the child's behaviour) on the way others respond to the child. For example, a child who is very active may induce family, friends, and teachers to provide opportunities for energetic play. In this way the predispositions of the genes can create an environment that correlates with these genotypic differences. The third type of correlation is an *active genotype-environment correlation*. This arises by the child seeking out environments and experiences that relate to their genetic propensities. For example, a sociable child will seek out the company of others and this will contrast with the environment sought by a more socially inhibited child.

The importance of this framework has been drawn out in a recent overview by Saltz (2019). In most of the work being summarised in this chapter, it will appear that psychology is drawing upon ideas and methods developed by biologists. The paper by Saltz shows the way studies in human behaviour genetics have developed the notions of r_{GE} and how these should now be applied in animal studies of wild nonhuman organisms. So this is a clear example of a reversal whereby research in psychology can inform research in biology.

The salience of these forms of r_{GE} changes with age. For example, Marceau et al. (2016) addressed the question of the extent to which r_{GE} influences the change in the quality of relationships between parent and child with age. They found that nonpassive gene-environment correlation (i.e. active and evocative r_{GE} combined) played a stronger role in adolescents in their late teens and that passive gene-environment correlation played a stronger role with younger adolescents (aged 10 and 11 years). These types of r_{GE} identified by Plomin et al. (1977) are illustrated in Fig. 3.2.

Interactions between genes and the environment (G × E) arise when the effect of an environmental risk is conditional on the person's genotype or vice versa (Caspi & Moffitt, 2006). Although G × E interactions are commonly studied, the mechanisms by which they arise are poorly understood (Belsky & Pluess, 2009). There is also substantial variation between traits in how often G × E occurs in a wide variety of species (Saltz et al., 2018), and it is proving difficult to identify G × E in studies using polygenic risk scores (Kandaswamy et al., 2022) (for details of these scores, see account below).

In commenting on the potential role of G × E in influencing behaviour, Rutter (2013) draws attention to likelihood that G × E is pervasive. It affects not just the vulnerability to adverse experience; rather genes influence the response to most environments. This notion underlies the differential susceptibility hypothesis. This

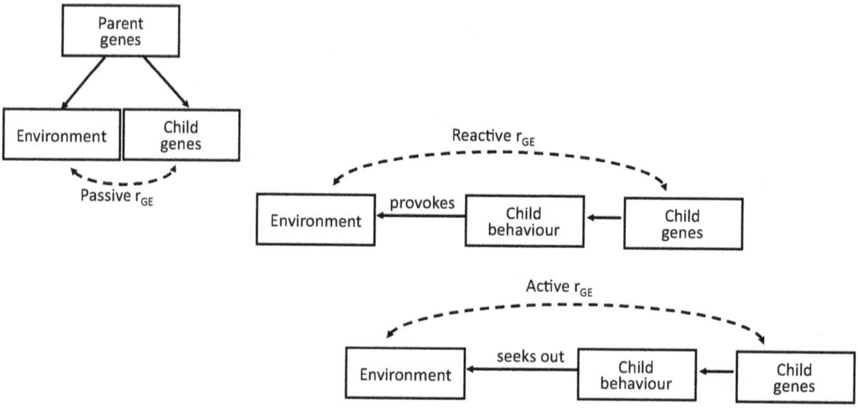

Fig. 3.2 Types of gene-environment correlation

is the suggestion that individuals vary in their vulnerability to the effects of experiences – both beneficial and adverse experiences (Belsky & Pluess, 2013). The same people will be more reactive than others to both positive and negative events and circumstances. There is evidence that genetic differences influence differential sensitivity to a range of experiences (Assary et al., 2021). It has been suggested that differential sensitivity may be an influence on a person's response to mental health treatment (Assary et al., 2023).

An illustration of how genes moderate the impact of an environmental risk is shown by a study on expressed emotion. The development of conduct problems in children with attention-deficit hyperactivity disorder (ADHD) is associated with mother's positive emotions expressed about their children. The children with ADHD whose mothers demonstrate a high level of positive emotion about their children are less likely to develop conduct problems (Taylor et al., 1996). Sonuga-Barke et al. (2009) showed that genes that are involved in the regulation of neurotransmitter systems moderate the vulnerability of children with ADHD to the development conduct problems when they experience a low level of maternal positively expressed emotion or a high level of negatively expressed emotion. The risk of developing conduct problems was related to the version of the dopamine D4 receptor gene and the serotonin transporter gene the children carried. It has also been demonstrated that the dopamine D4 receptor gene shows a G × E interaction with family risk factors in influencing reactions to marital conflict in children with ADHD (Martel et al., 2011). However studies on G × E interactions in relation to conduct problems were reviewed by Holz et al. (2018) who concluded that:

> conclusive indications of causal G × E patterns are largely lacking. Inconsistent findings, lack of replication and methodological limitations remain a major challenge. (Holz et al., 2018, p. 239)

Children-of-Twins (COT) Method A powerful tool for examining both genetic and environmental influences on behaviour across generations has emerged from studies of children born to parents who are twins [Children-of-Twins (COT) method]. The logic of the analysis of data from such families was first developed in the 1970s (Nance & Corey, 1976), but the method has only become more widely applied as suitably large samples of families of twins have become available (McAdams et al., 2014, 2018). The set of genetic correlations in the COT study is shown in Fig. 3.3. At the simplest level, children of a pair of MZ twins are just as closely related genetically to their uncles or aunts as they are to their parent (i.e. genetic correlation of 0.5). This means that if in a family with twin parents a child is more similar to their parent than their uncle/aunt, then this must be due to an effect arising from the nuclear family environment and not from genetic influences. These analyses have been taken further in the Extended Children-of-Twins (ECOT) model (Narusyte et al., 2008). This approach allows three mechanisms to be examined: direct phenotypic influence of parenting on child behaviour (controlling for both parental and child genotype), passive genotype-environment correlation, and evocative genotype-environment correlation.

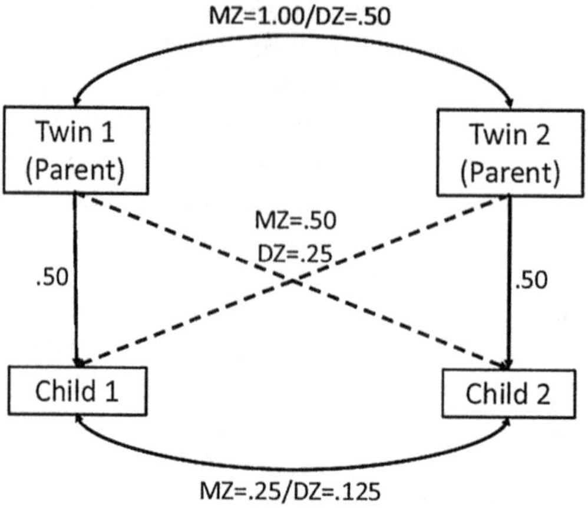

Fig. 3.3 Genetic correlations in Children-of-Twins (COT) studies. (Reproduced with the permission of the American Psychological Association from Fig. 1 in McAdams et al. (2014); permission conveyed through Copyright Clearance Center, Inc.)

An illustration of the power of ECOT approach is provided by Silberg et al. (2010). They examined the routes whereby parental depression influences child behaviour. Both depression and conduct problems in the child were found to be associated with parental depression. However the mechanisms producing these associations were distinct. Depression was transmitted by a direct environmental effect, i.e. exposure to a depressed parent. They note that other genetic factors seem to be responsible for the transmission of depression as the child approaches adulthood but in childhood depression in the child is a product of experiencing depression in the parent. For conduct problems in the child, both genetic and family environment effects were detected. This suggests that there is a genetically transmitted risk of depression in some children who show early conduct disorders. This study illustrates both the value of the ECOT design and the importance of a developmental approach to genetic influences on behaviour. These findings have been replicated in an independent sample and using a further extension of the CoT design – Multiple-Children-of-Twins-and-Siblings (MCOTS), which uses information from multiple children per mother (Gjerde et al., 2021).

Despite the developments in molecular genetics, heritability remains a key concept in behaviour genetics (Visscher et al., 2008). However, it has limitations in that although it provides an estimate of the relative magnitude of genetic and non-genetic factors within a population and a specific set of environmental circumstances, it cannot explain the differences between populations and environments. In addition, heritability is a measure of the aggregated effects of genetic differences and is not informative about the contributions of specific genes. For this molecular genetic studies are needed.

3.2 Molecular Genetics

Linkage Studies The early molecular genetic studies on behaviour used either linkage analysis or candidate gene association methods. DNA variants occur in about 0.1% of the base pairs that make up the genetic code. Most of these variants, known as alleles, do not act as a mutation, as they do not alter the gene's function. However they can act to show where in the DNA a gene effecting behaviour may be located. Linkage studies are based on the notion that a behavioural phenotype (e.g. inattention) will be inherited within a family along with specific variants in the structure of DNA. This linkage is unlikely to be between the behaviour and the gene it is influenced by but rather between the behaviour and a region of the DNA nearby to the gene. Studies on ADHD will be used to illustrate the application of molecular genetic methods to be described in this section.

A meta-analysis of linkage studies on ADHD identified 16q22–16q24 as a possible position where genes influencing ADHD might be found (Zhou et al., 2008). These positions are addressed for genes and refer to an area on a chromosome, in this case on the long arm (q) of chromosome 16 – the short arm is designated as "p". A weakness of linkage analyses is that they can only identify genes of large effect and, in the case of ADHD and most other behaviours, there are many genes involved and these are small effect.

Association Studies Association studies have greater power than linkage studies and so they can identify genes of smaller effect and be more precise as where a significant DNA variant may be located. The basic method in an association study is like any study of a risk factor. Association studies examine whether those people carrying a specific genetic variant are more likely to show the behaviour of interest compared to others that do not carry the variant. The initial application of association methods was to use candidate genes, that is, genes that are suggested by previous research to influence the behaviour. The early candidate-gene association studies on ADHD were reviewed in a meta-analysis by Gizer et al. (2009). Many of the candidate genes studied were involved in dopamine neurotransmitter systems. These were chosen since the drugs that treat ADHD target these systems. Gizer et al. (2009) found a number of genes influencing the dopamine system stood up to replications, e.g. the dopamine transporter gene and dopamine receptor genes D4 and D5.

However, in subsequent studies the candidate genes have not produced the results that were expected. These candidate genes were often those involved with catecholamine neurotransmitters such as dopamine. In a review Faraone and Larsson (2019) concluded that:

> Gene discovery for ADHD has succeeded but has left us with unexpected results. None of the genome-wide significant findings had been predicted a priori and a set of ADHD candidate genes, implicated primarily by the disorder's neuropharmacology, did not reach statistical significance. These findings challenge the idea that the core of ADHD's pathophysiology rests within the machinery of catecholaminergic transmission. (Faraone & Larsson, 2019, p. 569)

Subsequently more powerful association study methodologies have been developed. These are genome-wide association studies (GWASs). They are much more valuable in the analysis of highly polygenic behaviours. The technology used, genotyping microarrays, can measure thousands of genetic variants each of very small effect. These variants are not preselected, as in the candidate gene study. They are simply distributed as widely as possible over the genome. Using the GWAS approach, Demontis et al. (2019) identified 12 independent positions (loci) in the genome associated with ADHD. It is important to remember that GWAS does not identify genes but rather positions on chromosomes that are near to the genes involved.

This failure of the candidate gene approach is not restricted to ADHD. In a wide-ranging review of molecular genetic studies on psychiatric disorders, Duncan et al. (2019) concluded that:

> These modern genetic findings also demonstrate why candidate gene studies are no longer trusted by geneticists. Specifically, candidate gene studies nearly always hypothesized the wrong portions of the genome (and they may have always hypothesized the wrong variants), they hypothesized effect sizes larger than those that exist in nature. Further, candidate gene studies are methodologically inadequate in their ability to account for subtle differences in ancestry and relatedness, which can confound results. In sum, it is time to abandon candidate gene studies, and the results that they produced, in favor of the numerous highly reliable results that have emerged from GWAS. (Duncan et al., 2019, p. 1518)

Single-Nucleotide Polymorphisms (SNPs) Many genetic variants comprise just a change in one base pair in the DNA sequence. These single-nucleotide polymorphisms (SNPs) are very valuable in molecular genetic analyses even though they rarely influence gene expression. SNPs will be inherited alongside nearby genes that are functional, i.e. change the risk for behaviours. By mapping where specific patterns of SNPs occur, their association with the behaviour of interest can be tested. This then can lead to identification of loci where genes influencing the behaviour may be situated. However carrying a risk version of any one SNP has only a very small effect on a behaviour, which is almost invariably highly polygenic. The term "effect" here does not necessarily imply a causal relation to behaviour. The effect is shown by being predictive of behaviour. SNPs need to be analysed in very large samples with many thousands of participants. Care has to be taken that amidst this welter of results, false positives are avoided. This is achieved by the use of very stringent criteria of significance, e.g. $p < 0.000000005$.

A valuable approach in studies of behaviour is the production of aggregate measures based on SNP profiles. By adding together the effects of a large number of SNPs, the proportion of the variance explained by the genotype can be estimated – this is called SNP heritability or h^2_{SNP} (Yang et al., 2017). It has been a feature of molecular genetic studies on physical characteristics (e.g. height), illness (e.g. heart disease), and behaviour (e.g. autism) that h^2_{SNP} is much lower than h^2 estimated from the resemblance between relatives (e.g. from twin studies). This has been labelled the "missing heritability" problem. A number of explanations for this problem have been put forward (Owen & Williams, 2021). First is that h^2 from twin data is inflated by confounding from the shared environment. Second, h^2_{SNP} estimates do not take account of non-additive genetic effects, i.e. dominance and gene-gene interaction. Third, many risk alleles are missed in h^2_{SNP} estimates because their effects are too small or the risk alleles are too rare. Owen and Williams (2021) suggest that developments in molecular genetic methods support this last explanation; many causal variants in highly polygenic behaviours remain unidentified. These variants are likely to be uncovered by future whole-genome sequence analyses. It has also been suggested that the "missing heritability" problems may be false because more complex gene-environment interactions are overlooked (Genin, 2020). Shen and Feldman (2020) make an even more stringent critique of simple heritability estimates. They provide a model whereby genetic transmission is augmented by cultural transmission (Cavalli-Sforza & Feldman, 1973) and genetic nurturing (Kong et al., 2018) (see below). These factors, they suggest, make the interpretation of both h^2 and h^2_{SNP} problematic.

A more direct test of the relationship between h^2 and h^2_{SNP} was provided by Pettersson et al. (2019). They estimated h^2 of psychiatric disorders on the basis of similarities between members of a national sample of families comprising 4,408,646 siblings and maternal half siblings, i.e. born to the same mother but with different biological fathers. In the same study, h^2_{SNP} heritability estimates were obtained on a sample of 333,748 cases and controls. The study was based on very substantial samples for which psychiatric disorder had been identified on the basis of diagnostic criteria. As would expected from the discussion above, the h^2_{SNP} were lower than those based on the sibling data. However there were indications that the heritability estimates for different diagnoses were in a similar rank order. The highest sib study values of h^2 were obtained for ADHD (0.81) and for ASD (0.75). The respective h^2_{SNP} were 0.22 and 0.12. The findings indicated that quantitative genetic and molecular study estimates of heritability are somewhat robust across methods.

There were puzzling features of the initial application genome-wide association study (GWAS) methodology to behaviour problems. In the Twins Early Development Study (TEDS), no significant heritability based on analysis of DNA was found for behaviour problems (Trzaskowski et al., 2013). These null results for h^2_{SNP} were found on a general population sample of 2500 12-year-old twins on measures including the Strength and Difficulties Questionnaire (SDQ). For comparison the h^2 for the SDQ total score was around 0.40 for this sample. In a separate twin sample, Pappa et al. (2015) also found low h^2_{SNP}-based heritability for parental ratings on the Child Behavior Checklist (CBCL) internalising scale (0.12) and externalising scale (0.12).

The Trzaskowski et al. (2013) findings were replicated on an enlarged sample of twins from the TEDS study by Cheesman et al. (2017). They found h^2_{SNP} for behaviour problems to be very small and much lower than those estimated from twin data. This was not the case for cognitive and anthropometric measures for which twin heritability averaged 0.58 and SNP heritability averaged 0.28. They suggest therefore there is a need to revise the measurement of behaviour problems if they are going to be amenable to GWAS investigations. Cheesman et al. (2017) make a number of suggestions for the way behaviour problem data could be configured to increase the observed h^2_{SNP} heritability. These include using cross-rater composites, using data derived from stable overtime measures, and using multivariate genetic analyses to derive higher degrees of common genetic variance across measures. Cheesman et al. (2018) subsequently demonstrated that the use of repeated measures to obtain stable indices of emotional problems increased twin heritability (from 0.45 to 0.75) and SNP heritability (0.05–0.14) compared to that obtained from single measures at single time point.

A related use of SNPs is in the estimation of polygenic risk scores (PRS) (see Sect. 3.4). These are estimates of the likelihood that an individual will show a particular behaviour based on their genetic make-up. They are a sum of the number of risk variants in a person's DNA multiplied by the effect size of each variant in relation to the behaviour (Wray et al., 2020). PRS have become widely used to examine more directly the genetic correlation between behaviours and to test for gene-environment interactions (Harden & Koellinger, 2020).

Shared Genetic Risks A major insight from molecular genetic studies is the extent to which psychiatric and neurodevelopmental disorders share common genetic risks (Anttila et al., 2018). This is particularly the case for ADHD, bipolar disorder, major depressive disorders, and schizophrenia. Neuroticism also shares genetic risks with most psychiatric disorders. These findings provide further support for a transdiagnostic approach (for example see Eadeh et al., 2021, and discussion in Sect. 5.3). It is clear that the traditional Diagnostic and Statistical Manual (DSM) categorical approach to nosology does not identify conditions with, at the genetic level, distinct underlying pathologies.

It has emerged from GWAS studies that genes have multiple effects on complex traits such as behaviour. Watanabe et al. (2019) undertook a review of 4155 GWASs of 558 traits and examined the extent of pleiotropy, i.e. whether a gene influences more than one trait. They found that 90% of the loci on chromosomes identified in GWAS were associated with more than one trait. These loci are regions of the DNA that may or may not include the actual effective gene but which are at least closely associated with it. These results show that the large majority of complex traits, including behaviour, are highly polygenic and that almost all of these genes have pleiotropic effects whereby they influence more than one trait. The various mechanisms that are involved in pleiotropic genetic effects, especially how these relate to psychiatric disorders, are outlined in Lee et al. (2021).

These findings have led to the strong conclusion reached by Flint et al. (2020) that genes rarely have specific effects. Genes that are identified as being associated with one behaviour are also found to be involved in other behaviours. Furthermore they suggest that:

> Genetic action appears never to adhere to psychiatric nosology. (Flint et al., 2020, p. 122)

The emergence of evidence of common genetic influences on a wide range of psychiatric disorders has been taken a stage further by Schork et al. (2019). They have identified variants in genes expressed in early foetal development that are associated with psychiatric disorders. Some of these genes are known to be involved in the regulation of genes expressed in the neocortex in mid-gestation. They concluded that the results suggest that dysregulation, by common genetic variants, of genes that control neurodevelopment may result in general liability for many later psychiatric outcomes.

The substantial increase in the publication of studies using GWAS methodologies has been documented by Mills and Rahal (2019). They draw attention to need to extend the diversity of populations on which GWASs are conducted and therefore extend the range of people, in terms of ancestry, who can benefit from such investigations. In particular, in medically related studies, this would make salient findings on possible targeted treatments applicable to a broader section of the population in terms of ethnicity and race.

Genetic Nurture An additional complexity in gene-environment interplay was highlighted by Kong et al. (2018). They showed how non-transmitted alleles could have an influence on a child's phenotype via their impact on the nurturing provided by parents and relatives. Each parent only transmits half their genes to a child. The remaining non-transmitted genes can still have an effects on the child's development. They call this effect "genetic nurture". The environment created by the parents will be influenced by all their genes – both transmitted and non-transmitted. These alternative paths from the parent's genes to the child's behaviour are illustrated in Fig. 3.4.

The importance of this demonstration is that the observed effects found in GWAS do not necessarily reflect direct transmitted genetic effects alone. Kong et al. (2018) used educational attainment (EA) as the child characteristic and derived PRS separately from transmitted and non-transmitted alleles to demonstrate these effects. The effect of the non-transmitted alleles on EA was about one third of that obtained from transmitted alleles. This same research group developed an analysis method [relatedness disequilibrium regression (RDR)] that allowed the estimation of heritability that was independent of those environmentally carried effects of non-transmitted alleles (Young et al., 2018). They showed that by comparison with heritability estimates from twin pairs, the presence of the "genetic nurture" effects inflates the estimates from twins. For example, the h^2 from twin data for height was 0.81 and from the RDR method was 0.55. This method opens up a whole new set of insights into how genetic effects are transmitted within families, which is being fruitful in studies such as those on depression and anxiety (see Cheesman et al., 2020a, in Sect. 7.5).

The notion that there are multiple routes whereby parent genes can influence child outcome was taken further to examine prenatal genetic nurture by Armstrong-Carter et al. (2020). They examined both direct genetic effects (the influence of a person's genes) and social genetic effects (the indirect influences that other people's genes have through an impact on the shared environment). They established a gene-shared environment correlation between maternal genes associated with educational achievement and the quality of the child's prenatal environment. This social genetic

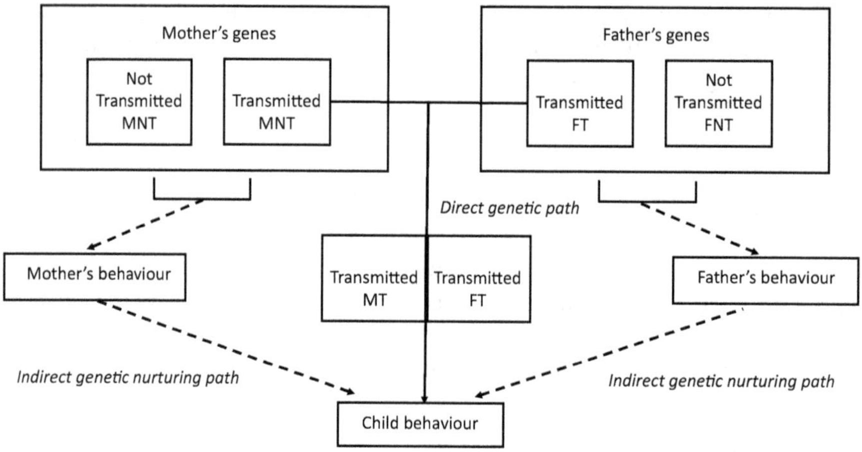

Fig. 3.4 Direct genetic and indirect genetic nurture effects on child behaviour. (Based on Fig. 1 in Kong et al. (2018))

route explained 30% of the covariance between maternal educational associated genetics and child early academic achievement even when direct genetic transmission had been controlled.

There are now a wide range of research designs and methods that have been developed to tease apart these complex mechanisms whereby parental characteristics can influence child behaviour (Branje et al. 2020; Jami et al., 2021). These designs include adoption and Children-of-Twins studies, matched pair designs (where just one sibling is exposed to the putative causal experience in the family), and molecular genetic studies. The following conclusions were reached in a review of such studies:

> Overall, reviewed studies showed reliable evidence of genetic transmission of depression, criminal behaviour, educational attainment, and substance use behaviours from parent-to-child. Additionally, cross-phenotype genetic overlap was observed in several instances; for example, parental depression, substance use, and educational attainment were all associated with offspring Externalising behaviours through genetic pathways… After accounting for genetic transmission, parental depression or anxiety were associated with offspring Internalising or Externalising behaviours through environmental pathways. For maternal exposures, these associations were related to concurrent maternal symptoms, with no long-lasting effect of prenatal depression or anxiety on offspring mental health. Other environmental associations and r_{GE} were observed for parent–offspring similarity in criminal behaviours, substance use behaviours, and educational attainment. In addition, positive and negative parenting behaviours held associations with offspring Internalising behaviours, Externalising behaviours, substance use behaviours, and educational attainment, with some evidence of r_{GE}. Finally, cross-lagged studies showed bidirectional associations between parenting traits and offspring behaviours, where parenting predicted offspring behaviours, and offspring behaviours predicted parenting. (Jami et al., 2021, p. 33)

These important conclusions could be drawn as the studies reviewed were able to control for genetic effects when investigating parental influences on their children's development. This is part of the broader picture that genetic studies have been just as informative about environmental effects as they have been about genetic effects per se.

Molecular Genetic Studies on G × E There has been a debate about the way the interaction between genetic and environmental influences (G × E) were conceptualised and analysed. This disagreement was between those who studied interaction between candidate genes and measured environment events and experiences (e.g. Caspi et al., 2003) and those for whom GWAS was the method of choice (e.g. Risch & Merikangas, 1996). This contrast of approaches was summarised by Duncan et al. (2014). One of the key areas of this disagreement was the genetics of depression in adults. There had been a history of claims of association between candidate genes and major depression in adults, but these were produced by relatively underpowered studies with small samples. The problem with underpowered studies is that, although the rate of false positives (type I error) is fixed, the rate of true positives is low. Consequently, a significant result is less likely to be a true positive in an underpowered study (Ioannidis, 2005).

In order to provide a resolution to the question of the role of candidate genes in major depression, Border et al. (2019) undertook an analysis of a number of large sample data sets (Ns from 62,138 to 443,2640). Their aim was summarised as follows:

> We focus on three lines of inquiry concerning how historical candidate genes may affect depression liability: (1) main effects of the most commonly studied candidate polymorphisms, (2) moderation of the effects of these polymorphisms by environmental exposures, and (3) main effects of common SNPs across each of the candidate genes. (Border et al., 2019, p. 378)

They found no clear evidence for candidate genes being associated with depression. Furthermore no gene-environment interactions were detected. They suggest that previous positive findings for candidate genes with respect to depression were false positives. They recommend depression research should abandon historical candidate genes and candidate gene-by-environment interaction hypotheses. The results of the Border et al. (2019) study do not necessarily mean that such interaction cannot be found for other psychological characteristics. However it seems like that advances in studying G × E will only be made by adopting well-powered GWAS approaches (Border & Keller, 2017).

The complex processes in gene-environment interplay have been extensively discussed by Mike Rutter (Rutter et al., 1997; Rutter, 2007; Rutter, 2015). He concludes that studies:

> …must move beyond the search for susceptibility genes 'for' specific mental disorders, must include a study of environmental risk factors, and must involve the study of the various forms of gene–environment interplay. Particularly as exemplified by epigenetic environmental effects on gene expression, and by G × E, it is not putting it too strongly to refer to the interplay as often (but certainly not always) involving gene–environment interdependence. (Rutter, 2007, p. 16)

Copy-Number Variants The account of the developments in molecular genetic methodology above has centred on frameworks looking for many genes of small effect. There are other genetic features that can have more major effects. One of these are rearrangements of the DNA sequence that can result in the deletion of DNA or the addition of extra sequences in the DNA. These mechanisms can produce copy-number variants (CNVs) where segments of DNA are found to vary in number between people. These CNVs have been found to be a major contributor to autism spectrum disorders (ASD). It has been estimated that CNVs contribute up to 40% of all cases of ASD (Yoon et al., 2021).

3.3 Epigenetics

Epigenetics is a set of processes that produce changes in gene function but not in the coding DNA sequence in the gene itself (for a review see Aristizabal et al., 2020). There are a number of ways these changes can be made. One of the most common in mammals is DNA methylation. Here a methyl group (CH_3) is added to bases (cytosine and adenine) in the DNA sequence. This usually results in the silencing of gene expression (i.e. reducing the gene activity). Another mechanism is the addition or removal of acetyl groups (CH_3CO) to histones, which are proteins associated with DNA. The addition and subtraction of acetyl groups acts to turn gene expression on and off.

Some of these epigenetic mechanisms act to allow cells to transmit information to its cellular descendants within an organism through cell division (mitosis). In this sense epigenetics simply refers to way genes act in concert through embryological development to form distinct tissues. A more contentious meaning of epigenetics is the transmission of information through meiosis, which could result in changes in subsequent generations. In addressing this possibility, it is important to distinguish intergenerational transmission (from parent to offspring) and transgenerational transmission (from parent to grandchild) (Heard & Martienssesn, 2014). This is necessary because in intergenerational transmission exposure to the original environmental trigger for epigenetic changes may be transmitted alongside the epigenetic changes themselves.

There is evidence for intergenerational transmission in both plants and animals, but there is a paucity of evidence for transgenerational transmission in mammals. As Heard and Martienssesn (2014) argue, this is for the very good reason that through evolution robust mechanisms have developed to ensure that most of these changes, which are very likely to be deleterious, are not propagated. Others, such as Dias et al. (2015), are more ready to accept that there is accumulating, but as yet unresolved, evidence that epigenetics may provide a mechanism for the non-genetic transmission of behavioural characteristics and learned behaviour across generations in animal studies.

One aspect of behaviour where there is some convergence in the evidence of transgenerational transmission is from animal and human studies of prenatal nicotine exposure and ADHD. Using a mouse model of ADHD-like behaviours, Buck et al. (2019) showed that an increase in ADHD-related behaviours in the mouse was related to nicotine exposure in the grandmother generation. In an earlier study, a similar transgenerational transmission of ADHD behaviours in the mouse was reported (Zhu et al., 2014). In both these studies, epigenetics was postulated as an explanation of the mechanism of transmission. This pattern of transmission of the effects of grandmother smoking to grandchild ADHD behaviour has been reported in a large sample of 53,635 of families in the USA (Yim et al., 2022). The effects of grandmaternal smoking during pregnancy on grandchild ADHD behaviours were only modest. Nevertheless, the authors suggest that epigenetic changes in the germline cells, i.e. through meiosis, is a possible explanation of the results.

It is of interest that it has also been suggested that grandmothers smoking during pregnancy is related to an increase in some features of autistic traits in their granddaughters and with a diagnosis of ASD in those where the mother did not smoke in pregnancy (Golding et al., 2017). Here too epigenetic changes in the germline cells were postulated as a possible mechanism of transmission. An alternative mechanism was suggested to be the transmission of damage to mitochondrial DNA produced by exposure to tobacco smoke during pregnancy.

To re-emphasise these epigenetic mechanisms involve the transmission of influences that are not carried by changes to the DNA sequences themselves but rather by other biochemical mechanisms such as DNA methylation. The latter alter gene expression but not the genes themselves.

The interplay between these epigenetic processes as they influence behaviour and health over different time scales has been outlined by Boyce et al. (2020). These epigenetic processes may be modified by environmental factors such as toxins but also by nutrition, stress, and smoking (Hanson & Skinner, 2016). A wide variety of influences early in life (pre- and postnatal) such as maternal diet and stress can have an enduring influences on behaviour (Tearne et al., 2015). These effects include increasing the risk of neurodevelopmental disorders via epigenetic mechanisms (Bale et al., 2010). These mechanisms may be particularly potent when regulating processes operating during episodes of brain reorganisation (Bacon & Brinton, 2021). Some of these long-term postnatal effects are created by influencing susceptibility to later experiences both positive and negative (Hartman & Belsky, 2018).

The role of antenatal stress on behavioural development has been the subject of an extensive range of research studies (Van den Bergh et al., 2020; Hartman & Belsky, 2018). The studies include the use of natural experiment designs such as that conducted by Simcock et al. (2017). They examined the later temperament of children whose mothers, when pregnant, were exposed to a disastrous flood in Queensland Australia. They found that the severity of the mother's prenatal stress in response to the flood was related to an increase in difficult temperament in the children at 6 months of age.

There is accumulating evidence that some of the effects of antenatal stress are mediated by epigenetic changes (Cao-Lei et al., 2020). One group of children that experience extreme perinatal stress are those born prematurely. A review of the evidence suggests that some of the adverse long-term effects of premature birth may be mediated via epigenetic mechanisms (Provenzi et al., 2018). However the implications of these findings for the care of premature infants are as yet unclear.

There are also epigenetic effects that mediate the impact of postnatal experiences on later behaviour. There are well-replicated findings that changes to DNA methylation can arise in children exposed to maltreatment and that these changes can endure into adulthood (Parade et al., 2021). A series of studies by Michael Meaney showed how maternal grooming behaviour in rats can have an influence on the behaviour of their offspring in adulthood and that this effect was mediated by modifications to gene expression, i.e. an epigenetic mechanism (Meaney, 2010). However this is not an example of a transgenerationally transmitted change in gene function (Isles, 2015). Parallel research on variation in maternal caregiving in humans suggests that some of the effects of the quality of maternal caregiving can contribute to behavioural development and this is at least partially explained by epigenetic changes (Provenzi et al., 2020).

A specific form of epigenetic marking is that associated with imprinting. Here gene expression in the child is influenced by the parent from which the gene was inherited. There are a number of rare behavioural syndromes that demonstrate imprinting, e.g. Angelman syndrome and Prader-Willi syndrome (Peters, 2014). It has been suggested that an imprinting mechanism was responsible for the transmission of social cognition abilities (Skuse et al., 1997), memory function (Bishop et al., 2000), and social anxiety (Hall et al., 2022) in girls with Turner's syndrome.

It has been found that differential epigenetic markers accumulate with age in MZ twins. These individuals have identical DNA and epigenetic markers, such as DNA methylations, at age 3 years. By 50 years striking differences in epigenetic markers have been found within twin pairs (Fraga et al., 2005). There is increasing evidence that such epigenetic markers may be associated with behavioural differences. Rijlaarsdam et al. (2021) found that patterns of DNA methylation were associated with scores on a general psychopathology factor in 10-year-old children. This was a specific association in that the correlations were not found with scores on internalising or externalising dimensions. An important feature of this study was that the findings were replicated in two independent samples. In addition there was evidence that these methylation differences were influenced by shared and non-shared environmental influences and not by genes. A model of how epigenetic factors influence psychological resilience to the effects of adverse and traumatic events has been developed by Smeeth et al. (2021).

It has proved very difficult to establish the presence of transgenerational transmission via epigenetic mechanisms in human behaviour and psychiatric disorders. Experimental studies with rodents (especially mice) have suggested that environmental influences can be transmitted across generations – see the example of prenatal nicotine exposure discussed above. Klengel et al. (2016) reviewed the literature on mouse models of inter- and transgenerational transmission of the risk of psychopathology. They conclude that:

> …a simple extrapolation of the results found in rodents to humans is not possible, and it remains speculative at the moment whether the biological inheritance of environmentally acquired marks is truly relevant for the development of psychiatric diseases in humans. (Klengel et al., 2016, p. 229)

A review of the possibility of epigenetic transgenerational transmission via fathers of behavioural traits carrying a risk of psychiatric disorders reached the following conclusion that:

> …further investigation is needed in order to demonstrate the occurrence of transgenerational inheritance via epigenetic alteration in the gametes. (Yeshurun & Hannan, 2019, p. 537)

3.4 Polygenic Risk Scores

Complex phenotypes, such as psychopathology, are influenced by a large number of genes, each of which contribute just a small part to the prediction of the phenotype. In these circumstances ways of aggregating information from a large number of genes are needed. Polygenic risk scores (PRS) are a means of using information from GWAS to achieve this.

PRS are derived to estimate the susceptibility of an individual to a particular behavioural variant based on their profile on a large number risk genes of small effect. They are calculated by multiplying the number of their risk alleles by the effect size of each allele on risk and then summing these products across all the risk genes (Martin et al., 2019). Wray et al. (2014, 2020) provide overviews of how polygenic scores are derived and how they have been applied to psychiatric and other complex phenotypes. A more extensive account of developments in the derivation of PRS and their implementation is given in Allegrini et al. (2022). The strengths and weaknesses of polygenic score methodology and their potential application in clinical practice have been outlined by Ronald (2020).

A key feature of PRS is that they provide a means of predicting the likely profile of traits a person may show. However they do not provide an explanation of the mechanisms whereby genes influence behaviour (Plomin & Von Stumm, 2022). Nevertheless they have the potential value of being able to predict which individuals are at risk of developing problems. As yet this prediction is not strong. The best performance by a PRS for child development is the explanation of 16% of the variance in educational achievement at age 16 years (Allegrini et al., 2019). Clearly the accuracy of the prediction from PRS needs to improve for it to be used to predict individuals at risk, but such an improvement is likely to be achieved from larger and better designed GWAS (Plomin & Von Stumm, 2022). One way to improve prediction from PRS is by combining data from different sources and time points. This was shown by Gidziela et al. (2021) who found that the ability of PRS to predict behaviour problems across childhood and adolescence was improved by using multiple PRS and measures aggregated across age and across rater. Nevertheless the variance explained was still very limited, i.e. 6%.

A feature of studies applying PRS to data on children is that PRS have been found to be rarely associated with specific psychopathologies alone. For example, PRS that are associated with either internalising or externalising behaviour are also associated with general psychopathology. However some PRS are associated with general psychopathology alone (Neumann et al., 2022). Evidence for specificity of

PRS associations has emerged from a study where PRS was analysed in conjunction with data on family history (Loughnan et al., 2022). Using data on 5204 children aged 9–11 years, it was found that a PRS for ADHD showed a specific association with ADHD when family history and PRS scores for other conditions were controlled. The same held for depression. The variance explained by the combination of PRS and family history was only a modest 7% of the variance in the total problems score of the CBCL. It is not clear whether the family history measure is indicative of genetic or environmental influences. However family history and the PRS explained both shared and unique variance in the behaviour scores. This suggests that family history may reflect environmental effects that act alongside and independently of genetic factors.

Evidence that PRS are related to general measures of psychopathology was obtained by Akingbuwa et al. (2020). They used pooled data from 7 longitudinal studies to obtain measures of psychopathology on 42,998 6- to 17-year-olds. Polygenic scores for individuals were constructed based on GWAS studies of adult disorders. Although small ($\beta = 0.023$ to 0.042), the associations between the PRS and childhood psychopathology were significant and stable across development. It was notable that the associations were not specific to any one type of psychopathology and may therefore be indicative of the action of a genetic-based general psychopathology factor in childhood (Allegrini et al., 2020).

The development of PRS methods has opened up many possibilities for examining environmental effects. These include using PRS as control measures in experiments and intervention studies and to more directly ascertain gene-environment interactions and correlations (Harden & Koellinger, 2020). However there are complexities to the interpretation of PRS that mean that they cannot be seen to be a pure measure of genetic influences. For example, Pingault et al. (2022) suggest the polygenic risk represented in a PRS may be mediated by exposure to environmental influences. They identify examples whereby PRS are associated with environmental exposures relevant to child development including maternal education, parenting, breastfeeding, or bullying victimisation. Under these circumstances it is not clear whether a relationship between a PRS and child behaviour is a direct effect of the genes or arises from r_{GE}.

The ability of PRS to make modest predictions about averages is not reflected in the accuracy with which predictions about individuals are made. This is well illustrated in Fig. 3.5 from Harden and Koellinger (2020), which uses data from Lee et al. (2018) on a PRS that predicts educational attainment:

> plotting .. PRS against actual years of schooling in a US sample of individuals with European ancestries. The relationship between the two variables is positive and statistically highly significant ($P = 2.2 \times 10^{-16}$, two-sided test). The PRS accounts for about 11% of the variance in the years of schooling after residualizing this variable for sex, birth year.....Yet we also see that, for almost any single value of the PRS, almost every level of actual education is observed. Even for PRS values that are 2 s.d. above or below the sample mean, we observe everything from high school drop-outs to people with PhDs". (Harden & Koellinger, 2020, p. 571)

These findings are a stark warning that it would not be appropriate to rely on PRS alone when predicting outcomes for individuals.

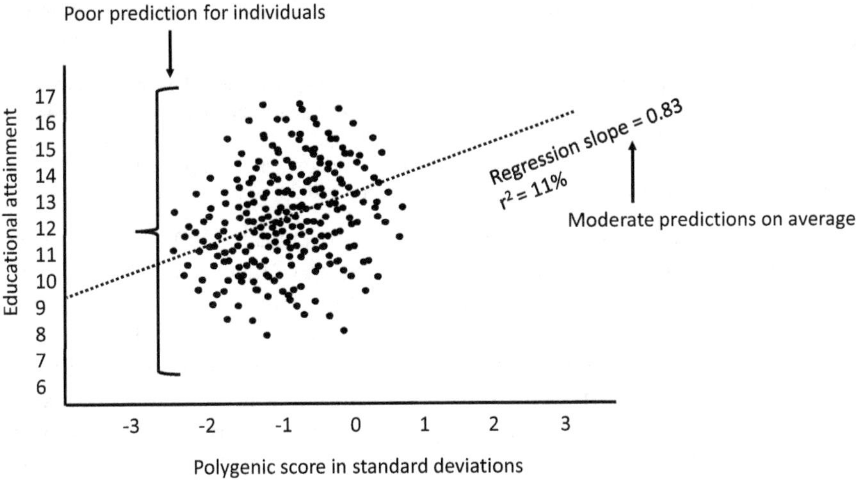

Fig. 3.5 Polygenic score for educational attainment plotted against years of education. (Adapted with the permission of Springer Nature BV from Fig. 1 in Harden and Koellinger (2020); permission conveyed through Copyright Clearance Center, Inc.)

Bolhuis et al. (2021) used PRS to test for gene-environment correlations between adversity in childhood and the risk of mental health problems in children. The PRS employed was that for schizophrenia. They found that a higher PRS was related to an increased exposure to childhood adversity. This association in part accounted for the association between PRS and child behaviour. They interpret their findings as indicating the action of either a passive or evocative gene-environment correlations (see Sect. 3.1). Either parents that pass on genetic risks also provide a more adverse environment (passive r_{GE}) or children's own actions lead to an increase in adversities (evocative r_{GE}).

This association between PRS and experiences and events is commonly found (Krapohl et al., 2017). As a consequence measured environmental risk factors may often reflect genetic influences. This means that a simple distinction between genetic and environmental risks becomes blurred. This is well illustrated in a study on education attainment by Cheesman et al. (2020b) that examined the relationship between PRS and education attainment in adopted children and in nonadopted children. The correlation between PRS and educational attainment is twice as high in the nonadoptees compared to the adoptees. This suggests that genetic influences on education attainment are in large measure mediated via the home environment. One approach to resolve these genotype-phenotype confounds is the use of family-based quasi-experimental research designs such as sibling comparisons, adoption, and intergenerational extended family studies. The value of such studies was reviewed by McAdams et al. (2023), and they concluded:

> genotype–phenotype associations are much like any other association – they may be causal in nature, but they may also be spurious, inflated, suppressed or partially or entirely confounded. Given this, the use of quasi-experimental methods to try to distinguish direct, causal genetic effects from non-causal associations is an extremely important step on the road to better understanding aetiology. (McAdams et al., 2023, p. 11)

A feature of many PRS studies is that they are derived from GWAS based on samples of unrelated individuals. Selzam et al. (2019) argue that such PRS predictions of trait outcomes are therefore a combination of directly transmitted effects from genes and others mediated by passive gene-environment correlations. Parents create environments for their children in part based on the parents' genotype. By this means the relationship between a trait and a PRS obtained in an unrelated set of people may include effects from passive gene-environment correlation and not from directly transmitted genes alone. Selzam et al. (2019) suggested that the difference in PRS scores between siblings will be independent of any such gene-environment correlations and also any environmental effects related to non-transmitted alleles (the nature of nurture – see Kong et al. (2018) in Sect. 3.2.). Such within family analyses also are independent of effects arising from population stratification and assortative mating.

Selzam et al. (2018) took the degree of unconfounding even further by using data from siblings that were DZ twins so that all shared environment effects are controlled such as the effects of pregnancy risk factors, parental age, and family income. By comparing the results of PRS predictions from analyses within families and for unrelated individuals, they were able to show that prediction of cognitive traits was about 60% higher in the independent sample than within families. This suggests an important role for gene-environment correlations. Once socio-economic status (SES) was taken into account, this difference was substantially reduced. Accordingly they conclude that SES is a major influence on cognitive traits via gene-environment correlations.

Plomin and von Stumm (2018) have shown how the study of genetic influences on IQ have been transformed by GWAS studies and PRS. It has been long established that IQ is highly heritable ($h^2 = 0.50$) and predicts important later educational attainment and well-being outcomes. Years of education is highly correlated with IQ and genes account for a substantial part of this association (Rietveld et al., 2014). This has created the possibility of studying years of education as a proxy for IQ in the large data sets required by GWAS. Plomin and von Strumm (2018) estimated that inherited genome sequence differences have to date accounted for 20% of the heritability of IQ. They suggest that the use of PRS will increase this proportion markedly in the near future. Evidence is also beginning to emerge that genes influencing years of education (as proxy for IQ) do so via a causal effect on brain volume (Lee et al., 2019).

The potential applications of PRS in clinical psychiatry have been appraised by Murray et al. (2021). They suggest that the application of PRS in routine clinical practice requires more clinical evaluation, but the time is not far off when they can be used to provide a foundation for building (with other risk factors) more accurate decisions about risk and the appropriateness of intervention. The limitations and potential of PRS have been outlined by Barker et al. (2022). They emphasise that predicting outcomes for individuals based on genetic risk alone is bound to be inadequate; see the above discussion of the Harden and Koellinger (2020) result. They argue that the essence of causality in psychopathology is the interplay between genes and the environment. However they argue that PRS can play an important role in identifying r_{GE} and G × E effects that gene-environment interplay entails.

A common feature of the current research in quantitative genetics, molecular genetics, and polygenic risk scores is that they converge on the notion that disorders are the extremes of normal variation (Plomin et al., 2009). Subsequent studies have supported the appropriateness of this framework applied, for example, to autism (Lundström et al., 2012; Robinson et al., 2016) and ADHD (Larsson et al., 2012).

3.5 Generalisations About the Findings from Behaviour Genetics

In 2000 Turkheimer postulated three "laws" of behaviour genetics. These were in fact broad generalisations of what had emerged from behaviour genetic research to that date. These laws were:

> First "Law" – "All human behavioural traits are heritable".
> Second "Law" – "The effect of being raised in the same family is smaller than the effect of genes".
> Third "Law" – "A substantial portion of the variation in complex human behavioural traits is not accounted for by the effects of genes or families".

He also has argued that the field must operate in the face of the "gloomy prospect". This is a term taken from Plomin and Daniels (1987) as follows:

> One gloomy prospect is that the salient environment might be unsystematic, idiosyncratic, or serendipitous events such as accidents, illnesses, or other traumas. … Such capricious events, however, are likely to prove a dead end for research. (Plomin & Daniels, 1987, p. 8)

Now a fourth "law" has been suggested by Chabris et al. (2015), which states:

> A typical human behavioral trait is associated with very many genetic variants, each of which accounts for a very small percentage of the behavioral variability. (Chabris et al., 2015, p. 304)

This "law" was proposed to accommodate the relative failure of candidate gene studies to replicate. Subsequent large-scale GWAS studies have reliably identified genes, but these are only of small effect.

An exercise to identify the core findings in behaviour genetics was undertaken by Plomin et al. (2016). They addressed the question of how robust behaviour genetic findings were to replication. They suggest that there are ten findings that have been robustly replicated

Finding 1. All psychological traits show significant and substantial genetic influence.

They suggest that the challenge is to find any adequately powered and replicated study that finds no genetic influences on a behavioural trait. This is the same as Turkheimer's first "law".

Finding 2. No traits are 100% heritable.

The range of heritabilities for behavioural traits is usually between 30 and 50%, but no studies approach the 100% figure.

Finding 3. Heritability is caused by many genes of small effect.

This is reflected in the difficulties of successfully replicating candidate gene studies and the findings from very large and therefore powerful GWAS studies that rarely identify genes that explain even 1% of the variation of behaviour in the population. This is the same of the Chabris et al. (2015) fourth "law".

Finding 4. Phenotypic correlations between psychological traits show significant and substantial genetic mediation.

This suggests that there are many groups of genes that have influences on multiple psychological characteristics. The demonstration that the p-factor (see Sect. 6.2) is highly heritable illustrates this "finding" for psychopathology (Waldman et al., 2016). This principle that there are generalist genes has been demonstrated also for cognitive abilities (Davis et al., 2009)

Finding 5. The heritability of intelligence increases throughout development.

This is a well-replicated and somewhat surprising finding. The expectation might be that as experience accumulates, the role of genetic influences might decrease. As far as IQ is concerned, this is not the case. For example, in a longitudinal study of a large pooled sample of 11,000 twins, h^2 was 49% at age 9 years, 55% at age 12 years, and 66% at age 17 years (Haworth et al., 2010). Why should this be? Haworth et al. (2010) suggest that it results from a gene-environment correlation whereby over time children select, modify, and create their own environments under the influence of their genes – an active r_{GE}. Thereby genes come to have greater effect with age by their influence on environments and experiences.

Finding 6. Age-to-age stability is mainly due to genetics.

This principle has been shown for both cognitive development and for behavioural differences. A meta-analysis of 15 longitudinal twin studies found that the increasing phenotypic stability in IQ with age was almost entirely mediated by genetic factors (Tucker-Drob & Briley, 2014). In a sample of twins studied between the ages 3 and 12 years, Bartels et al. (2004) found that, for both internalising and externalising behaviour, genes explained 43% and 60%, respectively, of the over-time stability in scores.

Finding 7. Most measures of the "environment" show significant genetic influence.

The reason being that many of the most salient environmental influences are provided by people who are genetically related to the child (passive r_{GE}) and are often selected or influenced by the child (active and evocative r_{GE}). These experiences are therefore an "out of the skin" pathway of genetic influences (Kendler & Baker, 2007)

Finding 8. Most associations between environmental measures and psychological traits are significantly mediated genetically.

An example of such mediation was found in a study by Pike et al. (1996), which showed a relationship between parental negativity towards the child and both depressive symptoms and antisocial behaviour in the child. They found that it was genetic factors that accounted for most of the correlation between measures of parental negativity and adolescent depressive symptoms and antisocial behaviour. This arose from a gene-environment correlation whereby both the environment experienced by the child and their own behaviours are influenced by the same genetic factors.

Finding 9. Most environmental effects are not shared by children growing up in the same family.

The question asked by Plomin and Daniels (1987) "Why are children from the same family so different from one another?" has been clearly answered in two ways. They are different, first because genes are so important for behavioural development but siblings only share 50% of their genes and second because the aspects of the environment that have a major influence are not those shared with other family members but rather are non-shared experiences. Family experiences are not unimportant but rather that the relevant experiences are specific to each child in the family.

Finding 10. Abnormal is normal.

There is a consistent finding that the factors influencing extreme behaviour, some of which would be labelled disorders, are simply the extremes of those operating over the range of normal behaviour. One behaviour genetic method for testing this is the DeFries and Fulker (DF) extremes analysis (DeFries & Fulker, 1985, 1988). This examines the differential regression to the mean of the MZ and DZ co-twins of twins who are extreme scorers (probands). If genetic factors are significant influences on extreme group membership, then the co-twins of DZ probands would regress to the mean to a greater extent than those of MZ probands. This difference can be used to estimate the magnitude of genetic effects on extreme group membership (called group heritability, h^2_g). If data have been obtained on a general population sample of twins, the regression analysis can be repeated for increasingly severe cut-offs for proband status. Changes in the size of genetic and of types of environmental influence can be compared to examine if any of these influences become more salient as severity is increased.

This method was used by Gjone et al. (1996) with general population sample of Norwegian twins to show that for attention-related problems, h^2_g remain constant as problem severity increased. Zavos et al. (2014) used the DeFries and Fulker approach and other methods to test for continuities in genetic factors across a range of severity of psychotic experiences. They showed that the same genetic and environmental factors influence both extreme, frequent psychotic experiences and milder, less frequent manifestations in adolescents. Robinson et al. (2011) showed that at varying degrees of extreme symptoms of autism traits, these were similar genetic aetiology across normal variation and the extremes. This is what Plomin et al. (2016) mean by "Abnormal is normal" – abnormality is just on the extreme end of a continuum of behaviour.

In a commentary on Plomin et al. (2016), Turkheimer provides a more sceptical view about the progress made by behaviour genetics. Nevertheless he comments that:

> Genetic influence is real and has profound methodological implications for how human behavior is studied. Even more important, when properly understood, behavior genetics frames a deep scientific question about the explanation of human behavior. (Turkheimer, 2016, p. 27)

Burt et al. (2019) have argued that to date behaviour genetics has been very successful at explaining "what is" but not "what could be". This refers to the way effective change could be implemented in part to better understand the causal relationships that underlie behaviour and in part to identify effective ways to intervene. They propose that an "experimental behaviour genetics" needs to be developed. A demonstration of this approach is provided by Burgoyne et al. (2020) in what they claim is the first randomised controlled trial incorporated into a twin study. They showed how a brief intervention to change attitude towards learning can change the relative magnitude of genetic and environmental influences on the participants' "mindset" motivation. After intervention the role of genetic influences was increased. They conclude that:

> the intervention appears to have augmented preexisting genetic variance, rather than activating novel genetic influences that were not present prior to the intervention. (Burgoyne et al., 2020, p. 11)

Although this limitation on the use of experimental designs might apply to human behaviour genetics, it ignores the long history of experimental behaviour genetic studies on animal models, especially that of the mouse (Bucan & Abel, 2002). A number of these mouse models have direct relevance to showing "what could be" in human behaviour. This is illustrated by the crucial place of mouse models in understanding the possible role of *SHANK* proteins in the development of autism spectrum disorders (Monteiro & Feng, 2017). This is just one of number of set of genes that are involved in the organisation of early stages of brain development the study of which is providing insight to the mechanisms underlying neurodevelopmental disorders such as autism (Courchesne et al., 2019).

3.6 Brain Imaging

There is an extensive range of methods for investigating the structure and functioning of the brain (Pine, 2006). These include measures of brain structure and volume [structural magnetic resonance imaging (sMRI)], of brain fibre pathway organisation [diffusion tensor imaging (DTI)], and of brain activity [functional magnetic resonance imaging (fMRI)], detailed millisecond resolution of activity in the cortex [magnetoencephalography (MEG)], detailed measures of cortical activity but with less good spatial resolution [event-related potentials (ERP)], and brain chemistry [magnetic resonance spectroscopy (MRS)].

There were initial expectations that using these methods studies of variation in normal patterns of brain growth and development would shed light into the origins of child psychiatric disorders (Marsh et al., 2008). However, with only a few exceptions, the applications of brain imaging techniques applied to the young infant have proved to be of limited value in identifying a biological underpinning for these disorders (Batalle et al., 2018; Gilmore et al., 2018). An exception is the study by Wee et al. (2017). They found modest correlations (0.25–0.32) between anatomical brain structure identified by DTI when the participants were neonates and internalising and externalising behaviours at 24 and 48 months of age. As yet this is an isolated finding that needs replicating.

Attempts to identify brain structure and function differences between those with a behavioural disorder and typically developing controls have also found but modest associations. Where group differences are found, magnetic resonance imaging (MRI) measures at the level of the individual are insufficiently discriminating and they cannot reliability aid diagnosis (Giedd et al., 2015; Milham et al., 2021).

There is emerging evidence of consistent but modest relationships between brain volumes and externalising problems in general population samples. Durham et al. (2021) investigated grey matter volumes (GMV) in relation to general psychopathology (p factor), internalising, conduct problems, and ADHD in 9607 children aged 9–10 years. There was an inverse relation between the general factor scores and GMV. This effect, although small, was also found for conduct problems and ADHD. However the specific internalising factor showed no significant relationship with regional GMV in this study. In a general population sample aged 12–19 years, externalising problems were also found to be related to thinner left insular and thinner right orbitofrontal cortex (Tanzer et al., 2021).

A meta-analysis of structural magnetic resonance imaging (sMRI) studies was conducted by Goodkind et al. (2015) to identify variations in regions of grey matter that were associated with psychiatric diagnoses. In addition they investigated the functional significance of the regions showing any volumetric differences from healthy controls. The findings suggest a broad range of psychiatric symptoms is associated with the integrity of an anterior insula and dorsal anterior cingulate. This region was shown to be involved in executive function deficits that were common across diagnoses. They suggested that although this shared neural substrate suggests common brain structural changes at some level, it is likely that these changes reflect a diverse set of aetiologies.

Based on a study of a number of psychiatric disorders in adults, Gong et al. (2019) have used sMRI to investigate possible common brain characteristics. They found that those with psychosis, unipolar depression, post-traumatic stress disorder, and compulsive-obsessive disorder had increased putamen volume compared to TD controls. The putamen is part of the dorsal striatum and has extensive interconnections with other parts of the brain including the cerebral cortex. Gong et al. (2019) concluded that increased putamen volume may reflect a transdiagnostic marker of familial vulnerability to psychopathology.

A very large International Consortium of over 1400 scientists have cooperated to pool data on brain imaging and the genetics of brain development. Based on data from this Consortium, the brain scans of 2264 participants with ADHD were obtained (Thompson et al., 2020). These showed significant differences from TD comparators in brain area volumes with small effect sizes (SMD < 0.15) in children. In adults with ADHD, none of the effect sizes were significantly greater than zero. Similarly small effect sizes were found in the pooled data from 1651 participants with ASD. It has been suggested that these small effect sizes might be false positives and disappear when more appropriate corrections, such as those for total brain volume, are applied (Williams et al., 2020). They found this effect in an analysis of the data in the Autism Brain Imaging Data Exchange data set (Di Martino et al., 2014).

A watershed publication from Marek et al. (2022) has demonstrated that there are major problems with brain-wide association studies (BWAS), which attempt to link individual difference in brain structure or function and behaviour. Based on a pooled sample of 50,000 participants, they found that:

> BWAS associations were smaller than previously thought, resulting in statistically underpowered studies, inflated effect sizes and replication failures at typical sample sizes. As sample sizes grew into the thousands, replication rates began to improve and effect size inflation decreased. More robust BWAS effects were detected for functional MRI (versus structural), cognitive tests (versus mental health questionnaires) and multivariate methods (versus univariate). Smaller than expected brain–phenotype associations and variability across population subsamples can explain widespread BWAS replication failures. In contrast to non-BWAS approaches with larger effects (for example, lesions, interventions and within-person), BWAS reproducibility requires samples with thousands of individuals. (Marek et al., 2022, p. 654)

Further complications have been identified that make the interpretation of the differences seen in MRI studies problematic. It is suggested these differences might arise from frequently occurring measurement artefacts that are correlated with other confounders such as body weight and medical comorbidities (Weinberger & Radulescu, 2016).

ADHD provides a good illustration of the inconsistencies in the findings for fMRI. Hart et al. (2013) undertook a meta-analysis of studies on fMRI with participants with ADHD. There was consistent evidence across studies of functional abnormalities in right hemispheric fronto-basal ganglia networks. There was some suggestion that long-term use of stimulant medication may normalise some of these activations. Subsequent meta-analyses of fMRI studies have produced conflicting results (Cortese et al., 2021; Sutcubasi et al., 2020). These inconsistencies arise both from differences in the type of meta-analysis used and the selection of studies to include. At present it would appear that fMRI has not yielded a clear picture of the differences in fMRI between those with ADHD and TD comparators.

This failure to find strong associations with brain measures for specific brain structures and measures of psychopathology has led to the exploration of whether a stronger relationship could be found by aggregating brain measures together in Neuroimaging Association Scores (NAS) (Axelrud et al., 2021). This procedure was developed to parallel the methods of polygenic risk scores used in genetic analyses. As yet only at an initial stage, this approach has identified predictors of p-factor scores (see Sect. 6.2) but only explains 1–3% of the variance. As the authors conclude:

> Our study indicates that combining several brain features into a single weighted score improves the replicability of psychopathology symptoms prediction, but effect sizes are still small. These findings suggest that the NAS could become a useful marker of general psychopathology, but that the effects of structures on psychopathology are weak. (Axelrud et al., 2021, p. 1093)

It has been argued that multivariate treatment of both the brain and the psychopathology measures provides an optimal approach to identify more robust findings (Genon et al., 2022). An example of such an approach is that of Modabbernia et al. (2021). They estimated common dimensions underlying variation in brain organisation and both psychopathology and environmental influences with correlations as large as 0.40 between these dimensions.

One aspect of behaviour in children that possibly shows more replicable associations with brain structure and function variation is psychopathy (see Sect. 8.1). Pujol et al. (2019) reviewed studies of those with psychopathy and TD individuals and found structural and functional differences in a number of brain regions. There is evidence for an association between callous traits (a component of psychopathy) and brain structure in a large sample from the general population. Bolhuis et al. (2019) found that childhood callous traits were associated with reduced global grey matter and decreases in cortical surface area and gyrification across several frontal and temporal areas.

A complication with studies of brain structure and function in relation to psychopathology arise from the effects of maltreatment (Teicher & Samson, 2016). Maltreatment is the most common potentially preventable factor associated with child psychiatric disorders (Green et al., 2010). Abuse and neglect have been found to be associated with structural and function brain changes (Teicher & Samson, 2016). Studies using fMRI have produced replicated evidence that early maltreatment can lead to changes in neurocognitive functioning (McCrory et al., 2017). These effects are shown in altered functioning in a threat processing, reward processing, emotion regulation, and executive control. These changes can be detected even in the absence of measured psychopathology and may reflect adaptations to early adverse environments.

This raises a potential confound in the brain studies of child psychopathology. Are the results of brain imaging studies of types of psychopathology identifying brain changes specific to the condition? Or are they picking up the enduring effects of prior maltreatment? Indeed the results presented by Danese et al. (2017) suggest an even earlier confounding factor. They analysed data from two large cohort studies to examine the relationship between being a victim of violence in childhood and impaired brain function. They found such a relationship in both studies but also that the relationship was largely explained by pre-existing cognitive vulnerabilities and non-specific effects of socio-economic disadvantage. Such findings require a reappraisal of the nature of the relationship between maltreatment and neurocognitive functioning.

The question of causality in the relationships between adverse experience, maltreatment, and brain development could only be truly addressed in an experiment. Obviously the random allocation to adverse experiences is not ethically acceptable. The closest route to such a design is via a natural experiment. The English Romanian Adoptees (ERA) study provides such a natural experiment. Children from Romanian orphanages were adopted by English families after having experienced between 3 and 41 months of severe deprivation. When these children were followed up into their adult years, it was found that, despite being subsequently cared for in an enrichening environment, they showed smaller total brain volumes and regional cortical alternations than nondeprived adoptees (Mackes et al., 2020). In turn these brain differences were related to lower general intelligence and higher hyperactivity scores in adulthood. The strongest evidence within this study that these effects on brain structure were causally related to early deprivation came from a dose-response relationship between the duration of deprivation and total brain volumes. The longer the period of deprivation, the smaller the total brain volumes. Even with such strong evidence, there remains the possibility that unmeasured and uncontrolled confounds are acting. This notwithstanding the ERA study provides the strongest evidence from human studies that adverse early experiences can cause sustained changes in brain structure and functioning.

The failure to clearly identify the underlying links between characteristics of the brain and psychopathology has been the subject of stringent critique from a network perspective (Borboom et al., 2019). The core of their commentary is that symptoms influence each other rather than showing a pattern of symptom associations arising from a common underlying cause embedded in the person's biology (see Sect. 2.5). A similar argument for the need to adopt an analysis "mutually reinforcing networks of causal mechanisms" to understand psychopathology was put forward by Kendler et al. (2011, p. 1143).

Borsboom et al. (2019) suggest this approach makes it implausible to suggest that either psychological or biological factors have primacy. Rather these two factors acting alongside external environmental mechanism produce complex interactions that preclude identifying a simple biological basis for psychopathology. This argument culminates in their assertion that:

> mental disorders are not brain disorders at all. (Borsboom et al., 2019 p. 2)

A more appropriate aphorism would be that *mental disorders are not merely brain disorders*.

3.7 Final Thoughts on the Biology of Behavioural Differences

The above account of the findings from contemporary genetic and brain imaging studies makes it clear that there is still much to be learned about the biological bases of behavioural variation in children. There are unresolved issues, for example, relating to cultural and genetic contributions to such individual differences. Research on behaviour genetics has been radically enhanced and extended by developments both in molecular genetics (Plomin & Viding, 2022) and in quantitative behaviour genetics, whose methods have retained their value in the post-genomic era (Harden, 2021). There is a recognition that quantitative genetic studies based on twin and family designs are complementary to GWAS studies (Friedman et al., 2021). This paper by Friedman et al. (2021) provides an excellent overview of quantitative and molecular genetic methods.

The history of the first 100 years of behaviour genetics has been reviewed by Plomin (2023) who emphasises the recent importance of the synthesis of quantitative and molecular genetic approaches as illustrated in Fig. 3.6. The key was the possibility provided by GWAS for the development of tools for what Plomin labels "behavioural genomics". GWAS produced genotypes that were associated with behavioural variation for individuals. These genotypes could be used, in the first component of behavioural genomics, to estimate quantitative genomic features such as SNP heritability and for analysis in genomic structural equation modelling (see Sect. 8.4 for an example of this approach). The latter applies quantitative genetic structural equation model fitting to estimates of SNP heritability and genetic correlations obtained from GWAS – a clear example is quantitative and molecular genetic coming together. As was described above in Sect. 3.4, GWAS genotypes provide the basis for the second component of behavioural genomics – PRS. These are predictors of behavioural traits that have a wide application in research studies as, once they have been initially validated, they have can be applied to analyse the effects on behaviour in new samples on which GWAS genotyping is available. The final component of behavioural genomics identified by Plomin is causal modelling (Pingault et al., 2018). The key here in causal modelling is to use GWAS genotypes in analyses that use experimental designs to attempt to deal with the confounding of genetic and environmental influences on behaviour. Examples of this are the genetic nurture methods developed by Kong et al. (2018) and illustrated in Fig. 3.4.

In a review of the considerable progress in psychiatric genetics that has been made in the previous decade, Sullivan and Geschwind (2019) suggest that it has become clear that there is a complex set of interdependent relationships that influence the expression of a risk gene. Such genes are often non-specific in their effects. The disorder that might arise is dependent on the impact of environmental factors and/or polygenic risk. They conclude that:

> Given that the genetic architectures of different psychiatric disorders often strongly overlap, we are challenged to re-evaluate and refine the diagnostic architectures of psychiatric disorders using fundamental genetic and neurobiological data. (Sullivan & Geschwind, 2019, p. 162)

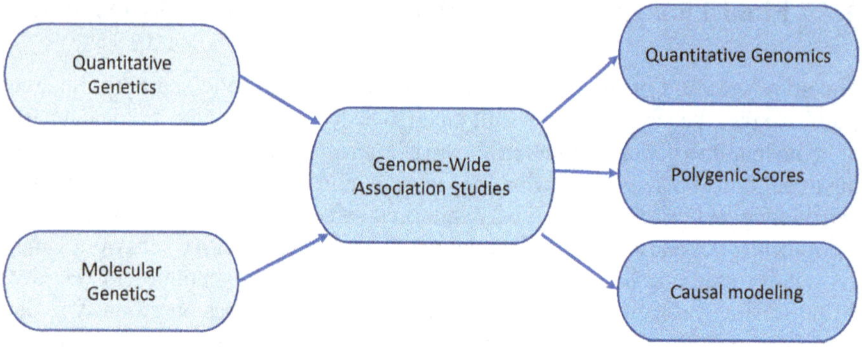

Fig. 3.6 Synthesis of the two worlds of genetics: from behaviour genetics to behavioural genomics. (Reproduced with the permission of Springer Nature BV from Fig. 1 Plomin (2023); permission conveyed through Copyright Clearance Center, Inc.)

A summary of molecular genetic studies on child psychopathology was produced by Akingbuwa et al. (2022). Their extensive meta-analysis of molecular genetic studies suggests that robustly associated genetic variants have been identified for childhood psychiatric conditions. These genetic variants appeared to explain comorbidity as well as stability across a range of psychiatric traits in childhood and across the lifespan. However there is a major difficulty in interpreting the results of molecular genetic studies; the welter of GWAS studies have identified thousands of loci that are associated with behavioural differences. The average effect of these GWAS loci is small. This gives rise to what has been called "the coherence problem". This arises because the genes linked to these loci have not been seen to provide, as yet, a coherent story about the underlying possible causal physiological mechanisms influencing behaviour (Reimers et al., 2019).

The imaging literature is also problematic in that it has yet to find strong and replicable associations between brain structure, brain function, and behaviour. This has led Gardner and Kleinman (2019) to argue that:

> there is no comprehensive biologic understanding of either the causes or the treatments of psychiatric disorders. (Gardner & Kleinman, 2019, p. 1697)

> New discoveries in genetics and neuroscience are exciting, yet they are still far from offering real help to real people in the hospital, clinic, and consulting room. Given the complexity of the human mind, this gap is not surprising. (Gardner & Kleinman, 2019, p. 1698)

Also that:

> Over the past half century, biologic research has come to largely replace all other forms of psychiatric research – psychosocial, cultural, public health, and community – which have thus been marginalized in spite of the useful knowledge these fields provide for everyday care of patients and prevention of mental illness. (Gardner & Kleinman, 2019, p. 1698)

Dumas-Mallet and Gonon (2020) suggest that this failure of neuroscience to make contributions that translate into clinical practice is not being disseminated to the general population. Moreover this bias influences the provision of treatments for mental illness in which neuroscience-based approaches overshadow psychotherapeutic and social approaches. The seemingly irreconcilable reductionist positions of both social and biological investigators have produced a "brainless" and "mindless" psychiatry, respectively (Decker, 2016; Frances, 2016). Frances (2016) reasserts the value of an integrated bio/psycho/social model as the best possible guide to clinical practice. As Rutter and Stevenson (2008) have argued, there has been an attempt to maintain such an integrated position in child psychiatry. Rutter (2010) identified Bronfenbrenner (1979) as being particularly influential in formulating an approach that considers child effects nested within family influences and these being embedded in communities. This par excellence is the bio/psycho/social model that Frances (2016) was seeking.

A good example of this multiple systems approach are the studies of callous-unemotional (CU) traits (Frick et al., 2014). Research on children and adolescents with severe conduct problems and elevated CU traits has shown distinct genetic, cognitive, emotional, biological, environmental, and personality characteristics that seem to implicate different aetiological factors underlying their behaviour problems relative to other youths with severe conduct problems. These wide-ranging investigations have resulted in effective treatments for conduct disorders, but these have different emphases depending on the mix of genetic and environmental influences thought to be acting. The shared environment has less of a role for those with CD and elevated CU traits. As a consequence the recommended treatments for those with elevated CU traits [referred to as limited prosocial emotions (LPE) in Fig. 3.7] differ from other children with conduct disorders (Fairchild et al., 2019).

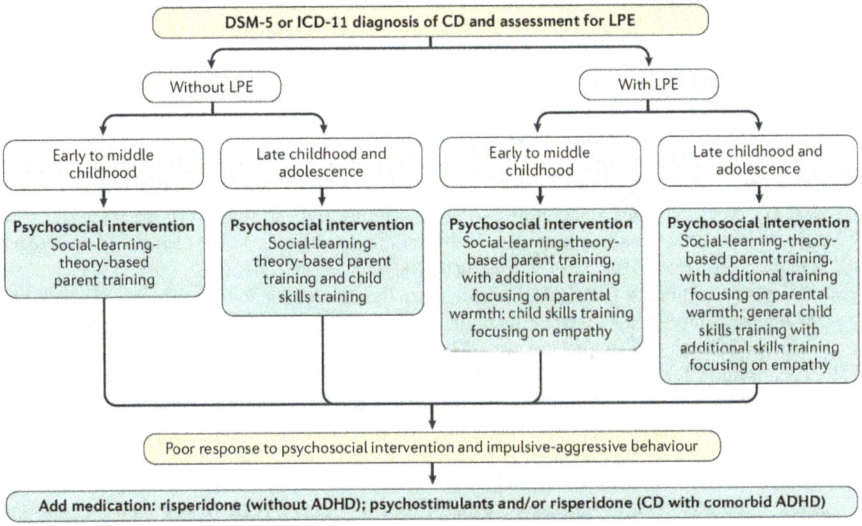

Fig. 3.7 Management of CD without comorbid disorders in different developmental periods. (Reproduced with the permission of Springer Nature from Fig. 1 Fairchild et al. (2019); permission conveyed through Copyright Clearance Center, Inc.)

References

Akingbuwa, W. A., Hammerschlag, A. R., Bartels, M., & Middeldorp, C. M. (2022). Systematic review: Molecular studies of common genetic variation in child and adolescent psychiatric disorders. *Journal of the American Academy of Child and Adolescent Psychiatry, 61*(2), 227–242. https://doi.org/10.1016/j.jaac.2021.03.020

Akingbuwa, W. A., Hammerschlag, A. R., Jami, E. S., Allegrini, A. G., Karhunen, V., Sallis, H., et al. (2020). Genetic associations between childhood psychopathology and adult depression and associated traits in 42998 individuals a meta-analysis. *JAMA Psychiatry, 77*(7), 715–728. https://doi.org/10.1001/jamapsychiatry.2020.0527

Allegrini, A. G., Baldwin, J. R., Barkhuizen, W., & Pingault, J.-B. (2022). Research review: A guide to computing and implementing polygenic scores in developmental research. *Journal of Child Psychology and Psychiatry*. https://doi.org/10.1111/jcpp.13611

Allegrini, A. G., Cheesman, R., Rimfeld, K., Selzam, S., Pingault, J. B., Eley, T. C., & Plomin, R. (2020). The p factor: Genetic analyses support a general dimension of psychopathology in childhood and adolescence. *Journal of Child Psychology and Psychiatry, 61*(1), 30–39. https://doi.org/10.1111/jcpp.13113

Allegrini, A. G., Selzam, S., Rimfeld, K., von Stumm, S., Pingault, J. B., & Plomin, R. (2019). Genomic prediction of cognitive traits in childhood and adolescence. *Molecular Psychiatry, 24*(6), 819–827. https://doi.org/10.1038/s41380-019-0394-4

Anttila, V., Bulik-Sullivan, B., Finucane, H. K., Walters, R. K., Bras, J., Duncan, L., et al. (2018). Analysis of shared heritability in common disorders of the brain. *Science, 360*(6395), 1313-+. https://doi.org/10.1126/science.aap8757

Aristizabal, M. J., Anreiter, I., Halldorsdottir, T., Odgers, C. L., McDade, T. W., Goldenberg, A., et al. (2020). Biological embedding of experience: A primer on epigenetics. *Proceedings of the National Academy of Sciences of the United States of America, 117*(38), 23261–23269. https://doi.org/10.1073/pnas.1820838116

Armstrong-Carter, E., Trejo, S., Hill, L. J. B., Crossley, K. L., Mason, D., & Domingue, B. W. (2020). The earliest origins of genetic nurture: The prenatal environment mediates the association between maternal genetics and child development. *Psychological Science, 31*(7), 781–791. https://doi.org/10.1177/0956797620917209

Assary, E., Krebs, G., & Eley, T. C. (2023). Practitioner review: Differential susceptibility theory: Might it help in understanding and treating mental health problems in youth? *Journal of Child Psychology and Psychiatry*. https://doi.org/10.1111/jcpp.13801

Assary, E., Zavos, H. M. S., Krapohl, E., Keers, R., & Pluess, M. (2021). Genetic architecture of environmental sensitivity reflects multiple heritable components: A twin study with adolescents. *Molecular Psychiatry, 26*(9), 4896–4904. https://doi.org/10.1038/s41380-020-0783-8

Axelrud, L. K., Simioni, A. R., Pine, D. S., Winkler, A. M., Pan, P. M., Sato, J. R., … Consortium, I. (2021). Neuroimaging Association Scores: Reliability and validity of aggregate measures of brain structural features linked to mental disorders in youth. *European Child and Adolescent Psychiatry, 30*, 1895–1906. https://doi.org/10.1007/s00787-020-01653-x

Bacon, E. R., & Brinton, R. D. (2021). Epigenetics of the developing and aging brain: Mechanisms that regulate onset and outcomes of brain reorganization. *Neuroscience and Biobehavioral Reviews, 125*, 503–516. https://doi.org/10.1016/j.neubiorev.2021.02.040

Bale, T. L., Baram, T. Z., Brown, A. S., Goldstein, J. M., Insel, T. R., McCarthy, M. M., . . . Nestler, E. J. (2010). Early life programming and neurodevelopmental disorders. Biological Psychiatry, 68(4), 314–319. https://doi.org/10.1016/j.biopsych.2010.05.028

Barker, E. D., Maughan, B., Allegrini, A., Pingault, J. B., & Sonuga-Barke, E. (2022). Editorial: Does the polygenic revolution herald a watershed in the study of GE interplay in developmental psychopathology? Some considerations for the special issue reader. *Journal of Child Psychology and Psychiatry, 63*(10), 1107–1110. https://doi.org/10.1111/jcpp.13692

Bartels, A., van den Oord, E., Hudziak, J. J., Rietveld, A. J. H., van Beijsterveldt, C. E. M., & Boomsma, D. I. (2004). Genetic and environmental mechanisms underlying stability and change in problem behaviors at ages 3, 7, 10, and 12. *Developmental Psychology, 40*(5), 852–867. https://doi.org/10.1037/0012-1649.40.5.852

Batalle, D., Edwards, A. D., & O'Muircheartaigh, J. (2018). Annual research review: Not just a small adult brain: Understanding later neurodevelopment through imaging the neonatal brain. *Journal of Child Psychology and Psychiatry, 59*(4), 350–371. https://doi.org/10.1111/jcpp.12838

Belsky, J., & Pluess, M. (2009). Beyond diathesis stress: Differential susceptibility to environmental influences. *Psychological Bulletin, 135*(6), 885–908. https://doi.org/10.1037/a0017376

Belsky, J., & Pluess, M. (2013). Beyond risk, resilience, and dysregulation: Phenotypic plasticity and human development. *Development and Psychopathology, 25*(4), 1243–1261. https://doi.org/10.1017/s095457941300059x

Bishop, D. V. M., Canning, E., Elgar, K., Morris, E., Jacobs, P. A., & Skuse, D. H. (2000). Distinctive patterns of memory function in subgroups of females with turner syndrome: Evidence for imprinted loci on the X-chromosome affecting neurodevelopment. *Neuropsychologia, 38*(5), 712–721. https://doi.org/10.1016/s0028-3932(99)00118-9

Bolhuis, K., Steenkamp, L. R., Blanken, L. M. E., Neumann, A., Jansen, P. R., Hillegers, M. H. J., et al. (2021). Schizophrenia polygenic risk is associated with child mental health problems through early childhood adversity: Evidence for a gene-environment correlation. *European Child and Adolescent Psychiatry.* https://doi.org/10.1007/s00787-021-01727-4

Bolhuis, K., Viding, E., Muetzel, R. L., El Marroun, H., Kocevska, D., White, T., et al. (2019). Neural profile of callous traits in children: A population-based neuroimaging study. *Biological Psychiatry, 85*(5), 399–407. https://doi.org/10.1016/j.biopsych.2018.10.015

Bonnevie, K. (1924). Studies on papillary patterns of human fingers. *Journal of Genetics, 15*, 1–23.

Border, R., Johnson, E. C., Evans, L. M., Smolen, A., Berley, N., Sullivan, P. F., & Keller, M. C. (2019). No support for historical candidate gene or candidate gene-by-interaction hypotheses for major depression across multiple large samples. *American Journal of Psychiatry, 176*(5), 376–387. https://doi.org/10.1176/appi.ajp.2018.18070881

Border, R., & Keller, M. C. (2017). Commentary: Fundamental problems with candidate gene-by-environment interaction studies – Reflections on Moore and Thoemmes (2016). *Journal of Child Psychology and Psychiatry, 58*(3), 328–330. https://doi.org/10.1111/jcpp.12669

Borsboom, D., Cramer, A. O. J., & Kalis, A. (2019). Brain disorders? Not really: Why network structures block reductionism in psychopathology research. *Behavioral and Brain Sciences, 42*. https://doi.org/10.1017/s0140525x17002266

Boyce, W. T., Sokolowski, M. B., & Robinson, G. E. (2020). Genes and environments, development and time. *Proceedings of the National Academy of Sciences of the United States of America, 117*(38), 23235–23241. https://doi.org/10.1073/pnas.2016710117

Branje, S., Geeraerts, S., de Zeeuw, E. L., Oerlemans, A. M., Koopman-Verhoeff, M. E., Schulz, S., et al. (2020). Intergenerational transmission: Theoretical and methodological issues and an introduction to four Dutch cohorts. *Developmental Cognitive Neuroscience, 45*. https://doi.org/10.1016/j.dcn.2020.100835

Bronfenbrenner, U. (1979). *The ecology of human development: Experiments by nature and design*. Harvard University Press.

Bucan, M., & Abel, T. (2002). The mouse: Genetics meets behaviour. *Nature Reviews Genetics, 3*(2), 114–123. https://doi.org/10.1038/nrg728

Buck, J. M., Sanders, K. N., Wageman, C. R., Knopik, V. S., Stitzel, J. A., & O'Neill, H. C. (2019). Developmental nicotine exposure precipitates multigenerational maternal transmission of nicotine preference and ADHD-like behavioral, rhythmometric, neuropharmacological, and epigenetic anomalies in adolescent mice. *Neuropharmacology, 149*, 66–82. https://doi.org/10.1016/j.neuropharm.2019.02.006

Burgoyne, A. P., Carroll, S., Clark, D. A., Hambrick, D. Z., Plaisance, K. S., Klump, K. L., & Burt, S. A. (2020). Can a brief intervention alter genetic and environmental influences on psychological traits? An experimental behavioral genetics approach. *Learning and Motivation, 72*. https://doi.org/10.1016/j.lmot.2020.101683

Burt, S. A. (2009). Rethinking environmental contributions to child and adolescent psychopathology: A meta-analysis of shared environmental influences. *Psychological Bulletin, 135*(4), 608–637. https://doi.org/10.1037/a0015702

Burt, S. A., Plaisance, K. S., & Hambrick, D. Z. (2019). Understanding "What Could Be": A call for “experimental behavioral genetics”. *Behavior Genetics, 49*(2), 235–243. https://doi.org/10.1007/s10519-018-9918-y

Cao-Lei, L., de Rooij, S., King, S., Matthews, S. G., Metz, G. A. S., Roseboom, T. J., & Szyf, M. (2020). Prenatal stress and epigenetics. *Neuroscience and Biobehavioral Reviews, 117*, 198–210. https://doi.org/10.1016/j.neubiorev.2017.05.016

Caspi, A., & Moffitt, T. E. (2006). Opinion – Gene-environment interactions in psychiatry: Joining forces with neuroscience. *Nature Reviews Neuroscience, 7*(7), 583–590. https://doi.org/10.1038/nrn1925

Caspi, A., Sugden, K., Moffitt, T. E., Taylor, A., Craig, I. W., Harrington, H., et al. (2003). Influence of life stress on depression: Moderation by a polymorphism in the 5-HTT gene. *Science, 301*(5631), 386–389. https://doi.org/10.1126/science.1083968

Cavalli-Sforza, L. L., & Feldman, M. W. (1973). Cultural versus biological inheritance – Phenotypic transmission from parents to children (a theory of effect of parental phenotypes on children’s phenotypes). *American Journal of Human Genetics, 25*(6), 618–637.

Chabris, C. F., Lee, J. J., Cesarini, D., Benjamin, D. J., & Laibson, D. I. (2015). The fourth law of behavior genetics. *Current Directions in Psychological Science, 24*(4), 304–312. https://doi.org/10.1177/0963721415580430

Cheesman, R., Eilertsen, E. M., Ahmadzadeh, Y. I., Gjerde, L. C., Hannigan, L. J., Havdahl, A., et al. (2020a). How important are parents in the development of child anxiety and depression? A genomic analysis of parent-offspring trios in the Norwegian Mother Father and Child Cohort Study (MoBa). *BMC Medicine, 18*(1). https://doi.org/10.1186/s12916-020-01760-1

Cheesman, R., Hunjan, A., Coleman, J. R. I., Ahmadzadeh, Y., Plomin, R., McAdams, T. A., et al. (2020b). Comparison of adopted and nonadopted individuals reveals gene-environment interplay for education in the UK Biobank. *Psychological Science, 31*(5), 582–591. https://doi.org/10.1177/0956797620904450

Cheesman, R., Purves, K. L., Pingault, J.-B., Breen, G., Rijsdij, F. K., Plomin, R., et al. (2018). Extracting stability increases the SNP heritability of emotional problems in young people. *Translational Psychiatry, 8*. https://doi.org/10.1038/s41398-018-0269-5

Cheesman, R., Selzam, S., Ronald, A., Dale, P. S., McAdams, T. A., Eley, T. C., & Plomin, R. (2017). Childhood behaviour problems show the greatest gap between DNA-based and twin heritability. *Translational Psychiatry, 7*. https://doi.org/10.1038/s41398-017-0046-x

Cortese, S., Aoki, Y. Y., Itahashi, T., Castellanos, F. X., & Eickhoff, S. B. (2021). Systematic review and meta-analysis: Resting-state functional magnetic resonance imaging studies of Attention-Deficit/Hyperactivity Disorder. *Journal of the American Academy of Child and Adolescent Psychiatry, 60*(1), 61–75. https://doi.org/10.1016/j.jaac.2020.08.014

Courchesne, E., Pramparo, T., Gazestani, V. H., Lombardo, M. V., Pierce, K., & Lewis, N. E. (2019). The ASD living biology: From cell proliferation to clinical phenotype. *Molecular Psychiatry, 24*(1), 88–107. https://doi.org/10.1038/s41380-018-0056-y

Danese, A., Moffitt, T. E., Arseneault, L., Bleiberg, B. A., Dinardo, P. B., Gandelman, S. B., et al. (2017). The origins of cognitive deficits in victimized children: Implications for neuroscientists and clinicians. *American Journal of Psychiatry, 174*(4), 349–361. https://doi.org/10.1176/appi.ajp.2016.16030333

Davis, O. S. P., Haworth, C. M. A., & Plomin, R. (2009). Learning abilities and disabilities: Generalist genes in early adolescence. *Cognitive Neuropsychiatry, 14*(4–5), 312–331. https://doi.org/10.1080/13546800902797106

Decker, H. S. (2016). Cyclical swings: The bete noire of psychiatry. *History of Psychology, 19*(1), 52–56. https://doi.org/10.1037/hop0000017

DeFries, J. C., & Fulker, D. W. (1985). Multiple-regresssion analysis of twin data. *Behavior Genetics, 15*(5), 467–473. https://doi.org/10.1007/bf01066239

Defries, J. C., & Fulker, D. W. (1988). Multiple-regression analysis of twin data- etiology of devaint scores versus individual-differences. *Acta Geneticae Medicae et Gemellologiae, 37*(3–4), 205–216. https://doi.org/10.1017/s0001566000003810

Demontis, D., Walters, R. K., Martin, J., Mattheisen, M., Als, T. D., Agerbo, E., et al. (2019). Discovery of the first genome-wide significant risk loci for attention deficit/hyperactivity disorder. *Nature Genetics, 51*(1), 63-+. https://doi.org/10.1038/s41588-018-0269-7

Di Martino, A., Yan, C. G., Li, Q., Denio, E., Castellanos, F. X., Alaerts, K., et al. (2014). The autism brain imaging data exchange: Towards a large-scale evaluation of the intrinsic brain architecture in autism. *Molecular Psychiatry, 19*(6), 659–667. https://doi.org/10.1038/mp.2013.78

Dias, B. G., Maddox, S. A., Klengel, T., & Ressier, K. J. (2015). Epigenetic mechanisms underlying learning and the inheritance of learned behaviors. *Trends in Neurosciences, 38*(2), 96–107. https://doi.org/10.1016/j.tins.2014.12.003

Dumas-Mallet, E., & Gonon, F. (2020). Messaging in biological psychiatry: Misrepresentations, their causes, and potential consequences. *Harvard Review of Psychiatry, 28*(6), 395–403.

Duncan, L. E., Pollastri, A. R., & Smoller, J. W. (2014). Mind the gap why many geneticists and psychological scientists have discrepant views about gene-environment interaction (GXE) research. *American Psychologist, 69*(3), 249–268. https://doi.org/10.1037/a0036320

Duncan, L. E., Ostacher, M., & Ballon, J. (2019). How genome-wide association studies (GWAS) made traditional candidate gene studies obsolete. *Neuropsychopharmacology, 44*(9), 1518–1523. https://doi.org/10.1038/s41386-019-0389-5

Durham, E. L., Jeong, H. J., Moore, T. M., Dupont, R. M., Cardenas-Iniguez, C., Cui, Z. X., et al. (2021). Association of gray matter volumes with general and specific dimensions of psychopathology in children. *Neuropsychopharmacology, 46*(7), 1333–1339. https://doi.org/10.1038/s41386-020-00952-w

Eadeh, H.-M., Markon, K. E., Nigg, J. T., & Nikolas, M. A. (2021). Evaluating the viability of neurocognition as a transdiagnostic construct using both latent variable models and network analysis. *Research on Child and Adolescent Psychopathology, 49*(6), 697–710. https://doi.org/10.1007/s10802-021-00770-8

Eaves, L. (2020). Birmingham and beyond. *Twin Research and Human Genetics, 23*(2), 68–71. https://doi.org/10.1017/thg.2020.27

Fairchild, G., Hawes, D. J., Frick, P. J., Copeland, W. E., Odgers, C. L., Franke, B., et al. (2019). Conduct disorder. *Nature Reviews Disease Primers, 5*. https://doi.org/10.1038/s41572-019-0095-y

Falconer, D. S. (1960). *Introduction to quantitative genetics*. Oliver and Boyd.

Faraone, S. V., & Larsson, H. (2019). Genetics of attention deficit hyperactivity disorder. Molecular Psychiatry, 24(4), 562–575. https://doi.org/10.1038/s41380-018-0070-0

Fisher, R. A. (1918). The correlation between relatives on the supposition of Mendelian inheritance. *Transactions of the Royal Society (Edinburgh), 52*, 399–433.

Fisher, R. A. (1919). The causes of human variability. *Eugenics Review, 10*, 213–220.

Fisher, R. A. (1930). *The genetical theory of natural selection*. Clarendon Press.

Flint, J., Greenspan, R. J., & Kendler, K. S. (2020). *How genes influence behaviour* (2nd ed.). Oxford University Press.

Fraga, M. F., Ballestar, E., Paz, M. F., Ropero, S., Setien, F., Ballestart, M. L., et al. (2005). Epigenetic differences arise during the lifetime of monozygotic twins. *Proceedings of the National Academy of Sciences of the United States of America, 102*(30), 10604–10609. https://doi.org/10.1073/pnas.0500398102

Frances, A. (2016). Entrenched reductionisms: The bete noire of psychiatry. *History of Psychology, 19*(1), 57–59. https://doi.org/10.1037/hop0000018

Frick, P. J., Ray, J. V., Thornton, L. C., & Kahn, R. E. (2014). Can callous-unemotional traits enhance the understanding, diagnosis, and treatment of serious conduct problems in children and adolescents? A comprehensive review. *Psychological Bulletin, 140*(1), 1–57. https://doi.org/10.1037/a0033076

Friedman, N. P., Banich, M. T., & Keller, M. C. (2021). Twin studies to GWAS: There and back again. *Trends in Cognitive Sciences, 25*(10), 855–869. https://doi.org/10.1016/j.tics.2021.06.007

Futuyma, D. J. (2017). Evolutionary biology today and the call for an extended synthesis. *Interface Focus, 7*(5). https://doi.org/10.1098/rsfs.2016.0145

Galton, F. (1876). The history of twins, as a criterion of the relative powers of nature and nurture. *The Journal of the Anthropological Institute of Great Britain and Ireland, 5*, 391–406.

Gardner, C., & Kleinman, A. (2019). Medicine and the mind – The consequences of psychiatry's identity crisis. *New England Journal of Medicine, 381*(18), 1697–1699. https://doi.org/10.1056/NEJMp1910603

Genin, E. (2020). Missing heritability of complex diseases: Case solved? *Human Genetics, 139*(1), 103–113. https://doi.org/10.1007/s00439-019-02034-4

Genon, S., Eickhoff, S. B., & Kharabian, S. (2022). Linking interindividual variability in brain structure to behaviour. *Nature Reviews Neuroscience, 23*(5), 307–318. https://doi.org/10.1038/s41583-022-00584-7

Gidziela, A., Rimfeld, K., Malanchini, M., Allegrini, A. G., McMillan, A., Selzam, S., et al. (2021). Using DNA to predict behaviour problems from preschool to adulthood. *Journal of Child Psychology and Psychiatry*. https://doi.org/10.1111/jcpp.13519

Giedd, J. N., Raznahan, A., Alexander-Bloch, A., Schmitt, E., Gogtay, N., & Rapoport, J. L. (2015). Child psychiatry branch of the National Institute of Mental Health longitudinal structural magnetic resonance imaging study of human brain development. *Neuropsychopharmacology, 40*(1), 43–49. https://doi.org/10.1038/npp.2014.236

Gilmore, J. H., Knickmeyer, R. C., & Gao, W. (2018). Imaging structural and functional brain development in early childhood. *Nature Reviews Neuroscience, 19*(3), 123–137. https://doi.org/10.1038/nrn.2018.1

Gizer, I. R., Ficks, C., & Waldman, I. D. (2009). Candidate gene studies of ADHD: A meta-analytic review. *Human Genetics, 126*(1), 51–90. https://doi.org/10.1007/s00439-009-0694-x

Gjerde, L. C., Eilertsen, E. M., Hannigan, L. J., Eley, T., Roysamb, E., Reichborn-Kjennerud, T., et al. (2021). Associations between maternal depressive symptoms and risk for offspring early-life psychopathology: The role of genetic and non-genetic mechanisms. *Psychological Medicine, 51*(3), 441–449. https://doi.org/10.1017/s0033291719003301

Gjone, H., Stevenson, J., & Sundet, J. M. (1996). Genetic influence on parent-reported attention-related problems in a Norwegian general population twin sample. *Journal of the American Academy of Child and Adolescent Psychiatry, 35*(5), 588–596. https://doi.org/10.1097/00004583-199605000-00013

Golding, J., Ellis, G., Gregory, S., Birmingham, K., Iles-Caven, Y., Rai, D., & Pembrey, M. (2017). Grand-maternal smoking in pregnancy and grandchild's autistic traits and diagnosed autism. *Scientific Reports, 7*. https://doi.org/10.1038/srep46179

Gong, Q. Y., Scarpazza, C., Dai, J., He, M. X., Xu, X., Shi, Y., et al. (2019). A transdiagnostic neuroanatomical signature of psychiatric illness. *Neuropsychopharmacology, 44*(5), 869–875. https://doi.org/10.1038/s41386-018-0175-9

Goodkind, M., Eickhoff, S. B., Oathes, D. J., Jiang, Y., Chang, A., Jones-Hagata, L. B., et al. (2015). Identification of a common neurobiological substrate for mental illness. *JAMA Psychiatry, 72*(4), 305–315. https://doi.org/10.1001/jamapsychiatry.2014.2206

Green, J. G., McLaughlin, K. A., Berglund, P. A., Gruber, M. J., Sampson, N. A., Zaslavsky, A. M., & Kessler, R. C. (2010). Childhood Adversities and Adult Psychiatric Disorders in the National Comorbidity Survey Replication I Associations With First Onset of DSM-IV Disorders. Archives of General Psychiatry, 67(2), 113–123. https://doi.org/10.1001/archgenpsychiatry.2009.186

Hall, S. S., Riley, M. J., Weston, R. N., Lepage, J. F., Hong, D. S., Jo, B., et al. (2022). Effects of X chromosome monosomy and genomic imprinting on observational markers of social anxiety in prepubertal girls with turner syndrome. *Journal of Autism Developmental Disorders, 52*(1), 16–27. https://doi.org/10.1007/s10803-021-04896-y

Hanson, M. A., & Skinner, M. K. (2016). Developmental origins of epigenetic transgenerational inheritance. *Environmental Epigenetics, 2*(1). https://doi.org/10.1093/eep/dvw002

Harden, K. P. (2021). "Reports of My Death Were Greatly Exaggerated": Behavior Genetics in the Postgenomic Era. In S. T. Fiske (Ed.), *Annual Review of Psychology, Vol 72* (Vol. 72, pp. 37–60).

Harden, K. P., & Koellinger, P. D. (2020). Using genetics for social science. *Nature Human Behaviour, 4*(6), 567–576. https://doi.org/10.1038/s41562-020-0862-5

Hart, H., Radua, J., Nakao, T., Mataix-Cols, D., & Rubia, K. (2013). Meta-analysis of functional magnetic resonance imaging studies of inhibition and attention in attention-deficit/hyperactivity disorder exploring task-specific, stimulant medication, and age effects. *JAMA Psychiatry, 70*(2), 185–198. https://doi.org/10.1001/jamapsychiatry.2013.277

Hartman, S., & Belsky, J. (2018). Prenatal programming of postnatal plasticity revisited-and extended. *Development and Psychopathology, 30*(3), 825–842. https://doi.org/10.1017/s0954579418000548

Haworth, C. M. A., Wright, M. J., Luciano, M., Martin, N. G., de Geus, E. J. C., van Beijsterveldt, C. E. M., et al. (2010). The heritability of general cognitive ability increases linearly from childhood to young adulthood. *Molecular Psychiatry, 15*(11), 1112–1120. https://doi.org/10.1038/mp.2009.55

Heard, E., & Martienssen, R. A. (2014). Transgenerational epigenetic inheritance: Myths and mechanisms. *Cell, 157*(1), 95–109. https://doi.org/10.1016/j.cell.2014.02.045

Holz, N. E., Zohsel, K., Laucht, M., Banaschewski, T., Hohmann, S., & Brandeis, D. (2018). Gene x environment interactions in conduct disorder: Implications for future treatments. *Neuroscience and Biobehavioral Reviews, 91*, 239–258. https://doi.org/10.1016/j.neubiorev.2016.08.017

Ioannidis, J. P. A. (2005). Why most published research findings are false. *PLoS Medicine, 2*(8), 696–701. https://doi.org/10.1371/journal.pmed.0020124

Isles, A. R. (2015). Neural and behavioral epigenetics; what it is, and what is hype. *Genes Brain and Behavior, 14*(1), 64–72. https://doi.org/10.1111/gbb.12184

Jami, E. S., Hammerschlag, A. R., Bartels, M., & Middeldorp, C. M. (2021). Parental characteristics and offspring mental health and related outcomes: A systematic review of genetically informative literature. *Translational Psychiatry, 11*(1). https://doi.org/10.1038/s41398-021-01300-2

Jinks, J. L., & Fulker, D. W. (1970). Comparison of biometrical genetical, MAVA, and classical approaches to the analysis of human behvaiour. *Psychological Bulletin, 73*(5), 311–349. https://doi.org/10.1037/h0029135

Kandaswamy, R., Allegrini, A., Nancarrow, A. F., Cave, S. N., Plomin, R., & von Stumm, S. (2022). Predicting alcohol use from genome-wide polygenic scores, environmental factors, and their interactions in young adulthood. *Psychosomatic Medicine, 84*(2), 244–250. https://doi.org/10.1097/psy.0000000000001005

Kendler, K. S., & Baker, J. H. (2007). Genetic influences on measures of the environment: A systematic review. *Psychological Medicine, 37*(5), 615–626. https://doi.org/10.1017/s0033291706009524

Kendler, K. S., Ohlsson, H., Lichtenstein, P., Sundquist, J., & Sundquist, K. (2019). The nature of the shared environment. *Behavior Genetics, 49*(1), 1–10. https://doi.org/10.1007/s10519-018-9940-0

Kendler, K. S., Zachar, P., & Craver, C. (2011). What kinds of things are psychiatric disorders? *Psychological Medicine, 41*(6), 1143–1150. https://doi.org/10.1017/s0033291710001844

Klengel, T., Dias, B. G., & Ressler, K. J. (2016). Models of intergenerational and transgenerational transmission of risk for psychopathology in mice. *Neuropsychopharmacology, 41*(1), 219–231. https://doi.org/10.1038/npp.2015.249

Kohn, M. (2004). *A reason for everything: Natural selection and the English imagination*. Faber and Faber.

Kong, A., Thorleifsson, G., Frigge, M. L., Vilhjalmsson, B. J., Young, A. I., Thorgeirsson, T. E., et al. (2018). The nature of nurture: Effects of parental genotypes. *Science, 359*(6374), 424–428. https://doi.org/10.1126/science.aan6877

Krapohl, E., Hannigan, L. J., Pingault, J. B., Patel, H., Kadeva, N., Curtis, C., et al. (2017). Widespread covariation of early environmental exposures and trait-associated polygenic variation. *Proceedings of the National Academy of Sciences of the United States of America, 114*(44), 11727–11732. https://doi.org/10.1073/pnas.1707178114

Laland, K. N., Uller, T., Fellman, M. W., Sterelny, K., Muller, G. B., Moczek, A., et al. (2015). The extended evolutionary synthesis: Its structure, assumptions and predictions. *Proceedings of the Royal Society B-Biological Sciences, 282*(1813). https://doi.org/10.1098/rspb.2015.1019

Larsson, H., Anckarsater, H., Rastam, M., Chang, Z., & Lichtenstein, P. (2012). Childhood attention-deficit hyperactivity disorder as an extreme of a continuous trait: A quantitative genetic study of 8,500 twin pairs. *Journal of Child Psychology and Psychiatry, 53*(1), 73–80. https://doi.org/10.1111/j.1469-7610.2011.02467.x

Lee, J. J., McGue, M., Iacono, W. G., Michael, A. M., & Chabris, C. F. (2019). The causal influence of brain size on human intelligence: Evidence from within-family phenotypic associations and GWAS modeling. *Intelligence, 75*, 48–58. https://doi.org/10.1016/j.intell.2019.01.011

Lee, J. J., Wedow, R., Okbay, A., Kong, E., Maghzian, O., Zacher, M., et al. (2018). Gene discovery and polygenic prediction from a genome-wide association study of educational attainment in 1.1 million individuals. *Nature Genetics, 50*(8), 1112-+. https://doi.org/10.1038/s41588-018-0147-3

Lee, P. H., Feng, Y. C. A., & Smoller, J. W. (2021). Pleiotropy and cross-disorder genetics among psychiatric disorders. *Biological Psychiatry, 89*(1), 20–31. https://doi.org/10.1016/j.biopsych.2020.09.026

Loughnan, R. J., Palmer, C. E., Makowski, C., Thompson, W. K., Barch, D. M., Jernigan, T. L., et al. (2022). Unique prediction of developmental psychopathology from genetic and familial risk. *Journal of Child Psychology and Psychiatry*. https://doi.org/10.1111/jcpp.13649

Lundström, S., Chang, Z., Rastam, M., Gillberg, C., Larsson, H., Anckarsater, H., & Lichtenstein, P. (2012). Autism spectrum disorders and autistic like traits similar etiology in the extreme end and the normal variation. *Archives of General Psychiatry, 69*(1), 46–52. https://doi.org/10.1001/archgenpsychiatry.2011.144

Lytton, H. (1977). Do parents create, or respond to, differences in twins? *Developmental Psychology, 13*(5), 456–459. https://doi.org/10.1037/0012-1649.13.5.456

Mackes, N. K., Golm, D., Sarkar, S., Kumsta, R., Rutter, M., Fairchild, G., et al. (2020). Early childhood deprivation is associated with alterations in adult brain structure despite subsequent environmental enrichment. *Proceedings of the National Academy of Sciences of the United States of America, 117*(1), 641–649. https://doi.org/10.1073/pnas.1911264116

Maes, H. H. M., Lapato, D. M., Schmitt, J. E., Luciana, M., Banich, M. T., Bjork, J. M., et al. (2023). Genetic and environmental variation in continuous phenotypes in the ABCD study ®. *Behavior Genetics, 53*(1), 1–24. https://doi.org/10.1007/s10519-022-10123-w

Maes, H. H., Neale, M. C., Kirkpatrick, R. M., & Kendler, K. S. (2021). Using multimodel inference/model averaging to model causes of covariation between variables in twins. *Behavior Genetics, 51*(1), 82–96. https://doi.org/10.1007/s10519-020-10026-8

Marceau, K., Knopik, V. S., Neiderhiser, J. M., Lichtenstein, P., Spotts, E. L., Ganiban, J. M., & Reiss, D. (2016). Adolescent age moderates genetic and environmental influences on parent-adolescent positivity and negativity: Implications for genotype-environment correlation. *Development and Psychopathology, 28*(1), 149–166. https://doi.org/10.1017/s0954579415000358

Marek, S., Tervo-Clemmens, B., Calabro, F. J., Montez, D. F., Kay, B. P., Hatoum, A. S., et al. (2022). Reproducible brain-wide association studies require thousands of individuals. *Nature, 603*(7902), 654-+. https://doi.org/10.1038/s41586-022-04492-9

Marsh, R., Gerber, A. J., & Peterson, B. S. (2008). Neuroimaging studies of normal brain development and their relevance for understanding childhood neuropsychiatric disorders. *Journal of the American Academy of Child and Adolescent Psychiatry, 47*(11), 1233–1251. https://doi.org/10.1097/CHI.0b013e318185e703

Martel, M. M., Nikolas, M., Jernigan, K., Friderici, K., Waldman, I., & Nigg, J. T. (2011). The dopamine receptor D4 gene (DRD4) moderates family environmental effects on ADHD. *Journal of Abnormal Child Psychology, 39*(1), 1–10. https://doi.org/10.1007/s10802-010-9439-5

Martin, A. R., Daly, M. J., Robinson, E. B., Hyman, S. E., & Neale, B. M. (2019). Predicting polygenic risk of psychiatric disorders. *Biological Psychiatry, 86*(2), 97–109. https://doi.org/10.1016/j.biopsych.2018.12.015

Mayo, O. (2009). Early research on human genetics using the twin method: Who really invented the method? *Twin Research and Human Genetics, 12*(3), 237–245. https://doi.org/10.1375/twin.12.3.237

McAdams, T. A., Cheesman, R., & Ahmadzadeh, Y. I. (2023). Annual research review: Towards a deeper understanding of nature and nurture: Combining family-based quasi-experimental methods with genomic data. *Journal of Child Psychology and Psychiatry*. https://doi.org/10.1111/jcpp.13720

McAdams, T. A., Hannigan, L. J., Eilertsen, E. M., Gjerde, L. C., Ystrom, E., & Rijsdijk, F. V. (2018). Revisiting the Children-of-Twins Design: Improving existing models for the exploration of intergenerational associations. *Behavior Genetics, 48*(5), 397–412. https://doi.org/10.1007/s10519-018-9912-4

McAdams, T. A., Neiderhiser, J. M., Rijsdijk, F. V., Narusyte, J., Lichtenstein, P., & Eley, T. C. (2014). Accounting for genetic and environmental confounds in associations between parent and child characteristics: A systematic review of Children-of-Twins studies. *Psychological Bulletin, 140*(4), 1138–1173. https://doi.org/10.1037/a0036416

McCrory, E. J., Gerin, M. I., & Viding, E. (2017). Annual research review: Childhood maltreatment, latent vulnerability and the shift to preventative psychiatry – The contribution of functional brain imaging. *Journal of Child Psychology and Psychiatry, 58*(4), 338–357. https://doi.org/10.1111/jcpp.12713

Meaney, M. J. (2010). Epigenetics and the biological definition of gene x environment interactions. *Child Development, 81*(1), 41–79. https://doi.org/10.1111/j.1467-8624.2009.01381.x

Merriman, C. (1924). The intellectual resemblance of twins. *Psychological Monographs, 33*, 1–58. https://doi.org/10.1037/h0093212

Milham, M. P., Vogelstein, J., & Xu, T. (2021). Removing the reliability bottleneck in functional magnetic resonance imaging research to achieve clinical utility. *JAMA Psychiatry, 78*(6), 587–588. https://doi.org/10.1001/jamapsychiatry.2020.4272

Mills, M. C., & Rahal, C. (2019). A scientometric review of genome-wide association studies. *Communications Biology, 2*. https://doi.org/10.1038/s42003-018-0261-x

Modabbernia, A., Janiri, D., Doucet, G. E., Reichenberg, A., & Frangou, S. (2021). Multivariate patterns of brain-behavior- environment associations in the adolescent brain and cognitive development study. *Biological Psychiatry, 89*(5), 510–520. https://doi.org/10.1016/j.biopsych.2020.08.014

Monteiro, P., & Feng, G. P. (2017). SHANK proteins: Roles at the synapse and in autism spectrum disorder. *Nature Reviews Neuroscience, 18*(3), 147–157. https://doi.org/10.1038/nrn.2016.183

Morton, N. E. (1974). Analysis of family resemblance. I. Introduction. *American Journal of Human Genetics, 26*, 318–330.

Murray, G. K., Lin, T., Austin, J., McGrath, J. J., Hickie, I. B., & Wray, N. R. (2021). Could polygenic risk scores be useful in psychiatry? A review. *JAMA Psychiatry, 78*(2), 210–219. https://doi.org/10.1001/jamapsychiatry.2020.3042

Nance, W. E., & Corey, L. A. (1976). Genetic models of analysis of data from families of identical-twins. *Genetics, 83*(4), 811–826. https://doi.org/10.1093/genetics/83.4.811

Narusyte, J., Neiderhiser, J. M., D'Onofrio, B. M., Reiss, D., Spotts, E. L., Ganiban, J., & Lichtenstein, P. (2008). Testing different types of genotype-environment correlation: An extended children-of-twins model. *Developmental Psychology, 44*(6), 1591–1603. https://doi.org/10.1037/a0013911

Neale, M. C., Hunter, M. D., Pritikin, J. N., Zahery, M., Brick, T. R., Kirkpatrick, R. M., et al. (2016). OpenMx 2.0: Extended structural equation and statistical modeling. *Psychometrika, 81*(2), 535–549. https://doi.org/10.1007/s11336-014-9435-8

Neumann, A., Jolicoeur-Martineau, A., Szekely, E., Sallis, H. M., O'Donnel, K., Greenwood, C. M. T., et al. (2022). Combined polygenic risk scores of different psychiatric traits predict general and specific psychopathology in childhood. *Journal of Child Psychology and Psychiatry, 63*(6), 636–645. https://doi.org/10.1111/jcpp.13501

Owen, M. J., & Williams, N. M. (2021). Explaining the missing heritability of psychiatric disorders. *World Psychiatry, 20*(2), 294–295. https://doi.org/10.1002/wps.20870

Pappa, I., Fedko, I. O., Mileva-Seitz, V. R., Hottenga, J.-J., Bakermans-Kranenburg, M. J., Bartels, M., et al. (2015). Single nucleotide polymorphism heritabiliiy of behavior problems in childhood: Genome-wide complex trait analysis. *Journal of the American Academy of Child and Adolescent Psychiatry, 54*(9), 737–744. https://doi.org/10.1016/j.jaac.2015.06.004

Parade, S. H., Huffhines, L., Daniels, T. E., Stroud, L. R., Nugent, N. R., & Tyrka, A. R. (2021). A systematic review of childhood maltreatment and DNA methylation: Candidate gene and epigenome-wide approaches. *Translational. Psychiatry, 11*(1). https://doi.org/10.1038/s41398-021-01207-y

Pearl, J., & Mackenzie, D. (2018). *The book of why: The new science of cause and effect*. Allen Lane.

Peters, J. (2014). The role of genomic imprinting in biology and disease: An expanding view. *Nature Reviews Genetics, 15*(8), 517–530. https://doi.org/10.1038/nrg3766

Pettersson, E., Lichtenstein, P., Larsson, H., Song, J., Agrawal, A., Borglum, A. D., et al. (2019). Genetic influences on eight psychiatric disorders based on family data of 4 408 646 full and half-siblings, and genetic data of 333 748 cases and controls. *Psychological Medicine, 49*(7), 1166–1173. https://doi.org/10.1017/s0033291718002039

Pike, A., McGuire, S., Hetherington, E. M., Reiss, D., & Plomin, R. (1996). Family environment and adolescent depressive symptoms and antisocial behavior: A multivariate genetic analysis. *Developmental Psychology, 32*(4), 590–603. https://doi.org/10.1037/0012-1649.32.4.590

Pine, D. S. (2006). A primer on brain imaging in developmental psychopathology: What is it good for? *Journal of Child Psychology and Psychiatry, 47*(10), 983–986. https://doi.org/10.1111/j.1469-7610.2006.01686.x

Pingault, J.-B., Allegrini, A. G., Odigie, T., Frach, L., Baldwin, J. R., Rijsdijk, F., & Dudbridge, F. (2022). Research review: How to interpret associations between polygenic scores, environmental risks, and phenotypes. *Journal of Child Psychology and Psychiatry, 63*, 1125–1139. https://doi.org/10.1111/jcpp.13607

Pingault, J. B., O'Reilly, P. F., Schoeler, T., Ploubidis, G. B., Rijsdijk, F., & Dudbridge, F. (2018). Using genetic data to strengthen causal inference in observational research. *Nature Reviews Genetics, 19*(9), 566–580. https://doi.org/10.1038/s41576-018-0020-3

Plomin, R. (2023). Celebrating a century of research in behavioral genetics. *Behavior Genetics, 53*(2), 75–84. https://doi.org/10.1007/s10519-023-10132-3

Plomin, R., & Daniels, D. (1987). Why are children in the same family so different from one another. *Behavioral and Brain Sciences, 10*(1), 1–16. https://doi.org/10.1017/s0140525x00055941

Plomin, R., DeFries, J. C., Knopik, V. S., & Neiderhiser, J. M. (2016). Top 10 replicated findings from behavioral genetics. *Perspectives on Psychological Science, 11*(1), 3–23. https://doi.org/10.1177/1745691615617439

Plomin, R., DeFries, J. C., & Loehlin, J. C. (1977). Genotype-environment interaction and correlation in analysis of human-behavior. *Psychological Bulletin, 84*(2), 309–322. https://doi.org/10.1037/0033-2909.84.2.309

Plomin, R., Haworth, C. M. A., & Davis, O. S. P. (2009). Common disorders are quantitative traits. *Nature Reviews Genetics, 10*(12), 872–878. https://doi.org/10.1038/nrg2670

Plomin, R., & Viding, E. (2022). Commentary: Will genomics revolutionise research on gene-environment interplay? *Journal of Child Psychology and Psychiatry*. https://doi.org/10.1111/jcpp.13687

Plomin, R., & von Stumm, S. (2018). The new genetics of intelligence. *Nature Reviews Genetics, 19*(3), 148–159. https://doi.org/10.1038/nrg.2017.104

Plomin, R., & von Stumm, S. (2022). Polygenic scores: Prediction versus explanation. *Molecular Psychiatry, 27*, 49–52. https://doi.org/10.1038/s41380-021-01348-y

Polderman, T. J. C., Benyamin, B., de Leeuw, C. A., Sullivan, P. F., van Bochoven, A., Visscher, P. M., & Posthuma, D. (2015). Meta-analysis of the heritability of human traits based on fifty years of twin studies. *Nature Genetics, 47*(7), 702-+. https://doi.org/10.1038/ng.3285

Provenzi, L., Brambilla, M., di Minico, G. S., Montirosso, R., & Borgatti, R. (2020). Maternal caregiving and DNA methylation in human infants and children: Systematic review. *Genes Brain and Behavior, 19*(3). https://doi.org/10.1111/gbb.12616

Provenzi, L., Guida, E., & Montirosso, R. (2018). Preterm behavioral epigenetics: A systematic review. *Neuroscience and Biobehavioral Reviews, 84*, 262–271. https://doi.org/10.1016/j.neubiorev.2017.08.020

Pujol, J., Harrison, B. J., Contreras-Rodriguez, O., & Cardoner, N. (2019). The contribution of brain imaging to the understanding of psychopathy. *Psychological Medicine, 49*(1), 20–31. https://doi.org/10.1017/s0033291718002507

Rao, D. C., Morton, N. E., & Yea, S. (1974). Analysis of family resemblance. II. A linear model for familial correlation. *American Journal of Human Genetics, 26*, 331–359.

Reimers, M. A., Craver, C., Dozmorov, M., Bacanu, S. A., & Kendler, K. S. (2019). The coherence problem: Finding meaning in GWAS complexity. *Behavior Genetics, 49*(2), 187–195. https://doi.org/10.1007/s10519-018-9935-x

Rende, R. D., Plomin, R., & Vandenberg, S. G. (1990). Who discovered the twin method? *Behavior Genetics, 20*(2), 277–285. https://doi.org/10.1007/bf01067795

Rietveld, C. A., Esko, T., Davies, G., Pers, T. H., Turley, P., Benyamin, B., et al. (2014). Common genetic variants associated with cognitive performance identified using the proxy-phenotype method. *Proceedings of the National Academy of Sciences of the United States of America, 111*(38), 13790–13794. https://doi.org/10.1073/pnas.1404623111

Rijlaarsdam, J., Barker, E. D., Caserini, C., Koopman-Verhoeff, M. E., Mulder, R. H., Felix, J. F., & Cecil, C. A. M. (2021). Genome-wide DNA methylation patterns associated with general psychopathology in children. *Journal of Psychiatric Research, 140*, 214–220. https://doi.org/10.1016/j.jpsychires.2021.05.029

Risch, N., & Merikangas, K. (1996). The future of genetic studies of complex human diseases. *Science, 273*(5281), 1516–1517. https://doi.org/10.1126/science.273.5281.1516

Robinson, E. B., Koenen, K. C., McCormick, M. C., Munir, K., Hallett, V., Happe, F., et al. (2011). Evidence that autistic traits show the same etiology in the general population and at the quantitative extremes (5%, 2.5%, and 1%). *Archives of General Psychiatry, 68*(11), 1113–1121. https://doi.org/10.1001/archgenpsychiatry.2011.119

Robinson, E. B., St Pourcain, B., Anttila, V., Kosmicki, J. A., Bulik-Sullivan, B., Grove, J., et al. (2016). Genetic risk for autism spectrum disorders and neuropsychiatric variation in the general population. *Nature Genetics, 48*(5), 552-+. https://doi.org/10.1038/ng.3529

Ronald, A. (2020). Editorial: Polygenic scores in child and adolescent psychiatry – Strengths, weaknesses, opportunities and threats. *Journal of Child Psychology and Psychiatry, 61*(5), 519–521. https://doi.org/10.1111/jcpp.13246

Rutter, M. (2007). Gene-environment interdependence. *Developmental Science, 10*(1), 12–18. https://doi.org/10.1111/j.1467-7687.2007.00557.x

Rutter, M. (2010). Child and adolescent psychiatry: Past scientific achievements and challenges for the future. *European Child and Adolescent Psychiatry, 19*(9), 689–703. https://doi.org/10.1007/s00787-010-0111-y

Rutter, M. (2013). Annual research review: Resilience – Clinical implications. *Journal of Child Psychology and Psychiatry, 54*(4), 474–487. https://doi.org/10.1111/j.1469-7610.2012.02615.x

Rutter, M. (2015). Some of the complexities involved in gene-environment interplay. *International Journal of Epidemiology, 44*(4), 1128–1129. https://doi.org/10.1093/ije/dyv054

Rutter, M., Dunn, J., Plomin, R., Simonoff, E., Pickles, A., Maughan, B., et al. (1997). Integrating nature and nurture: Implications of person-environment correlations and interactions for developmental psychopathology. *Development and Psychopathology, 9*(2), 335–364. https://doi.org/10.1017/s0954579497002083

Rutter, M., Moffitt, T. E., & Caspi, A. (2006). Gene-environment interplay and psychopathology: Multiple varieties but real effects. *Journal of Child Psychology and Psychiatry, 47*(3–4), 226–261. https://doi.org/10.1111/j.1469-7610.2005.01557.x

Rutter, M., & Stevenson, J. (2008). Developments in child and adolescent psychiatry over the last 50 years. In M. Rutter, D. Bishop, D. Pine, S. Scott, J. Stevenson, E. Taylor, & A. Thapar (Eds.), *Rutter's child and adolescent psychiatry* (pp. 3–17). Blackwell Publishing.

Saltz, J. B. (2019). Gene-environment correlation in humans: Lessons from psychology for quantitative genetics. *Journal of Heredity, 110*(4), 455–466. https://doi.org/10.1093/jhered/esz027

Saltz, J. B., Bell, A. M., Flint, J., Gomulkiewicz, R., Hughes, K. A., & Keagy, J. (2018). Why does the magnitude of genotype-by-environment interaction vary? *Ecology and Evolution, 8*(12), 6342–6353. https://doi.org/10.1002/ece3.4128

Schork, A. J., Won, H., Appadurai, V., Nudel, R., Gandal, M., Delaneau, O., et al. (2019). A genome-wide association study of shared risk across psychiatric disorders implicates gene regulation during fetal neurodevelopment. *Nature Neuroscience, 22*(3), 353-+. https://doi.org/10.1038/s41593-018-0320-0

Selzam, S., Coleman, J. R. I., Caspi, A., Moffitt, T. E., & Plomin, R. (2018). A polygenic p factor for major psychiatric disorders. Translational Psychiatry, 8. https://doi.org/10.1038/s41398-018-0217-4

Selzam, S., Ritchie, S. J., Pingault, J. B., Reynolds, C. A., O'Reilly, P. F., & Plomin, R. (2019). Comparing within- and between-family polygenic score prediction. *American Journal of Human Genetics, 105*(2), 351–363. https://doi.org/10.1016/j.ajhg.2019.06.006

Shen, H., & Feldman, M. W. (2020). Genetic nurturing, missing heritability, and causal analysis in genetic statistics. *Proceedings of the National Academy of Sciences of the United States of America, 117*(41), 25646–25654. https://doi.org/10.1073/pnas.2015869117

Siemens, H. (1924). *Die Zwillingspathologie*. Spiner-Verlag.

Silberg, J. L., Maes, H., & Eaves, L. J. (2010). Genetic and environmental influences on the transmission of parental depression to children's depression and conduct disturbance: An extended Children of Twins study. *Journal of Child Psychology and Psychiatry, 51*(6), 734–744. https://doi.org/10.1111/j.1469-7610.2010.02205.x

Simcock, G., Elgbeili, G., Laplante, D. P., Kildea, S., Cobham, V., Stapleton, H., et al. (2017). The effects of prenatal maternal stress on early temperament: The 2011 Queensland Flood Study. *Journal of Developmental and Behavioral Pediatrics, 38*(5), 310–321. https://doi.org/10.1097/dbp.0000000000000444

Skuse, D. H., James, R. S., Bishop, D. V. M., Coppin, B., Dalton, P., Aamodt-Leeper, G., et al. (1997). Evidence from Turner's syndrome of an imprinted X-linked locus affecting cognitive function. *Nature, 387*(6634), 705–708. https://doi.org/10.1038/42706

Smeeth, D., Beck, S., Karam, E. G., & Pluess, M. (2021). The role of epigenetics in psychological resilience. *Lancet Psychiatry, 8*(7), 620–629. https://doi.org/10.1016/s2215-0366(20)30515-0

Sonuga-Barke, E. J. S., Oades, R. D., Psychogiou, L., Chen, W., Franke, B., Buitelaar, J., et al. (2009). Dopamine and serotonin transporter genotypes moderate sensitivity to maternal expressed emotion: The case of conduct and emotional problems in attention deficit/hyperactivity disorder. *Journal of Child Psychology and Psychiatry, 50*(9), 1052–1063. https://doi.org/10.1111/j.1469-7610.2009.02095.x

Sullivan, P. F., & Geschwind, D. H. (2019). Defining the genetic, genomic, cellular, and diagnostic architectures of psychiatric disorders. *Cell, 177*(1), 162–183. https://doi.org/10.1016/j.cell.2019.01.015

Sutcubasi, B., Metin, B., Kurban, M. K., Metin, Z. E., Beser, B., & Sonuga-Barke, E. (2020). Resting-state network dysconnectivity in ADHD: A system-neuroscience-based meta-analysis. *World Journal of Biological Psychiatry, 21*(9), 662–672. https://doi.org/10.1080/15622975.2020.1775889

Tanzer, M., Derome, M., Morosan, L., Salaminios, G., & Debbane, M. (2021). Cortical thickness of the insula and prefrontal cortex relates to externalizing behavior: Cross-sectional and prospective findings. *Development and Psychopathology, 33*(4), 1437–1447. https://doi.org/10.1017/s0954579420000619

Taylor, E., Chadwick, O., Heptinstall, E., & Danckaerts, M. (1996). Hyperactivity and conduct problems as risk factors for adolescent development. *Journal of the American Academy of Child and Adolescent Psychiatry, 35*(9), 1213–1226. https://doi.org/10.1097/00004583-199609000-00019

Tearne, J. E., Allen, K. L., Herbison, C. E., Lawrence, D., Whitehouse, A. J. O., Sawyer, M. G., & Robinson, M. (2015). The association between prenatal environment and children's mental health trajectories from 2 to 14 years. *European Child and Adolescent Psychiatry, 24*(9), 1015–1024. https://doi.org/10.1007/s00787-014-0651-7

Teicher, M. H., & Samson, J. A. (2016). Annual research review: Enduring neurobiological effects of childhood abuse and neglect. *Journal of Child Psychology and Psychiatry, 57*(3), 241–266. https://doi.org/10.1111/jcpp.12507

Thompson, P. M., Jahanshad, N., Ching, C. R. K., Salminen, L. E., Thomopoulos, S. I., Bright, J., et al. (2020). ENIGMA and global neuroscience: A decade of large-scale studies of the brain in health and disease across more than 40 countries. *Translational Psychiatry, 10*(1). https://doi.org/10.1038/s41398-020-0705-1

Trzaskowski, M., Dale, P. S., & Plomin, R. (2013). No genetic influence for childhood behavior problems from DNA analysis. *Journal of the American Academy of Child and Adolescent Psychiatry, 52*(10), 1048–1056. https://doi.org/10.1016/j.jaac.2013.07.016

Tucker-Drob, E. M., & Briley, D. A. (2014). Continuity of genetic and environmental influences on cognition across the life span: A meta-analysis of longitudinal twin and adoption studies. *Psychological Bulletin, 140*(4), 949–979. https://doi.org/10.1037/a0035893

Turkheimer, E. (2000). Three laws of behavior genetics and what they mean. *Current Directions in Psychological Science, 9*(5), 160–164. https://doi.org/10.1111/1467-8721.00084

Turkheimer, E. (2016). Weak genetic explanation 20 years later: Reply to Plomin et al. *Perspectives on Psychological Science, 11*(1), 24–28. https://doi.org/10.1177/1745691615617442

Van den Bergh, B. R. H., van den Heuvel, M. I., Lahti, M., Braeken, M., de Rooij, S. R., Entringer, S., et al. (2020). Prenatal developmental origins of behavior and mental health: The influence of maternal stress in pregnancy. *Neuroscience and Biobehavioral Reviews, 117*, 26–64. https://doi.org/10.1016/j.neubiorev.2017.07.003

Visscher, P. M., Hill, W. G., & Wray, N. R. (2008). Heritability in the genomics era – Concepts and misconceptions. *Nature Reviews Genetics, 9*(4), 255–266. https://doi.org/10.1038/nrg2322

Waldman, I. D., Poore, H. E., van Hulle, C., Rathouz, P. J., & Lahey, B. B. (2016). External validity of a hierarchical dimensional model of child and adolescent psychopathology: Tests using confirmatory factor analyses and multivariate behavior genetic analyses. *Journal of Abnormal Psychology, 125*(8), 1053–1066. https://doi.org/10.1037/abn0000183

Watanabe, K., Stringer, S., Frei, O., Mirkov, M. U., de Leeuw, C., Polderman, T. J. C., et al. (2019). A global overview of pleiotropy and genetic architecture in complex traits. *Nature Genetics, 51*(9), 1339-+. https://doi.org/10.1038/s41588-019-0481-0

Wee, C. Y., Tuan, T. A., Broekman, B. F. P., Ong, M. Y., Chong, Y. S., Kwek, K., et al. (2017). Neonatal neural networks predict children behavioral profiles later in life. *Human Brain Mapping, 38*(3), 1362–1373. https://doi.org/10.1002/hbm.23459

Weinberger, D. R., & Radulescu, E. (2016). Finding the elusive psychiatric "Lesion" with 21st-century neuroanatomy: A note of caution. *American Journal of Psychiatry, 173*(1), 27–33. https://doi.org/10.1176/appi.ajp.2015.15060753

Williams, C. M., Peyre, H., Toro, R., Beggiato, A., & Ramus, F. (2020). Adjusting for allometric scaling in ABIDE I challenges subcortical volume differences in autism spectrum disorder. *Human Brain Mapping, 41*(16), 4610–4629. https://doi.org/10.1002/hbm.25145

Wray, N. R., Lee, S. H., Mehta, D., Vinkhuyzen, A. A. E., Dudbridge, F., & Middeldorp, C. M. (2014). Research review: Polygenic methods and their application to psychiatric traits. *Journal of Child Psychology and Psychiatry, 55*(10), 1068–1087. https://doi.org/10.1111/jcpp.12295

Wray, N. R., Lin, T., Austin, J., McGrath, J. J., Hickie, I. B., Murray, G. K., & Visscher, P. M. (2020). From basic science to clinical application of polygenic risk scores A primer. *JAMA Psychiatry*. https://doi.org/10.1001/jamapsychiatry.2020.3049

Wright, S. (1920). The relative importance of heredity and environment in determining the piebald pattern of Guinea-pigs. *Proceedings of the National Academy of Sciences USA, 6*, 320–332. https://doi.org/10.1073/pnas.6.6.320

Wright, S. (1921). Correlation and causation. *Journal of Agricultural Research, 20*, 557–585.
Wright, S. (1948). On the roles of directed and random changes in gene frequency in the genetics of populations. *Evolution; International Journal of Organic Evolution, 2*(4), 279–294. https://doi.org/10.2307/2405519
Yang, J., Zeng, J., Goddard, M. E., Wray, N. R., & Visscher, P. M. (2017). Concepts, estimation and interpretation of SNP-based heritability. *Nature Genetics, 49*(9), 1304–U1243. https://doi.org/10.1038/ng.3941
Yeshurun, S., & Hannan, A. J. (2019). Transgenerational epigenetic influences of paternal environmental exposures on brain function and predisposition to psychiatric disorders. *Molecular Psychiatry, 24*(4), 536–548. https://doi.org/10.1038/s41380-018-0039-z
Yim, G., Roberts, A., Ascherio, A., Wypij, D., Kioumourtzoglou, M.-A., & Weisskopf, M. G. (2022). Smoking during pregnancy and risk of attention-deficit/hyperactivity disorder in the third generation. *Epidemiology, 33*(3), 431–440. https://doi.org/10.1097/ede.0000000000001467
Yoon, S., Munoz, A., Yamrom, B., Lee, Y. H., Andrews, P., Marks, S., et al. (2021). Rates of contributory de novo mutation in high and low-risk autism families. *Communications Biology, 4*(1). https://doi.org/10.1038/s42003-021-02533-z
Young, A. I., Frigge, M. L., Gudbjartsson, D. F., Thorleifsson, G., Bjornsdottir, G., Sulem, P., et al. (2018). Relatedness disequilibrium regression estimates heritability without environmental bias. *Nature Genetics, 50*(9), 1304-+. https://doi.org/10.1038/s41588-018-0178-9
Zavos, H. M. S., Freeman, D., Haworth, C. M. A., McGuire, P., Plomin, R., Cardno, A. G., & Ronald, A. (2014). Consistent etiology of severe, frequent psychotic experiences and milder, less frequent manifestations A twin study of specific psychotic experiences in adolescence. *JAMA Psychiatry, 71*(9), 1049–1057. https://doi.org/10.1001/jamapsychiatry.2014.994
Zhou, K. X., Dempfle, A., Arcos-Burgos, M., Bakker, S. C., Banaschewski, T., Biederman, J., et al. (2008). Meta-analysis of genome-wide linkage scans of attention deficit hyperactivity disorder. *American Journal of Medical Genetics Part B-Neuropsychiatric Genetics, 147B*(8), 1392–1398. https://doi.org/10.1002/ajmg.b.30878
Zhu, J., Lee, K. P., Spencer, T. J., Biederman, J., & Bhide, P. G. (2014). Transgenerational transmission of hyperactivity in a mouse model of ADHD. *Journal of Neuroscience, 34*(8), 2768–2773. https://doi.org/10.1523/jneurosci.4402-13.2014

Chapter 4
Causal Analysis

There are a number of developments in methodology that have moved studies towards providing a clearer understanding of the factors producing individual differences in behaviour. The key distinction being examined in this chapter is that between an association and causation. Most of the studies in developmental psychopathology are observational or correlational – they do not have a manipulation of an independent variable, as is the case in an experiment. But isn't it commonplace to say that correlation is not causation? So how can causality be established from correlational/association data? This possibility is explained by Pearl (2010) as follows:

> A useful demarcation line that makes the distinction between associational and causal concepts crisp and easy to apply can be formulated as follows. An associational concept is any relationship that can be defined in terms of a joint distribution of observed variables, and a causal concept is any relationship that cannot be defined from the distribution alone. (Pearl, 2010, p. 77)

The distinction being made here is between estimates of association that simply describe the extent to which two factors co-occur and causal estimates that are based on additional information about the possible mechanisms giving rise to the association. The case for using methods that can attempt to identify causal influences from observation data in child development studies is clear (Foster, 2010; Miller et al., 2016).

Although establishing causality is a laudable and highly desirable goal, it is necessary to avoid being overconfident about achieving it. Coggon and Martyn (2005) provide a cautionary account of the limitations on establishing causality. There is the complexity that arises from whether a risk is a necessary and/or a sufficient cause. Smoking is a risk factor for lung cancer but is neither necessary nor sufficient for the development of lung cancer. Causes also need to be distinguished from other factors that might be predictive of a disease but are not causes but rather just markers. Coggon and Martyn (2005) give the example of yellow-stained fingers indicating a risk of lung cancer, but this is a marker not a cause – cleaning the fingers will not reduce the risk of developing this disease. Furthermore yellow-stained fingers

J. Stevenson, *Developmental Psychopathology*,
https://doi.org/10.1007/978-3-031-45787-6_4

might also arise from an exposure other than to tobacco smoke, e.g. excessive ingestion of carotenoids, the colouring in carrots. They argue that the fact that risk factors:

> …exist in a continuum in the population suggests that they are determined by the combination of factors, many of which might have only a small individual effect. This multiplicity means that complete understanding of causation is unlikely to be feasible, although it may be possible to identify some factors whose effects are large enough to offer scope for prevention. (Coggon & Martyn, 2005, p. 1436)

This characterisation of measures existing on a continuum and deriving from a multiplicity of factors each producing small effects is completely apposite for conceptualising the causes of variation in behaviour.

4.1 Randomised Controlled Trials

The randomised controlled trial (RCT) is often referred to as the "gold standard" for establishing causal relationships. The key feature of an RCT is that participants are allocated to alternative treatments or a control condition at random. This means that exposure to treatment will be unrelated to any possible confounds (but see discussion below of post-randomisation confounding). The effect of treatment on outcome will therefore be a true test of their causal relationship. Treatment in RCTs is usually an intervention to address a current dysfunction or, in the context of a preventive intervention, a possible adverse future outcome. In these cases the RCT will involve children with a condition or who are at high risk of developing a condition. Here there is every justification to conduct a study to establish the treatment efficacy. There is sometimes a question as to whether those in a control condition are being denied a beneficial treatment. There is a logical issue here in that until the RCT has been conducted, its efficacy is uncertain and the controls are not being denied a treatment of known benefit. Moreover it is often the case that those in the control condition will receive the treatment at the completion of the RCT. Often treatment as usual (TAU) is given to those in the control group. By giving TAU no one is denied access to orthodox treatment during the course of the trial.

It is more challenging to apply RCT methods to risk factors in the general population. Here the question is whether a potential risk factor has an adverse outcome and ethical constraints limit the scope for allocating children to a potential adverse risk factor. There are some contexts where this is possible especially where the effect of exposure is reversible. This is the case with dietary interventions. This will be illustrated by a pair of studies on food additives and hyperactivity.

There has been a long-standing concern that food additives, especially azo dye food colours, may exacerbate hyperactive behaviour in children (Feingold, 1975). Our research group at the University of Southampton conducted RCTs to determine whether artificial food additives had an impact on hyperactivity in young children from the general population.

The first study involved 3-year-old children living on the Isle of Wight (Bateman et al., 2004). The study design was a double-blinded placebo-controlled crossover drink-challenge trial. Double-blinded because the children, their families, and the psychologists assessing behaviour did not know which drink the children were receiving at any given time. Placebo-controlled because the drinks being taken could either contain the food additives or a placebo of fruit juices. The two drinks could not be differentiated on blind testing. The final feature of the design was that it was a crossover trial with the same children receiving the food additive and placebo drinks on subsequent weeks in a randomised sequence. This design provides a tight control on the possible effects of confounds.

There are two prime sources of complexity with a crossover trial. These are order effects and carry-over effects. These were tested for and there was no effect of whether the food additive drink was given first or second in the sequence (order effect). There was a washout period between the weeks with the challenges. In washout weeks the children had no drink challenge. There was no carry-over detected of an effect of the challenge before washout on the behaviour in the week after washout.

There were 277 3-year-old children in the study and their behaviour was monitored by testing in the clinic and with ratings by their parents. For the 4-week duration of the study, parents were asked to make sure that the children's diets did not contain the food additives that were of interest – artificial colouring (azo dyes) and a preservative, sodium benzoate. This means that any systematic changes in the children behaviour could only be attributed to the food challenges we were giving them. It was found that children's hyperactivity was 0.39 units higher in the weeks when they received the food additives challenges than when they received the placebo. Using the standard deviation of the scores in a baseline week before the challenges started (0.76), this difference gives an effect size as a standardised mean difference (SMD) = 0.39/0.76 = 0.51.

We had the opportunity to replicate this study on a second group of 3-year-olds and on a sample of 8-/9-year-olds living in Southampton (McCann et al., 2007). The basic elements of the design of this second study were the same as for Bateman et al. (2004): a randomised, double-blinded, placebo-controlled crossover trial with children from the general population. This second study had an added complexity of testing two different mixes of additives. The results however replicated the effect on 3-year-olds of the mix used in Bateman et al. (2004) and showed significant effect of a new mix on 8-/9-year-olds. McCann et al. (2007) concluded that it:

> provides evidence of deleterious effects of AFCA [artificial food colour and additives] on children's behaviour with data from a whole population sample, using a combination of robust objective measures with strong ecological validity, based partly on observations in the classroom and ratings of behaviour made independently by teachers and by parents in the different context of the home and applying double-blinded challenges with quantities of additives equal to typical dietary intakes. (McCann et al., 2007, p. 1566)

A feature of this RCT was that possible genetic moderators of the impact of food additives were tested. Azo dyes have been shown to provoke urticaria in some individuals, independent of whether or not they are aspirin sensitive, providing clinical evidence that artificial colours may result in histamine release. It was reasoned that histamine release and its effects on the central nervous system (CNS) may play a crucial role in mediating the effects of artificial food colours on attention-deficit hyperactivity disorder (ADHD) symptoms (Miller et al., 2022). For this reason a number of genetic polymorphisms were examined to see if they moderated the impact of food additives (Stevenson et al., 2010). They included genetic polymorphisms of histamine *N*-methyl transferase (*HNMT*) gene. Variants of this gene were found to modify the impact of additives on behaviour in both the 3- and 8-/9-year-olds. Demonstrating an association of the effect of food additives on behaviour with a plausible biological moderator adds supports to the conclusion that a causal relationship has been established. This finding is also an illustration of the principle that differential susceptibility to interventions may be missed if gene-environment interactions are not examined (Bakermans-Kranenburg & van IJzendoorn, 2015).

Of the available research methods appraised by Ohlsson and Kendler (2020) in their review of causal inference methods in psychiatric research, the RCT has the strongest case for establishing causality. It is the research design closest to the experiment in laboratory-based science. However this closeness to the laboratory experiment creates one of the main difficulties with the RCT. Experimental control increases the internal validity of the RCT, i.e. it provides a good test of whether the treatment variable influences the outcome in the sample studied. However this tight experimental control may detract from external validity, i.e. do the results generalise to other samples or to the population at large? (Cartwright, 2007).

Therefore there are limitations that need to be considered when considering the implications of findings from RCTs (Deaton & Cartwright, 2018).

> RCTs can play a role in building scientific knowledge and useful predictions but they can only do so as part of a cumulative program, combining with other methods, including conceptual and theoretical development, to discover not 'what works', but 'why things work'. (Deaton & Cartwright, 2018 p. 2)

So an RCT can, par excellence, identify whether a treatment can be effective but cannot by itself identify the likely mechanisms by which this is achieved. Moreover there may be features of an RCT that detract from the accuracy of its estimate of effectiveness.

> The chief advantage of the RCT is that it can, if well-conducted, give an unbiased estimate of an ATE [average treatment effect] in a study (trial) sample and thus provide evidence that the treatment caused the outcome in some individuals in that sample. Note that 'well-conducted' rules out all of the things that almost always occur in practice, including attrition, intentional lack of blinding or unintentional unblinding, and other post-randomization confounding and selection biases. (Deaton & Cartwright, 2018, p. 17)

These post-randomisation biases may arise, for example, from differential loss from the groups due to factors, such as subject demoralisation, in untreated groups. There are a number of ways of attempting to take such post-randomisation factors into account (Hernán et al., 2013). There is in addition the pervasive problem of adequate power. It is well recognised that studies with inadequate sample size and consequent low power are more likely to fail to identify a true effect, i.e. they produce false negatives. As Button et al. (2013) have shown, there are additional threats to the reliability of studies that arise from low power. The supposedly significant effects from studies with low power are often not true effects. When a small sample study does detect a true effect as significant, the estimate of the magnitude of this effect is likely to be exaggerated. These problems of small sample size are compounded by other factors such as bias (Ioannidis, 2005). Here bias is defined as "the combination of various design, data, analysis, and presentation factors that tend to produce [positive] research findings when they should not be produced".

These difficulties do not detract from the principle that the RCT represents the strongest test of a putative causal influence on behaviour. However there are major restrictions on the range of causal factors that can be tested in this way. Random allocation to risk exposure is simply not feasible and may be ethically unacceptable.

4.2 Moving from Associations to Causes

Ohlsson and Kendler (2020) discuss a number of ways methods can be applied to test for possible causal relationships. These are broadly described as RCTs, natural experiments, and statistical models. Why is establishing causality so important? They say:

> The observation of an association between a putative risk factor and a disorder provides a descriptive account of the world but gives no insights into the origins of that association or ways it might be altered. (Ohlsson & Kendler, 2020, p. 637)

It is the latter that is crucial if effective preventative interventions are to be developed. Efforts to influence a putative risk factor that is not causally related to an outcome will be of no consequence. Bzdok, Varoquaux, and Steyerberg (2021) put the case more strongly that "association is not prediction" is as important as the maxim that "correlation is not causation". The point being made here is that an association that holds for a difference between groups may not be accurate when a prediction based on this association is being made for an individual. Bzdok and Meyer-Lindednberg (2018) show how the methods in machine learning (see Sect. 2.8) can be used to enhance prediction in the individual case.

An example of the way an association at the group level does poorly as a predictor for the individual is the study by Baldwin et al. (2021). Adverse childhood experiences (ACEs) (see Sect. 7.4) were measured up to the age of 12 years in two large samples. These were physical abuse, sexual abuse, emotional abuse and neglect, physical neglect, domestic violence, parental antisocial behaviour, family history of substance abuse, family history of mental health problems, and parental separation or divorce. The outcomes were measures of physical and mental health in adulthood. Although at the level of the group higher ACE scores were associated with poorer health, when applied to individuals, the ACE scores were only marginally better than chance prediction. This was shown by area under the curve (AUC) values less than 0.60 – only marginally above the chance values of 0.50 (see Sect. 2.8 for an explanation of AUC).

When randomisation to a putative risk factor is not possible for ethical or real-world restrictions, natural experiments may provide an alternative route to testing causality (Thapar & Rutter, 2019; Wilson & Rhee, 2022). The possibility for natural experiments arises when circumstances lead to the opportunity to separate the effects of a putative cause from possible confounds. Rutter (2007) identifies 15 different types of natural experiment and appraises the strength and weakness of each. These natural experiments are usually highly reliant on genetically sensitive designs (see also Briley et al., 2018; Pingault et al., 2018; Sellers et al., 2022).

An example discussed by Rutter (2007) is that of the Children-of-Twins (COT) design (McAdams et al., 2014) (see Sect. 3.1). Here the offspring of parents who are either MZ or DZ twins are studied. The basis for this design is that since MZ twins are genetically identical and the child of one twin will be genetically related to their uncle or aunt to the same degree as to their own parent. That is, they will share an average of 50% of their genes. At the simplest level, an analysis can be made within the families of MZ twins. For a given characteristic (e.g. prosociality), if the correlation between a child and their parent is greater than the correlation between the child and their aunt/uncle, then there is evidence of an environmental effect, as the genetic contribution to these correlations is the same. McAdams et al. (2014) provide an extensive account of the ways of date from such families can be exploited to gain insights into the role and interplay between genetic and environmental influences on development.

Lynch et al. (2006) provided an example of a COT study. Their aim was to determine the causal relationship between harsh parenting and adverse outcome in children. The approach was based on the notion that if one member of an identical twin pair as a parent uses harsh physical punishment and the other parent does not, differences in the outcomes for their children can provide a test of a possible causal relationship. In such a case, most genetic and shared environmental confounding variables are controlled by definition. They found that restrained corporal punishment (defined as slapping or spanking) has only a small association with negative outcomes for children. By contrast harsh physical punishment did have significant associations with behavioural and emotional outcomes in the offspring. The tight control of potential confounds in this study strongly suggests that harsh physical punishment is causally related to adverse outcome in the child.

Other possibilities of using data from the study of twins to address the issue of causality have been presented by McAdams et al. (2021). These methods include multivariate structural equation models, co-twin control methods, direction of causation models (cross-sectional and longitudinal), and extended family designs used to assess intergenerational associations. D'Onofrio, Lahey, Turkheimer, and Lichtenstein (2013) provide a detailed breakdown of the advances and limitations of various family-based quasi-experimental natural experiments for examining genetic and environmental risks.

An example of using a family-based study was provided by Burt, Clark, and Neiderhiser (2022). Step-parents, especially fathers, are commonly found in the families of adolescents in the USA. These step-parents are not genetically related to the child but could transmit the risk for psychopathology via an environmental exposure. Burt et al. (2022) showed that paternal depression was associated with a range of problems in their adolescent stepchildren, including depression, regardless of whether or not fathers and their children were genetically related, i.e. the association held in families where the father was the biological parent and where he was a step-parent. This suggests an environmental risk that was found to be transmitted via father-child conflict.

There are a number of historically important definitive publications concerning the possibility demonstrating causal relationships in non-experimental studies, i.e. those where random allocation to risk is not possible. In epidemiology, Susser (1973) provided a landmark framework to approach this question using data from observational studies. Previously Hill (1965) had provided a set of nine "viewpoints" on what is needed to identify causality in relationships. These are #1. Strength of the association; #2. Consistency of the association; #3. Specificity of the association; #4. Temporality of the association; #5. Biological gradient, e.g. dose-response relationship; #6. Biological plausibility; #7. Coherence with other evidence; #8. Experiment; and #9. Analogy of other causal relationships. He suggests that #8 Experiment gives "the strongest support for the causation hypothesis". However he concludes that "None of my nine viewpoints can bring indisputable evidence for or against the cause-and-effect hypothesis and none can be required as a sine qua non".

Hill (1965) does not provide a detailed guide of the methodology to be used to applied tests for the application of the nine viewpoints [see Rothman and Greenland (2005) for a critique of Hill]. Here just three of the Hill viewpoints will be discussed.

Establishing causality requires a three-step process. The *first step* is to establish an association or correlation between the two variables. This of course is not straightforward. How large does an association have to be to indicate a possible causal relationship or does a correlation just have to be significantly different from zero (Hill's #1)? The *second step* is to examine the temporal precedence (Hill's #4). This is based on the assumption that a cause precedes an event and a consequence follows it in time. This is a necessary but not sufficient condition for causality to be present (Rothman & Greenland, 2005). This is where experimental studies (Hill's #8) have a crucial advantage over observational studies in that the timing of exposure to a putative cause can be controlled. In longitudinal studies, although exposure may not be under experimental control, the measurement of timing of events can be used to establish temporal precedence. However unlike experimental studies, where there is random allocation to exposure, non-experimental longitudinal designs cannot rule out the influence of an uncontrolled third variable. This leads to the need to address the *third step*, i.e. to establish that a relationship is non-spurious. That is that the relationship between two variables is not produced by the effect on each of third variable. This is the problem of confounds – an issue not discussed specifically by Hill (1965). Here things get very complicated (Davey Smith, 2019; Schwartz et al., 1999) (see Sect. 4.4 below).

4.3 Cross-Lagged Models

One of the most frequently used approaches to disentangling the direction of effects between measures is the use of longitudinal data (Collins, 2006). This approach is premised on the notion that cause must precede effect, and therefore in a longitudinal study, an early measurement is a candidate to be cause of later measurement but not vice versa. In making this assumption, it is important to take into account the time frame over which the causal effect is thought to take place (Gollob & Reichardt, 1987). There are three features that need to be considered. First, causes may take time to exert their effects. Has enough time elapsed for the effect to be apparent? Second, a variable can have an effect on itself. These autoregressive effects need to be estimated and taken into account in the analysis. Third, the size of an effect depends on the time interval. The time-lapse interval needs to be carefully considered when comparing effect sizes from different studies.

A simple two time-point measurement is represented in Fig. 4.1. The logic underlying the analysis of such a model is that the cross-lagged association between Time 1 and Time 2 is compared. If the relationship between *A*1 and *B*2 ("*s*") is significant and that between *B*1 and *A*2 ("*r*") is not significantly greater than zero, this indicates that *A* is causally related to *B* rather than vice versa. In the case where both cross-lagged relationships are significant, then the relative magnitude of paths "*s*" and "*r*" is estimated to judge which effect is greater.

The model in Fig. 4.1 also included the relationships between a measure and itself at an earlier time point, i.e. "*p*" and "*q*". These are autoregressive effects and reflect the extent to which a child with a high value on *A* at Time 1 is likely to have a higher value on *A* at Time 2 than other children. The cross-lagged path, e.g. "*s*", therefore represents the extent which the child's relative position on measure *B* at Time 2 is higher that would be expected from continuities since Time 1 alone, i.e. how much has *A* changed the child's relative position on *B*?

There are some other important features of Fig. 4.1. The correlation between the measures at Time 1 "*t*" needs to be included, although the direction of the causal

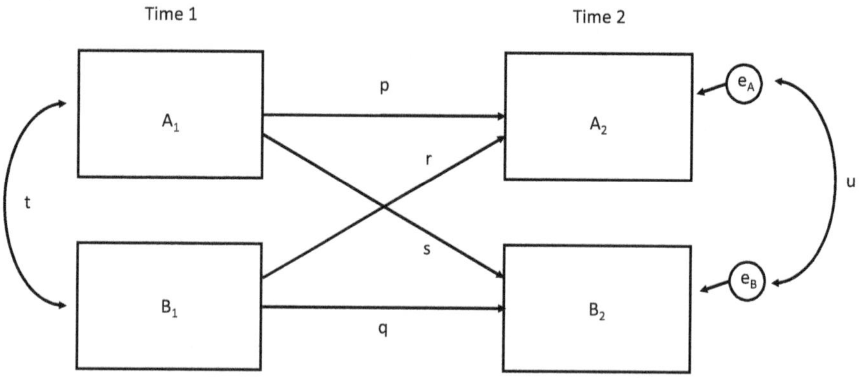

Fig. 4.1 Cross-lagged model

relationship between the Time 1 measures is not analysed. As was seen in Sect. 2.4 when a variable is dependent or being predicted, there will be part of the variance that remains unexplained. In Fig. 4.1 this error variance is indicated by the unmeasured latent variables "e_A" and "e_B". These error terms may themselves be correlated as indicated by the curved path "u".

The analysis and interpretation of cross-lagged path models was initially based on the comparison correlation coefficients (Kenny & Harackiewicz, 1979). However it came to be recognised that such approaches based on correlations may provide biased estimates (Rogosa, 1980). Latent variable models of longitudinal data were the preferred option as these can take into account time lags between causal effects, autoregressive effects, and the effects measurement error (Cole & Preacher, 2014). For an introduction to these cross-lagged panel models (CLPM), see Farrell (1994).

The results of such a cross-lagged analysis using latent variables are shown in Fig. 4.2. These data are from a longitudinal study of children with permanent childhood hearing loss (PCHL) (Stevenson et al., 2018). It had been shown in a meta-analysis that such children were vulnerable to the development of emotional and behavioural difficulties (EBD) (Stevenson et al., 2015). It was of concern to know whether the language comprehension difficulties experienced by these children (Pimperton et al., 2017) contributed to the development of EBD. Language comprehension was assessed at ages 8 and 16 years on a number of measures, and EBD was also assessed on multiple measures. Confirmatory factor analysis (see Sect. 2.4) was used to identify latent variables for language comprehension and for EBD at each age. Note that the measured variables are not presented in Fig. 4.2 – just the latent variables. The results as presented in Fig. 4.2 show the autoregressive coefficients for EBD as rated by teachers (0.50) and for language comprehension (0.87). There was little correlation between the unexplained variance in the latent variables (−0.09) at age 16 years. The correlation between the latent variables at age 8 years was −0.26, i.e. the less good the language comprehension, the greater the level of

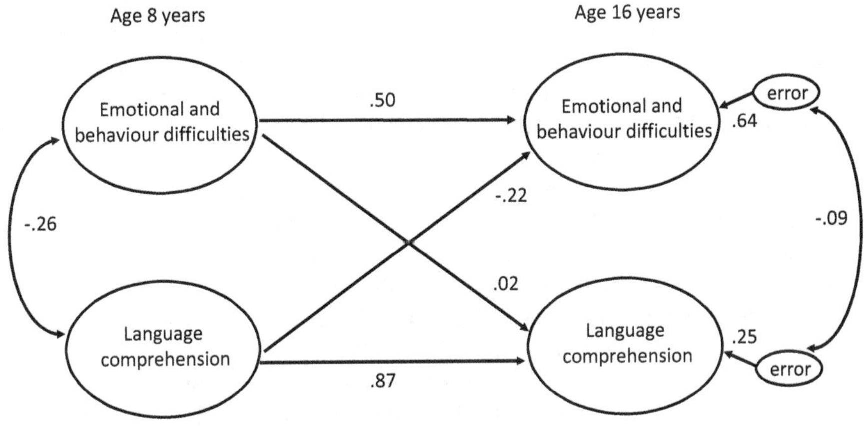

Fig. 4.2 Cross-lagged panel model (CLPM). (Adapted with the permission of John Wiley & Sons from Fig. 1 Stevenson et al. (2018); permission conveyed through Copyright Clearance Center, Inc.)

EBD. The key parameters in the analysis are the cross-lagged coefficients. These show that low language comprehension at age 8 years was associated with higher EBD scores at age 16 years $\beta = -0.22$ ($CI_{.95}$ –0.51 to −0.05). This effect was over and above the continuity in EBD scores between these two ages. The association between EBD at age 8 years and language comprehension at age 16 years was not significantly different from zero $\beta = 0.02$ ($CI_{.95}$ –0.15 to 0.18). These results suggest that language comprehension may influence the development of EBD in children with PCHL during their early teenage years.

When individuals are studied repeatedly over time, the longitudinal data can provide information on both within-person and between-person processes. When a child experiences discord between parents, this may lead to internalising problems in that child (a within-person effect). Children that experience more parental discord than other children may develop more internalising problems than other children (a between-person effect). Curran and Bauer (2011) provided the following example from medicine to illustrate the importance of this distinction:

> Empirical evidence has shown that an individual is more likely to experience a heart attack while exercising (i.e., the within-person effect), but at the same time people who exercise more tend to have a lower risk of heart attack (i.e., the between-person effect) (e.g., Curfman, 1993; Mittleman et al., 1993). Both the within person and between-person findings are valid, and each has direct public health relevance. However, generalizing the between-person effect to the individual would be an error of inference (e.g., the more you exercise the more likely you are to suffer a heart attack). (Curran & Bauer, 2011, p. 586)

It has come to be recognised that a cross-lagged analysis such as that shown in Fig. 4.1 is only able to identify between-person effects (Berry & Willoughby, 2017). A number of methods have been developed to allow the disaggregation of within- and between-person effects. These include autoregressive latent trajectory (ALT) models and latent curve models with structured residual (LCM-SR) (Curran et al., 2014), latent change models (Kievit et al., 2018), and the random intercepts cross-lagged panel model (RI-CLPM). These models and their associated analyses are complex and appraising studies that use them is challenging. However the strengths and weaknesses of the alternative models of cross-lagged data have been tested by Orth, Clark, Donnellan, and Robins (2021). They suggest that just two models provide optimal solutions – the CLPM when the interest is on between-person effects and the RI-CLPM when the focus is on within-person effects. The analysis presented in Fig. 4.2 is an example of CLPM.

An example of a study using the RI-CLPM approach is that of Halse, Steinsbekk, Hammar, and Wichstrøm (2022). They were able to show that in a sample of children studied from the age of 6 to 14 years, there were significant reciprocal causal relationships between executive function abilities and a range of psychiatric disorders including depression, anxiety, ADHD, and conduct disorder. By using the RI-CLPM approach, they could analyse the overtime relationships in the changes in the score of individual children on measures of psychiatric disorder symptoms were predicted by changes in executive function scores. Simultaneously the effects in the opposite direction could also be estimated, i.e. effects of changes in symptoms of disorders on changes in executive function scores. A feature of the RI-CLPM approach is that by using the child as their own control, there are automatic adjustments for time-invariant confounds both observed, e.g. gender and race, and unobserved. The results of the Halse et al. (2022) study were consistent with effects in both directions whereby symptoms of psychiatric disorders can have a negative impact on executive function performance and vice versa.

4.4 Dealing with Confounds

An illustration of the importance of dealing appropriately with confounders is shown by studies on the possibility that epidural anaesthesia might increase the risk of autism spectrum disorder (ASD). Qiu et al. (2020) examined the association between labour epidural analgesic (LEA) and ASD in a large cohort of 147,895 children. The rate of ASD in the LEA group was 1.9% and 1.3% in the non-LEA group. This gives a hazard ratio of 1.9/1.3 = 1.46. The authors controlled for the effects a number of known potential confounders, i.e. factor that might be related to LEA and that might themselves influence the risk of ASD. The confounders were:

> birth year, medical center, maternal age at delivery, parity, race/ethnicity, educational level, household income, history of comorbidity, diabetes during pregnancy, smoking during pregnancy, preeclampsia or eclampsia, prepregnancy body mass index, gestational weight gain, gestational age at delivery, and birth weight. (Qiu et al., 2020, p. E1)

Once these factors were adjusted, the hazard ratio of ASD in LEA vs non-LEA was reduced to 1.37 ($CI_{.95}$ 1.23–1.53). A control for the effects of unmeasured confounders was applied – the *E*-value (Haneuse et al., 2019) (see Sect. 4.11). They estimated the *E*-value for the HR of 1.37 to have a lower confidence of 1.76. This means that a potential confounder would have to be associated both with LEA and with ASD and need to increase the risk of ASD by a minimum of 1.76 to account for the observed HR. If the Qiu et al. (2020) finding holds, the demonstration of a causal link between LEA and ASD might have a major influence on obstetric practice and mothers' choice in managing labour. This could potentially be a repeat of the kind of controversy triggered by the paper by Wakefield et al. (1998) about the impact of measles-mumps-rubella vaccine on ASD. Here a "finding" of causal link was subsequently retracted but only after a substantially detrimental effect on rate of take-up of the vaccine. Do the Qiu et al. (2020) results stand up to scrutiny?

A subsequent study on LEA and ASD with a similar design by Wall-Wieler, Bateman, Hanlon-Dearman, Roos, and Butwick (2021) did not find a significantly increased risk once potential confounders were controlled HR = 1.08 ($CI_{.95}$ 0.97–1.20). One explanation for the difference in findings was that additional confounders were controlled in the second study, namely, induction of labour, labour dystocia (slow or protracted labour), and foetal distress. An important separate component of this second study was the use of LEA and non-LEA siblings to provide within family controls. This comparison also produced a non-significant result HR = 0.97 ($CI_{.95}$ 0.78–1.22).

In a stringent commentary on the Qiu et al. (2020) study, Carrier, Lavoie, and Zaphiratos (2021) suggest that although important confounders were controlled, residual and uncontrolled founders may have produce biased estimates that "cannot suggest causation".

> Adjusting for confounders is challenging, yet crucial to draw meaningful conclusions from retrospective studies. Otherwise, spurious correlations, thought to be causal, may lead to inappropriate health interventions, patient anxiety, or even costly interventions that do not benefit patients or healthcare providers. (Carrier et al., 2021, p. 279)

In an appraisal of the seemingly inconsistency from these two studies, Hanley, Ip, and Oberlander (2021) conclude that:

> women who choose to use LEA for pain relief during labour and delivery differ from women who choose to forego its use in ways that either may be factors in the development of ASD (e.g. genetics) or in ways that affect whether a child would be assessed and/or diagnosed for ASD (e.g. access to and feelings of trust in the medical system). We expect that these biological and contextual factors are both are at play. (Hanley et al., 2021, p. E1)

The key issue here is whether there are uncontrolled confounders that could produce an HR as large as 1.76 in the rate of ASD. In their commentary on the Qiu et al. (2020) study, Kern-Goldberger, Burris, and Levine (2021) identify a number of plausible candidates – namely:

> maternal and paternal history of psychiatric disorders, including anxiety and depression, were not included but have been linked to both epidurals as well as ASD. Furthermore, there are social and cultural differences between women who do and do not receive an epidural. Many of these differences also result in disparities with respect to timely evaluation and diagnosis of ASD, leading to ascertainment bias in the ASD outcome. (Kern-Goldberger et al., 2021, p. 537)

Fortunately the issue concerning LEA and ASD has now been resolved. Hegvik et al. (2022) conducted a study of nearly 4.5 million participants from Finland, Norway, and Sweden up to the age of 13 to 17 years. A key feature of the study was the possibility of using data on siblings to control for unmeasured within family confounds. They found that the putative effects of LEA were absent when this sibling's control data was taken into account.

The public health implications for both maternal and child health were so serious that the question of the link between LEA and ASD suggested by Qiu et al. (2020) needed to be addressed urgently by replications in other samples and with data sets able to control for wider set of possible confounds. Fortunately the increasing availability of well-characterised large population samples allowed these additional studies to be undertaken rapidly.

The conclusion reached by Hegvik et al. (2022) were:

> In the largest study of its kind, using total population data derived from three different countries, we did not find support for the hypothesis that exposure to labour epidural analgesia causes an increased risk of either offspring ASD or ADHD. In contrast to previous replication efforts, the current study was able to explicitly account for shared familial risks whilst being sufficiently large to estimate the associations with a high degree of precision. As the decision to use epidural analgesia in labor is unlikely to cause offspring neurodevelopmental disorders, there is no need to revise current clinical guidelines. (Hegvik et al., 2022, p. 5)

There are parallels here with studies on the possibility that caesarean delivery is associated with increased risk of neurodevelopmental disorders. Two systematic reviews and meta-analyses of this issue both indicated a possible increased risk of ASD. Zhang et al. (2019) reported an odds ratio (OR) = 1.33 ($CI_{.95}$ 1.25–1.41) and Curran et al. (2015) an OR = 1.23 ($CI_{.95}$ 1.07–1.40). In this case, OR is the ratio of likelihood that child will be ASD having had a caesarean delivery to the likelihood of being ASD having had a vaginal delivery. Both these systematic reviews concluded that the effects of residual confounding had not been controlled. This possibility was tested in a study of 1,179,341 term-birth singletons from a Swedish birth register (Zhang et al., 2021). They found that any supposed increased risk of ASD was explained by unmeasured familial confounding.

The issues concerning the interpretation and reporting of non-experimental studies raised by these studies on factors related to birth and the risk of neurodevelopmental conditions are discussed in a report that should be required reading for everyone conducting research. This is a report prepared by the Academy of Medical Sciences (2007) based on the findings of a working group chaired by Mike Rutter. The emphasis in the report is on how best to interpret non-experimental studies and to understand not only their limitations but also strengths, in indicating the possible role of environmental factors as causes of disease.

Directed Acyclic Graphs (DAGs) To address the question of confounders graphical tools for making explicit the relationships between variables have been developed (Bollen & Pearl, 2013; Chen & Pearl, 2015). These path diagrams are termed directed acyclic graphs (DAG) to which sets of rules for determining the presence of causal relationship can be applied (Pearl & Mackenzie, 2018). A graph is *directed* if all the paths imply a direction of causality. The graph is *acyclic* if it does not contain any closed feedback loops. The application of DAGs can be particularly helpful in understanding the effects of confounders (Greenland et al., 1999).

Rohrer (2018) provided a helpful introductory overview of the reasons for undertaking causal analyses based on DAGs. She also describes the way DAGs can be interpreted. Although these DAGs look like the model diagrams for structural equation models, they simply present the logical relationships between the variables being considered. There are various ways these variables can be investigated (by research design or by analysis), and their interpretation is not dependent on features such linear relationships or specific levels of measurement. The paths in a DAG are of three basic types: a causal chain (Fig. 4.3a), a fork (Fig. 4.3b), and an inverted fork (Fig. 4.3c). These can be added together to produce a DAG such as Fig. 4.3d. In Fig. 4.3d the causal effect of interest is between the independent variable (*D*) and dependent variable (*E*). However a simple correlational measure of the association between *D* and *E* will include a number of additional non-causal effects produced by confounders. The key to dealing with confounders is to eliminate "back-door paths". These non-causal connections are listed in Fig. 4.3d and only once these are controlled can the causal effect of *D* on *E* be estimated.

The key to conducting a causal analysis is to have a clear theory about the pattern of causal relationships between relevant measures and to make these explicit in a

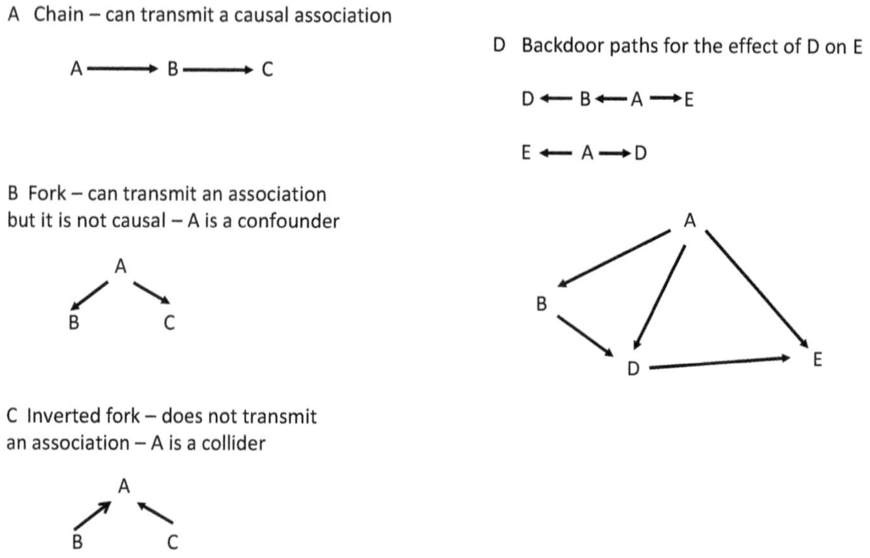

Fig. 4.3 DAG paths

DAG. There then needs to be a careful selection of which potential non-causal paths to control. This is illustrated in Fig. 4.4. In this example the causal relationship of interest is that between "conduct problems" and "marital discord". In Fig. 4.4a the association between them can be described by a correlation, but this does not establish causality, although such a correlation is a necessary condition for there to be a causal relationship. One valuable feature of many studies on child behaviour is that they have a longitudinal element. This provides a means to uncover the direction of a causal relationship in that the "values of a variable are caused only by values of prior variables" (Gollob & Reichardt, 1987). However simply having access to measures in a time series does not by itself lead to the demonstration of causal relationships (Hamaker et al., 2020). The longitudinal path from "marital discord at 7" and "conduct problems at 11" (Fig. 4.4b) may arise from the influence of a confounder. This is shown in Fig. 4.4c where "disruptive behaviour at 3" has detrimental effects on the relationship between the parents, as shown by "marital discord at 7", and both in turn influence "conduct problems at 11". To establish the "marital discord at 7" to "conduct problems at 11" relationship as causal requires the control of the effects of disruptive behaviour at 3 – but that may not be sufficient. As shown in Fig. 4.4d, there may be a third factor that influences all these measures of interest. "Poor housing conditions" may have an adverse effect on child behaviour and the marital relationship. This increases a number of back-door paths whose effects need to be controlled. The way these confounds are controlled may vary. The common effect of "disruptive behaviour at 3" may be best controlled statistically by treating it as a covariate. The effects of "poor housing" might be most appropriately addressed by dividing the sample into those in poor housing and those with

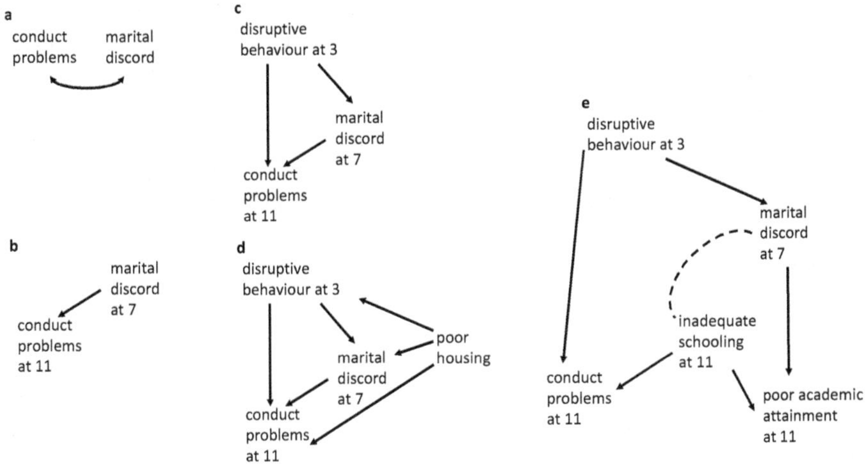

Fig. 4.4 Testing a causal model of the effect of marital discord on conduct problems

adequate housing and examining whether the "marital discord at 7" to "conduct disorder at 11" effect is maintained for both groups.

An illustration of why such controls need to be carefully planned is shown in Fig. 4.4e. If an approach is adopted where any associated third variable is controlled, there can be biasing consequences. A collider is a variable that is causally influenced by the variables of interest. In this case both "inadequate schooling at 11" and "marital discord at 7" can lead to poor "academic attainment at 11". "Poor academic attainment at 11" acts as a "collider", which is an example of an inverse fork (Fig. 4.3d). A control applied to a collider can result in the inadvertent opening of a spurious non-causal relationship in the DAG and consequently bias the estimate of causal effects on "conduct problems at 11". In Fig. 4.4e if "poor academic attainment at 11" was controlled by only including children that are doing well at school, this would open up a non-causal path between "marital discord at 7" and "conduct problems at 11" via "inadequate schooling at 11". This is represented by the non-causal dotted line between "inadequate schooling at 11" and "marital discord at 7". This would alter the estimate of the relationship between "conduct problems at 11" and "marital discord at 7". For a more extensive explanation of the problems raised by collider bias, see Rohrer (2018) and Pearl and Macknezie (2018). A specific form of collider bias can arise from sample selection or as a result of attrition. These can create specious relationships between measures (Munafò et al., 2018). Kline (2016) provides a detailed introduction to DAGs and their analysis using structural causal models.

A further illustration of the need to control for confounders is provided by Jaffee, Strait, and Odgers (2012). They addressed the question of how to identify risk factors that might be causally related to antisocial behaviour. The effects reported from observational studies were typically greater than those from studies that attempted to use natural experiments or quasi-experimental approaches. This suggests that a number of alternative processes rather than direct social causation might be at play. The first of these are genetic confounds where the relationship between a parental characteristic and the child reflects shared genetic influences rather than a socially transmitted effect. The second is reverse causation where the child's behaviour may lead to the risk factor rather than the other way round. The third is social selection where a child with a tendency of antisocial behaviour may select risk experiences, e.g. spending time with delinquent peers. The fourth is misidentification of risk factors where a supposed risk factor itself is not responsible for an effect on antisocial behaviour but is correlated with another factor that does increase risk.

Jaffee et al. (2012) found that when designs were adopted that controlled for these non-causal explanations, some of the putative causal effects disappeared, e.g. mothers smoking during pregnancy and parent alcohol use. For the majority of the putative social risk factors, including maltreatment, harsh and coercive discipline, divorce, maternal depression, parental antisocial behaviour, adolescent motherhood, peer deviance, and poverty, there was some evidence of social causation. However there is also some evidence for effects from familial confounding, reverse causation, and social selection.

4.5 Instrumental Variables

In addition to RCTs, other methods to test possible causality discussed by Ohlsson and Kendler (2020) include the use of instrumental variables, regression discontinuity and co-relative designs, and a range of statistical methods. Some of these methods will be described in turn starting with the instrumental variable approach (Hernán & Robins, 2006). The logic of this analysis is that an instrumental variable can be used to control for confounds. This is illustrated in Fig. 4.5 based on findings in Mojtabai and Crum (2013). What is of interest is the size of the causal effect of a risk factor (e.g. regular cigarette smoking) on a dependent variable (e.g. new-onset mood and anxiety disorders). This is path "b" in the diagram. The problem is that in a non-experimental study, there are confounds (observed and unobserved) that might be shared between the risk factor and the outcome. The analysis is based on a number of assumptions that allow this problem to be overcome.

The first assumption is that the instrumental variable is allocated "as-if" at random. It will therefore have zero correlation with potential confounds. In the Mojtabai and Crum (2013) example, the variation between American states in the tax on cigarettes should not be related to any other characteristics of the sample. The second assumption is that the instrumental variable is causally related to the risk factor (path "*a*"). In this case higher costs resulting from higher state taxes are related to lower rates of regular smoking. The third assumption is that the instrumental variable is not directly causally related to the outcome. Any correlation between these cigarette taxes and mood/anxiety disorders is mediated via the independent variable – regular cigarette smoking (i.e. via *a.b*) – and not by a direct influence. In this way the causal relationship between the risk factor and the outcome can be derived

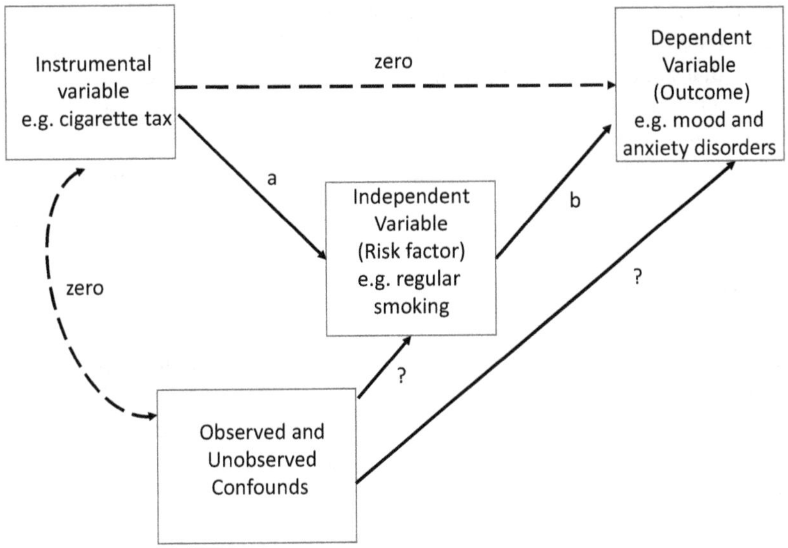

Fig. 4.5 Instrumental variable analysis model illustrated by variables used by Mojtabai and Crum (2013)

from the difference in the overall relationship between the instrumental variable and the outcome (*a.b*) and the relationship between the instrumental variable and the independent variable (*a*). Mojtabai and Crum (2013) were able to show that regular smoking was causally related to the recent onset mood and anxiety disorders and moreover that price increase is a potent influence on regular smoking and a possible route to improving mental health too.

Kendler et al. (2018) used this instrumental variable approach to identify the potential causal association between academic achievement at age 16 years and risk for drug abuse. The instrumental variable was month of birth. Within a year group academic achievement was consistently higher in the older than in the younger children. Importantly, as required by the logic of the instrumental analysis, month of birth was not associated with drug abuse risk when controlling for academic achievement. They showed that low academic achievement was related to drug abuse risk when the effects of month of birth were controlled. This suggests that academic achievement is potentially a causal factor for drug abuse risk.

In another example an instrumental variable approach was used to examine how preschool centre care quality causally impacts children's academic school readiness (Auger et al., 2014). This is a question of much interest to the field and one with important policy implications. Here the instrumental variable approach was applied to data from a controlled trial but where the quality of care itself was not under control by randomisation. They found that the quality of preschool care received by children has significant but only modest effects on children's academic school readiness (SMD = 0.03–0.14).

Instrumental variable analyses have a long history of being used in econometric studies. In studies of child behaviour, it is often challenging to identify available measures that could act as instrumental variables, since these need to be related to risk, are distributed as-if at random in the population, and are not directly causally related to outcome. However one variant of instrumental variable analysis is becoming more widely applied to child behaviour. This is Mendelian randomisation (MR).

4.6 Mendelian Randomisation

The key feature of MR is that it uses genetic variation that is randomly distributed in the population as an instrumental variable. The second of Mendel's laws of inheritance states that the inheritance of one trait is independent of (i.e. randomized with respect to) the inheritance of other traits. This holds as long the genes involved are on separate chromosomes. Lawlor, Harbord, Sterne, Timpson, and Davey Smith (2008) define MR as:

> a study that uses genetic variation that serves as a robust proxy for an environmentally modifiable exposure in order to make causal inferences about the outcomes of the modifiable exposure. (Lawlor et al., 2008, p. 1137)

In terms of Fig. 4.5, this genetic variation is an instrumental variable and exposure is the risk factor. Mendel's second law suggests that this genetic variation will be uncorrelated with potential confounds. However to act as an instrumental variable, two other conditions need to hold. The genetic variation needs to be related to the risk factor and must not be causally related to the outcome except via the risk factor.

Some of these natural experiments, such as Mendelian randomisation (MR), require very large sample sizes. With data on 3544 children from the Avon Longitudinal Study of Parents and Children (ALSPAC) study, MR has been employed to test for a causal relationship between mothers drinking alcohol during pregnancy and persistent conduct problems in the children (Murray et al., 2016). Even when adequate sample sizes are available, Mendelian randomisation may be prone to serious bias that arises from horizontal pleiotropy in the estimates of the size of causal effects (Verbanck et al., 2018). Horizontal pleiotropy arises in MR when the genetic variant selected as the instrumental variable is related to the outcome by an indirect route. This can arise, for example, from the genetic correlations that are repeatedly being found in GWAS (see Sect. 3.2) studies on behaviour.

There are a number of examples of the application of MR to examine causal factors on aspects of child development. Caramaschi et al. (2018) used MR to test whether maternal smoking during pregnancy increased the risk of autism in the child; they found no evidence that it did. In a sample of 1608 Chinese adolescents, Chao et al. (2017) applied MR to determine whether alcohol use by adolescents was causally related to internalising and externalising behaviour problems; they found no evidence of such an effect in relation to anxiety and depression. Within the externalising problems, alcohol use was seen to play a causal role in relation to aggression and attention problems but not to delinquency. Treur et al. (2021) applied a number of MR-related techniques to test for the possible bidirectional causal relationships between ADHD and substance use. They found that ADHD increases the likelihood of smoking initiation and heaviness of smoking among smokers, decreases the likelihood of smoking cessation, and increases the likelihood of cannabis initiation. There was only weak evidence that liability to ADHD increases alcohol dependence risk and little evidence for effects in the other direction for the effects of substance use on ADHD.

Artigas et al. (2020) also examined ADHD as a cause of cannabis use with MR methods. They used summary statistics from two large meta-analyses of genome-wide association studies of ADHD and of cannabis use. Both are partly determined by genetic factors and the study was undertaken to gain insights into the genetic overlap and causal relationship of these two behaviours. They found support for the notion that ADHD is causal for lifetime cannabis use, with a highly significant effect whereby cannabis use was nearly eight times more likely in individuals with ADHD in comparison to individuals without ADHD.

4.7 Regression Discontinuity Design

The pre-post design or regression discontinuity design is a natural experiment where the outcome measure is monitored over the time of change in a policy or by an intervention. There is no random allocation to treatment but rather an assumption that possible confounds would have continued as they were, if the change had not happened. Such an opportunity arose for Costello, Compton, Keeler, and Angold (2003) who were in the midst of conducting a longitudinal study of mental illness in children. A substantial proportion of the children in the study were from families of the Eastern Band of Cherokee Indians. In the middle of the study, these Indian families started to receive income from a gambling casino that had opened on their land. A number of families were thereby lifted out of poverty, whereas others were not. Although not randomly allocated, a change in circumstances (in this case additional family income) could be seen as robustly related to a change in the prevalence of conduct and oppositional defiant disorders (ODD) in children from poor families. Importantly other disorders, namely, anxiety and depression, were not affected. These findings argued for a causal benefit for some families from the windfall increase in income arising from a casino opening on an Indian reservation. Those families who were in poverty but were then raised out of it showed a reduction in conduct and ODD to the level of those in families who were never in poverty. This study showed that poverty was causally related to conduct disorders and ODD but not to internalising disorders.

4.8 Propensity Scores

One way to attempt to control risk factor groups on observed confounds, in the absence of randomisation, is to attempt to equate groups on a set of variables that are potential confounds. Confounds are variables that influence both risk and outcome. The values of these variables can be aggregated to form a propensity score (Rosenbaum & Rubin, 1983). The propensity score reflects the relationships between the possible confounds and exposure to risk. These scores are usually estimated using a logistic regression with risk/no risk as the dependent variable. The method is similar to that used in an analysis of covariance, but in that case, the effects of the covariates (potential confounds) on the outcome are taken into account rather than on the risk variable (see Chap. 8 in Tabachnick & Fidell, 2013).

The propensity scores can be used in a number of different ways in the subsequent analysis of the possibly unconfounded relationship between risk and outcome (Haukoos & Lewis, 2015). Lanza, Moore, and Butera (2013) provide a useful overview of the alternative uses of propensity score. The simplest of these is to create risk/no risk groups with pairs of individuals who are matched on their propensity scores. The groups matched in this way may be considered "as if" randomised. This matching process produces groups that are considered as "balanced" but may still be subject to the influence of unobserved covariates. Rosenbaum has developed sensitivity analyses to detect the extent to which a significant association found between observed variables could be due to unobserved confounding (Liu et al., 2013). These can be used to judge the confidence in the putative causal relationship identified in non-experimental studies.

Propensity score matching was used by Joyner and Beaver (2021) in the analysis of the putative causal association between maternal depression and internalising and externalising behaviours in children. A wide range of measures were available on a large longitudinally studied sample of children in the USA. Propensity scores were estimated using maternal characteristics (e.g. age and race), social support (e.g. satisfaction with quality of help with childcare), neighbourhood disadvantage (e.g. gangs and drug use in the locality), and adverse experience (e.g. partner's violent behaviour). The risk factor was maternal depression measured by a standardised DSM-based interview. The outcome of child behaviour was assessed using the CBCL. The initial association between maternal depression and internalising behaviour problems in the child was robust when propensity scores were applied. However the relationship with externalising behaviour was no longer significant. Rather than concluding that maternal depression is therefore causally related to internalising problems, Joyner and Beaver (2021) suggest that mothers who are depressed are more likely to detect symptoms in their children that are similar to their own and therefore this difference between internalising and externalising may be an artefact of shared method variance in the measurement of maternal and child mental health. Curiously Joyner and Beaver (2021) do not discuss the possibility of an uncontrolled genetic confound associated with maternal depression and, specifically, with internalising in the child.

A more stringent use of propensity scores to investigate the link between maternal depression and child behaviour was undertaken by Pelham et al. (2021). They equated groups of depressed and non-depressed mothers on propensity scores derived from 89 variables reflecting the broad family context. The initial significant association between maternal depression and internalising and externalising behaviour between age 4 and 14 years became much reduced after propensity score matching. The unadjusted associations gave effect sizes on mothers' ratings of SMD = 0.45, which fell to SMD = 0.07 after propensity score matching. Parallel reductions were seen in ratings by others such as teachers. They conclude that a substantial portion of the initial association between mothers' depression and later child behaviour problems is accounted for by confounding variables rather than a causal effect of depressive symptoms per se.

4.9 Direction Dependence Analysis

One of the statistical approaches to test for causality is direction dependence analysis (DDA). The core feature of this approach is that the higher-order moments (skew and kurtosis) of the distributions of variables and residuals in regression analyses will differ depending on the nature of the underlying causal model, i.e. if x causes y, y causes x, or x and y are associated via a third variable confound (Wiedermann & Li, 2018). The feasibility of applying DDA appropriately to data in applied settings has been doubted (Thoemmes, 2020) – but see the rejoinder from Wiedermann and Sebastian (2020). DDA has been applied to test for mediation of causal effects of Incredible Years Teacher Classroom Management programme on later academic competence in children aged 7 years. The findings from this study indicate that outcomes of the programme on student academic competence are mediated by student improvements in prosocial behaviour but not by changes in concentration problems or disruptive behaviour (Wiedermann et al., 2020).

4.10 Negative Control Exposure and Outcome

The logic of negative control outcomes and negative control exposure in nonrandomised or observational studies has been laid out by Dusetzina, Brookhart, and Maciejewski (2015). These control exposure and outcomes can be used to enhance the internal validity of nonrandomised studies (Thapar & Rutter, 2019). The reasoning here is that a negative control outcome should not show a significant difference between risk exposure groups in primary outcomes. The same holds for negative control exposures, which would not be expected to be related to outcome. Such a finding adds confidence in the validity of any treatment effects detected.

An example of a negative control exposure applied to child behaviour was a study by Langley, Heron, Smith, and Thapar (2012). They wanted to address the question of whether the association between maternal smoking in pregnancy and later ADHD in the child reflected a casual process. It is possible that such a causal link was mediated by an intrauterine effect. In that case there should be no association between ADHD and paternal smoking during pregnancy. If however the association arose from confounders, that could be genetic or family circumstances, then an association with paternal smoking might be found. They found that both maternal and paternal smoking during pregnancy were related to the later risk of ADHD in the child. The effect of paternal smoking remained when the effects of maternal smoking were taken into account. Importantly they conducted an analysis of families where neither mother nor father smoked but where the mother was exposed to smoke at her workplace during pregnancy. They found no relation between ADHD symptoms in the child and mother's exposure to passive smoking during pregnancy. This excludes the likelihood that paternal smoking links with ADHD were due to a passive smoking exposure for the mother. This pattern of results, using the negative exposure measure of paternal smoking, suggests that the effect of maternal smoking during pregnancy is not mediated by intrauterine effects but results from genetic or social confounding effects.

A classic negative control exposure is the use of a placebo treatment. This is administered in the same way as the active treatment but is not expected to have any causal impact on the outcome. A negative control outcome is one that shares the same potential source of bias as the primary outcome but for which there is no plausible causal connection with active treatment. The application of negative control outcomes in RCTs has been described by Arnold and Ercumen (2016). A sufficiently powered RCT analysed on an intention-to-treat basis should not be subject to bias. However differential attrition and unblinding of measurement can create bias. In these circumstances the use of negative control outcomes can be a useful test for residual bias in RCTs.

4.11 *E*-value

Dealing with confounders in observational studies is complex and can never be assumed to be complete. It is therefore valuable to understand what limits there might be on the scope of confounds to influence the results of a study. The *E*-value is a technique that quantifies the upper limit of the size of the effects of confounders (Haneuse et al., 2019; VanderWeele & Ding, 2017). This is a sensitivity analysis that identifies how strong the unmeasured confounding would have to be to invalidate the observed results. It is particularly valuable when applied to clinical trials where randomisation has not been possible.

The *E*-value is defined as:

> the minimum strength of association, on the risk ratio scale, that an unmeasured confounder would need to have with both the treatment and the outcome to fully explain away a specific treatment–outcome association, conditional on the measured covariates. (VanderWeele & Ding, 2017, p. 269)

This definition refers to effects being calculated as a risk ratio, but the application of *E*-estimates to other effect metrics is presented in Table 2 of VanderWeele and Ding (2017). The logic is that a large *E*-value suggests that effects detected in an observational study are unlikely to be an artefact produced by confounds. However the size of *E*-value depends on a number of factors, such as effect sizes. *E*-values will be small if the effect size is small and large if the effect size is large. Unlike the *p*-value the *E*-value is robust in that it will not be inflated by an increase in sample size. They can be calculated at the design stage of study in an analogous manner to power. This would indicate whether the covariates being applied in the study design are sufficiently strong to give an adequate control for confounds. An example of the use of the *E*-value is the study by Qiu et al. (2020) on labour epidural anaesthesia discussed above. The *E*-value has also been applied in a study of the impact of prenatal tobacco exposure on conduct disorder (CD) at age 15 years (Duko et al., 2021). This study found that the rates of CD symptoms in the child increased with the level of exposure to maternal smoking during pregnancy. The *E*-value suggested that the effects of uncontrolled confounders would have to be unfeasibly high to nullify the effects of maternal smoking on later conduct disorders in the child.

4.12 Causal Mediation Methods

> The counterfactual lies at the heart of causal inference—what would happen to an individual or clinician or organization if one changed its exposure to another condition or treatment? This counterfactual defines the effect of interest: the difference between what did happen and the counterfactual. A comparison of these ‘potential outcomes’ determines the effect of the exposure or treatment. One might be interested in the effect of growing up in a single-parent family on a child’s health and development. For a child growing up without his or her father, what his or her life would have been like had the father remained in the household is a counterfactual. (Foster, 2014, p. 803)

The use of counterfactuals is key to causal mediation methods. These methods are designed to identify which intermediary variables might be on the causal path from a treatment or risk factor to an outcome. They were developed based on the potential outcomes framework (Cuartas & McCoy, 2021).

These approaches have radically changed the methods of investigating mediation – see Pearl & Mackenzie (2018, chapter 9) for an account of how this approach was developed. MacKinnon, Valente, and Gonzalez (2020) argue that, although seemingly distinct, the regression (see Sect. 2.2) and causal mediation approaches have much in common. In the case where there is no interaction between a risk factor and a mediator, then the two methods will be concordant. However in the presence of such an interaction, the causal mediation approach tests for this directly and is more readily applicable to more complex cases such as non-linear relationships and categorical mediators and outcomes. For these reasons MacKinnon, Valente, and Gonzalez (2020) suggest that causal mediation analysis should be more widely adopted. The application of these methods is becoming easier with the development of software designed for causal mediation analysis. Valente, Rijnhart, Smyth, Muniz, and MacKinnon (2020) provide an overview of these packages and guidance on how to conduct and report this analysis.

An example of a causal mediation analysis is provided by Powell et al. (2020). They wanted to understand the mechanisms whereby by ADHD (risk variable) in childhood was associated with depression in adolescence (outcome variable). They used data on ADHD symptoms at 7.5 years and depressive symptoms at 17.5 years. They postulated that low academic attainment and peer relationship problems might mediate this relationship. The mediators were measured when the participants were aged 16 years. Possible confounding variables were sex, maternal age at birth, and maternal socio-economic status. These variables were possible confounders for the risk to mediator, mediator to outcome, and risk to outcome relationships and were therefore adjusted as covariates for each of these analyses. Using the causal mediation commands in STATA (see Valente et al., 2020, for details), they were able to identify the pure natural direct effect, total natural indirect effect, and percentage of the total effect that was mediated. These estimates are based on a counterfactual potential outcomes framework (Imai et al., 2010). Pure Natural Direct Effect is the direct (unmediated) effect of the risk variable on the outcome when the mediator takes the value it would take in the absence of risk. Total Natural Indirect Effect captures the mediated effect of the risk variable on the outcome that operates by changing the mediator. They found that both peer problem and academic attainment explained significant proportion of the effects of ADHD symptoms on later depression. The proportion of the total effect that was mediated by peer problems was 15% and by academic attainment was 20%.

4.13 Final Thoughts on the State of Knowledge About Testing Causation

> No single study, however beautifully designed, can unequivocally demonstrate causation. To improve our causal explanations, we would do best instead to opt for causal triangulation. (Krieger & Davey Smith, 2016, p. 1803)

The possibilities for testing causal relationships in epidemiological studies were reviewed by Ohlsson and Kendler (2020). They conclude that the randomised controlled trial is optimal for establishing causality but that it is not the only means for gaining traction on the question. A variety of methods can contribute (e.g. natural experiments and regression discontinuity designs) and much can be gained by using multiple methods to triangulate on possible causal mechanisms (Munafò & Davey Smith, 2018).

There are three broad types of study with distinct research goals (Hamaker et al., 2020). The goals are description, prediction, and causation. Each makes different demands on the rigour of the design of studies. "Descriptive studies" aim simply to identify the way groups differ on a set of measures or the extent to which these measures covary or correlate. "Predictive studies" require that an indicator be measured prior to an outcome. The aim is to establish the accuracy with which an outcome can be predicted, but there is no requirement that the mechanisms linking the predictor and outcome be known. Nevertheless "predictive studies" may be of value to identify individuals who may benefit from intervention (Larsson, 2021). Indeed many predictors may not be causally related to outcome. These are sometimes designated as "markers" in that they indicate a susceptibility to an outcome but only via a common association with a third factor. For example of testing for the presence of such a marker rather than a true cause, see Goodman, Simonoff, and Stevenson (1995). An intervention to change a marker would not necessarily change the outcome. For such a change to happen, a causal relationship needs to be established by an "explanatory study".

A case has been made that explanatory studies have shown that adverse childhood experiences (ACEs) are causally related to later poor mental health (Linden & LeMoult, 2022). They define ACEs as:

> severe negative environmental events that require significant emotional, cognitive, or neurobiological adaptation by an average child. ACEs may be chronic (e.g. prolonged separation from a caregiver) or involve single events. Common ACEs include parental incarceration, domestic violence, household mental illness/suicide, household alcohol and substance misuse, exposure to physical and sexual abuse, neighbourhood violence, bullying, discrimination, and parental death. (Linden & LeMoult, 2022, p. 1)

They argue that the strength of this causal relationship justifies the development of preventive and treatment interventions targeting children experiencing ACEs. Similarly Bourassa et al. (2022) argue that the effects of ACEs on health in midlife are mediated via later psychosocial adversities. Consequently preventive efforts should be directed to reduce the number of stressful life events people experience, reduce negative emotionality, reduce perceived stress, or improve health behaviours to offset the risk adverse outcomes in midlife. However a note of caution has been raised by Cuijpers, Smit, and Furukawa (2021). They show that at present the predictive strength of risk factors even, in combination, is too low and preventive interventions based on these are neither cost-effective nor ethical. The latter because too many people are labelled at risk who will not in fact develop a mental health problem. These problems stem from the inadequate specificity of risk indicators.

The focus of this chapter has been on the determination of plausible causal relations in non-experimental observational studies. Why is it so important to differentiate causality from association? Any attempt to act preventively will only be successful if an intervention is directed at a risk factor that is causally related to an adverse outcome. Given the desirability of prevention over treatment, establishing causes rather than associations becomes crucial.

Gordon (1983) distinguished between three types of preventive intervention:

> In summary, we propose to define prevention as measures adopted by or practiced on persons not currently feeling the effects of a disease, intended to decrease the risk that that disease will afflict them in the future. Prevention is classified into three levels on the basis of the population for whom the measure is advisable on cost-benefit analysis. Universal

measures are recommended for essentially everyone. Selective measures are advisable for population subgroups distinguished by age, sex, occupation, or other evident characteristics, but who, on individual examination, are perfectly well. Indicated measures are those that should be applied only in the presence of a demonstrable condition that identifies the individual as being at higher than average risk for the future development of a disease. (Gordon, 1983, p. 109)

The current state of prevention science as it is applied to child and youth mental health has been reviewed by Fusar-Poli et al. (2021). They argue that targeted prevention based on established causation and predictive risk factors for individuals addresses effort at those with the most to gain, but this is only a small proportion of the population. Universal approaches aim to shift the risk profile for the whole population and may therefore produce the greatest aggregate benefit. They argue that the most effective interventions are those aimed at the population as a whole.

Universal public health approaches targeting school climate or social determinants (demographic, economic, neighbourhood, environmental, social/cultural) of mental disorders hold the greatest potential for reducing the risk profile of the population as a whole. (Fusar-Poli et al., 2021, p. 200)

Grosz, Rohrer, and Thoemmes (2020) suggest that psychologists have been reluctant to draw explicit causal interpretations from the analysis of non-experimental data. Nonetheless psychologists make implicit reference to causality when presenting the results of their work. They suggest a four-step process that researchers could follow to incorporate a causal approach to their studies.

Step 1 requires the articulation of a clear causal question and a statement of the precise definition of the causal effect of interest. They suggest that "Translating the causal question into a hypothetical experiment and counterfactual thinking can help researchers do so because the counterfactual question 'What would happen to an individual if one changed the treatment?' lies at the heart of causal inference" (see Sect. 4.12). In the present context, the term risk factor replaces treatment.

Step 2 addresses how other variables relate to the putative causal variable (i.e. the risk factor) and outcome variable to identify potential confounders, colliders, mediators, and instrumental variables. This can be achieved most clearly by the use of a DAG (see Sect. 4.3).

Step 3 relates to how the causal effects can be identified and estimated, e.g. by multiple regression or the use of instrumental variables (see Sect. 4.4).

Step 4 examines how robust the model is by seeing how much the effect estimate would change if certain assumptions were violated, e.g. by E-value estimation (see Sect. 4.10).

Grosz et al. (2020) encourage the adoption of this series of steps to open up possibilities for examining causal processes as follows:

…we recommend that nonexperimental psychologists begin to talk openly about causal assumptions and causal effects. Only then can researchers take advantage of recent methodological advances in causal reasoning and analysis and develop a solid understanding of the underlying causal mechanisms that can inform future research, theory, and policymakers. (Grosz et al., 2020, p. 1243)

References

Academy of Medical Sciences. (2007). *Identifying the environmental causes of disease: How should we decide what to believe and when to take action? / an Academy of Medical Sciences working group report chaired by Michael Rutter*. Academy of Medical Sciences.

Arnold, B. F., & Ercumen, A. (2016). Negative control outcomes A tool to detect bias in randomized trials. *JAMA-Journal of the American Medical Association, 316*(24), 2597–2598. https://doi.org/10.1001/jama.2016.17700

Artigas, M. S., Sanchez-Mora, C., Rovira, P., Richarte, V., Garcia-Martinez, I., Pagerols, M., et al. (2020). Attention-deficit/hyperactivity disorder and lifetime cannabis use: Genetic overlap and causality. *Molecular Psychiatry, 25*(10), 2493–2503. https://doi.org/10.1038/s41380-018-0339-3

Auger, A., Farkas, G., Burchinal, M. R., Duncan, G. J., & Vandell, D. L. (2014). Preschool center care quality effects on academic achievement: An instrumental variables analysis. *Developmental Psychology, 50*(12), 2559–2571. https://doi.org/10.1037/a0037995

Bakermans-Kranenburg, M. J., & van Ijzendoorn, M. H. (2015). The hidden efficacy of interventions: Gene x Environment experiments from a differential susceptibility perspective. In S. T. Fiske (Ed.), *Annual Review of Psychology, 66*, 381–409.

Baldwin, J. R., Caspi, A., Meehan, A. J., Ambler, A., Arseneault, L., Fisher, H. L., et al. (2021). Population vs Individual prediction of poor health from results of adverse childhood experiences screening. *JAMA Pediatrics, 175*(4), 385–393. https://doi.org/10.1001/jamapediatrics.2020.5602

Bateman, B., Warner, J. O., Hutchinson, E., Dean, T., Rowlandson, P., Gant, C., et al. (2004). The effects of a double blind, placebo controlled, artificial food colourings and benzoate preservative challenge on hyperactivity in a general population sample of preschool children. *Archives of Disease in Childhood, 89*, 506–511. https://doi.org/10.1136/adc.2003.031435

Berry, D., & Willoughby, M. T. (2017). On the practical interpretability of cross-lagged panel models: Rethinking a developmental workhorse. *Child Development, 88*(4), 1186–1206. https://doi.org/10.1111/cdev.12660

Bollen, K. A., & Pearl, J. (2013). Eight myths about causality and structural equation models. In S. L. Morgan (Ed.), *Handbook of causal analysis for social research* (pp. 301–328). Springer.

Bourassa, K. J., Moffitt, T. E., Harrington, H., Houts, R., Poulton, R., Ramrakha, S., et al. (2022). Childhood adversity and midlife health: Shining a light on the black box of psychosocial mechanisms. *Prevention Science*. https://doi.org/10.1007/s11121-022-01431-y

Briley, D. A., Livengood, J., & Derringer, J. (2018). Behaviour genetic frameworks of causal reasoning for personality psychology. *European Journal of Personality, 32*(3), 202–220. https://doi.org/10.1002/per.2153

Burt, S. A., Clark, D. A., & Neiderhiser, J. M. (2022). Illuminating the origins of the intergenerational transmission of psychopathology with a novel genetically informed design. *Development and Psychopathology, 34*, 1756–1766. https://doi.org/10.1017/s0954579422000451

Button, K. S., Ioannidis, J. P. A., Mokrysz, C., Nosek, B. A., Flint, J., Robinson, E. S. J., & Munafo, M. R. (2013). Power failure: Why small sample size undermines the reliability of neuroscience. *Nature Reviews Neuroscience, 14*(5), 365–376. https://doi.org/10.1038/nrn3475

Bzdok, D., & Meyer-Lindenberg, A. (2018). Machine learning for precision psychiatry: Opportunities and challenges. *Biological Psychiatry-Cognitive Neuroscience and Neuroimaging, 3*(3), 223–230. https://doi.org/10.1016/j.bpsc.2017.11.007

Bzdok, D., Varoquaux, G., & Steyerberg, E. W. (2021). Prediction, not association, paves the road to precision medicine. *JAMA Psychiatry, 78*(2), 127–128. https://doi.org/10.1001/jamapsychiatry.2020.2549

Caramaschi, D., Taylor, A. E., Richmond, R. C., Havdahl, K. A., Golding, J., Relton, C. L., et al. (2018). Maternal smoking during pregnancy and autism: Using causal inference methods in a birth cohort study. *Translational Psychiatry, 8*. https://doi.org/10.1038/s41398-018-0313-5

Carrier, F. M., Lavoie, A., & Zaphiratos, V. (2021). Epidural analgesia during labour and autism risk: Getting lost on the causal path. *Canadian Journal of Anesthesia-Journal Canadien D Anesthesie, 68*(3), 277–284. https://doi.org/10.1007/s12630-020-01880-5

Cartwright, N. (2007). Are RCTs the gold standard? *BioSocieties, 2*, 11–20. https://doi.org/10.1017/S1745855207005029

Chao, M., Li, X. Y., & McGue, M. (2017). The causal role of alcohol use in adolescent externalizing and internalizing problems: A Mendelian randomization study. *Alcoholism-Clinical and Experimental Research, 41*(11), 1953–1960. https://doi.org/10.1111/acer.13493

Chen, B., & Pearl, J. (2015). Graphical tools for linear structural equation modeling, pp. 1–25. https://ftp.cs.ucla.edu/pub/stat_ser/r432.pdf

Coggon, D. I. W., & Martyn, C. N. (2005). Time and chance: The stochastic nature of disease causation. *Lancet, 365*(9468), 1434–1437. https://doi.org/10.1016/s0140-6736(05)66380-5

Cole, D. A., & Preacher, K. J. (2014). Manifest variable path analysis: Potentially serious and misleading consequences due to uncorrected measurement error. *Psychological Methods, 19*(2), 300–315. https://doi.org/10.1037/a0033805

Collins, L. M. (2006). Analysis of longitudinal data: The integration of theoretical model, temporal design, and statistical model. *Annual Review of Psychology, 57*, 505–528. https://doi.org/10.1146/annurev.psych.57.102904.190146

Costello, E. J., Compton, S. N., Keeler, G., & Angold, A. (2003). Relationships between poverty and psychopathology – A natural experiment. *JAMA-Journal of the American Medical Association, 290*(15), 2023–2029. https://doi.org/10.1001/jama.290.15.2023

Cuartas, J., & McCoy, D. C. (2021). Causal mediation in developmental science: A primer. *International Journal of Behavioral Development, 45*(3), 269–274. https://doi.org/10.1177/0165025420981640

Cuijpers, P., Smit, F., & Furukawa, T. A. (2021). Most at-risk individuals will not develop a mental disorder: The limited predictive strength of risk factors. *World Psychiatry, 20*(2), 224–225. https://doi.org/10.1002/wps.20852

Curfman, G. D. (1993). Is exercise beneficial – Or hazardous – To your heart. *New England Journal of Medicine, 329*(23), 1730–1731. https://doi.org/10.1056/nejm199312023292310

Curran, P. J., & Bauer, D. J. (2011). The disaggregation of within-person and between-person effects in longitudinal models of change. In S. T. Fiske, D. L. Schacter, & S. E. Taylor (Eds.), *Annual Review of Psychology, 62*, 583–619.

Curran, P. J., Howard, A. L., Bainter, S. A., Lane, S. T., & McGinley, J. S. (2014). The separation of between-person and within-person components of individual change over time: A latent curve model with structured residuals. *Journal of Clinical and Consulting Psychology, 82*(5), 879–894. https://doi.org/10.1037/a0035297

Curran, E. A., O'Neill, S. M., Cryan, J. F., Kenny, L. C., Dinan, T. G., Khashan, A. S., & Kearney, P. M. (2015). Research Review: Birth by caesarean section and development of autism spectrum disorder and attention-deficit/hyperactivity disorder: A systematic review and meta-analysis. *Journal of Child Psychology and Psychiatry, 56*(5), 500–508. https://doi.org/10.1111/jcpp.12351

D'Onofrio, B. M., Lahey, B. B., Turkheimer, E., & Lichtenstein, P. (2013). Critical need for family-based, quasi-experimental designs in integrating genetic and social science research. *American Journal of Public Health, 103*, 46–55. https://doi.org/10.2105/ajph.2013.301252

Davey Smith, G. (2019). Post-modern epidemiology: When methods meet matter. *American Journal of Epidemiology, 188*(8), 1410–1419. https://doi.org/10.1093/aje/kwz064

Deaton, A., & Cartwright, N. (2018). Understanding and misunderstanding randomized controlled trials. *Social Science & Medicine, 210*, 2–21. https://doi.org/10.1016/j.socscimed.2017.12.005

Dusetzina, S. B., Brookhart, M. A., & Maciejewski, M. L. (2015). Control outcomes and exposures for improving internal validity of nonrandomized studies. *Health Services Research, 50*(5), 1432–1451. https://doi.org/10.1111/1475-6773.12279

Duko, B., Pereira, G., Tait, R. J., Newnham, J., Betts, K., & Alati, R. (2021). Prenatal tobacco exposure and the risk of conduct disorder symptoms in offspring at the age of 14 years: Findings from the *Raine Study. Journal of Psychiatric Research, 142*, 1–8. https://doi.org/10.1016/j.jpsychires.2021.07.030

Farrell, A. D. (1994). Structural equation modeling with longitudinal data – Strategies for examining group-differences and reciprocal relationships. *Journal of Clinical and Consulting Psychology, 62*(3), 477–487. https://doi.org/10.1037/0022-006x.62.3.477

Feingold, B. F. (1975). Hyperkinesis and learning disabilities linked to artificial food flavors and colors. *American Journal of Nursing, 75*, 797–803.

Foster, E. M. (2010). Causal inference and developmental psychology. *Developmental Psychology, 46*(6), 1454–1480. https://doi.org/10.1037/a0020204

Foster, E. M. (2014). Mediation, identification, and plausibility: An illustration using Children's Mental Health Services. *Journal of Consulting and Clinical Psychology, 82*(5), 803–812. https://doi.org/10.1037/a0031980

Fusar-Poli, P., Correll, C. U., Arango, C., Berk, M., Patel, V., & Ioannidis, J. P. A. (2021). Preventive psychiatry: A blueprint for improving the mental health of young people. *World Psychiatry, 20*(2), 200–221. https://doi.org/10.1002/wps.20869

Gollob, H. F., & Reichardt, C. S. (1987). Taking account of time lags in causal-models. *Child Development, 58*(1), 80–92. https://doi.org/10.1111/j.1467-8624.1987.tb03492.x

Goodman, R., Simonoff, E., & Stevenson, J. (1995). The impact of child IQ, parent IQ and sibling IQ on child behavioural-deviance scores. *Journal of Child Psychology and Psychiatry and Allied Disciplines, 36*(3), 409–425. https://doi.org/10.1111/j.1469-7610.1995.tb01299.x

Gordon, R. S. (1983). An operational classification of disease prevention. *Public Health Reports, 98*(2), 107–109.

Greenland, S., Pearl, J., & Robins, J. M. (1999). Causal diagrams for epidemiologic research. *Epidemiology, 10*(1), 37–48. https://doi.org/10.1097/00001648-199901000-00008

Grosz, M. P., Rohrer, J. M., & Thoemmes, F. (2020). The taboo against explicit causal inference in nonexperimental psychology. *Perspectives on Psychological Science, 15*(5), 1243–1255. https://doi.org/10.1177/1745691620921521

Halse, M., Steinsbekk, S., Hammar, A., & Wichstrøm, L. (2022). Longitudinal relations between impaired executive function and symptoms of psychiatric disorders in childhood. *Journal of Child Psychology and Psychiatry*. https://doi.org/10.1111/jcpp.13622

Hamaker, E. L., Mulder, J. D., & van Ijzendoorn, M. H. (2020). Description, prediction and causation: Methodological challenges of studying child and adolescent development. *Developmental Cognitive Neuroscience, 46*. https://doi.org/10.1016/j.dcn.2020.100867

Haneuse, S., VanderWeele, T. J., & Arterburn, D. (2019). Using the E-value to assess the potential effect of unmeasured confounding in observational studies. *JAMA-Journal of the American Medical Association, 321*(6), 602–603. https://doi.org/10.1001/jama.2018.21554

Hanley, G. E., Ip, A., & Oberlander, T. F. (2021). Epidural analgesia and autism spectrum disorder risk – The challenges inherent in complex observational research. *JAMA Pediatrics, 175*(7), 675–677. https://doi.org/10.1001/jamapediatrics.2021.0382

Haukoos, J. S., & Lewis, R. J. (2015). The propensity score. *JAMA-Journal of the American Medical Association, 314*(15), 1637–1638. https://doi.org/10.1001/jama.2015.13480

Hegvik, T.-A., Klungsøyr, K., Kuja-halkola, R., Remes, H., Haavik, J., D'Onofrio, B. M., et al. (2022). Labor epidural analgesia and subsequent risk of offspring autism spectrum disorder and attention-deficit/hyperactivity disorder: A cross-national cohort study of 4.5 million individuals and their siblings. *American Journal of Obstetrics and Gynecology*. https://doi.org/10.1016/j.ajog.2022.08.016

Hernán, M. A., & Robins, J. M. (2006). Instruments for causal inference – An epidemiologist's dream? *Epidemiology, 17*(4), 360–372. https://doi.org/10.1097/01.ede.0000222409.00878.37

Hernán, M. A., Hernandez-Diaz, S., & Robins, J. M. (2013). Randomized trials analyzed as observational studies. *Annals of Internal Medicine, 159*(8), 560-+. https://doi.org/10.7326/0003-4819-159-8-201310150-00709

Hill, A. B. (1965). The environment and disease: Association or causation? *Journal of the Royal Society of Medicine, 58*, 295–300.

Imai, K., Keele, L., & Tingley, D. (2010). A general approach to causal mediation analysis. *Psychological Methods, 15*(4), 309–334. https://doi.org/10.1037/a0020761

Ioannidis, J. P. A. (2005). Why most published research findings are false. *PLoS Medicine, 2*(8), 696–701. https://doi.org/10.1371/journal.pmed.0020124

Jaffee, S. R., Strait, L. B., & Odgers, C. L. (2012). From correlates to causes: Can quasi-experimental studies and statistical innovations bring us closer to identifying the causes of anti-social behavior? *Psychological Bulletin, 138*(2), 272–295. https://doi.org/10.1037/a0026020

Joyner, B., & Beaver, K. M. (2021). Maternal depression and child and adolescent problem behaviors: A propensity score matching approach. *Psychiatric Quarterly, 92*, 655–674. https://doi.org/10.1007/s11126-020-09842-2

Kendler, K. S., Ohlsson, H., Fagan, A. A., Lichtenstein, P., Sundquist, J., & Sundquist, K. (2018). Academic achievement and drug abuse risk assessed using instrumental variable analysis and co-relative designs. *JAMA Psychiatry, 75*(11), 1182–1188. https://doi.org/10.1001/jamapsychiatry.2018.2337

Kenny, D. A., & Harackiewicz, J. M. (1979). Cross-lagged panel correlation- practice and promise. *Journal of Applied Psychology, 64*(4), 372–379. https://doi.org/10.1037/0021-9010.64.4.372

Kern-Goldberger, A. R., Burris, H. H., & Levine, L. D. (2021). Methodologic concerns with concluding a link between epidural and autism spectrum disorder. *JAMA Pediatrics, 175*(5), 536–537. https://doi.org/10.1001/jamapediatrics.2020.6692

Kievit, R. A., Brandmaier, A. M., Ziegler, G., van Harmelen, A. L., de Mooij, S. M. M., Moutoussis, M., et al. (2018). Developmental cognitive neuroscience using latent change score models: A tutorial and applications. *Developmental Cognitive Neuroscience, 33*, 99–117. https://doi.org/10.1016/j.dcn.2017.11.007

Kline, R. (2016). *Principles and practice of structural equation modelling* (4th ed.). Guilford Press.

Krieger, N., & Smith, G. D. (2016). The tale wagged by the DAG: Broadening the scope of causal inference and explanation for epidemiology. *International Journal of Epidemiology, 45*(6), 1787–1808. https://doi.org/10.1093/ije/dyw114

Langley, K., Heron, J., Smith, G. D., & Thapar, A. (2012). Maternal and paternal smoking during pregnancy and risk of ADHD symptoms in offspring: Testing for intrauterine effects. *American Journal of Epidemiology, 176*(3), 261–268. https://doi.org/10.1093/aje/kwr510

Lanza, S. T., Moore, J. E., & Butera, N. M. (2013). Drawing causal inferences using propensity scores: A practical guide for community psychologists. *American Journal of Community Psychology, 52*(3–4), 380–392. https://doi.org/10.1007/s10464-013-9604-4

Larsson, H. (2021). Causation and prediction in child and adolescent mental health research. *JCPP Advances, 1*(2), e12026.

Lawlor, D. A., Harbord, R. M., Sterne, J. A. C., Timpson, N., & Smith, G. D. (2008). Mendelian randomization: Using genes as instruments for making causal inferences in epidemiology. *Statistics in Medicine, 27*(8), 1133–1163. https://doi.org/10.1002/sim.3034

Linden, W., & LeMoult, J. (2022). Editorial Perspective: Adverse childhood events causally contribute to mental illness – we must act now and intervene early. *Journal of Child Psychology and Psychiatry, 63*(6), 715–719. https://doi.org/10.1111/jcpp.13541

Liu, W., Kuramoto, S. J., & Stuart, E. A. (2013). An introduction to sensitivity analysis for unobserved confounding in nonexperimental prevention research. *Prevention Science, 14*(6), 570–580. https://doi.org/10.1007/s11121-012-0339-5

Lynch, S. K., Turkheimer, E., D'Onofrio, B. M., Mendle, J., Emery, R. E., Slutske, W. S., & Martin, N. G. (2006). A genetically informed study of the association between harsh punishment and offspring behavioral problems. *Journal of Family Psychology, 20*(2), 190–198. https://doi.org/10.1037/0893-3200.20.2.190

MacKinnon, D. P., Valente, M. J., & Gonzalez, O. (2020). The correspondence between causal and traditional mediation analysis: The link is the mediator by treatment interaction. *Prevention Science, 21*(2), 147–157. https://doi.org/10.1007/s11121-019-01076-4

McAdams, T. A., Neiderhiser, J. M., Rijsdijk, F. V., Narusyte, J., Lichtenstein, P., & Eley, T. C. (2014). Accounting for genetic and environmental confounds in associations between parent and child characteristics: A systematic review of Children-of-Twins studies. *Psychological Bulletin, 140*(4), 1138–1173. https://doi.org/10.1037/a0036416

McAdams, T. A., Rijsdijk, F. V., Zavos, H. M. S., & Pingault, J.-B. (2021). Twins and causal inference: Leveraging nature's experiment. *Cold Spring Harbor Perspectives in Medicine, 11*(6). https://doi.org/10.1101/cshperspect.a039552

McCann, D., Barrett, A., Cooper, A., Crumpler, D., Dalen, L., Grimshaw, K., et al. (2007). Food additives and hyperactive behaviour in 3-year-old and 8/9-year-old children in the community: A randomised, double-blinded, placebo-controlled trial. *Lancet, 370*(9598), 1560–1567. https://doi.org/10.1016/s0140-6736(07)61306-3

Miller, P., Henry, D., & Votruba-Drzal, E. (2016). Strengthening causal inference in developmental research. *Child Development Perspectives, 10*(4), 275–280. https://doi.org/10.1111/cdep.12202

Miller, M. D., Steinmaus, C., Golub, M. S., Castorina, R., Thilakartne, R., Bradman, A., & Marty, M. A. (2022). Potential impacts of synthetic food dyes on activity and attention in children: A review of the human and animal evidence. *Environmental Health, 21*(1). https://doi.org/10.1186/s12940-022-00849-9

Mittleman, M. A., Maclure, M., Tofler, G. H., Sherwood, J. B., Goldberg, R. J., & Muller, J. E. (1993). Triggering of acute myocardial-infarction by heavy physical exertion – protection against triggering by regular exertion. *New England Journal of Medicine, 329*(23), 1677–1683. https://doi.org/10.1056/nejm199312023292301

Mojtabai, R., & Crum, R. M. (2013). Cigarette smoking and onset of mood and anxiety disorders. *American Journal of Public Health, 103*(9), 1656–1665. https://doi.org/10.2105/ajph.2012.300911

Munafò, M., & Davey Smith, G. (2018). Repeating experiments is not enough. *Nature, 553*(7689), 399–401. https://doi.org/10.1038/d41586-018-01023-3

Munafò, M. R., Tilling, K., Taylor, A. E., Evans, D. M., & Smith, G. D. (2018). Collider scope: When selection bias can substantially influence observed associations. *International Journal of Epidemiology, 47*(1), 226–235. https://doi.org/10.1093/ije/dyx206

Murray, J., Burgess, S., Zuccolo, L., Hickman, M., Gray, R., & Lewis, S. J. (2016). Moderate alcohol drinking in pregnancy increases risk for children's persistent conduct problems: Causal effects in a Mendelian randomisation study. *Journal of Child Psychology and Psychiatry, 57*(5), 575–584. https://doi.org/10.1111/jcpp.12486

Ohlsson, H., & Kendler, K. (2020). Applying causal inference methods in psychiatric epidemiology; A review. *JAMA Psychiatry, 77*, 637–644.

Orth, U., Clark, D. A., Donnellan, M. B., & Robins, R. W. (2021). Testing prospective effects in longitudinal research: Comparing seven competing cross-lagged models. *Journal of Personality and Social Psychology, 120*(4), 1013–1034. https://doi.org/10.1037/pspp0000358

Pearl, J. (2010). The foundations of causal inference. *Sociological Methodology, 40*(40), 75–149. https://doi.org/10.1111/j.1467-9531.2010.01228.x

Pearl, J., & Mackenzie, D. (2018). *The book of why: The new science of cause and effect*. Allen Lane.

Pelham, W. E., West, S. G., Lemery-Chalfant, K., Goodman, S. H., Wilson, M. N., Dishion, T. J., & Shaw, D. S. (2021). Depression in mothers and the externalizing and internalizing behavior of children: An attempt to go beyond association. *Journal of Abnormal Psychology, 130*(1), 60–77. https://doi.org/10.1037/abn0000640

Pimperton, H., Kreppner, J., Mahon, M., Stevenson, J., Terlektsi, E., Worsfold, S., et al. (2017). Language outcomes in deaf or hard of hearing teenagers who are spoken language users: Effects of universal newborn hearing screening and early confirmation. *Ear and Hearing, 38*(5), 598–610. https://doi.org/10.1097/aud.0000000000000434

Pingault, J. B., O'Reilly, P. F., Schoeler, T., Ploubidis, G. B., Rijsdijk, F., & Dudbridge, F. (2018). Using genetic data to strengthen causal inference in observational research. *Nature Reviews Genetics, 19*(9), 566–580. https://doi.org/10.1038/s41576-018-0020-3

Powell, V., Riglin, L., Hammerton, G., Eyre, O., Martin, J., Anney, R., et al. (2020). What explains the link between childhood ADHD and adolescent depression? Investigating the role of peer relationships and academic attainment. *European Child and Adolescent Psychiatry, 29*(11), 1581–1591. https://doi.org/10.1007/s00787-019-01463-w

Qiu, C. Y., Lin, J. C., Shi, J. X. M., Chow, T., Desai, V. N., Nguyen, V. T., et al. (2020). Association between epidural analgesia during labor and risk of autism spectrum disorders in offspring. *JAMA Pediatrics, 174*(12), 1168–1175. https://doi.org/10.1001/jamapediatrics.2020.3231

Rogosa, D. (1980). A critique of cross-lagged correlation. *Psychological Bulletin, 88*(2), 245–258. https://doi.org/10.1037/0033-2909.88.2.245

Rohrer, J. (2018). Thinking clearly about correlations and causation: Graphical causal models for observational data. *Advances in Methods and Practices in Psychological Science, 1*, 27–42.

Rosenbaum, P. R., & Rubin, D. B. (1983). The central role of the propensity score in observational studies for causal effects. *Biometrika, 70*(1), 41–55. https://doi.org/10.1093/biomet/70.1.41

Rothman, K. J., & Greenland, S. (2005). Causation and causal inference in epidemiology. *American Journal of Public Health, 95*, S144–S150. https://doi.org/10.2105/ajph.2004.059204

Rutter, M. (2007). Proceeding from observed correlation to causal inference the use of natural experiments. *Perspectives on Psychological Science, 2*(4), 377–395. https://doi.org/10.1111/j.1745-6916.2007.00050.x

Schwartz, S., Susser, E., & Susser, M. (1999). A future for epidemiology? *Annual Review of Public Health, 20*, 15–33. https://doi.org/10.1146/annurev.publhealth.20.1.15

Sellers, R., Riglin, L., Harold, G. T., & Thapar, A. (2022). Using genetic designs to identify likely causal environmental contributions to psychopathology. *Development and Psychopathology, 34*, 1653–1665. https://doi.org/10.1017/s0954579422000906

Stevenson, J., Sonuga-Barke, E. J. S., McCann, D., Grimshaw, K., Parker, K. M., Rose-Zerilli, M. J., et al. (2010). The role of histamine degradation gene polymorphisms in moderating the effects of food additives on children's ADHD symptoms. *American Journal of Psychiatry, 167*(9), 1108–1115. https://doi.org/10.1176/appi.ajp.2010.09101529

Stevenson, J., Kreppner, J., Pimperton, H., Worsfold, S., & Kennedy, C. (2015). Emotional and behavioural difficulties in children and adolescents with hearing impairment: A systematic review and meta-analysis. *European Child and Adolescent Psychiatry, 24*(5), 477–496. https://doi.org/10.1007/s00787-015-0697-1

Stevenson, J., Pimperton, H., Kreppner, J., Worsfold, S., Terlektsi, E., Mahon, M., & Kennedy, C. (2018). Language and reading comprehension in middle childhood predicts emotional and behaviour difficulties in adolescence for those with permanent childhood hearing loss. *Journal of Child Psychology and Psychiatry, 59*(2), 180–190. https://doi.org/10.1111/jcpp.12803

Susser, M. (1973). *Causal thinking in the health sciences*. Oxford University Press.

Tabachnick, B. G., & Fidell, L. S. (2013). *Using multivariate statistics* (6th ed.). Pearson.

Thapar, A., & Rutter, M. (2019). Do natural experiments have an important future in the study of mental disorders. *Psychological Medicine, 49*(7), 1079–1088. https://doi.org/10.1017/S0033291718003896

Thoemmes, F. (2020). The assumptions of direction dependence analysis. *Multivariate Behavioral Research, 55*(4), 516–522. https://doi.org/10.1080/00273171.2019.1608800

Treur, J. L., Demontis, D., Smith, G. D., Sallis, H., Richardson, T. G., Wiers, R. W., et al. (2021). Investigating causality between liability to ADHD and substance use, and liability to substance use and ADHD risk, using Mendelian randomization. *Addiction Biology*. https://doi.org/10.1111/adb.12849

Valente, M. J., Rijnhart, J. J. M., Smyth, H. L., Muniz, F. B., & MacKinnon, D. P. (2020). Causal mediation programs in R, Mplus, SAS, SPSS, and Stata. *Structural Equation Modeling-A Multidisciplinary Journal, 27*(6), 975–984. https://doi.org/10.1080/10705511.2020.1777133

VanderWeele, T. J., & Ding, P. (2017). Sensitivity analysis in observational research: Introducing the E-value. *Annals of Internal Medicine, 167*(4), 268-+. https://doi.org/10.7326/m16-2607

Verbanck, M., Chen, C.-Y., Neale, B., & Do, R. (2018). Detection of widespread horizontal pleiotropy in causal relationships inferred from Mendelian randomization between complex traits and diseases. *Nature Genetics, 50*(5), 693–698. https://doi.org/10.1038/s41588-018-0099-7

Wakefield, A. J., Murch, S. H., Anthony, A., Linnell, J., Casson, D. M., Malik, M., et al. (1998). RETRACTED: Ileal-lymphoid-nodular hyperplasia, non-specific colitis, and pervasive developmental disorder in children (Retracted article. See vol 375, pg 445, 2010). *Lancet, 351*(9103), 637–641. https://doi.org/10.1016/s0140-6736(97)11096-0

Wall-Wieler, E., Bateman, B. T., Hanlon-Dearman, A., Roos, L. L., & Butwick, A. J. (2021). Association of epidural labor analgesia with offspring risk of autism spectrum disorders. *JAMA Pediatrics, 175*, 698–705. https://doi.org/10.1001/jamapediatrics.2021.0376

Wiedermann, W., & Li, X. T. (2018). Direction dependence analysis: A framework to test the direction of effects in linear models with an implementation in SPSS. *Behavior Research Methods, 50*(4), 1581–1601. https://doi.org/10.3758/s13428-018-1031-x

Wiedermann, W., & Sebastian, J. (2020). Direction dependence analysis in the presence of confounders: Applications to linear mediation models using observational data. *Multivariate Behavioral Research, 55*(4), 495–515. https://doi.org/10.1080/00273171.2018.1528542

Wiedermann, W., Reinke, W. M., & Herman, K. C. (2020). Prosocial skills causally mediate the relation between effective classroom management and academic competence: An application of direction dependence analysis. *Developmental Psychology, 56*(9), 1723–1735. https://doi.org/10.1037/dev0001087

Wilson, S., & Rhee, S. H. (2022). Special Issue editorial: Leveraging genetically informative study designs to understand the development and familial transmission of psychopathology. *Development and Psychopathology, 34*(5), 1645–1652. https://doi.org/10.1017/s0954579422000955

Zhang, T., Sidorchuk, A., Sevilla-Cermeno, L., Vilaplana-Perez, A., Chang, Z., Larsson, H., et al. (2019). Association of cesarean delivery with risk of neurodevelopmental and psychiatric disorders in the offspring: A systematic review and meta-analysis. *JAMA Network Open, 2*(8). https://doi.org/10.1001/jamanetworkopen.2019.1023

Zhang, T., Brander, G., Mantel, A., Kuja-Halkola, R., Stephansson, O., Chang, Z., et al. (2021). Assessment of cesarean delivery and neurodevelopmental and psychiatric disorders in the children of a population-based Swedish birth cohort. *JAMA Network Open, 4*(3). https://doi.org/10.1001/jamanetworkopen.2021.0837

Chapter 5
Conceptualising Behavioural Differences

5.1 Behavioural Individuality

The term "behavioural individuality" (BI) was used by Thomas et al. (1963) in the title of a book on their New York study of temperament in childhood. This term is useful as it encompasses the notion of individual difference but is neutral with respect to pathology and to the origins of such differences and can be applied to both categories and dimensions. However there has not been a wide uptake of the term in subsequent research on children's behaviour. Indeed today the use of the phrase is largely restricted to studies on animal behaviour, particularly the behaviour of fish, for example, Baptista et al. (2020). However there are parallels between studies on BI in human and non-human primates. These were reviewed by von Borell et al. (2019). They showed that temperament-like features in non-human primates showed a similar degree of cross-situation and overtime stability of individual differences as are found in studies of children.

One of the benefits of studying BI in animals is the degree of experimental control that can be achieved. Bierbach et al. (2017) showed that for cloned genetically identical fish (the Amazon molly, *Poecilia formosa*), reared in identical conditions and in social isolation, there were still marked individual difference in behaviour. One possible reason for the emergence of BI under these circumstances was suggested by Linneweber et al. (2020). In a study of BI in walking behaviour in the fruit fly (*Drosophila melanogaster*) they showed that there was a link between variability in the development of the brain and the emergence of individuality in walking behaviour. The flies were from genetically identical strains but nevertheless showed individuality in their walking behaviour. This BI was produced by "non-heritable noise" during brain development. There was a link between this stochastic variation in brain wiring and behavioural individuality.

Such a process would produce non-shared environmental effects in quantitative behaviour genetic models (see Sect. 3.1). Tikhodeyev and Shcherbakova (2019)

J. Stevenson, *Developmental Psychopathology*,
https://doi.org/10.1007/978-3-031-45787-6_5

have suggested that the non-shared environment effects need to be divided into those external influences affecting an individual and internal random effects, such as those found by Linneweber et al. (2020), that takes place during individual development. They suggest that studies indicate that these internal non-shared environment effects make a much larger contribution to behavioural variation than the external non-shared environment effects. Frith (2019) has indicated the possible importance of these random influences on neurodevelopmental disorders. Mitchell (2007) and White (2019) have outlined how some of these chance stochastic processes during neurodevelopment might influence behaviour.

Gidziela et al. (2023) have examined how well measures of these external influences can account for the effects of the non-shared environment in studies of children's behaviour problems. They used data from the TEDS study and found that with the measures available of differential experiences of twins, based on parent report, they were unable to account for more than 3% of the variance attributable to the non-shared environment. They identify this as a "missing NSE gap" equivalent to the missing heritability problem (see Sect. 3.2).

In addition to chance events there is evidence that BI in animals is also influenced by genetic factors. Ayroles et al. (2015) found that genotypes showed wide difference in their propensity for variability. Earlier Kain et al. (2012) found that BI was present across all strains of fruit fly that they tested and suggest that it is a ubiquitous feature of animal behaviour. Bell et al. (2009) undertook a meta-analysis of the extent to which individual differences in behaviour were repeatable. Repeatability is the fraction of behavioural variation that is due to differences between individuals. Behaviours that show relatively low within-individual variance compared to high between-individual variance are more repeatable. In other words, when individuals behave consistently through time and when individuals behave differently from each other, then the behaviour is repeatable. With estimates from 114 studies of 98 species they found an average repeatability of significantly greater than zero, that is, 0.37: ($CI_{.95}$ 0.36 to 0.38). This is a strong indication that stable individual differences are a pervasive feature of behaviour wherever it is studied. There is a growing interest in individual differences in behaviour in biology both in terms of options for understanding the molecular genetic basis of behaviour (Bengston et al., 2018) and for studies of ecology and evolution (Dingemanse & Dochtermann, 2013; Reale et al., 2007).

These animal studies provide insights that need to be borne in mind when studying BI in children. For example, the notion that chance events in brain development ("non-heritable noise") can contribute to individual differences suggests a source of non-shared environmental influences in quantitative genetic analyses. These biological processes during development may not be obvious candidates for non-shared environmental effects, but their effect will appear in this "E" component of ACE modelling (see Sect. 3.1).

In the studies of BI in children the form of variation that is being considered is that arising between individuals – interindividual variation. There is a second form of variation – intraindividual variation. The study of the former is referred to as nomothetic, and the study of intraindividual variation as idiographic. Molenaar

(2004) argues that there is an important role for idiographic studies, based on time-series data obtained from repeated measurement of individuals, to accompany nomothetic studies. The potential value of this approach was shown in a study by Hankin et al. (2011). They found that the moderating effect of a particular genetic variant in the 5-HTTLPR gene induced the increase in depression (but not anxiety) in children in response to stress. This interaction between gene and stressor was only shown when the stress was measured idiographically. The distinction here being that the idiographic stress measurement considers stress in relation to the child's average level over time. The nomothetic measure examined stress exposure relative to that in the sample as a whole. It is beyond the scope of this book to consider the findings from the idiographic approach, although within-person repeated measures are employed in some of the studies discussed – for example, reaction time variability in children with attention-deficit hyperactivity disorder (ADHD) and autism spectrum disorder (ASD) (Karalunas et al., 2014). For a framework that attempts an integration of the idiographic and nomothetic approaches see Beltz et al. (2016). See Sect. 4.3 for a discussion of the related issue of between-person and within-person effects in the analysis of cross-lagged measures.

5.2 Behavioural Individuality and Temperament

Behavioural individuality in the young child was equated to temperamental differences in the original Thomas and Chess usage (Thomas & Chess, 1957). Such temperamental variation is couched in terms of difference in the child's style of observable behaviour, that is, how they behave. As we shall see below there has been a drift in the use of the term temperament so that it has been enlarged to incorporate individual differences in the mechanism underlying behaviour such as attention, cognition, and motivation, that is, why they behave.

Thomas and Chess developed a typology of temperament types based on the nine-dimensional scheme that had emerged in their interviews with parents (Birch et al., 1962; Thomas et al., 1968). These dimensions were activity level, rhythmicity, approach or withdrawal, adaptability, intensity of reaction, threshold of responsiveness, quality of mood, distractibility, and attention span and persistence. Based on these dimensions they identified three types of temperament. The first of these is the "easy" child who shows regular biological functioning, initial approach, adaptability, and positive mood. The second is the "difficult" child showing the opposite pattern: irregular functions, withdrawal, slow adaptability, and negative mood. The third is the "slow to warm up" child characterised as slow to adapt, have negative moods, and show low intensity of reactions.

The notion of personality covers a similar ground to temperament but includes additional elements of self-regulation. The distinction between the two was made by Rutter (1987) in the following way:

> … temperament is best viewed in terms of a relatively small number of simple, non-motivational, non cognitive, stylistic features of which emotionality, activity and sociability are the best validated. It is possible that these characteristics have fairly direct neurobiological correlates but this has yet to be demonstrated. By contrast, personality refers to the coherence of functioning that derives from how people react to their given attributes, how they think about themselves, and how they put these together into some form of conceptual whole. Rutter (1987), p. 454

Temperament is seen as quantitative differences between children. They can however be used to describe types, that is, qualitative differences, and at extremes can be considered dysfunctional. Graham et al. (1973) clarify these distinctions very well:

> It is generally agreed that it is useful to distinguish between personality and illness, or, on a more molecular level, between traits and symptoms. ….. [the] distinction between symptoms (which are stressful, inhibit adjustment, disrupt the normal continuity of behaviour, are experienced as alien to the personality, are transient, and may be idiosyncratic) and traits (which facilitate adjustment, are the "how" of behaviour, are dispositional, may be constitutionally determined, are relatively persistent, and are universally present in the population). Graham et al. (1973), p. 336

However, as will be discussed, this distinction between symptoms (of illness) and traits (of temperament) has been difficult to sustain with both tending to be persistent and both being influenced by constitutional factors.

How does behavioural individuality (BI) develop? This starts with antenatal influences. These will include genetic differences which will influence BI from the time they begin to shape brain development early in foetal development. There are also a number of antenatal effects on BI that are attributable to maternal nutrition and hormones. This range of biological factors is not independent of the social environment, for example, maternal hormone levels are changed by stressful experiences. The child is subsequently embedded in a set of influences in the context of the family and later broader social influences from peer groups and the like. This complex set of biological and experiential factors engage with each other. Boyce et al. (1998) define this social context for development as

> a set of interpersonal conditions, relevant to a particular behaviour or disorder and external to, but shaped and interpreted by, the individual child. Boyce et al. (1998), p. 143

For BI Thomas and Chess described part of this engagement as a "goodness of fit". This is the notion that certain features of BI are better suited to a particular family context than others. This fit does not mean that one feature of BI is better than another; rather certain BIs are suited to one family but not to another. Moreover this "goodness of fit" is not static. The family will influence the child, and the child will influence the family.

This latter process was brought to the fore by Bell (1968). He reviewed studies that purported to show the effects of parenting on the child. However this classic paper demonstrated that these relationships have to be seen as interactional with the effects of children on parents acting alongside the effects of parents on children.

Boyce et al. (1998) describe this process as follows:

> There is continuous *interplay* between features of the child and aspects of the social context in which the child is raised. This bidirectional transaction of context- upon-child and child-upon-context results in a continuous, mutually influential exchange between the developing individual and his or her social and physical environments. Boyce et al. (1998), p. 152

Transactional Model How then is it best to examine the joint effects of parent on child and child on the parent? Sameroff and Chandler (1975) took this notion of an interchange of effects a stage further in a transactional model. This model is based on the notion that that there is, as per Boyce et al. (1998) above, a continuous process of mutual influence between the child and the social context. This same transactional approach was proposed to account for the development of conduct problems in children and adolescents (Dodge & Pettit, 2003; Dodge et al., 2008). They posited that biological predispositions and the socio-cultural context mutually influenced each other and generated a series of experiences and responses that lead the child to be ill-equipped to deal with problematic social situations, other than by aggression.

The response of children to the experience of parental divorce and remarriage has also been formulated as a transactional model which emphasises the potential role of temperament as a moderator of the child's response to this stress (Hetherington et al., 1998). The complexities and importance of such transactions have been emphasised by Hinde (1992), particularly the effects of relationships on relationships. Such an approach

> … calls attention to the effects of interactions on interactions within a relationship and between relationships, so that a mother's marriage may affect (or be affected by) the mother-child relationship. Hinde (1992), p. 1025

Sameroff and MacKenzie (2003) identify the difficulties in trying to study a transactional system:

> These obstacles are theoretical (assessing dynamic system); logistic, (developing longitudinal studies with enough time points and large enough samples); and methodological, (assessing multiple interacting domains over time in order to identify points of qualitative change). Sameroff and MacKenzie (2003), p. 614

An early attempt to test a transactional model of mutual influences between mother and child measures was made by Hammen et al. (1990). The children were aged 8–16 years, and the study was longitudinal over a 6-month period. The model tested is shown in Fig. 5.1. They found that there was evidence that maternal functioning is related to the development of psychopathology in the child; the child's characteristics also contribute to maternal well-being in a cycle of negative mutual influence. A transactional model was similarly tested by Lansford et al. (2011). They used data from two longitudinal studies of children in middle childhood and adolescence to test for the bidirectional effects between parent's physical discipline and children's externalising behaviour. In both samples they found significant effects in both directions in a cross-lagged analysis (see Sect. 4.3). These studies

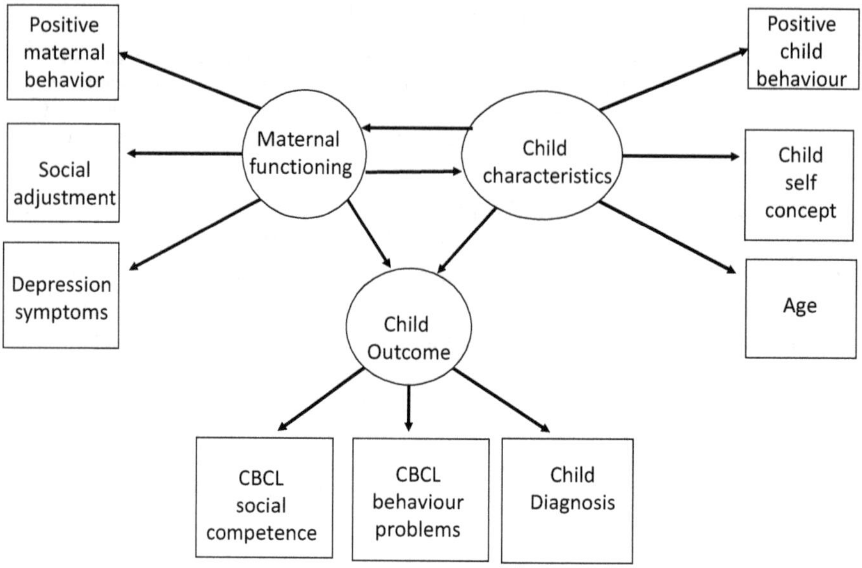

Fig. 5.1 Transactional model of maternal and child influences on psychopathology. (Adapted with the permission of American Psychological Association from Fig. 1 Hammen et al. (1990) *Developmental Psychology, 26*(1), 24–30; permission conveyed through Copyright Clearance Center, Inc.)

were not able to exclude the possibility that some of the relationships observed might arise from genetic influences shared by mother and child.

An example of the use of a genetically informative design to investigate bidirectional effects is that of Larsson et al. (2008). They used data from a longitudinally studied sample of 6230 twin pairs and employed a cross-lagged analysis as shown in Fig. 5.2. This analysis identified significant effects from the child's antisocial behaviour at age 4 acting to increase parental negativity when the child was aged 7 ($\beta = -0.15$). There was a similar sized effect ($\beta = 0.12$) of parental negativity when the child was aged 4 on antisocial behaviour at age 7 years. In these analyses the effects of possible shared genetic effects are taken into account. This study, and that of Lansford et al. (2011), suggests that the association between parenting and child antisocial behaviour is best explained by both parent-driven and child-driven effects. This conclusion is supported by findings on antisocial behaviour from a range of alternative research designs (Jaffee et al., 2012).

Speyer, Hall, Hang, Hughes, and Murray (2022) have shown the value of the application to transactional processes of autoregressive latent variable models with structural residuals outlined in Sect. 4.3. The importance of this method of analysis is that it can separate the effects of stable between-family differences from within-family changes over time. They found evidence for child-to-parent, parent-to-child, and parent-to-parent effects playing a role in the development of mental health difficulties for both parent and child.

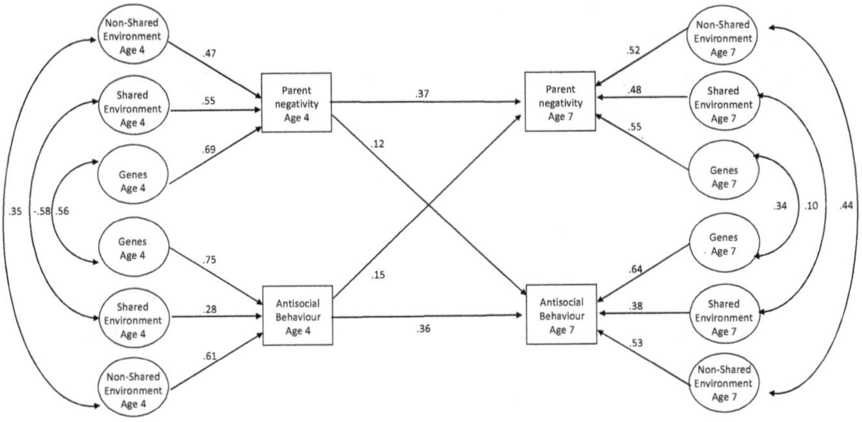

Fig. 5.2 Transactional model of parental and child influences on antisocial behaviour in a genetically informative study. (Adapted with the permission of Springer Nature BV from Fig. 2 Larsson et al. (2008). *Journal of Abnormal Child Psychology, 36*(5),633–645; permission conveyed through Copyright Clearance Center, Inc.)

In these studies of the mutual influences between parent and child there is a need to deal with the potential confound of passive gene–environment correlations (see Sect. 3.1). One study design that can avoid this confound is that of the longitudinal study of adoptive mothers and their adopted children. Roben et al. (2015) showed that the adoptive mothers' depressive symptoms when their adopted child was 9 months old increased the likelihood that the children reacted negatively to their mothers' negative behaviour when they were 18 months. This increase in the child's negative response was in turn predictive of higher levels of depressive symptoms on the adoptive mother 9 months later. Ahmadzadeh et al. (2019) used data from adoptive families to investigate the transactional process of transmission of anxiety symptoms between parent and child. They found that child anxiety symptoms at age 7 years predicted adoptive mothers' anxiety symptoms 1 year later. There was no evidence of mother-to-child or child-to-father effects. In both these studies the use of adopted children precluded a passive gene–environment correlation influencing the results.

Studies of bidirectional relationships between child and parents were reviewed by Paschall and Mastergeorge (2016). They acknowledged that some advances had been made but that many studies lacked the analytic methods and design features to provide clear evidence of the nature and strength of the transactional processes involved. In addition to the requirement for longitudinal studies, they identify the particular value of incorporating more advanced data analysis methods based on structural equation modelling and of adopting of genetically informative designs.

An example of the value of using structural equation modelling (see Sect. 2.5) is the study by Sokolovic et al. (2021). However they were only concerned with bidirectional effects over short time intervals in the context of mother–child discussions about recent conflicts. They used detailing codings of 5 minutes of discussion between mothers and children from two age groups. The younger children were between 5 and 9 years of age and the older sample between 7 and 13 years. Of central interest was the relation over 20-second time intervals between the extent of the mother's and child's constructiveness or destructiveness shown in the discussion. The bidirectional relationships were analysed using a dynamic structural equation modelling technique (Asparouhov et al., 2018). Mothers were not found to influence the balance of constructiveness and destructiveness children display from one 20-s interval to the next. By contrast children did influence their mothers' subsequent constructiveness. There was a difference between the way the mothers changed in relation to their children according to the age of the child. With their youngest children (i.e. age 7 or less), mothers were likely to offer more opposite responses (constructiveness following the child's destructiveness and vice versa). With their older children, mothers followed the child's lead and displayed more constructiveness or destructiveness in alignment with what their children had displayed in the previous interval.

A second example of the value of adopting structural equation modelling is the study by Xerxa et al. (2020) on the bidirectional relationships between parental separation, family conflicts, and child behaviour problems. The analysis included a method of the four-way decomposition of mediation and moderation (see Sect. 2.2) developed by VanderWeele (2014). This method can identify how much of an effect is mediated, how much is due to interaction, how much is due to both mediation and interaction together, and how much is due to neither. The data were obtained in a prospective study of a large general population sample of pregnant women and their families. The outcome measure of child behaviour problems was taken at ages 3, 5, and 9 years. They found that if parental separation occurs in families with low levels of conflict, parental separation does not relate to more child problem behaviour. They also showed that child problem behaviour has an influence in the opposite direction by fostering the persistence of family conflict.

Non-Shared Environment Genetically informative studies have resulted in major refinements of the way environmental influences on BI were understood. In behaviour genetic analysis it is rare to find heritabilities greater than 50%. This means that environmental influences must account for the remaining variance. This could either be factors that contribute to resemblance between siblings (the shared environment) or that contribute to differences between siblings (the non-shared environment). Plomin and Daniels (1987) reviewed this literature and came to the conclusion that the major environmental influences make children in a family different from, not similar to, one another. This influence is the non-shared environment.

Along with genes the effects of the non-shared environment will be to promote BI within families. This has been shown, for example, in relation to individual differences in positive qualities such as subjective well-being (SWB) and temperament positive affect (PA). In a twin and family study of SWB in adolescent and young adult twins, Bartels and Boomsma (2009) found that over half of the variance was attributable to the non-shared environment. Flom et al. (2018) examined PA based on both parent's report and direct observation of behaviour – a measure based on the frequency of smiles and/or laughter in structured episodes in the laboratory. In this study of 3-year-old twins both parent-rated and observed PA were influenced by genes. The observed PA was also substantially influenced by the non-shared environments. These studies indicate that experiences specific to the individual are promoting positive features of behaviour and emotions in children.

For measures of psychopathology once measurement error is taken into account the shared environment contributes little to explaining the variance. This conclusion was challenged by Burt (2009, 2014), who showed that for psychopathology in children a shared environment effect could be detected consistently. In her meta-analyses, the shared environment was significant for the main categories of psychopathology in children with the exception of attention-deficit/hyperactivity problems. However these shared environment effects were still less important (explaining 10–16% of the variance) than the non-shared environment (25–42% of the variance). In light of these findings, Plomin et al. (2016) concluded that "most environmental effects are not shared by children growing up in the same family" as one of the Top 10 Replicated Findings from Behavioural Genetics (see Sect. 3.5).

Temperament and Later Mental Health There is well-replicated evidence that aspects of early difficult temperament are risk factors for later mental problems in childhood (Rende, 1993), adolescence (Caspi et al., 1995; Leve et al., 2005), and into early adulthood (Bould et al., 2014).

The mechanisms that might mediate these relationships were investigated using measures of temperament at age 2 years and mental health at ages 21–23 years (Wu et al., 2022). They examined three possibilities. The first was that difficult temperament had a direct effect. The second was that these effects were in part mediated via an influence on a general psychopathology factor (see Sect. 6.6) in middle childhood. The third possibility was that the mediated effects were moderated by aspects of parenting during the preschool period. In this sample of 1892 children there was evidence of both a direct effect of difficult temperament on depressive symptoms in adulthood and of mediation via an intermediate general psychopathology factor. However there was no evidence that the features of parenting behaviour moderated these relationships. These findings were obtained using data from the Avon Longitudinal Study of Parents and Children (ALSPAC) cohort. Using this same data set Wu et al. (2022) were able to show that early difficult temperament was also a vulnerability factor for the failure to sustain engagement in education or the labour force in early adulthood.

5.3 Dimensions and Categories

The framing of BI as either temperament types or traits by Thomas et al. (1968) has parallels in other aspects of behavioural differences. Clark et al. (2017) discuss the alternative approaches to the classification of psychiatric disorder in DSM-5, ICD-11, and the National Institute of Mental Health's Research Domain Criteria (RDoC). DSM-5 stands for the Diagnostic and Statistical Manual of Mental Disorders (Fifth Edition) and is the dominant classificatory framework adopted in the United States. ICD-11 stands for the International Classification of Disease

(Eleventh Edition) produced by the World Health Organization. This provides a diagnostic classification of all aspects of health, not just mental health, that is adopted worldwide. The RDoC by contrast does not provide a diagnostic classification of mental health but instead focuses on the complex overlapping multidimensionality of mental illness. It is a framework that aims to situate mental health in the context of brain–behaviour relations across developmental and environmental contexts. DSM-5 and ICD-11 identify types, and RDoC identifies equivalents to traits.

Clark et al. (2017) suggest there are four key issues that present challenges to understanding and classifying mental disorder: aetiology, including the multiple causality of mental disorder; whether the relevant phenomena are discrete categories or dimensions; thresholds, which set the boundaries between disorder and non-disorder; and comorbidity, the fact that individuals with mental illness often meet diagnostic requirements for multiple conditions. These are all issues that apply equally to childhood mental disorders as they do to those in adults.

The impact of the RDoC on research into developmental psychopathology has been reviewed by Pacheco et al. (2022). They have shown that a move away from a symptom-based diagnostic framework to one more closely based on the biological and psychological mechanisms underlying mental illness is being reflected in the research being undertaken, specifically that funded by the National Institute of Mental Health in the United States. This is leading to both a greater emphasis on features of behaviour defined by their biology and on transdiagnostic problems. The transdiagnostic approach addresses the common behavioural features that underpin various diagnoses and attempts to identify the mechanisms operating to produce these features across conditions. Understanding the implications of RDoC for intervention and treatment of psychopathology is still at an early stage and as yet not fully understood.

There have been, and continue to be, radical changes to the theoretical frameworks adopted in studies in psychopathology. The time of all-encompassing theories, such as psychoanalysis, family therapy, attachment theory, and behaviourism, has passed and the science has moved on (Rutter & Stevenson, 2008). Although contributing to the development of subsequent more focussed theoretical formulations that were potentially falsifiable, these "big theories" have been superseded. This is despite attempts, for example, with psychoanalysis, to align thinking with developments in other branches of science (Kandel, 1999: Fonagy, 2003).

There are moves to understand adult psychiatric disorders in terms of dimensions rather than categories (e.g. Brown & Barlow, 2005; Widiger & Samuel, 2005). One of the most extensive examinations of the relationship between dimensional and categorical measures of psychopathology was undertaken by Taylor et al. (2019). They used data from a large population-based sample of 13,923 twin pairs. There were genetic correlations between the diagnostic categories and dimensional trait measures ranging from 0.31 to 0.69. They developed a range of polygenic risk scores (PRS) (see Sect. 3.4) for categorical disorders. These show strong relationships with the population trait measures. For example, at age 9 years the standardised regression coefficient for the prediction of ADHD trait score from the ADHD PRS was $\beta = 0.27$ ($CI_{.95}$ 0.21 to 0.33). The results suggest that that genetic factors associated with many psychiatric disorders are also associated with variation in less severe levels of characteristic traits throughout the general population. Consequently many psychiatric disorders are better characterised as continuous phenotypes rather than as categories.

The dimensional approach has been taken further in studies that examine the role of both genetic and environmental factors in mental health. Kendler et al. (2011) found that in a population of young adults that the organisation of common psychiatric disorders arose from genetic (not environmental) factors operating on internalising and externalising dimensions. Lahey et al. (2011) showed that these same dimensions underlie child and adolescent psychopathology and were primarily influenced by genetic liabilities.

There is a consequent need to develop scales that identify individual differences in behaviour across the full range. An example of this is the Extended Strengths and Weaknesses Assessment of Normal Behavior (E-SWAN) scales (Alexander et al., 2020). The scales were developed to assess behaviour variation that underpins panic disorder, social anxiety, major depression, and disruptive mood dysregulation disorder and build on an earlier dimensional measure of ADHD (Swanson et al., 2012).

An additional case for studying the full continuum of behavioural variation was made in relation to ADHD by Greven et al. (2018). They suggest this approach allows investigations to include the positive end of mental health rather than concentrating on deviations from the average towards pathology. Possible indicators of positive mental health can aid clinicians not least by identifying possible protective factors.

However there are good reasons not to consider categories and dimensions as competing frameworks for understanding behavioural differences (Zubin, 1967). Pickles and Angold (2003) concluded that much of the debate over categories and dimensions in psychopathology is misconceived. They argue that psychopathology is not observed directly. Instead research observes and studies its properties. Some of these properties are best considered dimensional and others categorical. The analogy they draw is with light. This is a phenomenon that has a duality. It can be considered as a wave or as particle. They say:

> When it comes to understanding refraction, a conception of light as behaving as a continuous wave turns out to be helpful, whereas particulate behaviour is more helpful conceptually for understanding reflection and energy transfer. In the same way, to understand depression, we find circumstances where it behaves as a dimension and circumstances where it behaves as a more discrete phenomenon. Pickles and Angold (2003), p. 547

They analysed the relationship between symptoms counts of puberty (Tanner scores) and counts of depression symptoms. These are both seemingly dimensional measures. However they conclude that the relationship between these two measures is most parsimoniously described as categorical. They emphasise that it is well known that if a genuine continuous relationship exists between two measures turning the measures into categories will lose power and underestimate the size of their relationship. They show that in the case of puberty and depressive symptoms the reverse is also true. Imposing a continuous metric on a categorical relationship may underestimate the strength of this relationship. They go on to argue that it will rarely be the case in psychopathology that one of the approaches, dimensional or categorical, will clearly be more appropriate than the other. Investigations therefore need to continue to consider both theoretical perspectives rather than considering this an all-or-none issue. A similar conclusion was reached earlier by Zubin (1967):

> The conflict between typology and dimensionality may be a pseudoconflict dependent upon the state of knowledge of the field. Zubin (1967), p. 398

Kagan (2018) takes the argument for categories further. He argues not just that categories may represent a better way to represent psychological characteristics but that there should be a routine attention to identified types in addition by features such as gender, class, and ethnicity. He argues that when this is done important differential risks are identified. So rather than controlling for the effects of these demographic variables they should be investigated as identifying kinds of individuals with distinctive patterns of relationship between risk and outcome. A demonstration of the complementarity between dimensional and categorical approaches is provided by Planalp and Goldsmith (2020). They used latent profile analysis (see Sect. 2.5) to identify types of children by their profiles on measures of temperament. They suggest that

> profiles also tend to highlight groups with extreme standing on any dimension of temperament in the profile. These extreme values may hold more functional significance than variants within the middle of the distribution. The argument is not that profile- based approaches should replace dimensional approaches but rather that the profile approach provides a needed complementary perspective. Planalp and Goldsmith (2020), p. e566

Coghill and Sonuga-Barke (2012) similarly argue that both dimensional and categorical approaches have value and that this will vary from disorder to disorder. They emphasise the importance of this dual approach especially in relation to the translation of scientific findings to clinical practice. They say:

> Where a dimensional model appears more appropriate, scientists and clinicians need to work together, rather than against each other as has often been the case in the past, to address and better understand the tensions and relationships between these dimensional disorders and the traditional categorical models. Coghill and Sonuga-Barke (2012), p. 485

There are methods of analysis of behaviours that can preserve the characteristics of both a continuum and a categorical model (Borsboom et al., 2016). These include factor mixture models (Lubke & Muthen, 2005) and grade-of-membership models (Woodbury et al., 1978). Factor mixture modelling has been shown to be able to identify relatively homogeneous sub-groups of children with ASD (Georgiades et al., 2013). They used continuum measures of “social communication deficits” and of “fixated interests and repetitive behaviours”. Based on the severity scores on these two dimensions three relatively homogeneous sub-groups were identified. It has been shown subsequently that sub-groups of children with ASD identified on the basis of these two dimensions have distinct neural circuitry and genetic profiles (Bertelsen et al., 2021). The conclusion from this study was that a blend of both continuum and categorical approaches may be the most appropriate way to examine the neural basis of variation in ASD.

There have been counter-arguments to Kagan (2018) that suggest that distinct categories are only found infrequently. Haslam et al. (2012) reviewed the literature that has examined whether the distinction categories (or taxa) are to be found in personality and in psychopathology. They concluded that latent categories are very rarely found in studies of either normal and abnormal personality. They are sometimes present in studies of psychopathology, including autism, but are infrequently present in studies of internalising and externalising behaviour. The strong trend in recent research supports the dimensional approach to psychopathology. A meta-analysis of categorical and dimensional measures of psychopathology showed that the use of continuous measures improved both reliability and validity (Markon et al., 2011). Indeed the increase in validity was sufficient to halve the sample size needed to achieve standard power requirements.

A framework for differentiating categories (taxa) and dimensions (factors) as the latent structure underlying psychopathology was developed by Meehl (1995). Based on this framework, Ruscio et al. (2007) developed a method (Comparison Curve Fit Index [CCFI]) to test whether a categorical or a dimension model best fitted the data. A comprehensive meta-analysis of studies using the CCFI method on a wide range of psychological domains, including psychopathology, has shown that the great majority of individual differences in psychological characteristics are best explained by underlying continua rather than categories (Haslam et al., 2020). The exception in this analysis was autism for which there were tentative indications in support of a categorical model. This is of interest given the findings Georgiades et al. (2013) and Bertelsen et al. (2021) discussed above.

These findings are supported by a study by Deserno et al. (2022). They applied the CCFI test to scores on children with ADHD and ASD and typically developing (TD) children. They found that a dimensional model best fitted the data for the ADHD and TD children. The opposite was the case for the ASD and TD children, where the data were more consistent with a categorical model.

For these reasons, with the possible exception of ASD, it is preferable to start research investigation of behavioural individuality and psychopathology with a dimensional model. It has been forcefully argued by Ben Lahey (2021) that there are additional reasons to abandon a categorical model of psychopathology. He suggests that there is an urgent need to move away from the binary diagnostic categories in a medical model of mental "illness" as is embodied in the DSM-5. The case for this reorientation made by Lahey (2021) is based on the following assertions:

1. There is no qualitative difference between normal and abnormal psychological functioning. Psychological problems are not illnesses but rather problematic ways of thinking, feeling, and behaving that lie on a continuum of severity.
2. There are no clear boundaries between types of psychological problems. These dimensions are often associated, and consequently people may experience problems in more than one dimension at any one time.

3. These psychological problems are not rare. At some time in their lives most people will experience problems.
4. The correlations between these problems reflect a hierarchically organised range of influences some of which have a generic effect and some that influence specific aspects of psychological functioning.
5. Although moderately stable these psychological problems can change over time and frequently show differences in stability in males and females.
6. These patterns of behaviour arise from the interplay of genes and experiences, and these factors operate in a similar way across the range of problem severity.

This account of the need to abandon the binary (ill/not ill) categoric system of DSM argues that not only does the dimensional approach more accurately reflect the findings in the scientific literature but also provides a more socially acceptable and less stigmatising view of psychological problems. For these reasons the dimensional framework endorsed by Lahey is the one that will be emphasised in the subsequent chapters of this book when discussing psychological problems in children and adolescents.

5.4 Characterising the Behaviour of Preschool Children

There is an unresolved issue regarding the way behavioural differences are conceptualised in the preschool child. As was discussed in Sect. 5.2 above, temperament differences are apparent from infancy onwards. What is less clear is how behaviour problems should be conceptualised in very young children. Should they be treated simply as a downward extension of the problems identified in older children? Or are there important distinct issues arising from developmental immaturity that make this approach inappropriate?

Campbell (2002) provides a helpful framework to consider the relative severity of the behaviour shown by a preschool child. She suggests that *worrisome* or *annoying behaviour* refers to typical and age-appropriate behaviour that may however concern some parents. An *age-specific problem behaviour* she takes to refer to an exaggeration in the frequency and/or intensity of typical behaviour to an upsetting degree, something which may or may not be a sign of more serious difficulty to come. *Symptomatic behaviour* designates a problem of probable clinical significance.

There has been a move towards developing clear diagnostic criteria for psychiatric problems in preschool children (Scheeringa et al., 2003). There is good evidence for the existence of psychopathology in 0–5-year-olds that conforms to the "conventional nosology" used in the DSM system. Scheeringa et al. (2003) suggests that this evidence is strongest for disruptive disorders – attention-deficit hyperactivity disorder (ADHD), oppositional-defiant disorder (ODD), and conduct disorder

Dimension	Illustrative clinical manifestations	
	DSM-IV symptom	Preschool manifestations
Aggression *Tendency to respond aggressively across a variety of contexts, ranging from expectable self-protection and mild aggressive teasing/play to severe violence*	'Uses a weapon to harm others' 'Often fights'	– Hits adults – Hurts others on purpose
Temper Loss *Overt expression and management of anger, ranging from normative mild-moderate expressions of anger in response to frustration to extreme dysregulated temper*	'Often loses temper' 'Often angry'	– Has destructive tantrums – Has trouble calming down when angry
Noncompliance *Resistance to, and failure to comply with, directives, rules and social norms, ranging from normative assertions of autonomy to pervasive and active disregard of rules/norms.*	'Often defies' 'Steals'	– Automatically resists when asked to do something – Is sneaky about rule breaking
Low Concern for Others *Active disregard of needs and feelings of others, including lack of guilt for transgressions and lack of empathy. Ranges normatively from mild insensitivity or disregard within contexts of stress or conflict to extreme and persistent disregard of others across a range of interactions and contexts*	'Is physically cruel' 'Forced sexual activity'	– Does not seem to care about pleasing others – Does not try to behave after being punished

Fig. 5.3 Illustration of developmental specification of behaviours within the core disruptive behaviour dimensions for the preschool period. (Reproduced with the permission of John Wiley & Sons from Table 1 Wakschlag et al. (2010) *Journal of Child Psychology and Psychiatry, 51*(1), 3–22; permission conveyed through Copyright Clearance Center, Inc.)

(CD) – and for major depressive disorder (MDD). Wakschlag et al. (2007) and Wakschlag et al. (2010) examined further the evidence for the categorising of disruptive disorders in the preschool child. They comment on the inappropriateness of viewing behaviour in this age as a downward extension of those seen in middle childhood and adolescence. They propose a fourfold set of core dimensions that characterise disruptive behaviour in the preschool period, and these are shown in Fig. 5.3.

They suggest that

> there is also widespread agreement that existing systems are insufficiently informed by developmental principles, imprecise in regard to discriminating underlying dimensions, minimally informative about the relation and boundaries between the broad range of normative misbehaviors and psychopathological forms of disruptive behavior, and of limited utility in explaining variation and continuity over the lifespan and in response to intervention. Wakschlag et al. (2010), p. 15

Gardner and Shaw (2008) concluded that there are considerable uncertainties over defining disorders in the preschool child. They adopt a broad classification into "disruptive problems" which include problems with oppositional behaviour and attentional deficits and "emotional problems" related to depression and anxiety. In addition they identify a group of problems related to feeding (infant, colic, failure to thrive, and food refusal). To these there are additional problems related to regulation such as those concerned with sleep (night settling and night waking). Others have argued that there is a similar structure for problems in both the preschool period and for older children, for example, Olino et al. (2014) – see Sect. 6.5 for a more extensive discussion of the studies on the structure of behaviour problems in the preschool period.

An early epidemiological study of behaviour problems in preschool children was undertaken by Richman et al. (1982). This study of 828 three-year-olds in the general population established the prevalence rate of mild problems to be 15%, of moderate severity to be 6% and, of severe problems to be 1%. These severity categories are to some extent arbitrary, but what was clear was that problematic behaviour was strongly linked with challenging family circumstances, such as those arising from inadequate housing. The methods used in this study were adopted at about the same time in another London-based study (Coleman et al., 1977) and in a rural American community (Earls, 1980). In both cases the rates of behaviour problems were similar to that found in Waltham Forest but slightly lower rates of overall problems in the American sample.

The Waltham Forest Study findings also suggested a strong reciprocal association between parent well-being and the young child's behaviour. The studies on the well-being of parents were reviewed by Nelson et al. (2014), who concluded

> … that the relationship between parenthood and well-being is highly complex. We propose that parents are unhappy to the extent that they encounter relatively greater negative emotions, magnified financial problems, more sleep disturbance, and troubled marriages. By contrast, when parents experience greater meaning in life, satisfaction of their basic needs, greater positive emotions, and enhanced social roles, they are met with happiness and joy. p. 846
> and
> parents' happiness appears to have critical implications for a wide range of children's outcomes. Nelson et al. (2014), p. 887

This review by Nelson et al. (2014) also brought out the impact of child temperament on parent well-being. They suggest that difficult temperament elevates negative emotions, reduces a parent's sense of competence, and affects marital satisfaction adversely. By contrast an easy temperament in a child can foster positive emotions and a feeling of competence in parents, especially fathers (Sirignano & Lachman, 1985). Clearly when studying behaviour in the young child is essential to consider the reciprocal effects of interactions between parental well-being and child behaviour.

This question of the importance of behaviour problems in the preschool child is put into context in a review by Vasileva et al. (2021). They conducted a meta-analysis of studies on 18,282 children under the age of 7 years. The pooled prevalence of mental disorders was 20.1% ($CI_{.95}$ 15.7 to 25.4) of which there are a significant number who needed appropriate treatment. Commenting on these findings, Fisher (2021) draws out the importance of early intervention to prevent the establishment of long-term disorder particularly for the group meeting the diagnostic criteria for two or more disorders where the estimated prevalence was 6.4% ($CI_{.95}$ 1.3 to 54.0). She points out that this sub-group is known to respond less well to treatment at later ages (Weisz et al., 2017).

5.5 Genetic Studies of Categories and Dimensions

The CCFI method developed by Ruscio et al. (2007), discussed above, tests category/dimension models based on the distribution of scores on symptom measures. A more direct route to test the distinction is the application of genetically informative research designs. These can determine whether categories, based on membership of groups that are at the extreme of a dimension, are more (or less) influenced by genetic factors than individual differences in the normal range.

The question of the relationship between trait-like measures of individual differences and categorical measures of deviance has been examined in a number of genetically informative studies. Colvert et al. (2015) used measures of autism spectrum disorder, a broad autism phenotype, and structured diagnostic assessment of autism with a large population sample of twins. They found that the spectrum and categorical disorder were primarily influenced by additive genetic factors with heritabilities of 0.56–0.95 and 0.76–0.95, respectively. They therefore concluded that the genetic factors influencing individual differences in autistic-like traits overlap considerably with those genetic factors influencing diagnoses of autism. Thus the spectrum model can be applied not just to common aspects of psychopathology but also to less prevalent conditions such as autism.

An early study of the possible differences in heritability for extreme scores and normal range heritability for behaviour problems showed that these heritabilities were similar (Graham & Stevenson, 1985). This analysis was based on ratings of behaviour on the Rutter scales (Elander & Rutter, 1996) by mothers, fathers, and teachers. The heritability of extreme scores roughly parallels the size of heritability of behavioural symptoms within the non-deviant range; in almost all cases these heritabilities were greater than zero. This, of course, does not necessarily mean that the same genetic influences are acting in the two cases. It was this finding that led Graham and Stevenson (1987) to propose that that ordinary, non-pathological behaviours, in extreme form, can be viewed as manifestations of emotional disorder, hyperactivity, and antisocial disorder. This is a version of what Nigg (2006) refers to as the spectrum/common cause model of the relationship between temperament and behaviour problems as follows:

> Normal and abnormal fall at different points on the same continuum, such that temperament is basically a subclinical manifestation of psychopathology, with shared etiological determinants. Nigg (2006), p. 405

DF Multiple Regression Method Twin data can be used to test directly whether the causes of extreme group membership differ from those producing individual difference in the normal range by using the DeFries and Fulker (1985) multiple regression method (DF). This identifies the extent to which genetic and environmental factors contribute to extreme group membership for a condition that can be measured on a continuum (see Sect. 3.5). It is based on the principle that if genetic factors are important, the co-twin of MZ in the extreme group (probands) will regress to the population mean less than the co-twins of DZ probands. To distinguish this type of heritability from that obtained in the wider general population (h^2) it is referred to as group heritability (h^2_g).

The DF method has been used to estimate h^2 and h^2_g for a number of behavioural differences in children. Deater-Deckard et al. (1997) compared h^2 and h^2_g for internalising and externalising behaviours in young adolescents. They found values that were very similar with h^2 slightly higher than h^2_g but not significantly so – mean $h^2 = 0.63$ and mean $h^2_g = 0.46$. Rende et al. (2006) used the DF regression approach to examine genetic and shared environment influence on persistent high levels and persistent low levels of depressive symptoms in adolescence. Significant genetic effects were found for both persistent and non-persistent low depression. Stevenson et al. (1992) tested the magnitude of genetic and environmental influences on individual differences and extreme fearfulness in twins aged 1–18 years. They found that genetic influences were stronger for fears that represented a threat to life, that is, fear of the unknown, fear of injury and small animals, and fear of danger. In each of these cases the values of h^2 and h^2_g were similar (h^2 = 0.0.46, 0.46, 0.34 and h^2_g = 0.50, 0.60 0.47, respectively). This DF method of analysis has been applied also to ADHD (e.g. Levy et al., 1997) and to cognitive abilities such as reading (e.g. DeFries et al., 1987). Martin et al. (2018) have reviewed the studies by applying the DF approach, and other methods, to test for shared genetic influences on psychiatric disorders and traits. They conclude that there is good evidence from twin and molecular genetic methods that certain child-onset neurodevelopmental disorders, such as ADHD and autism, are at the extreme ends of continuous distributions of population traits.

By varying the definition of extreme group membership it is possible to use twin data to test whether the contribution of genetic and environmental factors is greater or smaller as more extreme groups are identified. This approach has been applied to attention-related problems in a sample of Norwegian twins (Gjone et al., 1996). They divided the sample into pairs with a twin with a score of 0.5, 1.0, or 1.5 standard deviations above the mean, that is, with increasing degrees of attention problems. They found that there was no change in the size of genetic influences on attention problems across severity groups after accounting for the influence of possible confounders such as cerebral palsy, epilepsy, and low birth weight. This suggests that it is most parsimonious to consider severe problems of inattention as being caused simply by factors operating on differences in the normal range.

A method to provide a more detailed appraisal of changes in heritability across a spectrum was developed by Logan et al. (2012). This uses the basic DF regression approach and then applies a quantile regression method of analysis to estimate the magnitude of the effects of heritability and the shared environment at multiple percentile cut-offs within a continuous distribution. It provides a more powerful test of genetic effects and gives a more nuanced insight into any patterns of change in heritability across the range of scores. This method has subsequently been applied to reading ability (McGowan et al., 2019) and self-control (Schwartz et al., 2017). Frazier et al. (2014) used quantile regression to investigate the role of genetics and the shared environment in influencing quantitative measures of autism symptomology. They found that the dimensions of social communication and repetitive behaviour showed high heritability at the more extreme level of severity. Moreover these high scores on these two dimensions were influenced by a common set of genetic factors. To date quantile regression has not been applied to data on a broader range of behaviour problems.

Molecular Genetics The question of the relationships between normal variation and disorders can now be studied using molecular genetic techniques. Anttila et al. (2018) used findings from genome-wide association studies (GWAS) (see Sect. 3.2) to examine the extent of gene sharing between psychiatric and neurological disorders and neurocognitive quantitative phenotypes. They found an extensive degree of gene sharing between psychiatric disorders, for example, ADHD, anxiety disorders, depression, and schizophrenia, and quantitative characteristics. The same was not the case for neurological disorders which are more distinct genetically from each other and from the neurocognitive quantitative phenotypes. This finding supports the spectrum/common cause model for quantitative individual differences and mental and behavioural disorders.

Genetically informative studies are of wider relevance to the question of classifying individual differences in behaviour – not just the categorical/dimension distinction. The role of psychiatric genetic studies in the development of classification schemes is outlined in Smoller (2013) in a review with a particular focus on genetic influences that affect more than one condition. He addresses the question of what are the implications of two disorders having a shared genetic aetiology? He concludes that such pleiotropic effects are ubiquitous in psychiatric genetics and it is unlikely that specific genetic profiles will be found to distinguish psychiatric syndromes.

In a later broader review Smoller et al. (2019) address a number of important questions concerning studies of genetics and the structure of psychopathology. They identify two key principles that have emerged from recent psychiatric genetic research.

> (1) psychiatric disorders are highly polygenic, reflecting the contribution of hundreds to thousands of common variants of small effect and rare (often de novo) SNVs [single nucleotide variants] and CNVs [copy number variants]; (2) genetic influences on psychopathology commonly transcend the diagnostic boundaries of our clinical DSM nosology. At the level of genetic etiology, there are no sharp boundaries between diagnostic categories or between disorder and normal variation. Smoller et al. (2019), p. 417

This issue of genetics and the structure of psychopathology will be discussed at greater length in Sect. 6.8, where genetic influence on the p-factor is discussed.

5.6 Prosocial Behaviour

In the discussion of behavioural individuality so far there has been an emphasis on maladaptive and problematic behaviour. This needs to be counter-balanced by considering positive qualities of children's behaviour and the associated individual differences. These however have been the subject of far fewer studies.

The term prosocial behaviour refers to a number of behaviours with positive qualities that include helping, sharing, giving, co-operating, and responding to distress. The nature of prosocial behaviour changes during the early years. During the second year of life prosocial behaviour changes from being dependent on explicit communication to an understanding of others' emotions based on subtle cues (Svetlova et al., 2010). It is considered an aspect of competence in children. Such competencies are seen as a possible protective factor for children experiencing adversities (Garmezy et al., 1984) and are thought to be important for the subsequent development of meta-cognitive abilities and conscious awareness of mental states (Frith & Frith, 2012).

Penner et al. (2005) have described the way prosocial behaviour can be examined at a number of levels. The first they label the "meso" level and concerns the study of the prosocial interactions between people. The second ("micro" level) concerns individual differences in prosocial behaviour. The third ("macro" level) relates to prosocial behaviour shown in large groups and organisations. It is the micro level that is relevant here. In particular the role of genetic and environmental factors in the development of individual difference in prosocial behaviour.

There have been behaviour genetic studies that have addressed this question in relation to prosocial behaviour and competencies. Using the scales from the Infant-Toddler Social and Emotional Assessment (ITSEA) (Briggs-Gowan & Carter, 1998) with 1950 2-year-old twins, Saudino et al. (2008) found a lower heritability for the competence scale (boys $h^2 = 0.21$ and girls $h^2 = 0.15$) than for the behaviour problem scales ($h^2 = 0.46–0.56$). The reverse was found for the effects of the shared environment. These ranged from 0.25 to 0.34 for behaviour problems and boys = 0.73 and girls = 0.78 for the competence scale. A longitudinal study of 9424 twins from ages 2 to 7 years found that these shared environment effects on prosocial behaviour declined from 0.47 at 2 years to 0.03 at age 7 years (Knafo & Plomin, 2006). There was a concomitant increase in the size of genetic effects from 0.32 to 0.61.

There is evidence that one biological mechanism influencing prosocial behaviour is via increases in the level of the neuromodulator oxytocin (Shamay-Tsoory & Abu-Akel, 2016). Additional support for this mechanism comes from the finding that a genetic polymorphism rs53576 in the oxytocin rector gene (*OXTR*) may contribute the individual differences in prosocial behaviour (Tost et al., 2010). Wu and Su (2015) demonstrated a relationship in 3–5-year-olds between variants in OXTR and prosocial behaviour and theory of mind (see Sect. 10.2). A possible mechanism has been suggested by Wang et al. (2020). They found functional MRI changes for male homozygotes for the risk A allele in OXTR rs53576 compared with male G allele carriers. However based on a meta-analysis, there have been doubts about the importance of OXTR rs53576 and rs2254298 for social behaviour (Bakermans-Kranenburg & van Ijzendoorn, 2014). Many of the studies in this meta-analysis were of low power and the expected effect sizes were small. A subsequent systematic review identified a number of additional studies on OXTR variants and prosocial behaviour (Kohlhoff et al., 2022). The findings from the nine studies reviewed were mixed; some studies suggest a direct link between OXTR variants and prosocial behaviour, others indicated an interaction with factors such as maternal depression in influencing prosociality. The impact of variants in OXTR for prosocial behaviour must be considered uncertain.

What is the relationship between prosocial behaviour and behaviour problems? In a 20-year follow-up study of children initially studied when aged 8–12 years, Burt et al. (2008) found that higher social competencies were associated with fewer internalising problems at all ages. There was an initial negative relationship at age 10 years between social competence and externalising problems but not thereafter. Eisenberg et al. (2000) postulated that prosocial behaviour would be influenced by both the degree of negative emotionality and behavioural regulation. They found that in a sample of children followed from the preschool years, negative emotionality moderated the relation of behaviour regulation to prosocial behaviour. That is for children with high negative emotionality only, good behaviour regulation was related to a higher level of prosocial behaviour.

The relationship between prosocial behaviour and behaviour problems was examined in a longitudinal study of 160 children followed from age 5 to age 6 (Perren et al., 2007). The scores on the Strengths and Difficulties Questionnaire (SDQ) (see Sect. 2.4) completed by both teachers and parents were combined with the child's own reports of their behaviour obtained via the Berkeley Puppet Interview, which is a measure of a child's self-perception on the range of behaviours, feelings, and competencies (Measelle et al., 1998). This produced aggregated measures on conduct problems, hyperactivity, emotional symptoms, and prosocial behaviour at both ages. All four aspects of behaviour showed a moderate degree of stability with correlations ranging from 0.55 to 0.70. The overtime correlation of prosocial behaviour scores was 0.60. At age 5 there was a negative correlation between prosocial behaviour and conduct problems, hyperactivity and emotional problems. Prosocial behaviour at age 5 did not add to the prediction of these behaviour scores at age 6 years. However children with above-average emotional problems and prosocial scores at age 5 showed the highest level of emotional symptoms at age 6. A similar longitudinal study during adolescence found that those with a continuing profile of a high level of prosocial behaviour showed lower scores on externalising behaviour compared to those with a profile of low prosocial scores (Flynn et al., 2015).

A study of 4- and 5-year-olds showed that those at high risk of developing disruptive behaviour were less able than others to maintain positive engagement with people showing distress (Zahn-Waxler et al., 1995). At the same age externalising symptoms in children's ratings were associated with low levels of prosocial behaviour, whereas the opposite was found for internalising symptoms (Huber et al., 2019a). In a sample of 3–5-year-olds Hay et al. (2010) found the same relationship between conduct problems and low prosocial behaviour. However in this study this relationship disappeared once ADHD symptoms were controlled. They did not find a positive relationship between internalising symptoms and prosocial behaviour. Indeed the relationship between externalising symptoms and low prosocial behaviour seems to be a robust finding but that between internalising and prosocial behaviour is both more complex and less consistent in older children (Nantel-Vivier et al.,

2014) and in early childhood (Huber et al., 2019b). For example, a high level of internalising problems in adolescence was found in a sub-group of children with high prosocial behaviour at age 4 (Hay & Pawlby, 2003). This risk was particularly marked for boys showing high levels of early prosocial behaviour.

Reparative behaviours are one particular type of prosocial behaviour that includes helping, sharing, and comforting behaviours in addition to attempts to make amends, apologise, and own up to a wrongdoing (Tangney et al., 2007). There is evidence for three distinct trajectories of reparative behaviours (low, moderate, and high) across development in a 9-year longitudinal data set spanning from preschool through adolescence (Donohue et al., 2020). The group that showed enduring poor reparative prosocial skills included children who showed externalising behaviour and children who showed depression in the preschool period.

Starting at age 5–7 years, children and their families were studied for 6 years by McCoy et al. (2009). Over this time period their prosocial behaviour showed a high degree of stability. However the warmth of parenting and marital conflict had effects on prosocial behaviour (increasing and decreasing the level, respectively). In both cases the effects were mediated by influences on the child's emotional security. Xiao et al. (2019) investigated the relationship between children's anger and shyness at 3.5 years and their prosocial behaviour towards strangers 1 year later. They differentiated anger that was dispositional (a feature of temperament) and that was situationally tied to an unfair event. They found no relationship between dispositional anger and prosocial behaviour. Higher levels of situational anger were related to higher levels of prosocial behaviour 1 year later for children but only for children who were not shy.

These studies make it clear that prosocial behaviour should not be understood simply as the obverse of difficult or challenging antisocial behaviour. There are contrasting relationships between prosocial behaviour and internalising and externalising behaviour.

5.7 Final Thoughts on Conceptualising Behavioural Differences

How can these differences in perspectives be reconciled? Almost invariably when dimensions have been investigated, with the possible exception of ASD, they have been found to represent an appropriate way to present behavioural differences. However, even for ASD, a dimension formulation is apposite for many purposes (Happé & Frith, 2020). There are exceptions where a categorical framework identifies sub-groups with distinct characteristics in terms of the causes or outcomes of behaviour (Kagan, 2018). However these effects may best be considered as the moderation of the relationship between risk factors or developmental outcomes and behaviour rather than the basis for a categorical typology. It seems prudent therefore to investigate psychological problems using dimensional measures but also to test at a second stage for groups where the pattern of development may be distinct.

This approach is endorsed by Helena Kraemer, who writes wisely and cogently on methodology and data analysis. She argues that there are direct equivalencies between dimension and categorical frameworks for studying behaviour (Kraemer et al., 2004). However the two approaches have distinct advantages (Helzer et al., 2006). She suggests that that diagnostic categories are important in clinical contexts for communicating about mental illness but a dimensional approach provides a more powerful way to test the underlying nature of psychiatric illness. This dimensional approach is at the core of the multilevel hierarchical models which are the subject of the next chapter.

References

Ahmadzadeh, Y. I., Eley, T. C., Leve, L. D., Shaw, D. S., Natsuaki, M. N., Reiss, D., et al. (2019). Anxiety in the family: A genetically informed analysis of transactional associations between mother, father and child anxiety symptoms. *Journal of Child Psychology and Psychiatry, 60*(12), 1269–1277. https://doi.org/10.1111/jcpp.13068

Alexander, L. M., Salum, G. A., Swanson, J. M., & Milham, M. P. (2020). Measuring strengths and weaknesses in dimensional psychiatry. *Journal of Child Psychology and Psychiatry, 61*(1), 40–50. https://doi.org/10.1111/jcpp.13104

Anttila, V., Bulik-Sullivan, B., Finucane, H. K., Walters, R. K., Bras, J., Duncan, L., et al. (2018). Analysis of shared heritability in common disorders of the brain. *Science, 360*(6395), 1313-+. https://doi.org/10.1126/science.aap8757

Asparouhov, T., Hamaker, E. L., & Muthen, B. (2018). Dynamic structural equation models. *Structural Equation Modeling-A Multidisciplinary Journal, 25*(3), 359–388. https://doi.org/10.1080/10705511.2017.1406803

Ayroles, J. F., Buchanan, S. M., O'Leary, C., Skutt-Kakaria, K., Grenier, J. K., Clark, A. G., et al. (2015). Behavioral idiosyncrasy reveals genetic control of phenotypic variability. *Proceedings of the National Academy of Sciences of the United States of America, 112*(21), 6706–6711. https://doi.org/10.1073/pnas.1503830112

Bakermans-Kranenburg, M. J., & van Ijzendoorn, M. H. (2014). A sociability gene? Meta-analysis of oxytocin receptor genotype effects in humans. *Psychiatric Genetics, 24*(2), 45–51. https://doi.org/10.1097/YPG.0b013e3283643684

Baptista, V., Costa, E. F. S., Carere, C., Morais, P., Cruz, J., Cerveira, I., et al. (2020). Does consistent individual variability in pelagic fish larval behaviour affect recruitment in nursery habitats? *Behavioral Ecology and Sociobiology, 74*(6). https://doi.org/10.1007/s00265-020-02841-0

Bartels, M., & Boomsma, D. I. (2009). Born to be happy? The etiology of subjective well-being. *Behavior Genetics, 39*(6), 605–615. https://doi.org/10.1007/s10519-009-9294-8

Bell, A. M., Hankison, S. J., & Laskowski, K. L. (2009). The repeatability of behaviour: A meta-analysis. *Animal Behaviour, 77*(4), 771–783. https://doi.org/10.1016/j.anbehav.2008.12.022

Bell, R. Q. (1968). A reinterpretation of the direction of effects in studies of socialization. *Psychological Review, 75*(2), 81–95.

Beltz, A. M., Wright, A. G. C., Sprague, B. N., & Molenaar, P. C. M. (2016). Bridging the nomothetic and idiographic approaches to the analysis of clinical data. *Assessment, 23*(4), 447–458. https://doi.org/10.1177/1073191116648209

Bengston, S. E., Dahan, R. A., Donaldson, Z., Phelps, S. M., van Oers, K., Sih, A., & Bell, A. M. (2018). Genomic tools for behavioural ecologists to understand repeatable individual differences in behaviour. *Nature Ecology & Evolution, 2*(6), 944–955. https://doi.org/10.1038/s41559-017-0411-4

Bertelsen, N., Landi, I., Bethlehem, R. A. I., Seidlitz, J., Busuoli, E. M., Mandelli, V., et al. (2021). Imbalanced social-communicative and restricted repetitive behavior subtypes of autism spectrum disorder exhibit different neural circuitry. *Communications Biology, 4*(1). https://doi.org/10.1038/s42003-021-02015-2

Bierbach, D., Laskowski, K. L., & Wolf, M. (2017). Behavioural individuality in clonal fish arises despite near-identical rearing conditions. *Nature Communications, 8*. https://doi.org/10.1038/ncomms15361

Birch, H. G., Thomas, A., Chess, S., & Hertzig, M. E. (1962). Individuality in the development of children. *Developmental Medicine and Child Neurology, 4*, 370–379. https://doi.org/10.1111/j.1469-8749.1962.tb03192.x

Borsboom, D., Rhemtulla, M., Cramer, A. O. J., van der Maas, H. L. J., Scheffer, M., & Dolan, C. V. (2016). Kinds versus continua: A review of psychometric approaches to uncover the structure of psychiatric constructs. *Psychological Medicine, 46*(8), 1567–1579. https://doi.org/10.1017/s0033291715001944

Bould, H., Araya, R., Pearson, R. M., Stapinski, L., Carnegie, R., & Joinson, C. (2014). Association between early temperament and depression at 18 years. *Depression and Anxiety, 31*(9), 729–736. https://doi.org/10.1002/da.22294

Boyce, W. T., Frank, E., Jensen, P. S., Kessler, R. C., Nelson, C. A., Steinberg, L., & MacArthur Foundation Research Network on Psychopathology and Development. (1998). Social context in developmental psychopathology: Recommendations for future research from the MacArthur network on psychopathology and development. *Development and Psychopathology, 10*(2), 143–164. https://doi.org/10.1017/s0954579498001552

Briggs-Gowan, M. J., & Carter, A. S. (1998). Preliminary acceptability and psychometrics of the Infant-Toddler Social and Emotional Assessment (ITSEA): A new adult-report questionnaire. *Infant Mental Health Journal, 19*(4), 422–445. https://doi.org/10.1002/(sici)1097-0355(199824)19:4<422::aid-imhj5>3.0.co;2-u

Brown, T. A., & Barlow, D. H. (2005). Dimensional versus categorical classification of mental disorders in the fifth edition of the Diagnostic and Statistical Manual of Mental Disorders and beyond: Comment on the special section. *Journal of Abnormal Psychology, 114*(4), 551–556. https://doi.org/10.1037/0021-843x.114.4.551

Burt, K. B., Obradovic, J., Long, J. D., & Masten, A. S. (2008). The interplay of social competence and psychopathology over 20 years: Testing transactional and cascade models. *Child Development, 79*(2), 359–374. https://doi.org/10.1111/j.1467-8624.2007.01130.x

Burt, S. A. (2009). Rethinking environmental contributions to child and adolescent psychopathology: A meta-analysis of shared environmental influences. *Psychological Bulletin, 135*(4), 608–637. https://doi.org/10.1037/a0015702

Burt, S. A. (2014). Research Review: The shared environment as a key source of variability in child and adolescent psychopathology. *Journal of Child Psychology and Psychiatry, 55*(4), 304–312. https://doi.org/10.1111/jcpp.12173

Campbell, S. B. (2002). *Behavior problems in preschool children: Clinical and development issues*. The Guilford Press.

Caspi, A., Henry, B., McGee, R. O., Moffitt, T. E., & Silva, P. A. (1995). Temperamental origins of child and adolescent behavior problems - from age 3 to age 15. *Child Development, 66*(1). https://doi.org/10.1111/j.1467-8624.1995.tb00855.x

Clark, L. A., Cuthbert, B., Lewis-Fernandez, R., Narrow, W. E., & Reed, G. M. (2017). Three approaches to understanding and classifying mental disorder: ICD-11, DSM-5, and the National Institute of Mental Health's Research Domain Criteria (RDoC). *Psychological Science in the Public Interest, 18*(2), 72–145. https://doi.org/10.1177/1529100617727266

Coghill, D., & Sonuga-Barke, E. J. S. (2012). Annual Research Review: Categories versus dimensions in the classification and conceptualisation of child and adolescent mental disorders - implications of recent empirical study. *Journal of Child Psychology and Psychiatry, 53*(5), 469–489. https://doi.org/10.1111/j.1469-7610.2011.02511.x

Coleman, J., Wolkind, S., & Ashley, L. (1977). Symptoms of behavior disturbance and adjustment to school. *Journal of Child Psychology and Psychiatry, 18*(3), 201–209. https://doi.org/10.1111/j.1469-7610.1977.tb00432.x

Colvert, E., Tick, B., McEwen, F., Stewart, C., Curran, S. R., Woodhouse, E., et al. (2015). Heritability of autism spectrum disorder in a UK population-based twin sample. *JAMA Psychiatry, 72*(5), 415–423. https://doi.org/10.1001/jamapsychiatry.2014.3028

Deater-Deckard, K., Reiss, D., Hetherington, E. M., & Plomin, R. (1997). Dimensions and disorders of adolescent adjustment: A quantitative genetic analysis of unselected samples and selected extremes. *Journal of Child Psychology and Psychiatry, 38*(5), 515–525. https://doi.org/10.1111/j.1469-7610.1997.tb01538.x

DeFries, J. C., & Fulker, D. W. (1985). Multiple-regresssion analysis of twin data. *Behavior Genetics, 15*(5), 467–473. https://doi.org/10.1007/bf01066239

DeFries, J. C., Fulker, D. W., & Labuda, M. C. (1987). Evidence for a genetic etiology in reading-disability of twins. *Nature, 329*(6139), 537–539. https://doi.org/10.1038/329537a0

Deserno, M. K., Bathelt, J., Groenman, A. P., & Geurts, H. M. (2022). Probing the overarching continuum theory: Data-driven phenotypic clustering of children with ASD or ADHD. *European Child and Adolescent Psychiatry*. https://doi.org/10.1007/s00787-022-01986-9

Dingemanse, N. J., & Dochtermann, N. A. (2013). Quantifying individual variation in behaviour: Mixed-effect modelling approaches. *Journal of Animal Ecology, 82*(1), 39–54. https://doi.org/10.1111/1365-2656.12013

Dodge, K. A., Greenberg, M. T., Malone, P. S., & Conduct Problems Prevention Research Group. (2008). Testing an idealized dynamic cascade model of the development of serious violence in adolescence. *Child Development, 79*(6), 1907–1927. https://doi.org/10.1111/j.1467-8624.2008.01233.x

Dodge, K. A., & Pettit, G. S. (2003). A biopsychosocial model of the development of chronic conduct problems in adolescence. *Developmental Psychology, 39*(2), 349–371. https://doi.org/10.1037/0012-1649.39.2.349

Donohue, M. R., Tillman, R., & Luby, J. (2020). Early socioemotional competence, psychopathology, and latent class profiles of reparative prosocial behaviors from preschool through early adolescence. *Development and Psychopathology, 32*(2), 573–585. https://doi.org/10.1017/s0954579419000397

Earls, F. (1980). Prevalence of behavior problems in 3-year-old children - a cross-national replication. *Archives of General Psychiatry, 37*(10), 1153–1157. https://doi.org/10.1001/archpsyc.1980.01780230071010

Eisenberg, N., Fabes, R. A., Guthrie, I. K., & Reiser, M. (2000). Dispositional emotionality and regulation: Their role in predicting quality of social functioning. *Journal of Personality and Social Psychology, 78*(1), 136–157. https://doi.org/10.1037/0022-3514.78.1.136

Elander, J., & Rutter, M. (1996). Use and development of the Rutter parents' and teachers' scales. *International Journal of Methods in Psychiatric Research, 6*(2), 63–78. https://doi.org/10.1002/(sici)1234-988x(199607)6:2<63::aid-mpr151>3.3.co;2-m

Fisher, H. L. (2021). Editorial: 'The early bird catches the worm'—The need for even earlier intervention and targeted prevention for mental illnesses. *Journal of Child Psychology and Psychiatry, 62*(4), 369–371. https://doi.org/10.1111/jcpp.13407

Flom, M., Wang, M. J., Uccello, K. J., & Saudino, K. J. (2018). Parent- and observer-rated positive affect in early childhood: Genetic overlap and environmental specificity. *Behavior Genetics, 48*(6), 432–439. https://doi.org/10.1007/s10519-018-9924-0

Flynn, E., Ehrenreich, S. E., Beron, K. J., & Underwood, M. K. (2015). Prosocial behavior: Long-term trajectories and psychosocial outcomes. *Social Development, 24*(3), 462–482. https://doi.org/10.1111/sode.12100

Fonagy, P. (2003). Psychoanalysis today. *World Psychiatry : official journal of the World Psychiatric Association (WPA), 2*(2), 73–80. PMID: 16946899.

Frazier, T. W., Thompson, L., Youngstrom, E. A., Law, P., Hardan, A. Y., Eng, C., & Morris, N. (2014). A twin study of heritable and shared environmental contributions to autism. *Journal of Autism and Developmental Disorders, 44*(8), 2013–2025. https://doi.org/10.1007/s10803-014-2081-2

Frith, C. D., & Frith, U. (2012). Mechanisms of social cognition. In S. T. Fiske, D. L. Schacter, & S. E. Taylor (Eds.), *Annual review of psychology* (Vol. 63, pp. 287–313).

Frith, U. (2019). Flux of life. *Developmental Cognitive Neuroscience, 38*. https://doi.org/10.1016/j.dcn.2019.100669

Gardner, F., & Shaw, D. (2008). Behavioral problems of infancy and preschool children (0-5). In M. Rutter, D. Bishop, D. Pine, S. Scott, J. Stevenson, E. Taylor, & A. Thapar (Eds.), *Rutter's child and adolescent psychiatry* (Fifth ed.). Blackwell Publishing.

Garmezy, N., Masten, A. S., & Tellegen, A. (1984). The study of stress and competence in children - a building block for developmental psychopathology. *Child Development, 55*(1), 97–111. https://doi.org/10.2307/1129837

Georgiades, S., Szatmari, P., Boyle, M., Hanna, S., Duku, E., Zwaigenbaum, L., et al. (2013). Investigating phenotypic heterogeneity in children with autism spectrum disorder: A factor mixture modeling approach. *Journal of Child Psychology and Psychiatry, 54*(2), 206–215. https://doi.org/10.1111/j.1469-7610.2012.02588.x

Gidziela, A., Malanchini, M., Rimfeld, K., McMillan, A., Ronald, A., Viding, E., et al. (2023). Explaining the influence of non-shared environment (NSE) on symptoms of behaviour problems from preschool to adulthood: Mind the missing NSE gap. *Journal of Child Psychology and Psychiatry, 64*(5), 747–757. https://doi.org/10.1111/jcpp.13729

Gjone, H., Stevenson, J., & Sundet, J. M. (1996). Genetic influence on parent-reported attention-related problems in a Norwegian general population twin sample. *Archives of General Psychiatry, 35*(5), 588–596. https://doi.org/10.1097/00004583-199605000-00013

Graham, P., Rutter, M., & George, S. (1973). Temperamental characteristics as predictors of behavior disorders in children. *American Journal of Orthopsychiatry, 43*(3), 328–339. https://doi.org/10.1111/j.1939-0025.1973.tb00802.x

Graham, P., & Stevenson, J. (1985). A twin study of genetic influences on behavioral-deviance. *Journal of the American Academy of Child and Adolescent Psychiatry, 24*(1), 33–41. https://doi.org/10.1016/s0002-7138(09)60407-6

Graham, P., & Stevenson, J. (1987). Temperament and psychiatric-disorder - the genetic contribution to behavior in childhood. *Australian and New Zealand Journal of Psychiatry, 21*(3), 267–274. https://doi.org/10.1080/00048678709160922

Greven, C. U., Buitelaar, J. K., & Salum, G. A. (2018). From positive psychology to psychopathology: The continuum of attention-deficit hyperactivity disorder. *Journal of Child Psychology and Psychiatry, 59*(3), 203–212. https://doi.org/10.1111/jcpp.12786

Hammen, C., Burge, D., & Stansbury, K. (1990). Relationship of mother and child variables to child outcomes in a high-risk sample - a causal-modeling analysis. *Developmental Psychology, 26*(1), 24–30. https://doi.org/10.1037/0012-1649.26.1.24

Hankin, B. L., Jenness, J., Abela, J. R. Z., & Smolen, A. (2011). Interaction of 5-HTTLPR and idiographic stressors predicts prospective depressive symptoms specifically among youth in a multiwave design. *Journal of Clinical Child and Adolescent Psychology, 40*(4), 572–585. https://doi.org/10.1080/15374416.2011.581613

Happé, F., & Frith, U. (2020). Annual Research Review: Looking back to look forward - changes in the concept of autism and implications for future research. *Journal of Child Psychology and Psychiatry, 61*(3), 218–232. https://doi.org/10.1111/jcpp.13176

Haslam, N., Holland, E., & Kuppens, P. (2012). Categories versus dimensions in personality and psychopathology: A quantitative review of taxometric research. *Psychological Medicine, 42*(5), 903–920. https://doi.org/10.1017/s0033291711001966

Haslam, N., McGrath, M. J., Viechtbauer, W., & Kuppens, P. (2020). Dimensions over categories: A meta-analysis of taxometric research. *Psychological Medicine, 50*(9), 1418–1432. https://doi.org/10.1017/s003329172000183x

Hay, D. F., Hudson, K., & Liang, W. T. (2010). Links between preschool children's prosocial skills and aggressive conduct problems: The contribution of ADHD symptoms. *Early Childhood Research Quarterly, 25*(4), 493–501. https://doi.org/10.1016/j.ecresq.2010.01.003

Hay, D. F., & Pawlby, S. (2003). Prosocial development in relation to children's and mothers' psychological problems. *Child Development, 74*(5), 1314–1327. https://doi.org/10.1111/1467-8624.00609

Helzer, J. E., Kraemer, H. C., & Krueger, R. F. (2006). The feasibility and need for dimensional psychiatric diagnoses. *Psychological Medicine, 36*(12), 1671–1680. https://doi.org/10.1017/s003329170600821x

Hetherington, E. M., Bridges, M., & Insabella, G. M. (1998). What matters? What does not? Five perspectives on the association between marital transitions and children's adjustment. *American Psychologist, 53*(2), 167–184. https://doi.org/10.1037/0003-066x.53.2.167

Hinde, R. A. (1992). Developmental-psychology in the context of other behavioral-sciences. *Developmental Psychology, 28*(6), 1018–1029. https://doi.org/10.1037/0012-1649.28.6.1018

Huber, L., Plötner, M., & Schmitz, J. (2019a). Behavioral observation of prosocial behavior and social initiative is related to preschoolers' psychopathological symptoms. *PLoS One, 14*(11), e0225274–e0225274. https://doi.org/10.1371/journal.pone.0225274

Huber, L., Plötner, M., & Schmitz, J. (2019b). Social competence and psychopathology in early childhood: A systematic review. *European Child & Adolescent Psychiatry, 28*(4), 443–459. https://doi.org/10.1007/s00787-018-1152-x

Jaffee, S. R., Strait, L. B., & Odgers, C. L. (2012). From correlates to causes: Can quasi-experimental studies and statistical innovations bring us closer to identifying the causes of antisocial behavior? *Psychological Bulletin, 138*(2), 272–295. https://doi.org/10.1037/a0026020

Kagan, J. (2018). Kinds of individuals defined by patterns of variables. *Development and Psychopathology, 30*(4), 1197–1209. https://doi.org/10.1017/s095457941800055x

Kain, J. S., Stokes, C., & de Bivort, B. L. (2012). Phototactic personality in fruit flies and its suppression by serotonin and white. *Proceedings of the National Academy of Sciences of the United States of America, 109*(48), 19834–19839. https://doi.org/10.1073/pnas.1211988109

Kandel, E. R. (1999). Biology and the future of psychoanalysis: A new intellectual framework for psychiatry revisited. *American Journal of Psychiatry, 156*(4), 505–524. https://doi.org/10.1176/ajp.156.4.505

Karalunas, S. L., Geurts, H. M., Konrad, K., Bender, S., & Nigg, J. T. (2014). Annual Research Review: Reaction time variability in ADHD and autism spectrum disorders: Measurement and mechanisms of a proposed trans-diagnostic phenotype. *Journal of Child Psychology and Psychiatry, 55*(6), 685–710. https://doi.org/10.1111/jcpp.12217

Kendler, K. S., Aggen, S. H., Knudsen, G. P., Roysamb, E., Neale, M. C., & Reichborn-Kjennerud, T. (2011). The structure of genetic and environmental risk factors for syndromal and subsyndromal common DSM-IV Axis I and All Axis II disorders. *American Journal of Psychiatry, 168*(1), 29–39. https://doi.org/10.1176/appi.ajp.2010.10030340

Kohlhoff, J., Cibralic, S., Hawes, D. J., & Eapen, V. (2022). Oxytocin receptor gene (OXTR) polymorphisms and social, emotional and behavioral functioning in children and adolescents: A systematic narrative review. *Neuroscience and Biobehavioral Reviews, 135*. https://doi.org/10.1016/j.neubiorev.2022.104573

Knafo, A., & Plomin, R. (2006). Prosocial behavior from early to middle childhood: Genetic and environmental influences on stability and change. *Developmental Psychology, 42*(5), 771–786. https://doi.org/10.1037/0012-1649.42.5.771

Kraemer, H. C., Noda, A., & O'Hara, R. (2004). Categorical versus dimensional approaches to diagnosis: Methodological challenges. *Journal of Psychiatric Research, 38*(1), 17–25. https://doi.org/10.1016/s0022-3956(03)00097-9

Lahey, B. B. (2021). *Dimensions of psychological problems: Replacing diagnostic categories with a more science-based and less stigmatizing alternative*. Oxford University Press.

Lahey, B. B., Van Hulle, C. A., Singh, A. L., Waldman, I. D., & Rathouz, P. J. (2011). Higher-order genetic and environmental structure of prevalent forms of child and adolescent psychopathology. *Archives of General Psychiatry, 68*(2), 181–189. https://doi.org/10.1001/archgenpsychiatry.2010.192

Lansford, J. E., Criss, M. M., Laird, R. D., Shaw, D. S., Pettit, G. S., Bates, J. E., & Dodge, K. A. (2011). Reciprocal relations between parents' physical discipline and children's externalizing behavior during middle childhood and adolescence. *Development and Psychopathology, 23*(1), 225–238. https://doi.org/10.1017/s0954579410000751

Larsson, H., Viding, E., Rijsdijk, F. V., & Plomin, R. (2008). Relationships between parental negativity and childhood antisocial behavior over time: A bidirectional effects model in a longitudinal genetically informative design. *Journal of Abnormal Child Psychology, 36*(5), 633–645. https://doi.org/10.1007/s10802-007-9151-2

Leve, L. D., Kim, H. K., & Pears, K. C. (2005). Childhood temperament and family environment as predictors of internalizing and externalizing trajectories from ages 5 to 17. *Journal of Abnormal Child Psychology, 33*(5), 505–520. https://doi.org/10.1007/s10802-005-6734-7

Levy, F., Hay, D. A., McStephen, M., Wood, C., & Waldman, I. (1997). Attention-deficit hyperactivity disorder: A category or a continuum? Genetic analysis of a large-scale twin study. *Journal of the American Academy of Child and Adolescent Psychiatry, 36*(6), 737–744. https://doi.org/10.1097/00004583-199706000-00009

Linneweber, G. A., Andriatsilavo, M., Dutta, S. B., Bengochea, M., Hellbruegge, L., Liu, G., et al. (2020). A neurodevelopmental origin of behavioral individuality in the Drosophila visual system. *Science, 367*(6482), 1112-+. https://doi.org/10.1126/science.aaw7182

Logan, J. A. R., Petrill, S. A., Hart, S. A., Schatschneider, C., Thompson, L. A., Deater-Deckard, K., et al. (2012). Heritability across the distribution: An application of quantile regression. *Behavior Genetics, 42*(2), 256–267. https://doi.org/10.1007/s10519-011-9497-7

Lubke, G. H., & Muthen, B. (2005). Investigating population heterogeneity with factor mixture models. *Psychological Methods, 10*(1), 21–39. https://doi.org/10.1037/1082-989x.10.1.21

Markon, K. E., Chmielewski, M., & Miller, C. J. (2011). The reliability and validity of discrete and continuous measures of psychopathology: A quantitative review. *Psychological Bulletin, 137*(5), 856–879. https://doi.org/10.1037/a0023678

Martin, J., Taylor, M. J., & Lichtenstein, P. (2018). Assessing the evidence for shared genetic risks across psychiatric disorders and traits. *Psychological Medicine, 48*(11), 1759–1774. https://doi.org/10.1017/s0033291717003440

McCoy, K., Cummings, E. M., & Davies, P. T. (2009). Constructive and destructive marital conflict, emotional security and children's prosocial behavior. *Journal of Child Psychology and Psychiatry, 50*(3), 270–279. https://doi.org/10.1111/j.1469-7610.2008.01945.x

McGowan, D., Little, C. W., Coventry, W. L., Corley, R., Olson, R. K., Samuelsson, S., & Byrne, B. (2019). Differential influences of genes and environment across the distribution of reading ability. *Behavior Genetics, 49*(5), 425–431. https://doi.org/10.1007/s10519-019-09966-7

Measelle, J. R., Ablow, J. C., Cowan, P. A., & Cowan, C. P. (1998). Assessing young children's views of their academic, social, and emotional lives: An evaluation of the self-perception scales of the Berkeley puppet interview. *Child Development, 69*(6), 1556–1576. https://doi.org/10.2307/1132132

Meehl, P. E. (1995). Bootstraps taxometrics - solving the classification problem in psychopathology. *American Psychologist, 50*(4), 266–275. https://doi.org/10.1037/0003-066x.50.4.266

Mitchell, K. J. (2007). The genetics of brain wiring: From molecule to mind. *PLoS Biology, 5*(4), 690–692. https://doi.org/10.1371/journal.pbio.0050113

Molenaar, P. (2004). A manifesto on psychology as idiographic science: Bringing the person back into scientific psychology, this time forever. *Measurement, 2*, 201–218. https://doi.org/10.1207/s15366359mea0204_1

Nantel-Vivier, A., Pihl, R. O., Cote, S., & Tremblay, R. E. (2014). Developmental association of prosocial behaviour with aggression, anxiety and depression from infancy to preadolescence. *Journal of Child Psychology and Psychiatry, 55*(10), 1135–1144. https://doi.org/10.1111/jcpp.12235

Nelson, S. K., Kushlev, K., & Lyubomirsky, S. (2014). The pains and pleasures of parenting: When, why, and how is parenthood associated with more or less well-being? *Psychological Bulletin, 140*(3), 846–895. https://doi.org/10.1037/a0035444

Nigg, J. T. (2006). Temperament and developmental psychopathology. *Journal of Child Psychology and Psychiatry, 47*(3–4), 395–422. https://doi.org/10.1111/j.1469-7610.2006.01612.x

Olino, T. M., Dougherty, L. R., Bufferd, S. J., Carlson, G. A., & Klein, D. N. (2014). Testing models of psychopathology in preschool-aged children using a structured interview-based assessment. *Journal of Abnormal Child Psychology, 42*(7), 1201–1211. https://doi.org/10.1007/s10802-014-9865-x

Pacheco, J., Garvey, M. A., Sarampote, C. S., Cohen, E. D., Murphy, E. R., & Friedman-Hill, S. R. (2022). Annual Research Review: The contributions of the RDoC research framework on understanding the neurodevelopmental origins, progression and treatment of mental illnesses. *Journal of Child Psychology and Psychiatry, 63*(4), 360–376. https://doi.org/10.1111/jcpp.13543

Paschall, K. W., & Mastergeorge, A. M. (2016). A review of 25 years of research in bidirectionality in parent-child relationships: An examination of methodological approaches. *International Journal of Behavioral Development, 40*(5), 442–451. https://doi.org/10.1177/0165025415607379

Penner, L. A., Dovidio, J. F., Piliavin, J. A., & Schroeder, D. A. (2005). Prosocial behavior: Multilevel perspectives. *Annual Review of Psychology, 56*, 365–392. https://doi.org/10.1146/annurev.psych.56.091103.070141

Perren, S., Stadelmann, S., von Wyl, A., & von Klitzing, K. (2007). Pathways of behavioural and emotional symptoms in kindergarten children: What is the role of pro-social behaviour? *European Child and Adolescent Psychiatry, 16*(4), 209–214. https://doi.org/10.1007/s00787-006-0588-6

Pickles, A., & Angold, A. (2003). Natural categories or fundamental dimensions: On carving nature at the joints and the rearticulation of psychopathology. *Development and Psychopathology, 15*(3), 529–551. https://doi.org/10.1017/s0954579403000282

Planalp, E. M., & Goldsmith, H. H. (2020). Observed profiles of infant temperament: Stability, heritability, and associations with parenting. *Child Development, 91*(3), E563–E580. https://doi.org/10.1111/cdev.13277

Plomin, R., & Daniels, D. (1987). Why are children in the same family so different from one another. *Behavioral and Brain Sciences, 10*(1), 1–16. https://doi.org/10.1017/s0140525x00055941

Plomin, R., DeFries, J. C., Knopik, V. S., & Neiderhiser, J. M. (2016). Top 10 replicated findings from behavioral genetics. *Perspectives on Psychological Science, 11*(1), 3–23. https://doi.org/10.1177/1745691615617439

Reale, D., Reader, S. M., Sol, D., McDougall, P. T., & Dingemanse, N. J. (2007). Integrating animal temperament within ecology and evolution. *Biological Reviews, 82*(2), 291–318. https://doi.org/10.1111/j.1469-185X.2007.00010.x

Rende, R., Slomkowski, C., Lloyd-Richardson, E., Stroud, L., & Niaura, R. (2006). Estimating genetic and environmental influences on depressive symptoms in adolescence: Differing effects on higher and lower levels of symptoms. *Journal of Clinical Child and Adolescent Psychology, 35*(2), 237–243. https://doi.org/10.1207/s15374424jccp3502_7

Rende, R. D. (1993). Longitudinal relations between temperament traits and behavioral syndromes in middle childhood. *Journal of the American Academy of Child and Adolescent Psychiatry, 32*(2), 287–290. https://doi.org/10.1097/00004583-199303000-00008

Richman, N., Stevenson, J., & Graham, P. (1982). *Pre-school to school: A behavioural study.* Academic.

Roben, C. K. P., Moore, G. A., Cole, P. M., Molenaar, P., Leve, L. D., Shaw, D. S., et al. (2015). Transactional patterns of maternal depressive symptoms and mother-child mutual negativity in an adoption sample. *Infant and Child Development, 24*(3), 322–342. https://doi.org/10.1002/icd.1906

Ruscio, J., Ruscio, A. M., & Meron, M. (2007). Applying the bootstrap to taxometric analysis: Generating empirical sampling distributions to help interpret results. *Multivariate Behavioral Research, 42*(2), 349–386. https://doi.org/10.1080/00273170701360795

Rutter, M. (1987). Temperament, personality and personality-disorder. *British Journal of Psychiatry, 150*, 443–458. https://doi.org/10.1192/bjp.150.4.443

Rutter, M., & Stevenson, J. (2008). Developments in child and adolescent psychiatry over the last 50 years. In M. Rutter, D. Bishop, D. Pine, S. Scott, J. Stevenson, E. Taylor, & A. Thapar (Eds.), *Rutter's child and adolescent psychiatry* (pp. 3–17). Blackwell Publishing.

Sameroff, A., & Chandler, M. (1975). Reproductive risk and the continuum of caretaking casualty. In F. Horowitz, M. Hetherington, S. Scarr-Salapatek, & S. G (Eds.), *Review of child development research* (Vol. 4, pp. 187–244). University of Chicago Press.

Sameroff, A. J., & MacKenzie, M. J. (2003). Research strategies for capturing transactional models of development: The limits of the possible. *Development and Psychopathology, 15*(3), 613–640. https://doi.org/10.1017/s0954579403000312

Saudino, K. J., Carter, A. S., Purper-Ouakil, D., & Gorwood, P. (2008). The etiology of behavioral problems and competencies in very young twins. *Journal of Abnormal Psychology, 117*(1), 48–62. https://doi.org/10.1037/0021-843x.117.1.48

Scheeringa, M., Anders, T., Boris, N., Carter, A., Chatoor-Koch, I., Egger, H., et al. (2003). Research diagnostic criteria for infants and preschool children: The process and empirical support. *Journal of the American Academy of Child and Adolescent Psychiatry, 42*(12), 1504–1512. https://doi.org/10.1097/00004583-200312000-00018

Schwartz, J. A., Connolly, E. J., Nedelec, J. L., & Beaver, K. M. (2017). An investigation of genetic and environmental influences across the distribution of self-control. *Criminal Justice and Behavior, 44*(9), 1163–1182. https://doi.org/10.1177/0093854817709495

Shamay-Tsoory, S. G., & Abu-Akel, A. (2016). The social salience hypothesis of oxytocin. *Biological Psychiatry, 79*(3), 194–202. https://doi.org/10.1016/j.biopsych.2015.07.020

Sirignano, S. W., & Lachman, M. E. (1985). Personality-change during the transition to parenthood - the role of perceived infant temperament. *Developmental Psychology, 21*(3), 558–567. https://doi.org/10.1037/0012-1649.21.3.558

Smoller, J. W. (2013). Disorders and borders: Psychiatric genetics and nosology. *American Journal of Medical Genetics Part B-Neuropsychiatric Genetics, 162*(7), 559–578. https://doi.org/10.1002/ajmg.b.32174

Smoller, J. W., Andreassen, O. A., Edenberg, H. J., Faraone, S. V., Glatt, S. J., & Kendler, K. S. (2019). Psychiatric genetics and the structure of psychopathology. *Molecular Psychiatry, 24*(3), 409–420. https://doi.org/10.1038/s41380-017-0010-4

Sokolovic, N., Plamondon, A., Rodrigues, M., Borairi, S., Perlman, M., & Jenkins, J. M. (2021). Do mothers or children lead the dance? Disentangling individual and influence effects during conflict. *Child Development, 92*(2), E143–E157. https://doi.org/10.1111/cdev.13447

Stevenson, J., Batten, N., & Cherner, M. (1992). Fears and fearfulness in children and adolescents - a genetic-analysis of twin data. *Journal of Child Psychology and Psychiatry, 33*(6), 977–985. https://doi.org/10.1111/j.1469-7610.1992.tb00919.x

Svetlova, M., Nichols, S. R., & Brownell, C. A. (2010). Toddlers' prosocial behavior: From instrumental to empathic to altruistic helping. *Child Development, 81*(6), 1814–1827. https://doi.org/10.1111/j.1467-8624.2010.01512.x

Swanson, J. M., Schuck, S., Porter, M. M., Carlson, C., Hartman, C. A., Sergeant, J. A., et al. (2012). Categorical and dimensional definitions and evaluations of symptoms of ADHD: History of the SNAP and the SWAN rating scales. *The International Journal of Educational and Psychological Assessment, 10*(1), 51–70.

Tangney, J. P., Stuewig, J., & Mashek, D. J. (2007). Moral emotions and moral behavior. *Annual Review of Psychology, 58*, 345–372. https://doi.org/10.1146/annurev.psych.56.091103.070145

Taylor, M. J., Martin, J., Lu, Y., Brikell, I., Lundstrom, S., Larsson, H., & Lichtenstein, P. (2019). Association of genetic risk factors for psychiatric disorders and traits of these disorders in a Swedish population twin sample. *JAMA Psychiatry, 76*(3), 280–289. https://doi.org/10.1001/jamapsychiatry.2018.3652

Thomas, A., & Chess, S. (1957). An approach to the study of sources of individual differences in child behavior. *Journal of Clinical and Experimental Psychopathology, 18*(4), 347–357. PMID: 13481104.

Thomas, A., Chess, S., & Birch, H. (1968). *Temperament and behavior disorders in children*. New York University Press.

Thomas, A., Chess, S., Birch, H. G., Hertzig, M. E., & Korn, S. (1963). *Behavioral individuality in early childhood*. New York University Press.

Tikhodeyev, O. N., & Shcherbakova, O. V. (2019). The problem of non-shared environment in behavioral genetics. *Behavior Genetics, 49*(3), 259–269. https://doi.org/10.1007/s10519-019-09950-1

Tost, H., Kolachana, B., Hakimi, S., Lemaitre, H., Verchinski, B. A., Mattay, V. S., et al. (2010). A common allele in the oxytocin receptor gene (OXTR) impacts prosocial temperament and human hypothalamic-limbic structure and function. *Proceedings of the National Academy of Sciences of the United States of America, 107*(31), 13936–13941. https://doi.org/10.1073/pnas.1003296107

VanderWeele, T. J. (2014). A unification of mediation and interaction a 4-way decomposition. *Epidemiology, 25*(5), 749–761. https://doi.org/10.1097/ede.0000000000000121

Vasileva, M., Graf, R. K., Reinelt, T., Petermann, U., & Petermann, F. (2021). Research review: A meta-analysis of the international prevalence and comorbidity of mental disorders in children between 1 and 7 years. *Journal of Child Psychology and Psychiatry, 62*(4), 372–381. https://doi.org/10.1111/jcpp.13261

von Borell, C. J., Weiss, A., & Penke, L. (2019). Developing individual differences in primate behavior: The role of genes, environment, and their interplay. *Behavioral Ecology and Sociobiology, 73*(2). https://doi.org/10.1007/s00265-019-2633-8

Wakschlag, L. S., Briggs-Gowan, M. J., Carter, A. S., Hill, C., Danis, B., Keenan, K., et al. (2007). A developmental framework for distinguishing disruptive behavior from normative misbehavior in preschool children. *Journal of Child Psychology and Psychiatry, 48*(10), 976–987. https://doi.org/10.1111/j.1469-7610.2007.01786.x

Wakschlag, L. S., Tolan, P. H., & Leventhal, B. L. (2010). Research Review: 'Ain't misbehavin': Towards a developmentally-specified nosology for preschool disruptive behavior. *Journal of Child Psychology and Psychiatry, 51*(1), 3–22. https://doi.org/10.1111/j.1469-7610.2009.02184.x

Weisz, J. R., Kuppens, S., Ng, M. Y., Eckshtain, D., Ugueto, A. M., Vaughn-Coaxum, R., et al. (2017). What five decades of research tells us about the effects of youth psychological therapy: A multilevel meta-analysis and implications for science and practice. *American Psychologist, 72*(2), 79–117. https://doi.org/10.1037/a0040360

White, T. J. H. (2019). Brain development and stochastic processes during prenatal and early life: You can't lose it if you've never had it; but it's better to have it and lose it, than never to have had it at all. *Journal of the American Academy of Child and Adolescent Psychiatry, 58*(11), 1042–1050. https://doi.org/10.1016/j.jaac.2019.02.010

Widiger, T. A., & Samuel, D. B. (2005). Diagnostic categories or dimensions? A question for the diagnostic and statistical manual of mental disorders-fifth edition. *Journal of Abnormal Psychology, 114*(4), 494–504. https://doi.org/10.1037/0021-843x.114.4.494

Woodbury, M. A., Clive, J., & Garson, A. (1978). Mathematical typology - grade of membership technique for obtaining disease definition. *Computers and Biomedical Research, 11*(3), 277–298. https://doi.org/10.1016/0010-4809(78)90012-5

Wu, T. C. H., Meehan, A. J., Rijlaarsdam, J., Maughan, B., Fearon, P., & Barker, E. D. (2022). Developmental pathways from toddler difficult temperament to child generalized psychopathology and adult functioning. *Journal of Affective Disorders, 301*, 14–22. https://doi.org/10.1016/j.jad.2022.01.012

Wu, N., & Su, Y. J. (2015). Oxytocin receptor gene relates to theory of mind and prosocial behavior in children. *Journal of Cognition and Development, 16*(2), 302–313. https://doi.org/10.1080/15248372.2013.858042

Xerxa, Y., Rescorla, L. A., Serdarevic, F., Van Ijzendorn, M. H., Jaddoe, V. W., Verhulst, F. C., et al. (2020). The complex role of parental separation in the association between family conflict and child problem behavior. *Journal of Clinical Child and Adolescent Psychology, 49*(1), 79–93. https://doi.org/10.1080/15374416.2018.1520118

Xiao, S. X., Spinrad, T. L., & Eisenberg, N. (2019). Longitudinal relations of preschoolers' dispositional and situational anger to their prosocial behavior: The moderating role of shyness. *Social Development, 28*(2), 383–397. https://doi.org/10.1111/sode.12346

Zahn-Waxler, C., Cole, P. M., Welsh, J. D., & Fox, N. A. (1995). Psychophysiological correlates of empathy and prosocial behaviors in preschool-children with behavior problems. *Development and Psychopathology, 7*(1), 27–48. https://doi.org/10.1017/s0954579400006325

Zubin, J. (1967). Classification of the behavior disorders. *Annual Review of Psychology, 18*, 373–406. https://doi.org/10.1146/annurev.ps.18.020167.002105

Chapter 6
Hierarchical Models of Behaviour Differences

The case for a dimensional approach to psychopathology was made in Chap. 5. This is reinforced by studies that have investigated the characteristics of those who fall below the threshold for a categorical diagnosis. In relation to anxiety disorder Haller et al. (2014) showed, in a systematic review of studies on adults, that generalised anxiety disorder which falls below the threshold was nevertheless persistent and a debilitating condition. Similar findings emerged from a longitudinal study of sub-threshold depression in a cohort of children in New Zealand (Fergusson et al., 2005) and, for a variety of sub-threshold conditions, in a community-based sample of young adults in the United States (Shankman et al., 2009). The persistence of sub-threshold mental health conditions was studied specifically by Schreuder et al. (2021). In a sample of young adults they showed that stability is similar across symptom severity levels of mental health. They conclude

> that subthreshold psychopathology may resemble a stable state rather than a transient intermediate between mental health and psychiatric disorder. Schreuder et al. (2021), p. 1

This suggests that a dimensional framework for studying mental health is apposite since symptoms differ in severity and not in type. Similar conclusions were drawn in a study of sub-threshold attention-deficit hyperactivity disorder (ADHD) symptoms. There was no clear evidence of a point on the continuum of ADHD symptom severity where there was a sudden increase in impairment (Arildskov et al., 2021). This indicates that there is simply a linear increase in impairment as ADHD symptom severity increases. They conclude that in ADHD diagnoses the impairment assessment should be considered on a continuum and not on a binary judgement of impaired or not. In addition impairment should be appraised alongside an assessment of symptom severity and frequency.

These findings support the conclusions of Helzer et al. (2006) that, although diagnostic categories may be of value in clinical contexts for communicating about mental illness, a dimensional approach provides a better scientific formulation for

J. Stevenson, *Developmental Psychopathology*,
https://doi.org/10.1007/978-3-031-45787-6_6

understanding the underlying nature of psychiatric illness. This leads to the question of what are these dimensions and how they relate to each other. It is this issue that will be considered in the chapter.

6.1 Confirmatory Factor Analysis and Internalising and Externalising Factors

The early history of studies on the organisation of psychopathology symptoms in children was reviewed by Tom Achenbach in an account of the development of his measures of behaviour (Achenbach, 1966). Subsequently Achenbach (2020) provided a summary of the work by his group and others to extend and develop his measurement framework over the subsequent 50 years. In that landmark 1966 paper Tom Achenbach reports on an exploratory factor analysis (EFA) of symptoms from 300 female and 300 male child psychiatric patients. He identified two factors that he labelled "internalising" and "externalising" that have formed the cornerstone of the terminology and measures for child psychopathology subsequently developed by Achenbach and his colleagues. As this measurement framework developed and was applied to older age ranges additional scales and syndromes were identified, for example, thought problems.

The structure of behaviour problems in children has also been examined using confirmatory factor analysis (CFA) methods (see Sect. 2.4) and, for middle childhood and adolescence, a robust binary pattern of internalising and externalising behaviours has been found using a variety of measurement methods (e.g. Lahey et al., 2008). Alternative methods of analysis have also found the broad grouping of internalising and externalising; cluster analysis (see Sect. 2.3) was applied by Muratori et al. (2021) to identify groups with similar profiles on the Strength and Difficulties Questionnaire (SDQ) plus items measuring callous-unemotional traits (see Sect. 8.1). Using data from a sample of 2959 10–14-year-olds they found four distinct profiles. One comprising those with no problems (42%), one with subthreshold hyperactivity (33%), and then two clusters with predominantly internalising (19%) and predominantly externalising (7%) problems, respectively.

CFAs have also replicated this broad internalising (emotional disorders) and externalising (disruptive disorders) distinction for preschool children. For example, Strickland et al. (2011) conducted CFAs on checklist data from 796 4-year-old children on problem behaviour from the Early Child Symptom Inventory (ECI-4). For emotional disorders the best-fit model included the following factors: social phobia, separation anxiety disorder, generalised anxiety disorder, and major depressive disorder. Three further factors were identified for disruptive disorders – ADHD – inattentive type, ADHD-hyperactive/impulsivity type, and oppositional-defiant disorder. Despite differences in sampling and in the measurement of behaviour, the results obtained by Strickland et al. (2011) were broadly similar to those found in an earlier study on preschool children by Sterba et al. (2007).

The question that will now be addressed is how these dimensions of behaviour relate to each other? Are they independent or are they associated, and if so, what is the pattern of these associations?

There are a number of alternative ways models of the dimensions of psychopathology can be constructed. These alternatives are illustrated in Fig. 6.1. The simplest is where the items of behaviour are linked by a single factor (Fig. 6.1a). A more complex model is one that has a number of separate group factors which are themselves correlated (Fig. 6.1b). A model that combines these two is shown in Fig. 6.1c. This has a general factor that accounts for the tendency of all behaviours to co-occur and separate uncorrelated group factors that accommodate the additional relationships found within more homogeneous subgroups, for example, internalising and externalising behaviours; this is a bifactor model. The final alternative is a higher-order factor model (Fig. 6.1d). This replaces the correlations in the correlated group factor model with a superordinate general factor. Over the past decade or so there has been a vigorous debate about which is the most appropriate way to model the pattern of associations between behaviours.

6.2 Bifactor Analysis and the p-Factor

There has been a re-emergence of interest in bifactor analysis. This is a method of structural analysis, first developed by Holzinger and Swineford (1937), and seeks to identify group factors that account for covariance in relatively homogeneous subgroups of symptoms (or behaviours or disorders). It also identifies a general factor that explains the additional tendency for all symptoms to relate to each other, whatever sub-group they may belong to (see Fig. 6.1c). This terminology of group factors and a general factor will be used here to describe the results from studies whatever other terminology the authors may have used. This consistency avoids confusion and was recommended by Reise in his seminal 2012 paper on the rediscovery of bifactor analysis.

The bifactor model is fitted to the correlation (variance/covariance) matrix between the items. The items can be responses to questions about behaviour from a questionnaire or interview measure, scale scores, or diagnostic categories. The bifactor approach was first applied to measures of psychopathology in adults (e.g. Lahey et al., 2012; Patrick et al., 2007) and subsequently to measures in adolescence (e.g. Patalay et al., 2015; Tackett et al., 2013) and in middle childhood (e.g. Lahey et al., 2015; Martel et al., 2017). In all these cases, the bifactor model provided the best fit for the data.

Overfitting However there are concerns over whether the bifactor model overfits the data and thereby always provides the best-fitting model (Greene et al., 2019; Greene et al., 2022). Overfitting occurs when the analysis starts to explain error rather than true variance in the data (Bonifay, Lane, & Reise, 2017). In addition there are uncertainties over the interpretation of the group factors in the bifactor

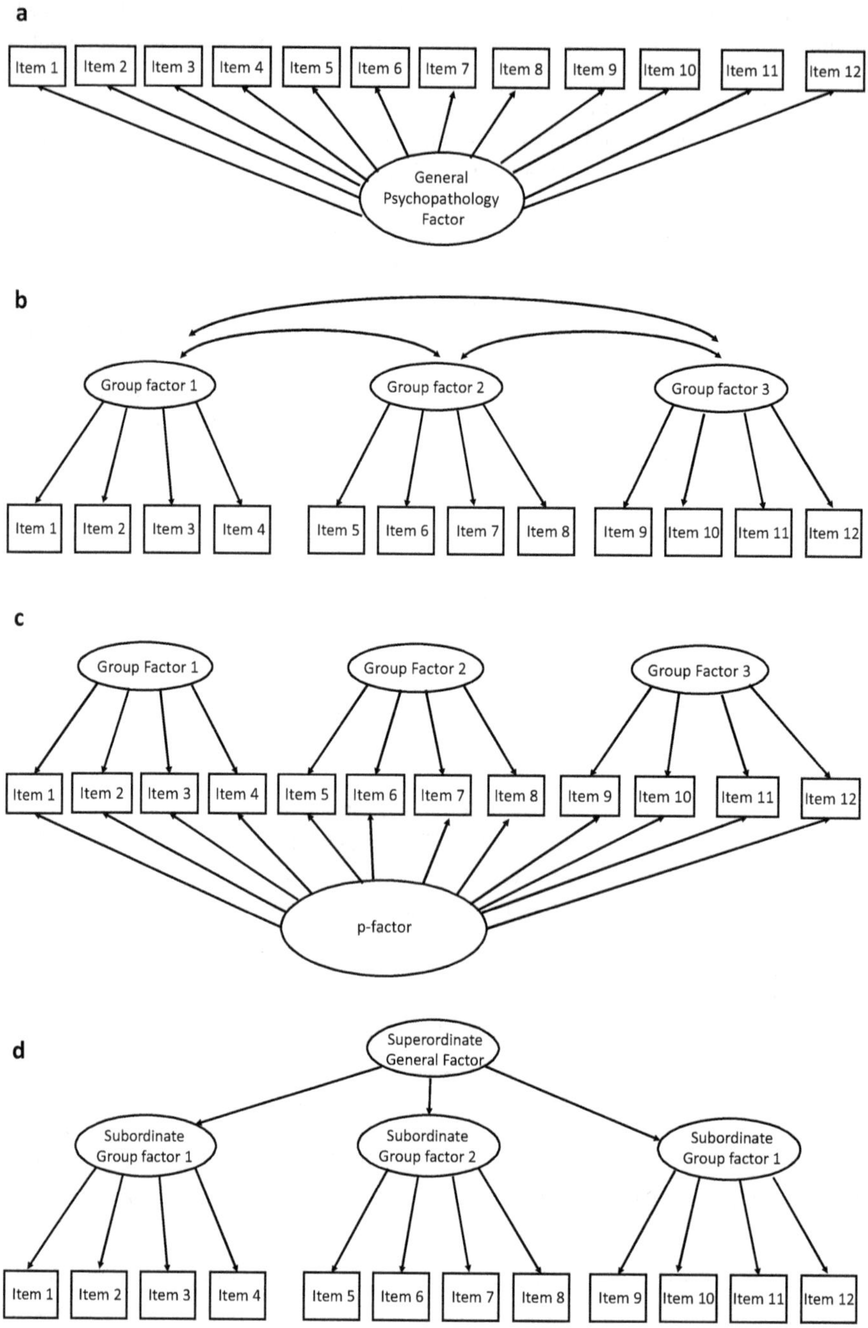

Fig. 6.1 (**a**) Single-factor model. (**b**) Correlated group factor model. (**c**) Bifactor model. (**d**) Higher-order factor model

analysis (Conway et al., 2019). Conway et al. (2019) suggest that as the general factor explains most of the variance in behaviour and the group factors may reflect "nuisance" residual variance and consequently are of little predictive utility. These issues have been reviewed by Sellbom and Tellegen (2019), who recommend that before adopting a bifactor solution as the optimal representation of the relationship between a set of measures, additional ancillary tests be estimated, not just model fit, and that there be a strong a priori reason to expect such a general factor to be found. Importantly they strongly endorse the importance of examining the relationship between the general and group factors and external validating measures.

Ancillary Tests There are a number of these ancillary tests that can be used to evaluate bifactor models (Rodriguez et al., 2016). These are measures that assess psychometric features such as scale reliability, for example, coefficient omega. Omega indicates whether a substantial portion of the variance in the items is explained by the general and group factors. Omega hierarchical estimates the extent to which the general factor explains variance which is independent of the group factor. Rodriguez et al. (2016) also recommended additional indicators to determine whether a bifactor model is an improvement on a simpler single-factor solution, for example, explained common variance (ECV) and percentage uncontaminated correlation (PUC).

GPF and the p-Factor The terminology in these model-fitting analyses aimed at determining the optimal solution for the structure of psychopathology has become confusing. The term "p-factor" was applied by Caspi et al. (2014) to the general factor loading on all behaviours where general factor and uncorrelated group factors have been extracted using a bifactor model. It should be noted that in some bifactor analysis studies the group factors have been allowed to correlate, which may make the interpretation of the group factors more problematic (Reise, 2012). The term "general psychopathology factor" (GPF) has been used to refer to the higher-order factor obtained in a variety of analyses, including hierarchical models and bifactor analysis (Markon, 2019). It has also been used for higher-order factors derived from other analytic methods such as the bass-ackwards method (e.g. see Kim & Eaton, 2015; Michelini et al., 2019).

Here the term GPF will be used in this generic sense and the term p-factor will be limited to refer to a general factor that has been identified using a bifactor analysis. The confusion arises as the term p-factor is sometimes applied to the general factor identified in a range of analyses rather than just a bifactor. Maintaining the reference of p-factor to the general factor extracted by bifactor analysis is important, not least in relation to the group factors. In a bifactor analysis these group factors are independent of each other and are unrelated to the p-factor. Consequently studies looking at characteristics that might be associated with these group factors are doing so for a measure that is "pure". This feature of group factor score from a bifactor analysis has come to be labelled "p-free" (Caspi et al., 2023). This p-free status means that any risk or outcome measure associated with the p-free factor score arises from processes specifically linked to this factor and not from associations with psychopathology in general.

In an analysis of data on psychopathology in early adulthood from the Dunedin longitudinal study Caspi et al. (2014) found that the bifactor model (Fig. 6.1c) fitted the data better than either a correlated factor model (Fig. 6.1b) or a higher-order factor model (Fig. 6.1d). As a final test Caspi et al. (2014) tested whether a single factor (Fig. 6.1a) would fit the data. They found that it did not and concluded that the p-factor alone does not account for the association between the measures of psychopathology. The group factors are an essential component.

6.3 Higher-Order Models

There are a number of ways higher-order models such as that in Fig.6.1d have been formulated. One that has become central to recent research efforts is the Hierarchical Taxonomy of Psychopathology (HiTOP) which has been proposed by a large consortium of researchers. Their objectives as laid out on the group's webpage are as follows and details about the HiTOP approach are given in the next section:

> … to advance the classification of psychopathology to maximize its usefulness for research and clinical practice. The HiTOP aims to address limitations of traditional nosologies, such as the DSM-5 and ICD-10, including arbitrary boundaries between psychopathology and normality, often unclear boundaries between disorders, frequent disorder co-occurrence, heterogeneity within disorders, and diagnostic instability.
> https://renaissance.stonybrookmedicine.edu/HITOP/AboutHiTOP (accessed 5 August 2023)

HiTOP A higher-order model approach has informed an innovative formulation for the taxonomy of psychopathology – the Hierarchical Taxonomy of Psychopathology (HiTOP) (Kotov et al., 2017; Ruggero et al., 2019; Waszczuk et al., 2020). HiTOP attempts to move the classification of psychopathology away from a reliance on categories to one that is based on dimensional measures of pathology (Krueger et al., 2018). This HiTOP model has been largely applied to adult psychopathology, but the group factors from the HiTOP of "internalising" and "disinhibited externalising" can clearly be identified in childhood. The thought disorder spectra in HiTOP need to be examined more extensively to establish if they have an equivalence in childhood. There is an unresolved issue of the place of neurodevelopmental disorders, such as ASD and ADHD, in the HiTOP framework (Stanton et al., 2021). However it has been shown that the broad structure of internalising and externalising group factors holds in a similar manner in those with autism and non-autistic individuals (Rodriguez-Seijas et al., 2020).

Conway, Forbes, South et al. (2021) have produced a detailed guide and tutorials on the use of HiTOP in research. This provides an excellent introduction to the application of this approach to the dimensional analysis of psychopathology – sometimes labelled as a transdimensional dispositional approach. The need to address the question of the relationship between components of psychopathology was re-affirmed in a large Danish study. Using Danish national health register data on almost six million people, Plana-Ripoll et al. (2019) showed that comorbidity within mental disorders is pervasive, and the risk of showing multiple disorders persists over time.

The formulation of psychopathology under HiTOP is not without its critics, for example, Haeffel et al. (2022a,b). These critics suggest that it is of little, if any, relevance to clinical practice, and moreover it is atheoretical in that there is no rationale, apart from co-occurrence, for grouping dimensions together. Accepting that HiTOP is a work in progress, DeYoung et al. (2022) counter this critique by showing the way in which the framework has been validated against external criteria. They argue that, although based on observed co-occurrences between symptoms rather than an understanding of aetiology, this does not preclude it being of value in guiding diagnosis and treatment. Indeed they say this approach may be preferable in the absence of adequate knowledge about aetiology.

Causal Hierarchical Models The hierarchical approach exemplified by HiTOP is based on an analysis of correlations between phenotypic measures. This has been extended by Lahey et al. (2011), and Lahey et al. (2017) include an examination of the role of putative causal genetic and environmental factors in producing the pattern of association observed between psychopathology symptoms in children and adults. The hierarchical causal taxonomy attempts to identify the relationships between the shared experiential and genetic influences on psychopathology to account for the observed correlations between phenotypic measures. The approach applies a method of analysing data on twin resemblance (see Sect. 3.1) to identify genetic, shared, and non-shared influences not simply on the measures of psychopathology, but on the latent general and group factors that underlie them.

The results from Lahey et al. (2011) suggest that non-specific (general) influences, especially genetic, act to produce correlations between group factors, such as internalising and externalising. Non-shared environmental factors that are particular to the individual are significant for specific symptoms rather than having a general influence. In this analysis there was no evidence of shared environmental influences on psychopathology. This model of generalist genes and specialist environments was reviewed by Rhee et al. (2015) in the context of other behaviour genetic studies on comorbidity. They concluded that

> First, studies support distinguishing internalizing from externalizing disorders from the preschool years to adulthood. Second, research also supports the model of generalist genes and specialist environments, with disorder-specific influences being mostly non-shared environmental influences. Third, negative emotionality is a heritable common underlying feature explaining the overlap between internalizing and externalizing disorders. Fourth, although evidence is less consistent, daring is a heritable broadband-specific underlying feature that distinguishes externalizing from internalizing disorders. Rhee et al. (2015), p. 29

These conclusions have been replicated in subsequent studies, although there is a suggestion that the reversed effects of specialist genes and generalist environments may have a role to play in the development of internalising and externalising problems in adolescence (Marceau & Neiderhiser, 2022). The relationship between the HiTOP model and this more ambitious hierarchical causal taxonomy has been summarised by Lahey et al. (2021).

Higher-Order Factor vs p-Factor There is a clear distinction between the HiTOP hierarchical model and the p-factor model based on a bifactor analysis. The general factor is at the top of a hierarchy of factors in HiTOP (Fig. 6.1d), whereas the p-factor has bottom-up influences on all behaviours (Fig. 6.1c). This contrast was tested in a study of adult psychopathology by Hyland et al. (2021). They concluded that a higher-order representation of the general factor, as described in HiTOP, appears to be a more appropriate way to conceptualise this general dimension of psychopathology than the p-factor bifactor approach. This study was based on a sample of adults who had experienced a traumatic life event, and consequently the generalisability of this result must be in doubt.

In summary, these results suggest that a solution with a general factor and internalising and externalising group factors is found across age groups from middle childhood upwards, using different methods of structural equation modelling and different measures of psychopathology. The structure of psychopathology in the preschool child will be considered in Sect. 6.5.

6.4 Is the p-Factor Real or an Artefact of Bifactor Analysis?

There are concerns that there may be artefacts from the bifactor model analysis that lead to it showing a better fit than alternative plausible models (Markon, 2019). Watts et al. (2019) have argued that stringent appraisals of the bifactor model suggest that the p-factor approach does not explain more of the variance than more parsimonious correlated group factor models (see Fig. 6.1b). Their argument hinges on three "tests" –first, the general factor should be roughly equally weighted on the symptoms; second, the group factors should have robust reliabilities; and third, the bifactor model should explain more of the variance in external criteria.

In their analysis of psychopathology symptoms measured by the Emory Combined Rating Scale (Waldman et al., 1998) on 2498 4–17-year-olds, Watts et al. (2019) found that in their models the p-factor varied in the loading on symptoms and a model that constrained these weights to be equal fitted significantly less well than an unconstrained model. The reliability of the group factors in bifactor models was less good than in the alternative models, but in general the reliabilities were adequate. However the bifactor model was as good, if not better, at predicting external criteria than the alternative models. The external criteria used were a range of measures, namely the Antisocial Process Screening Device (Frick & Hare, 2001), the EAS Temperament Survey for Children (Buss & Plomin, 1984), and the Reactive-Proactive Aggression Scale (Dodge & Coie, 1987).

Watts et al. (2020) take the critique of the p-factor further.

They argue that there are four major issues with the status of the p-factor that emerge when model (i.e. the results of the statistical analysis) and theory (i.e. the explanation of the nature of the factors) are distinguished. First, simply establishing good model fit does not itself indicate good validity. Second, most explanations of the p-factor are weak theories in that they are "narrative and imprecise descriptions" and do not make unique and distinctive predictions that are not also predicted by other theories. Third, the p-factor is "ill-defined and even protean" – by that they mean that the constitution of the p-factor varies considerably depending on the set of indicators being used. It is therefore difficult to replicate across studies. Fourth, although often considered to reflect causal mechanisms the p-factor is derived from latent variable models and these do not reveal causality.

A resolution of these disagreements has been proposed by Forbes et al. (2021). This group undertook an analysis of two longitudinal waves of nationally representative data on adults from the United States (n = 43,093 and n = 34,653) based on the following models: a count of diagnoses, single-factor, correlated factor, higher-order, and bifactor models. They found that a single-factor model did not capture the shared variance in the data and multidimensional models were needed. Whatever the model the general factor showed good reliability and validity. However the group factors in the bifactor model did not show good validity or reliability. The authors concluded with three recommendations. First, fit indices should not be used in isolation when choosing between different models. Second, the reliability of latent variables needs to be tested. Third, the interpretation of the unique effects of group factors should be made warily whatever model is being considered.

These findings, combined with those from Conway et al. (2019) and Rosenstrom et al. (2019), suggest that it is a hierarchical factor solution and the bifactor models provide very similar solutions. Indeed Conway et al. (2019) found that the factor scores in the bifactor and second-order factor in a hierarchical solution correlate at $r = 0.97$. Rosenstrom et al. (2019) argue that a general factor in psychopathology as a higher-order factor influencing internalising, externalising, and thought disorder offers scientific advantages as a "measurable construct instead of an unexplained correlation"; the latter being exemplified by Fig. 6.1b.

It is important to recognise that different factor solutions may be preferable for different purposes. As Moore et al. (2020) argue, the bifactor model is particularly valuable when the goal is to identify both common and unique correlates of the dimensions of psychopathology. On the surface, bifactor and higher-order factor models are similar in defining general and specific factors of psychopathology, but they actually differ in important ways. Tests of associations of factor scores with external variables – such as clinical outcomes, risk factors, and neurobiological variations – of the two models are necessarily different in form and meaning (Lahey et al., 2021). The crucial difference is that in the bifactor model the general and group factors are uncorrelated with each other and therefore distinct independent associations with external variables can be tested.

p-Factor and Risks An example of the value of the bifactor model is given by the systematic investigation of the correlates of the p-factor and the group factors internalising and externalising undertaken by Brislin et al. (2022). The data were from 10,000 9- and 10-year-olds in the Adolescent Brain Cognitive Development (ABCD) study. The associated measures were grouped as follows: social diversity, impulsivity, fear/distress, and general neurocognition (an aggregate score on a number of cognition tasks). They found that the first three were all positively related to the p-factor and general neurocognition was negatively correlated. Social adversity was unrelated to internalising and positively related to externalising. Impulsivity was negatively related to internalising but positively related to externalising – the opposite pattern was found for fear/distress. Finally general neurocognition was positively related to internalising and unrelated to externalising. The Brislin et al. (2022) study provides a demonstration of the potential of p-factor analysis to identify underlying influences on behaviour that have distinct associations with risk factors.

p-Factor and Outcomes There have been a number of longitudinal studies examining the nature and later significance of the GPF in children and adolescents. Pettersson et al. (2018) obtained data on the mental health of 16,806 twin children aged 9 and 12 years. They were able to link these with data on adverse outcomes in adolescence, including psychiatric diagnoses, drug prescriptions, court convictions, and "failure to achieve eligibility for beginning high school, which can occur due to either prior excess school absence or low grades". They found that the risk of adverse outcomes in adolescence was determined largely by the GPF.

Child psychopathology was assessed between 4 and 8 years in three independent birth cohorts using a range of diagnostic and questionnaire-based measures, and multiple informants (Sallis et al., 2019). They derived models that included a GPF and group factors of internalising and externalising. The association between scores of these factors and outcomes in later adolescence and early adulthood was estimated. The outcomes included mental health, problem drinking, criminal activity, and educational attainment. They found that the GPF was the best predictor of outcome. The internalising factor also predicted later anxiety and depression.

The importance of the GPF for outcomes in mid-life was established by Hoffmann et al. (2023) in a follow-up of the Isle of Wight Study (see Sect. 8.3) cohort into their mid-40s. They found that GPF scores based on parents' and teachers' ratings of behaviour were associated with a range of adverse psychosocial outcomes some 30 years after the behaviour ratings were made.

Generalisability A crucial issue in judging the value of hierarchical models is whether the structure and the associated characteristics of the factor scores generalise across different samples. Hoffmann et al. (2022) have shown that the p-factor characteristics are reproduced across 11 bifactor models of CBCL items derived by different research groups on different samples. The models were similar in fit and broadly congruent in their psychometric properties across studies. They conclude that p-factor solutions are robust across studies, methods, and samples.

It has been suggested that an alternative formulation of the bifactor approach may provide more robust solutions that generalise across samples. This is the S-1 bifactor model (Eid et al., 2017). Under this model a subset of measures are used to identify the general factor. Using this S-1 approach with measures of ADHD and oppositional deficient disorder symptoms, Burns et al. (2020) were able to produce a structure that showed convergent and discriminant validity across sources of ratings. A problem with the S-1 bifactor approach is that it necessarily removes a subset of behaviours to identify the general factor. This may aid the production of interpretable group factors but leaves the general factor equated with a subset of indicators, thereby making the interpretation of the general factor problematic (Greene et al., 2022).

There are two additional issues related to generalisability. There is a largely under-investigated question of the general applicability of the GPF across cultures. A review of whether measures of child and adolescent psychopathology had been assessed for their validity and suitability for use across cultures was undertaken by Stevanovic et al. (2017). They identified 26 scales where information on such cross-cultural measurement invariance was available. They concluded that none of the scales had strong evidence in support of their use cross-culturally.

There have been few studies concerning cross-cultural measurement invariance in hierarchical models. In one such study, He and Li (2021) examined hierarchical models for psychopathology measures in African American ($n = 3088$) and European American ($n = 5147$) samples aged 8–21 years. The model fitting produced similar results in both groups, and they suggest that the hierarchical factor structure of psychopathology may be robust to racial–ethnic differences. Cicero and Ruggero (2021) have endorsed the importance of the issue of establishing factorial invariance across racial and ethnic groups. They also suggested that a wider range of measures needs to be tested, in particular for dimensional approaches. There is also a need to extend the range of populations being studied.

An extensive examination of the applicability of the p-factor model to the behavioural development of young children was undertaken by Avinun et al. (2022). They used data from a longitudinally studied sample of over 2000 twins between the ages of 3 and 13 years. The availability of data on twins allowed the effects of the factors of genetics and the shared environment to be estimated. They found that a structure of p-factor and p-free internalising and externalising factors was present from age 3 years onwards. A shared environment effect was only found for the p-free externalising factor. All the factors showed marked genetic influences which were largely stable. Analyses of early-life experiences explained little of the variance in any of the factors. An important feature of the study was that the participants were all Hebrew-speaking Israeli families. The findings therefore extend the range of ethnicities for which the p-factor has been found.

The second further issue related to generalisability is that most of the studies on the p-factor with children and adolescents have been based on samples of children from the general population. There may therefore be concerns over the applicability of the findings to children referred to clinics and receiving a clinical diagnosis. A study on two groups of around 1000 referred children and referred adolescents was undertaken to address this issue (Gomez et al., 2019). Using data from a diagnostic interview with the parent, they found that the bifactor model with a p-factor and internalising and externalising group factors provided the optimum model for both age groups. As in other studies the reliability (see Sect. 6.2) of the p-factor was higher than the two group factors.

In summary, the bifactor analysis produces reproducible results in children and adolescents that replicate across different studies using different methods. There are few studies that examine whether similar factor structures emerge from studies on samples from different ethnic groups.

6.5 Is There a General Psychopathology Factor (GPF) in the Behaviour of Preschool Children?

There have been a limited number of studies applying higher-order or bifactor analysis to measures of the behaviour of preschool children. Some of these have been restricted to a subset of behaviours. For example, in a group of referred preschool children aged 3.5–5.5 years Geeraerts et al. (2015) found that a bifactor model produced the best fit to a measure of symptoms of dysregulation. Using a measure, solely of anxieties and fears, Spence et al. (2001) found a second-order factor structure, such as that in Fig. 6.1b, to be the best fit for the data from a large sample of 2.5–6.5-year-olds rated by mothers or by fathers. The high covariation between factors measuring social phobia, separation anxiety, generalised anxiety, obsessive-compulsive disorder, and fear of physical injury was best explained by their loading onto a single higher-order factor of anxiety in general. The structure of these anxiety symptoms in the preschool child is similar to that found in older children (Muris et al., 1999).

There have also been p-factor analyses of measures based on a wider range of behaviours with the preschool child. Using scores of the Infant –Toddler Social and Emotional Assessment (ITSEA) from 1- to 3-year-olds, Carter et al. (2003) found the best fit to be a total problem model. This included a p-factor loading on all symptoms and three group factors labelled "externalising", "internalising", and "dysregulation". In this analysis the group factors were allowed to correlate. Olino et al. (2014) applied a bifactor analysis to the symptoms from the Preschool Age Psychiatric Assessment (PAPA) (Egger & Angold, 2004) measured in 3-year-olds. The optimal fit was obtained with two group factors (internalising and externalising) and a general factor that loaded on all symptoms, apart from phobia. In addition, a substantial correlation (r = 0.36) was found between depression and inattention – this is an association specific to these two symptoms that is not explained by the general factor. The results of this analysis are presented in Fig. 6.2.

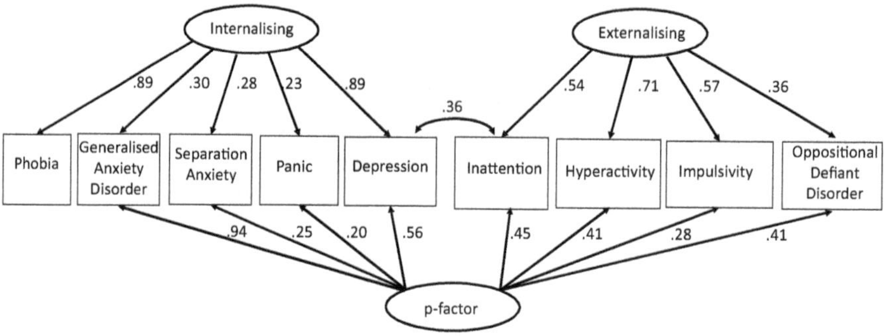

Fig. 6.2 Bifactor model of preschool age psychopathology. (Adapted with the permission of Springer Nature BV from Fig. 1 Olino et al. (2014). *Journal of Abnormal Child Psychology, 42*(7), 1201–1211; permission conveyed through Copyright Clearance Center, Inc.)

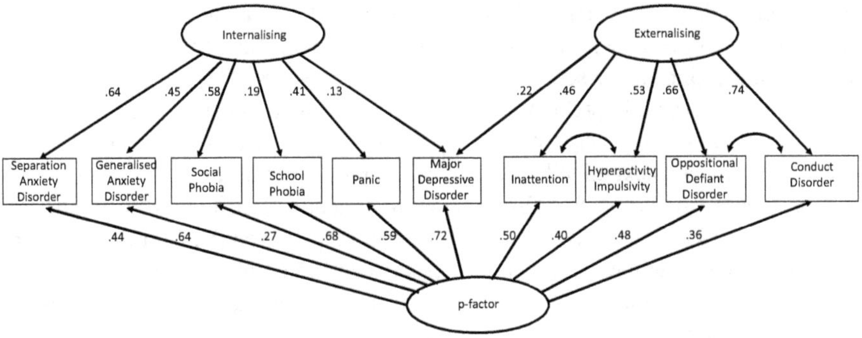

Fig. 6.3 Bifactor model of psychopathology in 5–11-year–olds. (Adapted with the permission of John Wiley & Sons from Fig. 1 Lahey et al. (2015). *Journal of Child Psychology and Psychiatry, 56*(4), 415–422; permission conveyed through Copyright Clearance Center, Inc.)

For comparison the results from an older age group (5–11-year-olds) of the bifactor analysis by Lahey et al. (2015) are presented in Fig. 6.3. It should be noted that these data were obtained for girls only. There are some differences in the disorders included in the analyses in Figs. 6.2 and 6.3. Conduct is included as a separate disorder in the older children, and phobias are divided into social and school phobias. The methods used to measure psychopathology were different – the PAPA in Olino et al. (2014) and the Child Symptom Inventory-4 in Lahey et al. (2015). These differences notwithstanding there are clear parallels between the results for children in the preschool and middle childhood periods. There is a p-factor at both ages which loads on all disorders (with the exception of phobia in the preschool group). The same two group factors are present – internalising and externalising. At both ages there are additional associations between major depressive disorder and externalising disorders. At 5–11 years major depressive disorders load on externalising and for the preschool children there is a residual correlation between depression and inattention. It should be noted for the older children there are correlations between residual inattention and hyperactivity/impulsivity and between oppositional-defiant disorder and conduct disorder.

The relationship between the general and group factors in preschool children (aged 3–4 years) and behaviour in preadolescence (aged 9–12 years) was examined by Michelini et al. (2022). The analysis replicated a hierarchical structure for behaviour in the preschool period. The general factor identified was predictive of behaviours in preadolescence with the group factors explaining additional variance. The findings add to the recognition of the potential importance of identifying profiles on hierarchical factors in the preschool period to inform the selection of potential targets for early innervation and prevention.

Wade et al. (2021) have produced an innovative analysis of the influences on psychopathology factors in young children. They studied a general population sample of 501 Canadian children and families followed from birth to 3 years of age. They found that a latent bifactor model incorporating the p-factor and internalising and externalising group factors provided the best child psychopathology item correlations. They then examined how a family socialisation model of the impact of maternal education and family income/assets measured at birth might influence p-factor and group factor scores measured at age 3 years. These effects might be both direct or via family process variables, such as maternal depression, sensitivity, and sibling relationship negativity. The possible role of mediation via child cognitive factors was also examined. They found a direct effect of lower maternal education on higher p-factor scores. Both maternal education and family income/assets had indirect effects on the p-factor via maternal responsiveness. Correlations were found between a number of maternal measures and internalising, but the evidence was less strong for the mediated effects on internalising and externalising group factor scores. The study provides a good example of the way p-factor analysis can identify the effects of family factors on psychopathology in general and more specific influences on internalising and externalising. However the design of the study did not allow for control of confounds by possible genetic influences to be made.

The results from the studies reviewed above indicate that the structure of the psychopathologies in the preschool period can be formulated as broadly equivalent to the general psychopathology model that is found in older children.

Bifactor Analyses in Adults and Children A somewhat different pattern emerges from the application of bifactor analysis to data on psychopathology in adulthood. For example Fig. 6.4 presents the model found by Lahey et al. (2012) for a large sample of adults in the United States, where general p-factor is present. Here the internalising group factor is split between distress and fears. As in children a single externalising group factor was found. There is evidence that a thought disorder group factor can also be found in bifactor analyses of data from adults (Caspi et al., 2014).

Levin-Aspenson et al. (2021) have reviewed the p-factor research in adulthood but also briefly comment on studies with children and adolescents. They suggest that in childhood there are differences between studies in the behaviours loading most highly on the p-factor. Some found internalising and inattentiveness to predominate (Olino et al., 2014; Olino et al., 2018). By contrast others have found externalising and ASD-related behaviours load more highly (Hankin et al., 2017; Martel et al., 2017; Neumann et al., 2016; Pettersson et al., 2018). They suggest that the variation between studies in the way psychopathology has been measured makes it even more difficult to draw conclusions about the most salient features of the p-factor in adolescence. However, they tentatively suggest that externalising behaviours feature more strongly in child and adolescent studies than they do in studies on adults.

The potential value of a hierarchical model in the design and planning of prevention approaches was developed by Forbes et al. (2019). Their developmental approach is reproduced in Fig. 6.5. This suggests age-related foci for intervention from the preschool period through to adulthood. In this model interventions centred on the p-factor are concentrated in the preschool period.

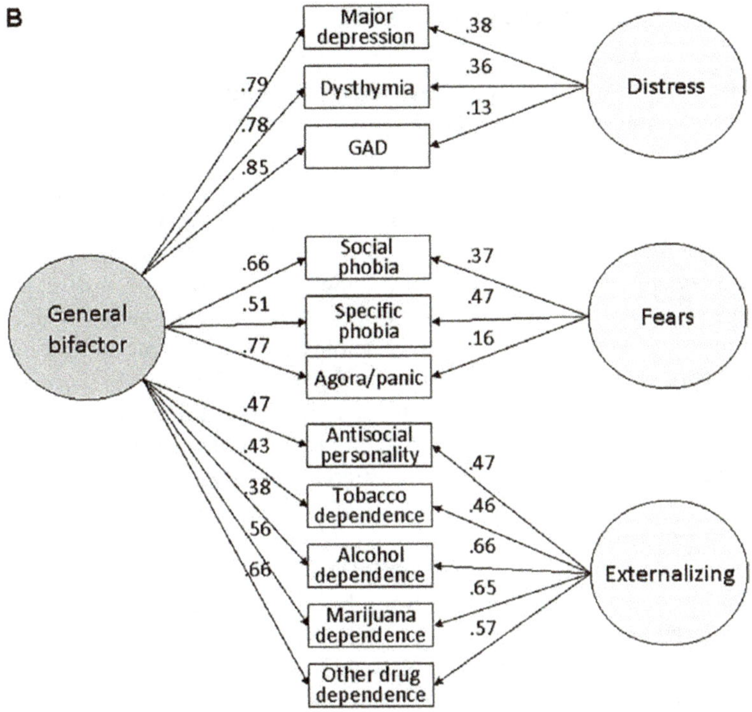

Fig. 6.4 Bifactor model of psychopathology in adults. (Reproduced with the permission of American Psychological Association from Fig. 1B Lahey et al. (2012). *Journal of Abnormal Psychology, 121*(4), 971–977; permission conveyed through Copyright Clearance Center, Inc.)

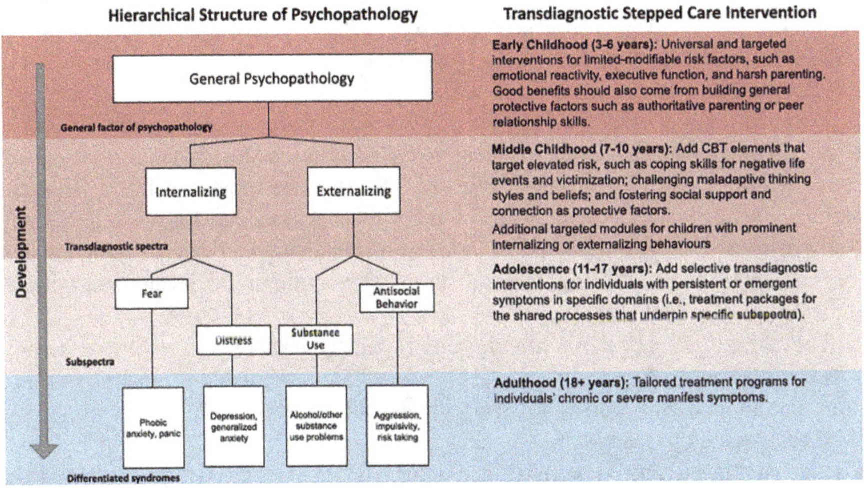

Fig. 6.5 Example of a developmentally informed and transdiagnostic stepped care approach to intervention, paired with examples of elements drawn from the Hierarchical Taxonomy of Psychopathology (HiTOP) model. (Reproduced with the permission of Elsevier Science & Technology Journals from Fig. 2 Forbes et al.. (2019). *Behaviour Research and Therapy, 119*, 103411; permission conveyed through Copyright Clearance Center, Inc.)

6.6 The Development of the p-Factor

In this section on development the terminology is based on studies using a bifactor analysis but applies equally to the development of the general factor in higher-order models.

An understanding of the development of the p-factor is lacking. There are two processes that have been proposed. The first possible process is dynamic mutualism whereby the p-factor is a product of the interactions between symptoms that influence and mutually reinforce each other (see Sect. 2.5 on Network analysis). Under this mechanism the p-factor is *not* seen as acting to generate a general risk of psychopathology. Rather it arises because symptoms are linked to one another from the causal relationships between them. By direct contrast, differentiation is premised on the idea that over time the effects of common influences accumulate to produce a set of underlying latent factors. One of these influences a general liability to develop psychopathology and the other a more differentiated set of group factors (Sterba et al., 2010). Under the differentiation model the p-factor is seen as a cause in common for all behaviours.

There have been a number of longitudinal studies that have investigated developmental aspects of the p-factor model from the preschool age onwards. Olino et al. (2018) re-assessed the sample studied by Olino et al. (2014) some 3 years later to examine the stability of the bifactor solution. The bifactor model provided an adequate fit for the data at age 6 years. There was homotypic stability for the p-factor and internalising and externalising group factors. McElroy et al. (2018) used a bifactor model with data on the Child Behavior Checklist (CBCL) for 1253 children to examine the longitudinal stability of general and group factors from 2 years of age up to the age of 14 years. They found that bifactor models fitted the symptom data well at all ages and that the p-factor explained most of the symptom variance at all ages (60–71%). They also found evidence in the overtime associations between the general and group factors in support of both dynamic mutualism and p-differentiation.

Based on a study of 2228 adolescents followed from age 11 to 26 years, Richards et al. (2022) also concluded that neither differentiation nor dynamic mutualism explained the pattern of results. Instead the results were more consistent with the action of shared risk factors. However there are suggestions from a longitudinal study between the ages of 14 and 21 years of internalising and externalising behaviour in 2450 girls that dynamic mutualism may be acting in the development of the p-factor (Choate et al., 2022).

The stability of both p-factor and group factors (internalising and externalising) was investigated by Snyder et al. (2017) in a longitudinally studied sample of children and adolescents aged 9–17 years when first assessed. After 18 months they were reassessed on a range of behaviour questionnaires including the CBCL. They found that the p-factor (r = 0.81) and internalising (r = 0.71) and externalising (r = 0.72) group factors all exhibited strong stability across 18 months.

The development of the p-factor in a sample of 1572 children was studied on eight occasions between the ages of 7 and 16 years by Murray et al. (2016). They tested which of the two models of development would best explain the changes in the p-factor over time. They suggested that the developmental consequences of the two processes will be different. Mutual dynamism, as proposed by Caspi et al. (2014), would result in the gradual increase in the strength of the general p-factor and a related decline in the strength of group factors (i.e. internalising and externalising). By contrast p-differentiation should lead to a gradual strengthening of the influence of the group factors and a concomitant decline in the role of the general p-factor. The results of the Murray et al. (2016) study were

> The relative strength of the p-factor and specific factors varied within a relatively narrow range over this time period and did not show an overall systematic increase or decrease with time. Such trajectories are not consistent with simple versions of a dynamic mutualism process of p-factor growth over time which would predict an increasingly strong p-factor with time. Nor are they consistent with p-differentiation: a process of increasing specificity in the expression of a general liability for psychopathology. Rather, our results suggest that from the point at which children enter school until adolescence, the extent to which a diversity of psychopathological behaviours within and between domains are co-morbid remains quite constant. Murray et al. (2016), p. 1588

These studies with data relevant to the question of the development of the p-factor have failed to give any clear evidence in favour of either process. At present it therefore appears that the p-factor is relatively stable and does not show the developmental pattern of change in the loadings on the p-factor and group factors predicted by either dynamic mutualism or p-differentiation.

6.7 What Does the GPF Represent?

Conway et al. (2019) tested the correlated factor, bifactor, and higher-order factor models as ways of representing the HiTOP model of mental health. The analysis was based on a data set of 25,000 students who were seeking mental health support. They found that a bifactor model, a higher-order, and a correlated factors model fitted the data equally well. They suggest that the bifactor analysis produced a model that was less easily interpreted. In particular the group factors that remain after the shared variance has been captured in the p-factor do not conform to an expected pattern. They conclude that these group factors from the bifactor analysis may reflect "nuisance" variance only. Importantly they found that scores derived from a bifactor analysis and from the second-order factor (GPF) in the higher-order model are very highly correlated with $r = 0.97$. They conclude that the HiTOP approach to the formation of mental illness is to be preferred to a categorical approach since the HiTOP transdiagnostic model was successful in predicting criterion validity measures and that categorical diagnoses added little to the explained variance. In relation to the result of the hierarchical approach, they say

> ... we caution that the validity and interpretation of the p-factor remains a pressing, unresolved issue for psychopathology researchers. Researchers have argued that it reflects negative emotionality or general distress that sets the stage for the full spectrum of mental health problems (e.g., Tackett et al., 2013). Alternately, it could represent a unitary outcome of mental illness, akin to the concept of demoralization proposed as a hallmark of all types of psychopathology (Tellegen et al., 2003). That is, the p-factor could represent dysfunction that occurs as a common endpoint for various mental disorders (Widiger & Oltmanns, 2017). Conway et al. (2019), p. 738

Here they are using the term p-factor to refer to either a higher-order factor (GPF) or the p-factor in the bifactor model. In either case Conway et al. (2019) suggest that an understanding of the validity and interpretation of this GPF should be a priority for work in this field.

There are various possibilities for the interpretation of the GPF . The original paper introducing the term p-factor by Caspi et al. (2014) suggested that

> ... it may represent low-to-high psychopathology severity. The higher a person scores on the p-factor, the worse that person fares on indicators tapping severity, duration of disorder, extent of sequential comorbidity, adult life impairment, childhood developmental history, family history of liability to psychiatric illness, and brain function from early life to midlife. Caspi et al. (2014), p. 131

As Conway et al. (2019) noted above, Tackett et al. (2013) suggested that the general factor in a bifactor analysis reflects negative emotionality. This interpretation is supported by Class et al. (2019), who found parent-rated negative emotionality measured in childhood and adolescence -predicted scores of the GPF based on self-reported symptoms in early adulthood. Moreover there was a high degree of stability in the general factor over a 12-year period. There is also some evidence to suggest that the p-factor in preschool and middle childhood is a reflection of dysregulation that arises from a combination of high negative emotionality and low executive control (Phillips et al., 2022). There is a similar suggestion from Carver et al. (2017) that poor constraint over reactions to emotion underlies the p-factor.

There are studies being undertaken to improve an understanding of the GPF and what it might represent by way of psychological processes influencing psychopathology in general. Brandes et al. (2019) investigated the association between the p-factor and neuroticism in children aged 7–13 years of age. They found that a bifactor solution fitted best both to the psychopathology measures (CBCL and Diagnostic Schedule for Children) and measures of neuroticism, including the Inventory of Children's Individual Differences–Short (Deal et al., 2007) and temperament questionnaires developed by Rothbart and colleagues. The p-factor captures much of the same variance as general trait neuroticism/negative affectivity. Furthermore, the externalising group factor in this model is strongly correlated with specific variance in trait irritability, whereas the internalising group factor may also have a high correlation with specific variance in the trait fearfulness.

Shields et al. (2019) examined which components of self-regulation might be closely associated with the p-factor in a sample aged between 8 and 18 years. Self-regulation reflects the ability to manage emotions and behaviours over time and contexts, allowing individuals to inhibit impulsive responses and carry out goal-directed activities. The two components studied were executive function (EF), which they defined as top-down mental control mechanisms tied to goal-directed behaviour, self-control, and self-regulation abilities, and effortful control (EC), defined as a temperament trait indexed by planfulness, error detection, dominant response inhibition, and non-dominant response activation. They suggest that the correlation between EF and EC measures in children is low and therefore may be independently related to the p-factor. They found that the p-factor was associated with both EF and EC but only modestly. The p-factor largely accounted for associations between EF and EC with internalising and externalising behaviour. The correlation between the p-factor and EC was greater ($r = -0.38$) than that with EF ($r = -0.16$). However they could not exclude that this might be due to shared method variance between the psychopathology and EC measures – both assessed by parents. This was not the case for EF which was assessed using experimental tasks.

There are a number of facets of cognitive function that have been shown to be related to GPF scores including executive function (e.g. Castellanos-Ryan et al., 2016; Romer & Pizzagalli, 2021) and IQ (e.g. Caspi et al., 2014). Kramer et al. (2023) have shown that a latent variable measuring processing speed is also strongly related to p-factor scores in adolescents. The association with processing speed remained significant when general cognitive ability was controlled, suggesting a specific processing speed/p-factor association. A similar result was found in a study of adults (Haywood et al., 2022).

Rosenstrom et al. (2019) summarised four ways in which researchers have tried to identify the source of the influence of the GPF. The first was a life history strategy model put forward by Del Giudice (2014a, b), whereby the GPF is seen to reflect reactions to a general dimension of environmental stress.

The second was a balance in fast and slow cognitive processes (Carver et al., 2017). Here those whose functioning is relatively dominated by a fast reflexive system are highly reactive to emotions as a result of genetics, neurobiology, temperament, and personality. They are more vulnerable to psychopathology than those who are less reactive to emotions and who are more likely to use a reflective response mode. Under this model the GPF represents individual differences in the extent to which cognitions are dominated by fast reflexive processes.

The third formulation concerns the integrity of the nervous system and was postulated in the initial p-factor study (Caspi et al., 2014). In the early years the lack of brain integrity is shown by neurological soft signs, impairments in receptive language development, and deficits on standard IQ tests. This brain integrity measure taken in childhood correlated −0.16 with the p-factor score measured longitudinally.

The fourth formulation is based on a more direct measure of brain integrity. For example, there is a relationship between GPF scores and indicators of inefficient intrinsic functional brain connectivity in the visual cortex (Elliott et al., 2018). As yet there is no consensus on the processes that might be involved, but Rosenstrom et al. (2019) argue that the GPF representing a single shared measurable source presents considerable advantages in the search for possible causal effects over an unexplained association in the correlated factor model.

It is possible that the p-factor represents a common outcome of mental illness rather than a common cause (Conway et al., 2019). Smith et al. (2020) reviewed the studies on the GPF. They concluded that the most plausible explanation is that it represents an index of impairment that relates to the duration and intensity of mental health treatment. This is the case for both adults and children.

The answer to the question headed in this section – "What does the GPF represent?" – is, disappointingly, that there is as yet no clear evidence for which formulation of the GPF is most plausible. However see the discussion of Caspi et al. (2023) below in Sect. 6.9.

6.8 Does the GPF Carry Genetic Influences?

There is accumulating evidence that there are genetic influences on psychopathology that transcend diagnostic boundaries (Geschwind & Flint, 2015; Pettersson et al., 2016). The general and group factor scores arising in bifactor analyses have been examined to determine how well they relate to possible causes of a general psychopathology propensity.

Quantitative Genetic Analyses Waldman et al. (2016) extended the bifactor approach to test for genetic and environmental influences on both group factors and the general factor using data from a sample of 6–17-year-old twins. They found that genes explained 43% of the variance in the general factor and 65% and 19% of the variance in the group factors, externalising and internalising, respectively. The corresponding values for the influence shared environmental influences were 25%, 16%, and 44%. These results suggest that during childhood and adolescence genes and the shared environment each have a moderate effect on the propensity to develop psychopathology symptoms.

Allegrini et al. (2020) have subsequently examined genetic and environmental influences on GPF models in a longitudinal study of 7026 twin pairs. They replicated the finding of a significant role of genetic influence on the GPF, with genes explaining between 44% and 60% of the variance in the factor ages 7, 9, 12, and 16 years. The shared environmental influences on the general factors ranged between 26% and 46% of the variance and the non-shared between 10% and 14% across these age groups.

A model that aligns the current understanding of genetic influences on psychopathology with observed patterns of co-occurrence among mental disorders was proposed by Waszczuk et al. (2020). They argue that the evidence suggests that genetic influences do not fit traditional psychiatric diagnoses, and that an alternative classification approach, such as the HiTOP model, is more likely to facilitate the search for molecular genetic variants linked to mental illness. Waszczuk et al. (2021) suggest that the co-occurrence of depression, conduct, and hyperactivity symptoms across adolescence arises from common genetic influences. This indicates that the GPF is influenced by genes, and this influence is stable over time.

Selzam et al. (2018) used four different methods to obtain genetic correlations between psychiatric disorders in adults. Applying a principal component analysis to these correlations separately for all four methods, a general first component was identified that explained between 20% and 60% of the variance. This provides strong support for the notion that there is a general genetically influenced GPF contributing to psychopathology.

Similar findings were obtained by Grotzinger et al. (2019), who identified a genetic general factor influencing psychopathology in two samples of young children under the age of 7 years. Internalising, externalising, ADHD, and self-regulation problems are all loaded onto this GPF. The GPF was found to have a heritability of 0.63 and 0.46 in the two samples. They also found that in both samples the GPF was negatively correlated (−0.21 and −0.34) with a general cognitive factor. They conclude that the GPF and general cognitive factor association is a product of genetic and shared environmental factors acting on both in the first years of life.

Harden et al. (2020) used data from 1913 twin children (mean age 13 years) taking part in the Texas Twin Project to investigate the possible role of cognitive factors (IQ and executive function) in influencing general risk for psychopathology. The latent factors underlying these two aspects of cognition were highly heritable (h^2 = 0.86–0.92). The genetic correlations between the latent cognitive measures and the GPF underlying psychopathology were robust (−0.20 to −0.38). These negative correlations indicate that the low scores of executive function and IQ measures were related by genetic mechanisms to high scores of the risk for general psychopathology.

Polygenic Risk Scores An important advance in understating the possible mechanism relating genetic risk to the p-factor was made in a study by Pat et al. (2022) that used the large Adolescent Brain Cognitive Development (ABCD) data set from a sample representative of the general population (Garavan et al., 2018). They examined which psychological characteristics (punishment sensitivity, reward sensitivity, and general cognitive ability, g) might mediate the association between a number of PRS (see Sect. 3.4) and p-factor scores in 4814 9–10-year-olds. The PRS were constructed for a liability to develop a number of disorders. They found the effects on p-factor score of PRS associated with major depressive disorder (MDD) and ADHD PRS were both partially mediated by general cognitive abilities. In addition the effect of the MDD PRS on p-factor scores was also partially mediated by punishment sensitivity. By contrast it was reward sensitivity that contributed additionally to the mediation of ADHD PRS scores of the p-factor.

PRS were used by Riglin et al. (2020) to examine the genetic influences on the full range of psychopathology in a cohort at age 7 and 13 years. The PRS were based on data from a number of large consortia of databases. The PRS were then used to predict psychopathology measures from the Avon Longitudinal Study of Parents and Children (ALSPAC). They found that the PRS for schizophrenia and ADHD are associated with a p-factor, and this association persists from early- to mid-childhood age. Riglin et al. (2020) conclude that, using genetic liability, a unidimensional perspective for psychopathology can be found. However there are also specific types of genetic psychopathology risk that emerge later in childhood.

Using PRS for 14 risk factors, including educational attainment, intelligence, smoking initiation, antisocial behaviour, and anxiety, Jansen et al. (2021) found a number of relationships between a psychiatric diagnosis and individual PRS scores. When the PRS were combined in multivariate analysis they were able to explain 5.9% of the variance in psychiatric caseness, with the PRS for education attainment and smoking initiation making the largest contribution to the prediction. The results suggest that psychopathology in children is influenced by a wide variety of genetic risk factors, with optimal prediction being obtained by pooling these risk factors together. These multiple risks act in concert to create a risk via the GPF.

Molecular Genetics Studies are also starting to identify the genetic contribution to the GPF at the molecular level. Neumann et al. (2016) estimated the cumulative effect of single-nucleotide polymorphisms (SNPs) on GPF scores in a sample of 2000 6–8-year-olds. It was found that these genetic differences accounted for 38% of the variance in GPF scores. This GPF was associated with lower IQ, higher negative affectivity, and lower effortful control, but not with surgency.

Using a pooled sample of 38,418 school-aged children from 20 population-based cohort studies, Neumann et al. (2022) were able to obtain an h^2_{SNP} of 5% (see Sect. 3.2) for total psychiatric problems – a proxy indicator for the GPF. These genetic effects on the total score were shared with common psychiatric disorders but not with autism. There were moderate genetic correlations between the GPF and intelligence, educational attainment, well-being, smoking, and body fat.

Biological Basis of GPF There is evidence that high p-factor scores are related to reduced grey matter volume of the visual association cortex and alterations in the white matter pathways within the cerebello-thalamo-cortical circuit (Romer et al., 2018). These findings were replicated in a separate sample from the Dunedin study (Romer et al., 2021). Reduced white matter volumes were found to be related to both general and group factor scores, specifically conduct problems and ADHD, in a sample of 9607 children aged 9–10 years (Durham et al., 2021).

Patel et al. (2021) conducted a study of the shared neurobiology underlying variation in cortical thickness in six disorders (attention-deficit/hyperactivity disorder, autism spectrum disorder, bipolar disorder, major depressive disorder, obsessive-compulsive disorder, and schizophrenia). The data were obtained from neuroimaging a total of 12,721 cases and 15,600 comparison participants. The results implicated atypical development in pyramidal cells (and dendrites) as increasing a general vulnerability to mental illness via a GPF. This pathophysiology may involve both prenatal and postnatal processes. The participants in this study were aged between 2 and 89 years.

Brain structure was investigated in a younger sample aged 9–10 years by Mewton et al. (2022). They did not find a significant relation at this age between cortical thickness and GPF score. However they did find lower cortical volume and surface area to be transdiagnostic biomarkers for general psychopathology in preadolescence.

Using data from the Philadelphia Neurodevelopmental Cohort, Kaczkurkin et al. (2018) found that those with a high p-factor score showed elevated perfusion in several brain regions, including the right dorsal anterior cingulate cortex (ACC) and left rostral ACC. In the same cohort of 11–23-year-olds overall psychopathology was associated with globally reduced grey matter volume (Kaczkurkin et al., 2019). Functional brain differences have been found to be associated with p-factor scores, for example, reduced activation of the executive system (Shanmugan et al., 2016).

6.9 The Significance of the GPF

One benefit of the higher-order model and the p-factor model is the possibility of homing in on causality. The alternative correlated group factor models leave unexplained *how* these correlations between group factors arise – what are the mechanisms producing their association? On these grounds hierarchical factor models would be preferred as they identify an influence that can possibly explain the origin of the correlations that are left unaccounted for in the correlated group factors model (Fig. 6.1b). Moreover it provides the means for deriving a measure that can be used to test for relationships with putative external causal influences. The advantage of the bifactor model over the higher-order model is that the p-factor and group factors are unrelated to each other. This allows separate tests to be made of the causes that have general effects and those with more specific influences on behaviour.

Trauma and the p-Factor The role of types of trauma in influencing scores of the p-factor was investigated by Lewis et al. (2021). Specifically they were concerned to differentiate the results of single isolated traumas and more complex traumas in influencing psychopathology at age 18 years. They defined complex trauma exposure as (a) a traumatic experience that involved (b) multiple events that were (c) interpersonal assaults or threats and (d) that occurred in childhood or adolescence. Examples of complex trauma include repeated child abuse, severe bullying, and witnessing neighbourhood violence. By contrast non-complex traumas involved a single event or non-interpersonal events only such as one-off assault, an accident, and learning about the sudden death of a parent. They also examined the role of pre-existing vulnerabilities from childhood. These included internalising and externalising symptoms at age 5 years, IQ score at age 5 years, proportion of family members with a history of mental illness, family socio-economic status, and sex.

They found that these pre-existing vulnerabilities were associated with the risk of experiencing complex traumas. Complex trauma was associated with an increased risk of psychopathology as indicated, for example, by higher p-factor scores. Complex trauma was also associated with a lowered cognitive functioning in early adulthood. However when the effects of childhood vulnerabilities were taken into account the relationship with cognitive functioning was much reduced. This same control did not eradicate the relationship between the experience of complex trauma and later psychopathology. The results demonstrate the need to take into account both the nature of trauma and the response to trauma in order to understand the mechanisms that might lead to later psychopathology.

p-Factor and Gene–Environment Correlations Sprooten et al. (2021) have argued that there are equivalences to the p-factor derived from phenotypic associations and the general factors in genetic and neuroimaging studies. They suggest that although the nature of the associations between these phenotypic, genetic, and neural general factors is unknown, there is an important role for a complex of gene–environment correlations to explain these inter-relationships. They argue that in all three realms (phenotype, genetic, and neural) the p-factors show consistent associations with environmental measures that are heritable. These measures include household income, years of education, and welfare benefit use – see, for example, the results reported by Trzaskowski et al. (2014) and Hill et al. (2016). Sprooten et al. (2021) draw the following general conclusion:

> … general dimensions of psychopathology and genetic liability for psychopathology reflect a dense web of mutually reinforcing traits that propagate throughout development, via the environment and the brain, in conferring risk for psychiatric disorders. Sprooten et al. (2021), p. 6

p-Factor Score Change as a Treatment Outcome The potential benefit of the analysis of p-factor scores in treatment studies was shown by Constantinou et al. (2019). They conducted a trial comparing the effects of multisystemic therapy with those of "management as usual" on antisocial behaviour in adolescents. They employed a model of behaviour that included a p-factor identified in a bifactor analysis and group factors reflecting anxiety, mood, antisocial behaviour, and inattention. They found that treatment resulted in reduced scores of the p-factor and the antisocial factor. By contrast the scores of the anxiety group factor increased under treatment. They postulate that the latter represents a return to a more typical level of fearfulness, this being characteristically reduced in adolescents with severe conduct problems. They conclude that a bifactor model is useful for distinguishing general and specific changes under treatment that are obscured in the usual analyses of symptom scores.

p-Factor and Lifetime Risk It is well established that about half of the population will develop a psychiatric disorder at some time in their life (Kessler et al., 2005). Caspi et al. (2020) have gone on to show that mental disorder life histories shift among different successive disorders. This means that an assessment of mental well-being at a single time is insufficient. Rather the emphasis should be on the flux and dynamics of mental health across the life span. Where there is stability of risk for some form of psychiatric disorder it was carried by the p-factor. They found that "brain health" was one influence on the p-factor score. This was measured at age 3 years as a composite measure derived from a 45-minute examination that included assessments by a paediatric neurologist; standardised tests of cognitive function, receptive language, and motor skills; and examiners' ratings of emotional and behavioural regulation. It was related to the participants' p-factor score ($r = -0.16$) – the general psychopathology factor measured across the life span. Caspi et al.

(2020) conclude that these findings imply that there should be less reliance on diagnosis-specific research and clinical protocols.

One such alternative clinical protocol is that of the transdiagnostic clinical staging model for the planning of treatment for adolescents (Shah et al., 2020). The transdiagnostic approach is based on considering the person as located along a multidimensional and evolving continuum of illness and not the categorical approach based on single discrete disorders (see also the framework from Forbes et al. (2019) in Fig. 6.5). A transdiagnostic modular cognitive-behavioural therapy (CBT) programme has been shown to outperform "management as usual" for youth with emotional and behavioural problems (Jeppesen et al., 2021). This randomised clinical trial of 396 children and adolescents aged 6–16 years found that parent-reported SDQ scores were significantly reduced for transdiagnostic modular CBT compared with "management as usual". The authors conclude that

> this pragmatic study adds to the growing evidence that the wide-scale implementation of transdiagnostic modular CBT in nonspecialist care settings provides timely indicated prevention and quality care for help-seeking youth. Jeppesen et al. (2021), p. e2

Caspi et al. (2023) An important overview of the state of play in p-factor research was produced by Caspi et al. (2023). They provide an outline of the history behind their seminal paper (Caspi et al., 2014) in which they labelled the general factor from a bifactor analysis, the p-factor. They identify a number of crucial issues related to the derivation and interpretation of structural equation models of psychopathology dimensions. Analyses of data at 18 years of age from a longitudinal study of just over 1000 twin pairs born in England and Wales (Moffit & E-Risk Study Team, 2002) were used to address these issues.

The first issue is how is it best to identify a general factor. There are a number of alternative that have been shown in Fig. 6.1: single-factor model (Fig. 6.1a), correlated factor model (Fig. 6.1b), bifactor model (Fig. 6.1c), and higher-order factor model (Fig. 6.1d). They found that the single-factor model consistently had the poorest fit and the bifactor model had the best fit.

The second issue is whether the bifactor approach overfits the data (see Sect. 6.2) and thereby artefactually provides the best fit. Caspi et al. (2023) examined a number of alternative indicators of the psychometric performance of the bifactor analyses. They found that as well as fitting well on traditional measures, such as RMSEA and CFI (see Sect. 2.5), the p-factor had a good reliability but not the group factors.

The third issue is that of the introduction of modifications to the core bifactor model such as correlation between the group factors or the presence of behaviours which do not load onto a group factor but just on the p factor. They found that modifications made to the bifactor model did not detract from the reliable identification of the p-factor.

The fourth issue is that of interpreting the group factors in the bifactor analysis. There has been some confusion over the terminology with group factors in a hierarchal model and in a bifactor model receiving the same label. They suggest that the group factors in a bifactor analysis should be labelled "p-free" to show that they do not correlate with the general factor. They found that p-free factors sometimes have shown low reliably and their interpretation may be moot. Nevertheless they suggest that an analysis of the association between p-free factor scores and a wide range of child, family, and social measures showed that the p-free scores were an index of "pure" disorders. By this they mean that they allow the study of one disorder while controlling for all other disorders.

The final issue addressed by Caspi et al. (2023) is just what the p-factor represents. Does it capture shared causal influences on all aspects of psychopathology and, if so, what are these? They showed that the p-factor indeed did capture these shared risks and that, drawing on findings from the Dunedin study (Poulton et al., 2023), higher scores of the p-factor are associated with earlier onset, longer persistence, and a wider range of disorders into middle adulthood. As to what constitutes "p" they say:

> ... we hypothesize that p represents the disordered form and content of thought that permeates practically every disorder dimension. Examples include not only delusions and hallucinations but also difficulty in dealing with uncertainty; difficulty in making decisions; irrational fears, worries, and rumination; intrusive thoughts and memories; unhelpful schemas; reexperiencing trauma; dissociative states; beliefs that something terrible will happen if a behavior is not performed; body image disturbances; hostile attributions made in response to ambiguous social situations; and attributing failure to internal, stable, and global causes. Caspi et al. (2023), p. 24

6.10 p-Factor or GPF: Which One to Choose?

Bornovalova et al. (2020) provide an excellent overview of the issues that relate to the interpretation of bifactor models in psychopathology. They compare the value of the bifactor approach to that of the hierarchical and the correlated factor approaches. The closing paragraph in this paper is worth reproducing in full:

> To close, we reiterate that statistical modeling cannot make fundamental limitations of data disappear. The questions that data can address are a function of the research design, not the model chosen to analyze them. Cross-sectional relationships among indicators cannot speak to developmental processes regardless of the type of model (bifactor or network) or indicator (behavioral symptoms or biological variables) used. The appropriate level of analysis for psychopathology (e.g., symptoms, disorders, spectra, p factor) is a question best addressed empirically—for example, by comparing genetic and neurobiological correlates of individual symptoms versus broader factors (van Bork et al., 2017; Zald & Lahey, 2017)—or pragmatically—for example, do components from one model yield stronger predictions of clinically relevant outcomes than components from another model? Paired with rigorous research designs that can rule out methodological confounds, such as longitudinal and multi-informant designs, bifactor modeling can be a useful tool for investigating the nature of psychopathology constructs (broad and narrow) and their mechanisms, development, and responsiveness to treatment. Bornovalova et al. (2020), p. 24

Lahey et al. (2021) also provided an overview of the current state of knowledge concerning hierarchical models of psychopathology. They conclude that the evidence suggests that there is a general factor influencing all measures and specific factors with more limited effects. There are many familial influences with pleiotropic effects reflected in the general factor and these stem from both genes and the shared environment. Person-specific experiences (i.e. non-shared environment) have an impact on the specific factors. They argue that the models based on a second-order factor and the bifactor model often provide general factors that are highly correlated and in this sense may be interchangeable. However the bifactor model provides a general factor and group factors that are independent of each other whereas those from the second-order model are correlated. This means that the bifactor solution is better suited to testing correlates of group factors that are independent of the general factor.

Lahey et al. (2021) also address the concerns that have been raised about the fit of bifactor models (Markon, 2019) and their replicability (Watts et al., 2019). In relation to fit, it is their view that differentiating among well-fitting models on the basis of fit alone is inappropriate. Rather the onus should be on testing the external validity and utility of the models. They suggest that longitudinal studies have provided strong evidence that all factors in bifactor models are replicable over time. On these grounds they endorse the bifactor model of a general and group factors as an optimal basis for examining the neurobiological correlates and clinical implications of hierarchical dimensions of psychopathology.

6.11 Final Thoughts on Hierarchical Factor Models

The final verdict on how best to represent the structure of psychopathology cannot rest on psychometric analyses alone. The similarities between the alternative representations in terms of fit for data mean that some additional criteria will be needed. For the models implying a common cause, that is, latent variable models, and the specifically the p-factor model, validation from external sources is needed. This has primarily centred on a search for biological associations. The commonality of the basis of a number of psychiatric conditions is becoming clear from a variety of sources. This is leading to the notion that there are transdiagnostic characteristics that can identify neural alterations that are associated with broad risk factors for psychopathology (Barch, 2020). Such findings converge with the results of studies applying model-fitting studies to symptoms that suggest a common GPF underlying psychopathology. These developments have implications for the early identification of children and adolescents at risk for psychiatric illness (Raballo & Poletti, 2020).

The aphorism that "all models are wrong but some are useful" (Box, 1979, p. 202) is very apposite here. Taking Box's aphorism a little further – "all models are wrong but different models may be useful for different purposes". As Greene et al. (2019) conclude:

> … it must be recognized that biases in relative fit indices do not invalidate favored models or imply that alternative models are more valid. Converging lines of evidence support the utility of a general factor of psychopathology, as this dimension can be postulated even without reference to superior fit. ………the choice between correlated factors (or higher-order) and bifactor models can be made on practical grounds where the study aims justify the modeling approach. The former is most effective at identifying clusters of variables that are positively interrelated, whereas the latter is most effective at decomposing indicators' variance into that which is shared versus unique. Greene et al. (2019), p. 759

Levy (2020) suggests that

> In sum, the p-factor captures what has been known in the field for a while now – the overlap in symptomatology, within-category heterogeneity, lack of category-specific developmental course, shared common and rare mutations, true pleiotropy and mixed neuroimaging results, point to diffuse, sometimes non-existent, boundaries among neurodevelopmental disorders (NDD), and possibly other childhood disorders as well. Levy (2020), p. 2

The question of extending the p-factor/transdiagnostic framework to neurodevelopmental disorders raised by Levy (2020) will be addressed in Chap. 10.

There is an interesting historical footnote to the work on the p-factor. Caspi and Moffitt (2018) draw attention to the suggestion of Jones (1946) that there may a general factor underlying psychological problems. This insight is illustrated by the following quotations:

> … there may be an innate factor akin to the General Intelligence G, the nature of which it still remains to be elucidate, but which may be of cardinal importance….to attain the balanced mentality that is our ideal.
> and
> … if such a factor can ever be isolated it may prove to have a physiological basis which will bring us back to the often neglected problems of heredity. Jones (1946), p. 10

This shows that not only did Ernest Jones predict the presence of a general factor underlying psychological problems but also that this vulnerability would be influenced by genetic differences between people.

References

Achenbach, T. M. (1966). The classification of children's psychiatric symptoms: A factor-analytic study. *Psychological Monographs, 80*(7), 1–37. https://doi.org/10.1037/h0093906

Achenbach, T. M. (2020). Bottom-up and top-down paradigms for psychopathology: A half-century odyssey. *Annual Review of Clinical Psychology, 16*, 1–24. https://doi.org/10.1146/annurev-clinpsy-071119-115831

Allegrini, A. G., Cheesman, R., Rimfeld, K., Selzam, S., Pingault, J. B., Eley, T. C., & Plomin, R. (2020). The p factor: Genetic analyses support a general dimension of psychopathology in childhood and adolescence. *Journal of Child Psychology and Psychiatry, 61*(1), 30–39. https://doi.org/10.1111/jcpp.13113

Arildskov, T. W., Sonuga-Barke, E. J. S., Thomsen, P. H., Virring, A., & Ostergaard, S. D. (2021). How much impairment is required for ADHD? No evidence of a discrete threshold. *Journal of Child Psychology and Psychiatry*. https://doi.org/10.1111/jcpp.13440

Avinun, R., Knafo-Noam, A., & Israel, S. (2022). The general psychopathology factor from early to middle childhood: Longitudinal genetic and risk analyses. *Journal of Psychopathology and Clinical Science, 131*(7), 705–715. https://doi.org/10.1037/abn0000780

Barch, D. M. (2020). What does it mean to be transdiagnostic and how would we know? *American Journal of Psychiatry, 177*(5), 370–372. https://doi.org/10.1176/appi.ajp.2020.20030243

Bonifay, W., Lane, S. P., & Reise, S. P. (2017). Three concerns with applying a bifactor model as a structure of psychopathology. *Clinical Psychological Science, 5(1)*, 184–186. https://doi.org/10.1177/2167702616657069

Bornovalova, M. A., Choate, A. M., Fatimah, H., Petersen, K. J., & Wiernik, B. M. (2020). Appropriate use of bifactor analysis in psychopathology research: Appreciating benefits and limitations. *Biological Psychiatry, 88*(1), 18–27. https://doi.org/10.1016/j.biopsych.2020.01.013

Box, G. E. P. (1979). Robustness in the strategy of scientific model building. In R. L. Launer & G. N. Wilkinson (Eds.), *Robustness in statistics*. Academic.

Brandes, C. M., Herzhoff, K., Smack, A. J., & Tackett, J. L. (2019). The p factor and the n factor: Associations between the general factors of psychopathology and neuroticism in children. *Clinical Psychological Science, 7*(6), 1266–1284. https://doi.org/10.1177/2167702619859332

Brislin, S. J., Martz, M. E., Joshi, S., Duval, E. R., Gard, A., Clark, D. A., et al. (2022). Differentiated nomological networks of internalizing, externalizing, and the general factor of psychopathology ('p factor') in emerging adolescence in the ABCD study. *Psychological Medicine, 52*(14), 3051–3061. https://doi.org/10.1017/s0033291720005103

Burns, G. L., Geiser, C., Servera, M., Becker, S. P., & Beauchaine, T. P. (2020). Application of the bifactor S-1 model to multisource ratings of ADHD/ODD Symptoms: An appropriate bifactor model for symptom ratings. *Journal of Abnormal Child Psychology, 48*(7), 881–894. https://doi.org/10.1007/s10802-019-00608-4

Buss, A., & Plomin, R. (1984). *Temperament: Early developing personality traits*. Lawrence Erlbaum.

Carter, A. S., Briggs-Gowan, M. J., Jones, S. M., & Little, T. D. (2003). The Infant-Toddler Social and Emotional Assessment (ITSEA): Factor structure, reliability, and validity. *Journal of Abnormal Child Psychology, 31*(5), 495–514. https://doi.org/10.1023/a:1025449031360

Carver, C. S., Johnson, S. L., & Timpano, K. R. (2017). Toward a functional view of the p factor in psychopathology. *Clinical Psychological Science, 5*(5), 880–889. https://doi.org/10.1177/2167702617710037

Caspi, A., & Moffitt, T. E. (2018). All for one and one for all: Mental disorders in one dimension. *American Journal of Psychiatry, 175*(9), 831–844. https://doi.org/10.1176/appi.ajp.2018.17121383

Caspi, A., Houts, R. M., Belsky, D. W., Goldman-Mellor, S. J., Harrington, H., Israel, S., et al. (2014). The p factor: One general psychopathology factor in the structure of psychiatric disorders? *Clinical Psychological Science, 2*(2), 119–137. https://doi.org/10.1177/2167702613497473

Caspi, A., Houts, R. M., Ambler, A., Danese, A., Elliott, M. L., Hariri, A., et al. (2020). Longitudinal assessment of mental health disorders and comorbidities across 4 decades among participants in the Dunedin Birth Cohort Study. *JAMA Network Open, 3*(4). https://doi.org/10.1001/jamanetworkopen.2020.3221

Caspi, A., Houts, R. M., Fisher, H. L., Danese, A., & Moffitt, T. E. (2023). The general factor of psychopathology (p): Choosing among competing models and interpreting p. *Clinical Psychological Science*. https://doi.org/10.1177/21677026221147872

Castellanos-Ryan, N., Briere, F. N., O'Leary-Barrett, M., Banaschewski, T., Bokde, A., Bromberg, U., et al. (2016). The structure of psychopathology in adolescence and its common personality and cognitive correlates. *Journal of Abnormal Psychology, 125*(8), 1039–1052. https://doi.org/10.1037/abn0000193

Choate, A. M., Bornovalova, M. A., Hipwell, A. E., Chung, T., & Stepp, S. D. (2022). The general psychopathology factor (p) from adolescence to adulthood: Exploring the developmental trajectories of p using a multi-method approach. *Development and Psychopathology*, 1–19. https://doi.org/10.1017/s0954579422000463

Cicero, D., & Ruggero, C. (2021). Commentary– Opening a can of worms: The importance of testing the measurement invariance of hierarchical models of psychopathology – A commentary on He and Li (2020). *Journal of Child Psychology and Psychiatry, 62*(3), 299–302. https://doi.org/10.1111/jcpp.13353

Class, Q. A., Van Hulle, C. A., Rathouz, P. J., Applegate, B., Zald, D. H., & Lahey, B. B. (2019). Socioemotional dispositions of children and adolescents predict general and specific second-order factors of psychopathology in early adulthood: A 12-year prospective study. *Journal of Abnormal Psychology, 128*(6), 574–584. https://doi.org/10.1037/abn0000433

Constantinou, M. P., Goodyer, I. M., Eisler, I., Butler, S., Kraam, A., Scott, S., et al. (2019). Changes in general and specific psychopathology factors over a psychosocial intervention. *Journal of the American Academy of Child and Adolescent Psychiatry, 58*(8), 776–786. https://doi.org/10.1016/j.jaac.2018.11.011

Conway, C. C., Mansolf, M., & Reise, S. P. (2019). Ecological validity of a quantitative classification system for mental illness in treatment-seeking adults. *Psychological Assessment, 31*(6), 730–740. https://doi.org/10.1037/pas0000695

Conway, C. C., Forbes, M. K., South, S. C., & HiTOP Consortium. (2021). A hierarchical taxonomy of psychopathology (HiTOP) primer for mental health researchers. *Clinical Psychological Science*. https://doi.org/10.1177/21677026211017834

Deal, J. E., Halverson, C. F., Jr., Martin, R. P., Victor, J., & Baker, S. (2007). The inventory of children's individual differences: Development and validation of a short version. *Journal of Personality Assessment, 89*(2), 162–166. https://doi.org/10.1080/00223890701468550

Del Giudice, M. (2014a). An evolutionary life history framework for psychopathology. *Psychological Inquiry, 25*(3–4), 261–300. https://doi.org/10.1080/1047840x.2014.884918

Del Giudice, M. (2014b). A tower unto heaven: Toward an expanded framework for psychopathology. *Psychological Inquiry, 25*(3–4, 394),–413. https://doi.org/10.1080/1047840x.2014.925339

DeYoung, C. G., Kotov, R., Krueger, R. F., Cicero, D. C., Conway, C. C., Eaton, N. R., et al. (2022). Answering questions about the hierarchical taxonomy of psychopathology (HiTOP): Analogies to whales and sharks miss the boat. *Clinical Psychological Science, 10*(2), 279–284. https://doi.org/10.1177/21677026211049390

Dodge, K. A., & Coie, J. D. (1987). Social-information-processing factors in reactive and proactive aggression in childrens peer groups. *Journal of Personality and Social Psychology, 53*(6), 1146–1158. https://doi.org/10.1037/0022-3514.53.6.1146

Durham, E. L., Jeong, H. J., Moore, T. M., Dupont, R. M., Cardenas-Iniguez, C., Cui, Z. X., et al. (2021). Association of gray matter volumes with general and specific dimensions of psychopathology in children. *Neuropsychopharmacology, 46*(7), 1333–1339. https://doi.org/10.1038/s41386-020-00952-w

Egger, H. L., & Angold, A. (2004). The preschool age psychiatric assessment (PAPA): A structured parent interview for diagnosing psychiatric disorders in preschool children. In R. DelCarmen-Wiggins & A. Carter (Eds.), *Handbook of infant, toddler and preschool mental health assessment* (pp. 223–243). Oxford University Press.

Eid, M., Geiser, C., Koch, T., & Heene, M. (2017). Anomalous results in G-factor models: Explanations and alternatives. *Psychological Methods, 22*(3), 541–562. https://doi.org/10.1037/met0000083

Elliott, M. L., Romer, A., Knodt, A. R., & Hariri, A. R. (2018). A connectome-wide functional signature of transdiagnostic risk for mental illness. *Biological Psychiatry, 84*(6), 452–459. https://doi.org/10.1016/j.biopsych.2018.03.012

Fergusson, D. M., Horwood, L. J., Ridder, E. M., & Beautrais, A. L. (2005). Subthreshold depression in adolescence and mental health outcomes in adulthood. *Archives of General Psychiatry, 62*(1), 66–72. https://doi.org/10.1001/archpsyc.62.1.66

Forbes, M. K., Rapee, R. M., & Krueger, R. F. (2019). Opportunities for the prevention of mental disorders by reducing general psychopathology in early childhood. *Behaviour Research and Therapy, 119*, 103411. https://doi.org/10.1016/j.brat.2019.103411

Forbes, M. K., Greene, A. L., Levin-Aspenson, H. F., Watts, A. L., Hallquist, M., Lahey, B. B., et al. (2021). Three recommendations based on a comparison of the reliability and validity of the predominant models used in research on the empirical structure of psychopathology. *Journal of Abnormal Psychology, 130*(3), 297–317. https://doi.org/10.1037/abn0000533

Frick, P. J., & Hare, R. D. (2001). *The antisocial process screening device (ASPD)*. MultiHealth Systems.

Garavan, H., Bartsch, H., Conway, K., Decastro, A., Goldstein, R. Z., Heeringa, S., et al. (2018). Recruiting the ABCD sample: Design considerations and procedures. *Developmental Cognitive Neuroscience, 32*, 16–22. https://doi.org/10.1016/j.dcn.2018.04.004

Geeraerts, S. B., Deutz, M. H. F., Dekovic, M., Bunte, T., Schoemaker, K., Espy, K. A., et al. (2015). The Child Behavior Checklist dysregulation profile in preschool children: A broad dysregulation syndrome. *Journal of the American Academy of Child and Adolescent Psychiatry, 54*(7), 595–602. https://doi.org/10.1016/j.jaac.2015.04.012

Geschwind, D. H., & Flint, J. (2015). Genetics and genomics of psychiatric disease. *Science, 349*(6255), 1489–1494. https://doi.org/10.1126/science.aaa8954

Gomez, R., Stavropoulos, V., Vance, A., & Griffiths, M. D. (2019). Re-evaluation of the latent structure of common childhood disorders: Is there a general psychopathology factor (P-Factor)? *International Journal of Mental Health and Addiction, 17*(2), 258–278. https://doi.org/10.1007/s11469-018-0017-3

Greene, A. L., Eaton, N. R., Li, K. Q., Forbes, M. K., Krueger, R. F., Markon, K. E., et al. (2019). Are fit indices used to test psychopathology structure biased? A simulation study. *Journal of Abnormal Psychology, 128*(7), 740–764. https://doi.org/10.1037/abn0000434

Greene, A. L., Watts, A. L., Forbes, M. K., Kotov, R., Krueger, R. F., & Eaton, N. R. (2022). Misbegotten methodologies and forgotten lessons from Tom Swift's Electric Factor Analysis Machine: A demonstration with competing structural models of Psychopathology. *Psychological Methods*. https://doi.org/10.1037/met0000465

Grotzinger, A. D., Cheung, A. K., Patterson, M. W., Harden, K. P., & Tucker-Drob, E. M. (2019). Genetic and environmental links between general factors of psychopathology and cognitive ability in early childhood. *Clinical Psychological Science, 7*(3), 430–444. https://doi.org/10.1177/2167702618820018

Haeffel, G. J., Jeronimus, B. F., Fisher, A. J., Kaiser, B. N., Weaver, L. J., Vargas, I., et al. (2022a). HiTOP is not an improvement over the DSM. *Clinical Psychological Science, 10*(2), 285–290. https://doi.org/10.1177/21677026211068873

Haeffel, G. J., Jeronimus, B. F., Kaiser, B. N., Weaver, L. J., Soyster, P. D., Fisher, A. J., et al. (2022b). Folk classification and factor rotations: Whales, sharks, and the problems with the Hierarchical Taxonomy of Psychopathology (HiTOP). *Clinical Psychological Science, 10*(2), 259–278. https://doi.org/10.1177/21677026211002500

Haller, H., Cramer, H., Lauche, R., Gass, F., & Dobos, G. J. (2014). The prevalence and burden of subthreshold generalized anxiety disorder: A systematic review. *BMC Psychiatry, 14*. https://doi.org/10.1186/1471-244x-14-128

Hankin, B. L., Davis, E. P., Snyder, H., Young, J. F., Glynn, L. M., & Sandman, C. A. (2017). Temperament factors and dimensional, latent bifactor models of, child psychopathology: Transdiagnostic and specific associations in two youth samples. *Psychiatry Research, 252*, 139–146. https://doi.org/10.1016/j.psychres.2017.02.061

Harden, K. P., Engelhardt, L. E., Mann, F. D., Patterson, M. W., Grotzinger, A. D., Savicki, S. L., et al. (2020). Genetic associations between executive functions and a general factor of psychopathology. *Journal of the American Academy of Child and Adolescent Psychiatry, 59*(6), 749–758. https://doi.org/10.1016/j.jaac.2019.05.006

Haywood, D., Baughman, F. D., Mullan, B. A., & Heslop, K. R. (2022). What accounts for the factors of psychopathology? An investigation of the neurocognitive correlates of Internalising, Externalising, and the p-Factor. *Brain Sciences, 12*(4). https://doi.org/10.3390/brainsci12040421

He, Q., & Li, J. (2021). Factorial invariance in hierarchical factor models of mental disorders in African American and European American youths. *Journal of Child Psychology and Psychiatry, 62*(3), 289–298. https://doi.org/10.1111/jcpp.13243

Helzer, J. E., Kraemer, H. C., & Krueger, R. F. (2006). The feasibility and need for dimensional psychiatric diagnoses. *Psychological Medicine, 36*(12), 1671–1680. https://doi.org/10.1017/s003329170600821x

Hill, W. D., Hagenaars, S. P., Marioni, R. E., Harris, S. E., Liewald, D. C. M., Davies, G., et al. (2016). Molecular genetic contributions to social deprivation and household income in UK Biobank. *Current Biology, 26*(22), 3083–3089. https://doi.org/10.1016/j.cub.2016.09.035

Hoffmann, M. S., Moore, T. M., Axelrud, L. K., Tottenham, N., Zuo, X. N., Rohde, L. A., et al. (2022). Reliability and validity of bifactor models of dimensional psychopathology in youth. *Journal of Psychopathology and Clinical Science, 131*(4), 407–421. https://doi.org/10.1037/abn0000749

Hoffmann, M. S., Evans-Lacko, S., Collishaw, S., Knapp, M., Pickles, A., Shearer, C., & Maughan, B. (2023). Parent- and teacher-reported associations from adolescent bifactor models of psychopathology: An outcome-wide association study of 26 outcomes in mid-life. *Journal of Child Psychology and Psychiatry, 64*(3), 345–483. https://doi.org/10.1111/jcpp.13707

Holzinger, K., & Swineford, F. (1937). The bifactor method. *Psychometrika, 2*, 41–54.

Hyland, P., Murphy, J., Shevlin, M., Bentall, R. P., Karatzias, T., Ho, G. W. K., et al. (2021). On top or underneath: Where does the general factor of psychopathology fit within a dimensional model of psychopathology? *Psychological Medicine, 51*(14), 2422–2432. https://doi.org/10.1017/s003329172000104x

Jansen, A. G., Jansen, P. R., Savage, J. E., Kraft, J., Skarabis, N., Polderman, T. J. C., & Dieleman, G. C. (2021). The predictive capacity of psychiatric and psychological polygenic risk scores for distinguishing cases in a child and adolescent psychiatric sample from controls. *Journal of Child Psychology and Psychiatry, 62*(9), 1079–1089. https://doi.org/10.1111/jcpp.13370

Jeppesen, P., Wolf, R. T., Nielsen, S. M., Christensen, R., Plessen, K. J., Bilenberg, N., et al. (2021). Effectiveness of transdiagnostic cognitive-behavioral psychotherapy compared with management as usual for youth with common mental health problems a randomized clinical trial. *JAMA Psychiatry, 78*(3), 250–260. https://doi.org/10.1001/jamapsychiatry.2020.4045

Jones, E. (1946). A valedictory address. *International Journal of Psychoanalysis, 27*, 7–12.

Kaczkurkin, A. N., Moore, T. M., Calkins, M. E., Ciric, R., Detre, J. A., Elliott, M. A., et al. (2018). Common and dissociable regional cerebral blood flow differences associate with dimensions of psychopathology across categorical diagnoses. *Molecular Psychiatry, 23*(10), 1981–1989. https://doi.org/10.1038/mp.2017.174

Kaczkurkin, A. N., Park, S. S., Sotiras, A., Moore, T. M., Calkins, M. E., Cieslak, M., et al. (2019). Evidence for dissociable linkage of dimensions of psychopathology to brain structure in youths. *American Journal of Psychiatry, 176*(12), 1000–1009. https://doi.org/10.1176/appi.ajp.2019.18070835

Kessler, R. C., Berglund, P., Demler, O., Jin, R., & Walters, E. E. (2005). Lifetime prevalence and age-of-onset distributions' of DSM-IV disorders in the national comorbidity survey replication. *Archives of General Psychiatry, 62*(6), 593–602. https://doi.org/10.1001/archpsyc.62.6.593

Kim, H., & Eaton, N. R. (2015). The hierarchical structure of common mental disorders: Connecting multiple levels of comorbidity, bifactor models, and predictive validity. *Journal of Abnormal Psychology, 124*(4), 1064–1078. https://doi.org/10.1037/abn0000113

Kotov, R., Krueger, R. F., Watson, D., Achenbach, T. M., Althoff, R. R., Bagby, R. M., et al. (2017). The Hierarchical Taxonomy of Psychopathology (HiTOP): A dimensional alternative to traditional nosologies. *Journal of Abnormal Psychology, 126*(4), 454–477. https://doi.org/10.1037/abn0000258

Kramer, E., Willcutt, E. G., Peterson, R. L., Pennington, B. F., & McGrath, L. M. (2023). Processing speed is related to the general psychopathology factor in youth. *Research on Child and Adolescent Psychopathology*. https://doi.org/10.1007/s10802-023-01049-w

Krueger, R. F., Kotov, R., Watson, D., Forbes, M. K., Eaton, N. R., Ruggero, C. J., et al. (2018). Progress in achieving quantitative classification of psychopathology. *World Psychiatry, 17*(3), 282–293. https://doi.org/10.1002/wps.20566

Lahey, B. B., Rathouz, P. J., Van Hulle, C., Urbano, R. C., Krueger, R. F., Applegate, B., et al. (2008). Testing structural models of DSM-IV symptoms of common forms of child and adolescent psychopathology. *Journal of Abnormal Child Psychology, 36*(2), 187–206. https://doi.org/10.1007/s10802-007-9169-5

Lahey, B. B., Van Hulle, C. A., Singh, A. L., Waldman, I. D., & Rathouz, P. J. (2011). Higher-order genetic and environmental structure of prevalent forms of child and adolescent psychopathology. *Archives of General Psychiatry, 68*(2), 181–189. https://doi.org/10.1001/archgenpsychiatry.2010.192

Lahey, B. B., Applegate, B., Hakes, J. K., Zald, D. H., Hariri, A. R., & Rathouz, P. J. (2012). Is there a general factor of prevalent psychopathology during adulthood? *Journal of Abnormal Psychology, 121*(4), 971–977. https://doi.org/10.1037/a0028355

Lahey, B. B., Rathouz, P. J., Keenan, K., Stepp, S. D., Loeber, R., & Hipwell, A. E. (2015). Criterion validity of the general factor of psychopathology in a prospective study of girls. *Journal of Child Psychology and Psychiatry, 56*(4), 415–422. https://doi.org/10.1111/jcpp.12300

Lahey, B. B., Krueger, R. F., Rathouz, P. J., Waldman, I. D., & Zald, D. H. (2017). A hierarchical causal taxonomy of psychopathology across the life span. *Psychological Bulletin, 143*(2), 142–186. https://doi.org/10.1037/bul0000069

Lahey, B. B., Moore, T. M., Kaczkurkin, A. N., & Zald, D. H. (2021). Hierarchical models of psychopathology: Empirical support, implications, and remaining issues. *World Psychiatry, 20*(1), 57–63. https://doi.org/10.1002/wps.20824

Levin-Aspenson, H. F., Watson, D., Clark, L. A., & Zimmerman, M. (2021). What is the general factor of psychopathology? Consistency of the p factor across samples. *Assessment, 28*(4), 1035–1049. https://doi.org/10.1177/1073191120954921

Levy, Y. (2020). Commentary: Time to reconceptualize ASD? Comments on Happé and Frith (2020) and Sonuga-Barke (2020). *Journal of Child Psychology and Psychiatry, 62*(8), 1042–1044. https://doi.org/10.1111/jcpp.13345

Lewis, S. J., Koenen, K. C., Ambler, A., Arseneault, L., Caspi, A., Fisher, H. L., et al. (2021). Unravelling the contribution of complex trauma to psychopathology and cognitive deficits: A cohort study. *British Journal of Psychiatry, 219*(2), 448–455. https://doi.org/10.1192/bjp.2021.57

Marceau, K., & Neiderhiser, J. (2022). Generalist genes and specialist environments for adolescent internalizing and externalizing problems: A test of severity and directionality. *Development and Psychopathology, 34*(1), 379–386. https://doi.org/10.1017/s0954579420001108

Markon, K. E. (2019). Bifactor and hierarchical models: Specification, inference, and interpretation. In T. Widiger & T. D. Cannon (Eds.), *Annual review of clinical psychology, Vol 15* (Vol. 15, pp. 51–69). Annual Reviews.

Martel, M. M., Pan, P. M., Hoffmann, M. S., Gadelha, A., do Rosario, M. C., Mari, J. J., et al. (2017). A general psychopathology factor (P Factor) in children: Structural model analysis and external validation through familial risk and child global executive function. *Journal of Abnormal Psychology, 126*(1), 137–148. https://doi.org/10.1037/abn0000205

McElroy, E., Belsky, J., Carragher, N., Fearon, P., & Patalay, P. (2018). Developmental stability of general and specific factors of psychopathology from early childhood to adolescence: Dynamic mutualism or p-differentiation? *Journal of Child Psychology and Psychiatry, 59*(6), 667–675. https://doi.org/10.1111/jcpp.12849

Mewton, L., Lees, B., Squeglia, L. M., Forbes, M. K., Sunderland, M., Krueger, R., et al. (2022). The relationship between brain structure and general psychopathology in preadolescents. *Journal of Child Psychology and Psychiatry, 63*(7), 734–744. https://doi.org/10.1111/jcpp.13513

Michelini, G., Barch, D. M., Tian, Y., Watson, D., Klein, D. N., & Kotov, R. (2019). Delineating and validating higher-order dimensions of psychopathology in the Adolescent Brain Cognitive Development (ABCD) study. *Translational Psychiatry, 9*. https://doi.org/10.1038/s41398-019-0593-4

Michelini, G., Gair, K., Tian, Y., Miao, J. J., Dougherty, L. R., Goldstein, B. L., et al. (2022). Do general and specific factors of preschool psychopathology predict preadolescent outcomes? A transdiagnostic hierarchical approach. *Psychological Medicine*, 1–10. https://doi.org/10.1017/s003329172200246x

Moffitt, T. E., & E-Risk Study Team. (2002). Teenaged mothers in contemporary Britain. *Journal of Child Psychology and Psychiatry, 43*(6), 727–742. https://doi.org/10.1111/1469-7610.00082

Moore, T. M., Kaczkurkin, A. N., Durham, E. L., Jeong, H. J., McDowell, M. G., Dupont, R. M., et al. (2020). Criterion validity and relationships between alternative hierarchical dimensional models of general and specific psychopathology. *Journal of Abnormal Psychology, 129*(7), 677–688. https://doi.org/10.1037/abn0000601

Muratori, P., Paciello, M., Castro, E., Levantini, V., Masi, G., Milone, A., et al. (2021). At-risk early adolescents profiles in the community: A cluster analysis using the Strengths and Difficulties Questionnaire. *Psychiatry Research, 305*, 114209. https://doi.org/10.1016/j.psychres.2021.114209

Muris, P., Merckelbach, H., Schmidt, T., & Mayer, B. (1999). The revised version of the Screen for Child Anxiety Related Emotional Disorders (SCARED-R): Factor structure in normal children. *Personality and Individual Differences, 26*(1), 99–112. https://doi.org/10.1016/S0191-8869(98)00130-5

Murray, A. L., Eisner, M., & Ribeaud, D. (2016). The development of the general factor of psychopathology 'p Factor' through childhood and adolescence. *Journal of Abnormal Child Psychology, 44*(8), 1573–1586. https://doi.org/10.1007/s10802-016-0132-1

Neumann, A., Pappa, I., Lahey, B. B., Verhulst, F. C., Medina-Gomez, C., Jaddoe, V. W., et al. (2016). Single nucleotide polymorphism heritability of a general psychopathology factor in children. *Journal of the American Academy of Child and Adolescent Psychiatry, 55*(12), 1038–1045. https://doi.org/10.1016/j.jaac.2016.09.498

Neumann, A., Nolte, I. M., Pappa, I., Ahluwalia, T. S., Pettersson, E., Rodriguez, A., et al. (2022). A genome-wide association study of total child psychiatric problems scores. *PLoS One, 17*(8). https://doi.org/10.1371/journal.pone.0273116

Olino, T. M., Dougherty, L. R., Bufferd, S. J., Carlson, G. A., & Klein, D. N. (2014). Testing models of psychopathology in preschool-aged children using a structured interview-based assessment. *Journal of Abnormal Child Psychology, 42*(7), 1201–1211. https://doi.org/10.1007/s10802-014-9865-x

Olino, T. M., Bufferd, S. J., Dougherty, L. R., Dyson, M. W., Carlson, G. A., & Klein, D. N. (2018). The development of latent dimensions of psychopathology across early childhood: Stability of dimensions and moderators of change. *Journal of Abnormal Child Psychology, 46*(7), 1373–1383. https://doi.org/10.1007/s10802-018-0398-6

Pat, N., Riglin, L., Anney, R., Wang, Y., Barch, D. M., Thapar, A., & Stringaris, A. (2022). Motivation and cognitive abilities as mediators between polygenic scores and psychopathology in children. *Journal of the American Academy of Child and Adolescent Psychiatry, 61*(6), 782-+. https://doi.org/10.1016/j.jaac.2021.08.019

Patalay, P., Fonagy, P., Deighton, J., Belsky, J., Vostanis, P., & Miranda, W. (2015). A general psychopathology factor in early adolescence. *British Journal of Psychiatry, 207*(1), 15–22. https://doi.org/10.1192/bjp.bp.114.149591

Patel, Y., Parker, N., Shin, J., Howard, D., French, L., Thomopoulos, S. I., et al. (2021). Virtual histology of cortical thickness and shared neurobiology in 6 psychiatric disorders. *JAMA Psychiatry, 78*(1), 47–63. https://doi.org/10.1001/jamapsychiatry.2020.2694

Patrick, C. J., Hicks, B. M., Nichol, P. E., & Krueger, R. F. (2007). A bifactor approach to modeling the structure of the psychopathy checklist-revised. *Journal of Personality Disorders, 21*(2), 118–141. https://doi.org/10.1521/pedi.2007.21.2.118

Pettersson, E., Larsson, H., & Lichtenstein, P. (2016). Common psychiatric disorders share the same genetic origin: A multivariate sibling study of the Swedish population. *Molecular Psychiatry, 21*(5), 717–721. https://doi.org/10.1038/mp.2015.116

Pettersson, E., Lahey, B. B., Larsson, H., & Lichtenstein, P. (2018). Criterion validity and utility of the general factor of psychopathology in childhood: Predictive associations with independently measured severe adverse mental health outcomes in adolescence. *Journal of the American Academy of Child and Adolescent Psychiatry, 57*(6), 372–383. https://doi.org/10.1016/j.jaac.2017.12.016

Phillips, E. M., Brock, R. L., James, T. D., Nelson, J. M., Espy, K. A., & Nelson, T. D. (2022). Empirical support for a dual process model of the P-Factor: Interaction effects between preschool executive control and preschool negative emotionality on general psychopathology. *Journal of Psychopathology and Clinical Science, 131*(8), 817–829. https://doi.org/10.1037/abn0000777

Plana-Ripoll, O., Pedersen, C. B., Holtz, Y., Benros, M. E., Dalsgaard, S., de Jonge, P., et al. (2019). Exploring comorbidity within mental disorders among a Danish national population. *JAMA Psychiatry, 76*(3), 259–270. https://doi.org/10.1001/jamapsychiatry.2018.3658

Poulton, R., Guiney, H., Ramrakha, S., & Moffitt, T. E. (2023). The Dunedin study after half a century: Reflections on the past, and course for the future. *Journal of the Royal Society of New Zealand, 53*, 446–465. https://doi.org/10.1080/03036758.2022.2114508

Raballo, A., & Poletti, M. (2020). Advances in early identification of children and adolescents at risk for psychiatric illness. *Current Opinion in Psychiatry*. https://doi.org/10.1097/yco.0000000000000652

Reise, S. P. (2012). The rediscovery of bifactor measurement models. *Multivariate Behavioral Research, 47*(5), 667–696. https://doi.org/10.1080/00273171.2012.715555

Rhee, S. H., Lahey, B. B., & Waldman, I. D. (2015). Comorbidity among dimensions of childhood psychopathology: Converging evidence from behavior genetics. *Child Development Perspectives, 9*(1), 26–31. https://doi.org/10.1111/cdep.12102

Richards, J. S., Hartman, C. A., Ormel, J., & Oldehinkel, A. J. (2022). Continuity of psychopathology throughout adolescence and young adulthood. *Journal of Clinical Child & Adolescent Psychology*. https://doi.org/10.1080/15374416.2022.2042695

Riglin, L., Thapar, A. K., Leppert, B., Martin, J., Richards, A., Anney, R., et al. (2020). Using genetics to examine a general liability to childhood psychopathology. *Behavior Genetics, 50*(4), 213–220. https://doi.org/10.1007/s10519-019-09985-4

Rodriguez, A., Reise, S. P., & Haviland, M. G. (2016). Evaluating bifactor models: Calculating and interpreting statistical indices. *Psychological Methods, 21*(2), 137–150. https://doi.org/10.1037/met0000045

Rodriguez-Seijas, C., Gadow, K. D., Rosen, T. E., Kim, H., Lerner, M. D., & Eaton, N. R. (2020). A transdiagnostic model of psychiatric symptom co-occurrence and autism spectrum disorder. *Autism Research, 13*(4), 579–590. https://doi.org/10.1002/aur.2228

Romer, A. L., & Pizzagalli, D. A. (2021). Is executive dysfunction a risk marker or consequence of psychopathology? A test of executive function as a prospective predictor and outcome of general psychopathology in the adolescent brain cognitive development study (R). *Developmental Cognitive Neuroscience, 51*. https://doi.org/10.1016/j.dcn.2021.100994

Romer, A. L., Knodt, A. R., Houts, R., Brigidi, B. D., Moffitt, T. E., Caspi, A., & Hariri, A. R. (2018). Structural alterations within cerebellar circuitry are associated with general liability for common mental disorders. *Molecular Psychiatry, 23*(4), 1084–1090. https://doi.org/10.1038/mp.2017.57

Romer, A. L., Knodt, A. R., Sison, M. L., Ireland, D., Houts, R., Ramrakha, S., et al. (2021). Replicability of structural brain alterations associated with general psychopathology: Evidence from a population-representative birth cohort. *Molecular Psychiatry, 26*(8), 3839–3846. https://doi.org/10.1038/s41380-019-0621-z

Rosenstrom, T., Gjerde, L. C., Krueger, R. F., Aggen, S. H., Czajkowski, N. O., Gillespie, N. A., et al. (2019). Joint factorial structure of psychopathology and personality. *Psychological Medicine, 49*(13), 2158–2167. https://doi.org/10.1017/s0033291718002982

Ruggero, C. J., Kotov, R., Hopwood, C. J., First, M., Clark, L. A., Skodol, A. E., et al. (2019). Integrating the hierarchical taxonomy of psychopathology (HiTOP) into clinical practice.

Journal of Consulting and Clinical Psychology, 87(12), 1069–1084. https://doi.org/10.1037/ccp0000452

Sallis, H., Szekely, E., Neumann, A., Jolicoeur-Martineau, A., van Ijzendoorn, M., Hillegers, M., et al. (2019). General psychopathology, internalising and externalising in children and functional outcomes in late adolescence. *Journal of Child Psychology and Psychiatry, 60*(11), 1183–1190. https://doi.org/10.1111/jcpp.13067

Schreuder, M. J., Wigman, J. T. W., Groen, R. N., Wichers, M., & Hartman, C. A. (2021). On the transience or stability of subthreshold psychopathology. *Scientific Reports, 11*(1). https://doi.org/10.1038/s41598-021-02711-3

Sellbom, M., & Tellegen, A. (2019). Factor analysis in psychological assessment research: Common pitfalls and recommendations. *Psychological Assessment, 31*(12), 1428–1441. https://doi.org/10.1037/pas0000623

Selzam, S., Coleman, J. R. I., Caspi, A., Moffitt, T. E., & Plomin, R. (2018). A polygenic p factor for major psychiatric disorders. *Translational Psychiatry, 8*. https://doi.org/10.1038/s41398-018-0217-4

Shah, J. L., Scott, J., McGorry, P. D., Cross, S. P. M., Keshavan, M. S., Nelson, B., et al. (2020). Transdiagnostic clinical staging in youth mental health: A first international consensus statement. *World Psychiatry, 19*(2), 233–242. https://doi.org/10.1002/wps.20745

Shankman, S. A., Lewinsohn, P. M., Klein, D. N., Small, J. W., Seeley, J. R., & Altman, S. E. (2009). Subthreshold conditions as precursors for full syndrome disorders: A 15-year longitudinal study of multiple diagnostic classes. *Journal of Child Psychology and Psychiatry, 50*(12), 1485–1494. https://doi.org/10.1111/j.1469-7610.2009.02117.x

Shanmugan, S., Wolf, D. H., Calkins, M. E., Moore, T. M., Ruparel, K., Hopson, R. D., et al. (2016). Common and dissociable mechanisms of executive system dysfunction across psychiatric disorders in youth. *American Journal of Psychiatry, 173*(5), 517–526. https://doi.org/10.1176/appi.ajp.2015.15060725

Shields, A. N., Reardon, K. W., Brandes, C. M., & Tackett, J. L. (2019). The p factor in children: Relationships with executive functions and effortful control. *Journal of Research in Personality, 82*. https://doi.org/10.1016/j.jrp.2019.103853

Smith, G. T., Atkinson, E. A., Davis, H. A., Riley, E. N., & Oltmanns, J. R. (2020). The general factor of psychopathology. In T. Widiger & T. D. Cannon (Eds.), *Annual review of clinical psychology* (Vol. 16, pp. 75–98).

Snyder, H. R., Young, J. F., & Hankin, B. L. (2017). Strong homotypic continuity in common psychopathology-, Internalizing-, and Externalizing-Specific Factors over time in adolescents. *Clinical Psychological Science, 5*(1), 98–110. https://doi.org/10.1177/2167702616651076

Spence, S. H., Rapee, R., McDonald, C., & Ingram, M. (2001). The structure of anxiety symptoms among preschoolers. *Behaviour Research and Therapy, 39*(11), 1293–1316. https://doi.org/10.1016/s0005-7967(00)00098-x

Sprooten, E., Franke, B., & Greven, C. U. (2021). The P-factor and its genomic and neural equivalents: An integrated perspective. *Molecular Psychiatry*. https://doi.org/10.1038/s41380-021-01031-2

Stanton, K., DeLucia, E. A., Brown, M. F. D., & McDonnell, C. G. (2021). Advancing understanding of the classification of broad autism phenotype and attention-deficit/hyperactivity disorder symptom dimensions within the Hierarchical Taxonomy of Psychopathology. *Personality and Mental Health, 15*(2), 113–123. https://doi.org/10.1002/pmh.1498

Sterba, S., Egger, H. L., & Angold, A. (2007). Diagnostic specificity and nonspecificity in the dimensions of preschool psychopathology. *Journal of Child Psychology and Psychiatry, 48*(10), 1005–1013. https://doi.org/10.1111/j.1469-7610.2007.01770.x

Sterba, S. K., Copeland, W., Egger, H. L., Costello, E. J., Erkanli, A., & Angold, A. (2010). Longitudinal dimensionality of adolescent psychopathology: Testing the differentiation hypothesis. *Journal of Child Psychology and Psychiatry, 51*(8), 871–884. https://doi.org/10.1111/j.1469-7610.2010.02234.x

Stevanovic, D., Jafari, P., Knez, R., Franic, T., Atilola, O., Davidovic, N., et al. (2017). Can we really use available scales for child and adolescent psychopathology across cultures? A systematic review of cross-cultural measurement invariance data. *Transcultural Psychiatry, 54*(1), 125–152. https://doi.org/10.1177/1363461516689215

Strickland, J., Keller, J., Lavigne, J. V., Gouze, K., Hopkins, J., & LeBailly, S. (2011). The structure of psychopathology in a community sample of preschoolers. *Journal of Abnormal Child Psychology, 39*(4), 601–610. https://doi.org/10.1007/s10802-011-9487-5

Tackett, J. L., Lahey, B. B., van Hulle, C., Waldman, I., Krueger, R. F., & Rathouz, P. J. (2013). Common genetic influences on negative emotionality and a general psychopathology factor in childhood and adolescence. *Journal of Abnormal Psychology, 122*(4), 1142–1153. https://doi.org/10.1037/a0034151

Tellegen, A., Ben-Porath, Y. S., McNulty, J. L., Arbisi, P. A., Graham, J. R., & Kaemmer, B. (2003). *MMPI–2 restructured clinical scales: Development, validation, and interpretation*. University of Minnesota Press.

Trzaskowski, M., Harlaar, N., Arden, R., Krapohl, E., Rimfeld, K., McMillan, A., et al. (2014). Genetic influence on family socioeconomic status and children's intelligence. *Intelligence, 42*, 83–88. https://doi.org/10.1016/j.intell.2013.11.002

van Bork, R., Epskamp, S., Rhemtulla, M., Borsboom, D., & van der Maas, H. L. J. (2017). What is the p-factor of psychopathology? Some risks of general factor modeling. *Theory & Psychology, 27*(6), 759–773. https://doi.org/10.1177/0959354317737185

Wade, M., Plamondon, A., & Jenkins, J. M. (2021). A family socialization model of transdiagnostic risk for psychopathology in preschool children. *Research on Child and Adolescent Psychopathology*. https://doi.org/10.1007/s10802-021-00789-x

Waldman, I. D., Rowe, D. C., Abramowitz, A., Kozel, S. T., Mohr, J. H., Sherman, S. L., et al. (1998). Association and linkage of the dopamine transporter gene and attention-deficit hyperactivity disorder in children: Heterogeneity owing to diagnostic subtype and severity. *American Journal of Human Genetics, 63*(6), 1767–1776. https://doi.org/10.1086/302132

Waldman, I. D., Poore, H. E., van Hulle, C., Rathouz, P. J., & Lahey, B. B. (2016). External validity of a hierarchical dimensional model of child and adolescent psychopathology: Tests using confirmatory factor analyses and multivariate behavior genetic analyses. *Journal of Abnormal Psychology, 125*(8), 1053–1066. https://doi.org/10.1037/abn0000183

Waszczuk, M. A., Eaton, N. R., Krueger, R. F., Shackman, A. J., Waldman, I. D., Zald, D. H., et al. (2020). Redefining phenotypes to advance psychiatric genetics: Implications from Hierarchical Taxonomy of Psychopathology. *Journal of Abnormal Psychology, 129*(2), 143–161. https://doi.org/10.1037/abn0000486

Waszczuk, M. A., Zavos, H. M. S., & Eley, T. C. (2021). Why do depression, conduct, and hyperactivity symptoms co-occur across adolescence? The role of stable and dynamic genetic and environmental influences. *European Journal of Child and Adolescent Psychiatry, 30*, 1013–1025. https://doi.org/10.1007/s00787-020-01515-6

Watts, A. L., Poore, H. E., & Waldman, I. D. (2019). Riskier tests of the validity of the bifactor model of psychopathology. *Clinical Psychological Science, 7*(6), 1285–1303. https://doi.org/10.1177/2167702619855035

Watts, A. L., Lane, S. P., Bonifay, W., Steinley, D., & Meyer, F. A. C. (2020). Building theories on top of, and not independent of, statistical models: The case of the p-factor. *Psychological Inquiry, 31*(4), 310–320. https://doi.org/10.1080/1047840x.2020.1853476

Widiger, T. A., & Oltmanns, J. R. (2017). The general factor of psychopathology and personality. *Clinical Psychological Science, 5*(1), 182–183. https://doi.org/10.1177/2167702616657042

Zald, D. H., & Lahey, B. B. (2017). Implications of the hierarchical structure of psychopathology for psychiatric neuroimaging. *Biological Psychiatry: Cognitive Neuroscience and Neuroimaging, 2*(4), 310–317. https://doi.org/10.1016/j.bosc.2017.02.003

Chapter 7
Internalising Problems

7.1 Clarifying Terminology

The paper by Achenbach in 1966 was a watershed in the development of measurement of behavioural variation in children. There have been a number of prior studies providing analyses of the variety of behavioural symptoms shown by children that produced classifications (e.g. Jenkins & Hewitt, 1944). There were also prior applications of factor analysis to measures of child problem behaviour (Digman, 1963; Peterson, 1961). The most extensive of these was the Behavioral Classification Project (Dreger et al., 1964). However it was Achenbach (1966) who applied factor analysis to data from a symptom checklist, which was the basis of the later Child Behavior Checklist (CBCL), and the resulting framework has had a lasting influence. This was 1 year before the first of the Rutter Scales was published (Rutter, 1967). The latter were designed as a simple questionnaire for use in screening or in surveys. The Achenbach scales were designed initially to classify the behaviours of child psychiatric patients and were accordingly more extensive in the behaviours covered and more time consuming to complete than the scales produced by Rutter. The relative merits of these scales were appraised by Goodman and Scott (1999) based on the CBCL and the Strength and Difficulties Questionnaire (SDQ), which evolved from the Rutter scales. It is clear that both the longer (CBCL) and the shorter (SDQ) questionnaires have their merits and are useful for measuring behaviour but are optimal for different applications.

The CBCL and its related questionnaires provide measures of broadband groupings of internalising and externalising problems. Although internalising had been a concept in psychoanalysis, the use of the terms by Tom Achenbach was explained as follows:

> The label is not intended to carry dynamic implications. It means only that the symptoms at the Externalizing end describe conflict with the environment, while those at the other end describe problems within the self. (Achenbach, 1966, p. 10)

J. Stevenson, *Developmental Psychopathology*,
https://doi.org/10.1007/978-3-031-45787-6_7

To illustrate the behaviours that are subsumed under domains of internalising (peer problems and emotional problems) and externalising (hyperactivity-inattention problems and conduct problems), the items in the original five-factor format of the SDQ are listed below – see Goodman (2001) for details of the psychometric properties of the SDQ. The SDQ is used as it is a more succinct summary of the internalising and externalising behaviours than the CBCL.

Prosocial behaviour
Considerate of other people's feelings
Shares readily with other children (treats, toys, pencils, etc.)
Helpful if someone is hurt, upset, or feeling ill
Kind to younger children
Often volunteers to help others (parents, teachers, other children)
Hyperactivity-inattention problems
Restless, overactive, cannot stay still for long
Constantly fidgeting or squirming
Easily distracted, concentration wanders
Thinks things out before acting (reversed)
Sees tasks through to the end, good attention span (reversed)
Emotional symptoms
Often complains of headaches, stomach-aches, or sickness
Many worries, often seems worried
Often unhappy, down-hearted, or tearful
Nervous or clingy in new situations, easily loses confidence
Many fears, easily scared
Conduct problems
Often has temper tantrums or hot tempers
Generally obedient, usually does what adults request (reversed)
Often fights with other children or bullies them
Often lies or cheats
Steals from home, school or elsewhere
Peer problems
Rather solitary, tends to play alone
Has at least one good friend (reversed)
Generally liked by other children (reversed)
Picked on or bullied by other children
Gets on better with adults than with other children

A confirmatory factor analysis of the SDQ suggested that internalising and externalising problems could be appropriately extracted by aggregating the emotional problems and peer problem scales and the behaviour problem and hyperactivity problem scales, respectively (Goodman et al., 2010). The prosocial scale is a distinct factor of behaviour that is outside the internalising/externalising framework. Subsequent studies of the use of the SDQ with 3–5-year-old children rated by teachers and parents found that both the original five-factor solution (Dahlberg et al., 2019) and the second-order internalising and externalising factors (three-factor solution) (Ezpeleta et al., 2013) could be captured in the scores for these preschool children. It should be noted that the three-factor solution did not fit as well as the five-factor solution in the Croft et al. (2015) study of preschool children. However the absolute fit of the three-factor solution was good (RMSEA = 0.028), which is lower than the 0.06 recommended as the maximum RMSEA for good fit by Hu and Bentler (1999).

The version of the Achenbach scales for ages 1.5–5 years also identifies the second-order factors of internalising and externalising. A model of child psychopathology that includes a general factor (p-factor) and group factors of internalising and externalising has been shown to be an optimal fit to data for preschoolers (Olino et al., 2014), those in middle childhood (Lahey et al., 2015), and adolescents (Tackett et al., 2013). This represents convergent evidence that it is appropriate to summarise behaviours into internalising and externalising problems plus a general factor and apply the framework to children across a wide age range.

A terminology was suggested by Gardner and Shaw (2008) of a broad classification of problems in the preschool child into "disruptive problems", which include problems with oppositional behaviour and attentional deficits, and "emotional problems" related to depression and anxiety. These groupings are analogous to internalising and externalising problem terms used for older children and maybe more appropriately descriptive for this young age group. However the terms internalising and externalising have been adopted pervasively in studies of children of all ages, including the preschool child, and will be used here.

7.2 Structure of Internalising Problems

The behaviours and feelings most commonly associated with internalising problems are those related to anxiety, depression, and fearfulness.

Zahn-Waxler et al. (2000) provided a historical overview of the development in the understanding of anxiety and depression in children and summarised the state of knowledge at the beginning of the twenty-first century. They drew attention to the fact that it was only recently (to 2000) that anxiety and depression were recognised as being present in children. The situation has now changed so markedly that Collishaw et al. (2010) reported that twice as many young people reported frequent feelings of depression or anxiety in 2006 as in 1986. The effect was particularly marked for girls. It was not possible to identify the possible reasons for this increase. It should be noted that this data was obtained from rating scales and did not refer to diagnoses. The Global Burden of Diseases, Injuries, and Risk Factors Study 2015 (Vos et al., 2016), which examines the impact of physical, sensory, and mental disorders on well-being on a global basis, found that in middle childhood conduct and anxiety disorders were in the top 10 causes of disability. In adolescents and young adults (aged between 15 and 39 years) depression and anxiety disorders were in the top 10 causes in these age groups too.

The structure of anxiety, depression, and fearfulness will be considered in turn.

Anxiety To illustrate the structure of anxiety a widely used self-report measure of anxiety in children will be described – the Spence Children's Anxiety Scale (Spence, 1998). In a confirmatory factor analysis (CFA) of anxiety items, Spence found that a six-factor structure with a higher-order general factor fitted the data well. The six latent factors were identified as panic/agoraphobia, separation anxiety, social phobia, physical injury fears, obsessive-compulsive disorder, and generalised anxiety. These six factors were closely associated with correlations ranging from $r = 0.55$ to 0.91. As this suggests, a model with a second-order general anxiety factor fitted the data well (Comparative Fit Index, CFI = 0.96).

In considering these internalising problems there is a need to take age-related changes into account. For example, there is a question about whether the pattern of anxiety symptoms shown by preschoolers is equivalent to that found in older children and adults. Spence et al. (2001) investigated this issue in a sample of 2–6-year-olds and found that a five-factor solution provided a good fit. These factors – social phobia, separation anxiety, generalised anxiety, obsessive-compulsive disorder, and fears of physical injury – were consistent with DSM-IV diagnostic categories of anxiety disorders. These factors were correlated with each other, and a model with a general second-order factor fitted the data well (CFI = 0.94). This study suggested that in preschoolers, although separate facets of anxiety can be found, these components of anxiety are not strongly differentiated and discrete anxiety subtypes are not found.

Egger and Angold (2006) reviewed the evidence concerning internalising problems in preschoolers. In the few general population samples for which data were available the prevalence of anxiety problems was 9% and of depression was up to 2%. Studies are now being conducted on the influences on the development and outcome of internalising in the preschool years. For example, a close relationship has been established between maternal internalising and child internalising between the ages of 3 and 6 years (Zhou & Buss, 2021), and depression has been shown to have high stability from the preschool period through adolescence (Gaffrey et al., 2018).

Depression Depression is a common but often unrecognised problem in adolescence (Thapar et al., 2012) and one which can have a markedly adverse on current well-being. It may also result in continuing difficulties, including an elevated risk of suicide (Hawton & van Heeringen, 2009). The treatment of adolescent depression with both pharmacological and psychological interventions is an important component of suicide prevention (Zalsman et al., 2016). An important overview of the state of knowledge about depression, including its impact on child development, has been produced by Herrman et al. (2022). This overview places particular emphasis on the need for prevention and action to mitigate its adverse effects on children and other family members.

The items from the Short Mood and Feelings Questionnaire (SMFQ) (Messer et al., 1995) will be used to illustrate the range of symptoms that are used to assess depression in children. The 13 items are miserable, didn't enjoy, so tired, restless, no good, cried a lot, concentrate, hate self, bad person, lonely, nobody loves, never as good, and everything wrong. Messer et al. (1995) found that a CFA clearly indicated that a single factor explained the correlations between these items. This single-factor structure has been replicated in extensive subsequent studies (for a review see Schlechter et al., 2023).

Fearfulness It is common to find depression, anxiety, and fearfulness co-occurring in children and adolescents. Fearfulness is the aspect of internalising that has been least studied in isolation. Of course experiencing fear is a normal reaction to a real or imagined threat, and this needs to be differentiated from phobias or pathological fears (Gullone, 2000). These "normal" fears show a pattern whereby they become less common and severe with age. Fears experienced by young children relate to their immediate experiences. In later childhood fears become more directed to anticipated events and more general situations or events.

A widely used measure of fears in children is the Fear Survey Schedule for Children – Revised (FSSC-R) (Ollendick, 1983). In the original report on the FSSC-R on 8–11-year-old children a five-factor solution was obtained. The five factors were "fear of failure and criticism", "fear of the unknown", "fear of injury and small animals", "fear of danger and death", and "medical fears". Subsequent CFAs have found that that at this age this five-factor structure provided a good fit on RMSEA (0.04) and a marginally good fit on the CFI (0.85) (Bokhorst et al., 2008). This same study showed that social fears became more differentiated after the age of 9, and accordingly a seven-factor solution was more appropriate. Using a shortened version of the FSSC-R, Muris et al. (2014) also replicated the five-factor solution. These factors were substantially correlated in a non-clinical sample of children and adolescents, with correlations ranging between 0.41 and 0.79.

Some of the most common fears in young children are those associated with night-time such as fear of the dark, sleeping alone, monsters, or ghosts. These may be experienced at some time by nearly 75% of children (Lewis et al., 2021). Common adverse consequences of these fears are night-time waking, disrupted sleep, and separation difficulties. A potentially valuable approach to dealing with night-time fears is the simple expedient of reading with the child. The books being read should provide guidance on the reduction of anxiety and the modelling of effective behaviour. In a small initial demonstration study of nine children this intervention has been shown to be effective for some children (Lewis et al., 2015). A subsequent RCT of a sample of 64 children with night-time fears and co-sleeping with parents gave further evidence of its effectiveness (El Rafihi-Ferreira et al., 2018). In this RCT bibliotherapy was augmented by the use of a doll to facilitate sleeping independently. The intervention produced significant improvements in the children's sleep symptoms, but also in anxiety level, fearfulness, and daytime behaviours.

Association Between Internalising Symptoms Ghandour et al. (2019) examined the prevalence of diagnosed anxiety and depression in children and adolescents in the United States. This was a large-scale survey that generated data of 43,283 children in the general population. The prevalence of diagnosed depression was found to be 3% and anxiety was 7%. For both conditions the prevalence increased with age; the prevalence rates being almost twice as high at 12–17 years than at 6–11 years. Anxiety and depression were very commonly found together, with 74% of those diagnosed with depression showing concurrent anxiety and 33% of those diagnosed with anxiety being concurrently depressed. The mechanisms leading to this co-occurrence are discussed by Cummings et al. (2014).

As an illustration of the gap between the number in the population with internalising problems and the number receiving a diagnosis, the rate of diagnosed depression and anxiety in 12–17-years-olds was found to be 6% and 10%, respectively (see Table 1 in Ghandour et al., 2019). These rates can be compared with the figures of 14% (mood disorders) and 32% (anxiety disorders) for 13–18-year-olds found in a study of the prevalence of disorders in a representative sample of adolescents in the United States (Merikangas et al., 2010). There are many children and adolescents in the population with internalising disorders that are undiagnosed and consequently are likely to be untreated.

A meta-analysis of 242 studies on adults found that shame was strongly associated with depression ($r = 0.43$) (Kim et al., 2011). Shame has also been found to be related to anxiety even when depressive symptoms were controlled and vice versa, with shame being associated with depression when anxiety was controlled. An important development has been the clarification of the distinction between shame and guilt, with the former being more closely associated with depression. Shame is characterised as a pervasive negative evaluation of the self and guilt being directed towards a specific action. Shame is accompanied by emotions such as anger, anxiety, and self-disgust, whereas guilt elicits sorrow and empathy.

The relationships between shame, anxiety, and depression in adolescence were studied in a genetically informative longitudinal study by Nikolic et al. (2022). In this age group shame was moderately to strongly associated with both concurrent depression and anxiety ($r = 0.60$) but only with increased depression, and not anxiety, over the subsequent 2 years. Shame was moderately heritable, and these genetic factors were primarily responsible for the association with depression and anxiety. There were also substantial non-shared environmental influences on shame, and these explained most of the relation with subsequent increases in depression. This suggests that shame represents a significant factor contributing to the association between depression and anxiety.

7.3 Stability of Internalising Problems

Stability of Internalising Problems in General Doering et al. (2022) undertook a longitudinal study of 4492 twins between the ages of 9 and 15 years. They found only a modest association between internalising symptoms measured at these two ages. Internalising measures at 9 years only explained 15% of the variance in internalising at 15 years. They conclude that these findings suggest that childhood and adolescent internalising behaviours are at least partially distinct.

Gutman and McMaster (2020) followed a sample of over 17,000 UK children from the age of 3–14 years. They wanted to establish whether the age-related changes over this period were different for boys and girls. They identified three trajectories for the pooled sample of boys and girls, with two relatively stable groups showing either high (9% of the sample) or low probabilities of internalising problems (66%) and a group with a rising trajectory (25%). For girls in this group these internalising problems continued to rise, but levelled off for boys from age 11. There were a number of characteristics that differentiated these trajectory groups. Boys and girls in the increasing and high-probability groups were more likely to report a number of problematic outcomes, including high body mass index, self-harm, low mental well-being, depressive symptoms, and low educational motivation, than the low group. Girls on the increasing trajectory also reported more cigarette and cannabis use and early sexual activity at age 14 compared to girls on the low trajectory.

The role of genetic and environmental factors in producing stability and change in emotional and behaviour problems in children and adolescents was examined by Hannigan et al. (2017). They identified 58 studies that were informative on this question. They found that stability was primarily influenced by genetic factors, though shared environmental factors play some role, albeit a small one. Change was found to be influenced both by genetic factors and non-shared environmental influences.

Stability of Anxiety The prevalence and continuities of anxiety were investigated in a longitudinal study of 1041 children from early childhood (4–6 years) through middle childhood (8–10 years) to adolescence (12–14 years) by Steinsbekk et al. (2022). Over this time period about 10% of children experienced an anxiety disorder. Although anxiety disorders are found in childhood, those shown in early childhood generally did not predict later anxiety symptoms. By middle childhood anxiety symptoms are more stable and more predictive of anxiety in adolescence. They conclude that middle childhood may be particularly important for preventive and treatment interventions. There is evidence that there are strong genetic effects on the continuity of anxiety symptoms during middle childhood (Trzaskowski et al., 2012).

An appraisal of the changes in the prevalence of anxiety disorders between 9 and 26 years was made by Copeland et al. (2014). In this longitudinal study of 1420 participants there was a U-shaped pattern with high levels of separation anxiety in childhood and panic, agoraphobia, and generalised anxiety featuring in young adulthood. There was a slightly higher rate of disorders in females, but this was only significant for those over the age of 15 years.

Stability of Depression In the adolescent years depression has been found to carry a substantial risk of depression in adulthood (Fryers & Brugha, 2013; Johnson et al., 2018). For example, Fombonne et al. (2001) found that 75% of adolescents with depression showed depression in their adult years. However there has been an outstanding question as to whether depression in children before puberty presents an early stage of depression that will last into adolescence and beyond or whether it is a distinct condition with its own course. Sands et al. (2022) conducted a systematic review to investigate this issue. The limited evidence from the 17 relevant publications they traced suggests that this early-onset pattern of symptoms was associated with an enduring risk of later depression and that prepubertal internalising systems more generally also predicted later anxiety disorders. They note that these associations with disorders in adulthood were less strong than those found for depression in adolescence.

The relationship between anxiety and depression in children between the ages of 4 and 5 years was studied by Lavigne et al. (2015). They found a relatively high correlation (over 0.75) between measures of anxiety between the ages of 4, 5, and 6 years and a slightly lower stability for depression (over 0.50). Moreover they found that both anxiety and depression were associated with higher levels of one another in the subsequent year. This relationship was also studied over middle childhood by Tanguay-Garneau et al. (2020). They found that anxiety and depression were associated between the ages of 6 and 12 years. Depressive symptoms were more stable than those of anxiety. Depression had a more marked impact than anxiety on later depression and anxiety.

The stability of the combined symptoms of anxiety and depression was studied in a cohort sequential study of 49,524 twins over a 25-year period (Nivard et al., 2015). This design is achieved by studying twin pairs for 25 years with repeated assessment of symptoms of anxiety and depression. The twins were aged between 3 and 38 years when first assessed. During adolescence there was a significant increase in scores and higher scores in females emerging over this period. Heritability was high in childhood (over 0.60) and decreased to 0.3–0.40 during adulthood. Phenotypic correlations across ages were $r = 0.5$ in childhood, $r = 0.6$ in adolescence, $r = 0.7$ in young adults, and $r = 0.8$ in adults. Longitudinal stability was mainly determined by genetic factors.

Lussier et al. (2021) used molecular genetic data to create polygenic risk scores (PRS) to investigate possible changes in the genes associated with depression in children studied longitudinally from age 4 to 17 years. They found that different trajectories of depressive symptomatology were predictable from PRS, with these scores being closely related to early-adolescent-onset depression. The Lussier et al. (2021) study was based on the Avon Longitudinal Study of Children and Parents (ALSPAC) sample. In the same sample Rice et al. (2019) found that very early-onset depression (i.e. before the age of 12 years) was associated with PRS for ADHD and with neurodevelopmental traits such as language difficulties.

It has been suggested, based on a network analysis (see Sect. 2.6), that depressed mood and worry at age 10 years may be particularly strong influences on other symptoms of psychopathology, including externalising behaviours, that develop subsequently in adolescence (Funkhouser et al., 2021).

Stability of Fears The variation between children in the development of fear symptoms between the ages of 4 and 11 years has been identified by Broeren et al. (2013). There were two developmental trajectories found for fears. The first was a mainly stable level of fears which was followed by most children. There was a small group of both boys and girls where there was an increasing then decreasing level of fears with a peak at around 8 years of age.

The question of the relationship between high levels of fearfulness in the early years and later anxiety was addressed by Buss (2011). She followed a general population sample of 24-month-old children each year for 3 years. The study found that being fearful in situations that are relatively low in threat (i.e. are predictable and controllable and in which children have many coping resources) is an early precursor to risk for anxiety development as measured by parental and teacher reports of children's anxiety in kindergarten.

7.4 Risk Factors for Internalising Problems

Gender The most consistent risk factor associated with internalising problems in children is gender (Zahn-Waxler et al., 2008). The excess of problems in girls is found for anxiety (Lewinsohn et al., 1998), depression (Kuehner, 2017), and fearfulness (McLean & Anderson, 2009). This excess increases with age into adolescence, and the gender difference persists into adulthood.

Salk et al. (2017) produced two major meta-analyses on gender differences in depression in nationally representative samples from over 90 different nations. The first examined studies of diagnosed depression, and the second, studies using measures of symptoms of depression. The effect of gender on depression diagnoses gave an effect size of OR = 1.95. The corresponding effect size for the higher mean depression symptoms in girls was SMD = 0.27. There were strong age effects on these effect sizes, with a peak at age 16 (SMD = 0.47) for both diagnoses and depression symptoms. This gender effect started to emerge by the age of 12 years.

Hyde et al. (2008) developed an integrated model of factors influencing the emergence of gender imbalance in the rate of depression. They called this model ABC (affective, biological, cognitive), and it took the form of vulnerability-stress model. These three ABC components (affective – e.g. temperament; biological – e.g. pubertal hormones; and cognitive – e.g. ruminating repetitively and passively about the negative emotions) produce a vulnerability which leads to depression when stresses, such as negative life events, are experienced. The components of the model are experienced more often by females in terms of both vulnerabilities (e.g. temperament, cognitive style) and stressors (e.g. child sexual abuse). The ABC model was revised and extended to include a broader range of social and cultural factors such as structural gender inequality and media exposure (Hyde & Mezulis, 2020). They conclude that any one of the factors associated with the increased risk for depression in girls is unlikely to have a large effect. The evidence suggests that many influences act in concert to generate the greater susceptibility to depression in girls and that different individuals have different vulnerabilities and experience different adversities.

Parenting and the Family Environment Parenting has been considered to be a major influence on anxiety in children as the following makes clear:

> Traditional models of childhood anxiety sought to explain the development of anxiety in terms of single main effects and focused primarily on the broad parenting dimensions of acceptance versus rejection and psychological granting of autonomy versus psychological control. (McLeod et al., 2007b, p. 155)

However, when these authors undertook a meta-analysis of the findings from 47 studies on the association between aspects of parenting and child anxiety, they found only a weak association. Differences in parenting behaviour accounted for only 4% of the variance in child anxiety, with parental control being more strongly associated than parental rejection. They conclude that an understanding of the origins of child anxiety will have to be based on a wider range of factors than just parenting.

McLeod et al. (2007a) also produced a meta-analysis of findings on aspects of parenting that are related to depression. Their findings paralleled the above meta-analysis on parenting and anxiety. They found that parenting accounted for a modest 8% of the variance in child depression. Parental control was not as strongly related to childhood depression as parental rejection. As with anxiety these findings indicated that a wider range of factors other than parenting are involved in creating vulnerability to depression. The search for specific associations between particular childhood adversities and depression has been disappointing (Kessler et al., 2001).

This search is made more complex by the interplay of gene and environment influences. Lau and Eley (2008) showed how two childhood adversities, negative life events and maternal punitive discipline, were linked by both gene–environment correlations (r_{GE}) and gene–environment interaction (G × E). Twin and sibling data on adolescents indicated that those at genetic risk for depression may be exposed to increased social adversity (r_{GE}) and more susceptible to developing symptoms in response to these risks (G × E).

Experiences in families and in particular aspects of parental care have been extensively examined as possible influences on internalising problems in younger children. For example, Bayer et al. (2012) investigated the risk factors for internalising in a general population sample of 733 Australian children during the preschool period. The strongest predictors of internalising behaviours at 5 years of age were harsh discipline, maternal stress, having no older siblings, single parenthood, and maternal substance misuse. Between them these factors explained 22% of the variation in internalising behaviours.

Across a range of styles of parenting, the results of studies examining the relationship between child depression and anxiety have been mixed (Allmann et al., 2022). However reliable associations have been reported between parental anxiety and internalising problems in children. It is essential to separate out the effects of exposure of the child to parental anxiety from an association that may arise from the genetic relationship between parent and child. Ahmadzadeh et al. (2021) undertook a systematic review and meta-analysis of studies that were able to use genetically informative designs to separate out these two effects. They identified eight publications that were based on various designs (adoption, sibling comparison, children of twins, or in vitro fertilisation) that could achieve such a separation of effects. With genetic factors controlled there was no residual association between prenatal parental anxiety and internalising in the child. The effects of exposure to parental anxiety postnatally were significant but small ($r = 0.13$).

It has been demonstrated that high levels of parental criticism are experienced by children with internalising behaviours. It is important to distinguish the direction of effects. Does parental criticism lead to internalising behaviour or does internalising increase parental criticism? The former seems to be the most likely effect. However the plausibility of child-to-parent effects has been shown by the fact that the improvements in parenting have been found to follow from the treatment of adolescent anxiety (Silverman et al., 2009, 2021),

An additional possible consideration is the role of genetic factors that may influence both parental criticism and internalising in the child. The Children of Twins (COT) design is able to ascertain the nature of relationships between parent and child characteristics once genetic factors are controlled (see Sect. 3.1) (Ahmadzadeh et al., 2022). In this study they were able to show that the relationship between parental criticism and child internalising was maintained once the effects of genetics had been controlled. However the study was unable to determine the direction of effects between these two factors.

Rodrigues et al. (2021) undertook a meta-analysis of studies concerning the relationship between paternal sensitivity and child development. They considered sensitive parenting as involving the reading subtle affective and cognitive cues of children and, in turn, responding in a manner that is sensitive, stimulating, or both. They did not identify a significant relationship with children's internalising problems and only a very small relationship with externalising problems $r = -0.08$ ($CI_{.95}$ -0.14 to -0.03). Similar significant but small relationships have been found with maternal sensitivity and internalising problems (Kok et al., 2013). These relationships were found in two longitudinal studies and provide consistent evidence for only a modest association between sensitivity and internalising problems across time.

Sullivan et al. (2022) investigated whether aspects of parenting mediated the relationship between socio-economic risks and child behaviour. Socio-economic cumulative risk was measured by summing dichotomised variables based on family income, household use of public assistance, parental education, single-parent status, and teenage parenthood. They found that both positive and negative parenting accounted for the relationship between socio-economic cumulative risk and externalising problems. However these features of parenting did not play a role in the association of socio-economic risks with internalising problems.

Hudson et al. (2019) investigated the relationship between early anxiety symptoms, inhibited temperament, and maternal overinvolvement and later anxiety in the child. They found an interaction between inhibited temperament and maternal overinvolvement such that behaviourally inhibited preschoolers had higher anxiety symptoms at age 12, only when exposed to maternal overinvolvement at age 4. The increased risk of anxiety in inhibited children was reduced when mothers showed low levels of overinvolvement at age 4.

The evidence from these studies is that the relationship between measures of parenting and the family environment and internalising in children and adolescents is only modest. Moreover when studies have been able to take genetic influences into account these effects are further reduced.

Life Events The landmark studies of George Brown and colleagues (e.g. Brown & Harris, 1978) demonstrated the importance of life events for the onset of depression in adult women. A crucial issue is whether such an association arises from depression being a response to an adverse life event or whether the behaviour associated with depression leads to the adverse events. A third possibility is that of a third factor having an influence on both the life event and depression.

One way to attempt to differentiate the first two of these processes is to distinguish between adverse life events that arise independently of the action of the person and those that might be dependent on the person's behaviour (Brown et al., 1973; Sandberg et al., 1993). Examples of independent adverse life events include a close friend's family moving out of the neighbourhood and the death of a relative. Examples of dependent adverse life events are doing poorly in a test at school and having an argument with a sibling.

The validity of the classification of life events in this manner was tested by Kendler et al. (1999) in a twin study. They showed that dependent (but not independent) life events were heritable and therefore any dependent life event/depression association may be subject to a gene–environment correlation. The importance of excluding dependent life events in investigating the causal influences on depression in adolescence was shown by Boardman et al. (2011). The association between dependent (but not independent life events) was largely explained by common genetic factors.

A second distinction is that between threat and loss events. In a sample of young women, Finlay-Jones and Brown (1981) showed that threat or danger events in the previous year were associated with the onset of anxiety. However in the case of the onset of depression it was loss events that showed an association. For children loss events include the loss by death or by separation of a relative, loss of status at school, and the loss of a cherished idea, for example, break-up of a friendship.

Adopting this framework of dependent/independent and threat/loss for classifying life events, Eley and Stevenson (2000) examined the association of different types of life event and chronic stresses with anxiety and depression in children. They excluded dependent life events and were able to control for family confounds by testing the association with anxiety and depression in discordant twin pairs where, for example, one twin showed depression and their co-twin did not. They were not able to control completely for possible genetic confounds. This would have been possible by limiting the analysis to discordant MZ pairs but the modest sample size available required the inclusion of discordant DZ pairs too. However this possible genetic confound will have been limited by the analysis of just independent life events. Using this approach they were able to replicate Finlay-Jones and Brown (1981) finding a specific association of threat events with anxiety and loss events with depression in children aged between 8 and 16 years. This pattern of associations was subsequently replicated by Williamson et al. (2005) in a study of 6–12-year-old children.

Adverse Childhood Experiences There are a number of risks that have been aggregated under the rubric of adverse childhood experiences (ACE). These include childhood physical abuse; household substance abuse; childhood sexual abuse; household mental illness; exposure to domestic violence; emotional, psychological,

or verbal abuse; parental separation or divorce; and household criminality and neglect. These experiences in isolation have been shown to increase the risk of behaviour problems in children. However there is a recognition that these experiences do not occur in isolation and children usually experience more than one (Rutter & Sandberg, 1992). There is replicated evidence that there is a linear increase in the risk of adverse later physical and mental health outcomes with increase in the number of ACEs (Anda et al., 2006; Hughes et al., 2017).

When considering risk it is clear that multiple risks have a bigger impact on children than single risks alone. However there are a number of factors, such as social deprivation, that result in a child being likely to experience a number of adverse risks. The strengths and weaknesses of alternative methods of measuring cumulative multiple risks are discussed by Evans et al. (2013). They argue that simple cumulative risk indices are appropriate and valuable methods for measures of multiple risks. In such a cumulative risk measure a count is made of the number of high risks a child experiences. This approach has been shown to be predictive of a wide range of developmental outcomes. It has advantages over more complex multivariate approaches in that it avoids statistical complexities of the correlations and interactions between risks and is parsimonious in expressing cumulative risk as a single number.

However caution has to be urged before using the aggregated ACE measures routinely to screen the population for risk (Anda et al., 2020). In particular they stress that although ACE scores are predictive at the population level, their accuracy in predicting outcomes from multiple risks for individuals is weak. An additional concern is that a simple aggregation of the number of ACEs produces a score that ignores important interactions between specific adverse experiences (Briggs et al., 2021). This is illustrated in Fig. 7.1, where the risk of adult psychopathology associated with poverty and sexual abuse shows a synergistic interaction. The effect of the

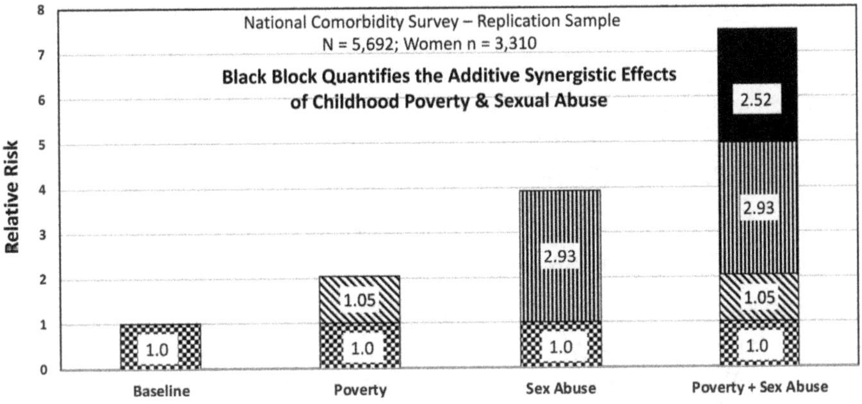

Fig. 7.1 Additive synergy between childhood poverty and sexual abuse for complex adult psychopathology in women. (Reproduced with the permission of the American Psychological Association from Figure 1 Briggs et al. (2021); permission conveyed through Copyright Clearance Center, Inc.)

two risk factors, when experienced together, is greater than the combination of risks for the two separate experiences. Consequently these ACE scores should be treated with caution as the basis on which to make decisions about services, treatment, or care of individuals (Finkelhor, 2018).

An extensive analysis of the relationships between ACEs and internalising and externalising problems was undertaken by Bevilacqua et al. (2021). They studied 8823 members of a UK cohort and measured ACEs before the age of 3 years and behaviour up to the age of 14 years. To address the above concerns over the use of aggregated ACE scores, they analysed the ACE–behaviour relationship in three distinct ways. The first was based on individual ACEs, the second used an ACE summation score, and the third was based on identifying clusters of ACEs using latent class analysis (see Sect. 2.5). They found that the association between ACEs and child behaviour was apparent from age 3 years onwards. The ACE scores showed a dose–response relationship with internalising, externalising, and prosocial behaviour. The individual ACEs associated with internalising problems were parental discord and parental depression. For externalising behaviour, physical punishment and harsh parenting were the ACEs most strongly related. The application of latent class clustering failed to identify interpretable clusters. These results suggest that it is valuable to examine both individual ACEs and the summed ACE score in predicting the development of later psychopathology.

By contrast a study of 8572 children from the ALSPAC study did find ACE clusters using latent class analysis (Lacey et al., 2022). These clusters were "low ACEs" (comprising 55% of children), "parental separation and mother's mental health problems" (18%), "parental mental health problems, convictions, and separation" (15%), "abuse and mental health problems" (6%), and "poly adversity" (6%). The poly adversity cluster had experienced parental separation, interparental violence, physical and emotional abuse, parental mental health problems, and parental alcohol problems. Cluster membership was strongly related to poverty. For example the odds ratio for being in the poly adversity cluster was OR = 9.15 ($CI_{.95}$ 5.77 to 14.51) compared to the low ACE cluster when the child had experienced poverty.

It is not clear why, using the same data set, Lacey et al. (2022) could identify ACE clusters using LCA and Bevilacqua et al. (2021) could not. Lacey et al. (2022) do not present findings on the relationship between cluster membership and psychopathy that could complement the results from Bevilacqua et al. (2021). However a study of a large sample of Danish children ($N = 2198$) at risk of abuse also examined clusters of ACEs identified by LCA (Haahr-Pedersen et al., 2021). They found different latent classes for males and females. The classes based on ACEs differed internalising and externalising scores but the effect sizes were very small.

Social Deprivation Adversity and social deprivation have been shown to be associated with psychopathology in children and adolescents (McLaughlin et al., 2012). The factors that might lead to this link have been shown to include, for example, poor language development (e.g. Miller et al., 2021). What is less clear is just what features of early adverse experiences might be instigating this vulnerability. Phillips et al. (2023) investigated whether the unpredictability of early-life experiences or the deprivation of positive experiences might play a role. Unpredictability was measured as the frequency of changes in caregivers' romantic partners, residential changes, and caregiver job losses. Deprivation was assessed using the following subscales of the Early Childhood Home Observation for the Measurement of the Environment (Bradley et al., 2001): learning materials, language stimulation, physical environment, parental responsivity, and academic stimulation. Phillips et al. (2023) tested whether the influence of these early experiences on later psychopathology might be mediated via effects on executive function during the preschool period. They measured executive function (they used the term "executive control") using a battery developed by James et al. (2016). They found that deprivation, not unpredictability, uniquely predicts p-factor scores in later adolescence. In this study the effects of deprivation were carried by impaired executive function which was discernible during the preschool years.

The association of psychopathology with poverty and other indicators of socio-economic status in the United States was examined by Peverill et al. (2021). They undertook a meta-analysis based on a pooled sample of 26,715 participants aged 3–19 years. Small-to-moderate associations with child psychopathology were found for low family income (SMD = 0.19), low parental education (SMD = 0.25), poverty status (SMD = 0.25), and receipt of public assistance (SMD = 0.32). When examined separately the association with socio-economic status was slightly larger for externalising (SMD = 0.28) than for internalising (SMD = 0.22). The study could not identify the mechanisms that underlie this association. They suggest that these might include lack of access to resources that support cognitive, social, emotional, and physical development; greater exposure to trauma and violence; cumulative exposure to stressors; and differences in family processes and functioning.

The specific effect of exposure to community violence was examined by Fowler et al. (2009). Community violence ranged from the less severe but pervasive forms of violence on the streets, such as drug deals or robberies, which are common in urban areas, to the most extreme forms of neighbourhood violence, including witnessing stabbings and shootings or being the victim of such acts. The effect size for internalising was SMD = 0.54 ($CI_{.95}$ 0.44 to 0.47) and for externalising SMD = 0.63 ($CI_{.95}$ 0.61 to 0.65). The relationship with externalising was greater for adolescents than for children, and the reverse was the case for internalising.

Bullying There is evidence that victims of bullying are likely to show signs of internalising such as depression, loneliness, generalised and social anxiety, and low global and social self-worth. Hawker and Boulton (2000) conducted a meta-analysis on the effects of peer victimisation on adjustment. The effect sizes ranged from $r = 0.45$ for depression (SMD = 1.0) to $r = 0.25$ (SMD = 0.52) for anxiety measures. These effect sizes were somewhat inflated by shared method variance as the child reports on their own experience of being bullied and on their own behaviour. For studies that avoided the problem of shared method variance the effect sizes were lower but were statistically significant ($p < 0.001$); $r = 0.29$ (SMD = 0.60) for depression and $r = 0.19$ (SMD = 0.39) for anxiety.

The Hawker and Boulton (2000) meta-analysis was based on cross-sectional studies. A subsequent meta-analysis by Reijntjes et al. (2010) was restricted to longitudinal studies. They found that internalising problems function as both antecedents and consequences of peer victimisation. Peer victimisation predicts an increase in internalising problems $r = 0.18$ ($CI_{.95}$ 0.12 to 0.24), and internalising problems were found to predict an increase in peer victimisation $r = 0.08$ ($CI_{.95}$ 0.01 to 0.16). They conclude that these reciprocal influences suggest a vicious cycle that contributes to the high stability of peer victimisation. This suggestion is supported by the results of a longitudinal twin study which also demonstrated the role of social isolation as an intermediary between the experience of peer victimisation and subsequent internalising (Morneau-Vaillancourt et al., 2023).

Singham et al. (2017) used a population-based cohort study using a twin-difference design with a large sample of 11,108 twins to estimate the size of the impact of bullying on internalising. The twin-difference design method aims to control for environmental and genetic sources of confounding by comparing the outcome in twin pairs where one twin is exposed to a risk factor (in this case bullying) and the other is not. The twin pairs were studied between the ages of 11 and 16 years. They found evidence that childhood exposure to bullying directly contributes to a number of internalising problems, including anxiety, depression, paranoid thoughts, and cognitive disorganisation. However this direct influence was reduced after 5 years. The authors suggest that

> in addition to primary prevention aiming to stop childhood exposure to bullying, secondary preventive interventions should support resilience processes and address prior vulnerabilities in children exposed to bullying. (Singham et al., 2017, p. 1113)

The effectiveness of school-based anti-bullying interventions to reduce internalising symptoms is only modest. Guzman-Holst et al. (2022) undertook a meta-analysis of 22 studies examining this question. They found a very small effect size of SMD = 0.06 ($CI_{.95}$ 0.03 to 0.10) of anti-bullying interventions on reducing internalising symptoms.

Language Development There is well-replicated evidence that early developmental features of language development are related to behaviour problems in children. Delayed language development was one of the strongest risk factors in an epidemiological study of behaviour problems in 3-year-old children (Stevenson et al., 1985). It may be that child language development is critical for helping children to learn and modulate their own emotions and behaviours, as well as recognise and interpret the emotional displays of and internal states of mind of others (Salmon et al., 2016).

Three meta-analyses have been reported on the issue of the relationship between atypical language development and behaviour problems in young children. Hentges et al. (2021) undertook a meta-analysis of the association between language skills and internalising and externalising in 139 samples of children. These associations were either measured contemporaneously or with the language skills measured at an earlier age than behaviour. Despite this requirement, the data were essentially correlational and the direction of effects could not be determined. The effect sizes for the relationship between language ability and behaviour were similar for internalising SMD = 0.23 ($CI_{.95}$ 0.19 to 0.28) and externalising SMD = 0.22 ($CI_{.95}$ 0.18 to 0.20). There was a greater effect size for boys than girls for externalising. Similar results were reported in a meta-analysis of 51 studies on children with language and learning disorders (Donolato et al., 2022) but with slightly larger effect sizes for externalising SMD = 0.42 ($CI_{.95}$ 0.34 to 0.49) than internalising SMD = 0.36 ($CI_{.95}$ 0.29 to 0.43) problems. A similar pattern was reported in a meta-analysis by Yew and O'Kearney (2013). Using a categorical outcome measure of behaviour they found in 19 longitudinal studies that children with specific language impairment were more likely than TD children to show clinical levels of emotional problems risk ratio, RR = 1.84 ($CI_{.95}$ 1.04 to 3.25), and behaviour problems, RR = 2.26 ($CI_{.95}$ 1.6 to 3.08).

A detailed examination of the nature of these relationships between degrees of language impairment and behaviour was produced by Goh, Griffiths, Norbury, and the SCALES Team (2021). They found that both emotional and conduct problems were more common in children with language disorder even when the effects of non-verbal ability and social disadvantage were controlled. These associations were particularly marked for those with the most severe language deficit.

Prenatal and Perinatal Risks Premature birth is a factor that has a wide range of impacts on children's development including behaviour. A meta-analysis based on 1556 children born prematurely and 1720 children born at term was undertaken by Bhutta et al. (2002). Prematurity was defined at birth before 37 weeks' gestation. They found that there was an 11-point difference in IQ ($CI_{.95}$ 9.2 to 12.5), with the preterm children having lower IQs and that IQ was correlated with gestational age within the preterm group. Both internalising and externalising problems were more common in preterm children, and a diagnosis of ADHD was more likely in preterm children with a relative risk of 2.63 ($CI_{.95}$ 1.85 to 3.78).

A systematic review and meta-analysis have suggested that a range of prenatal, perinatal, and postnatal exposures are significantly associated with depression in children (Su et al., 2021). Those factors presenting significant risks were low birth weight, premature birth, small gestational age, maternal education, socio-economic status, having younger parents (<20 years), having older parents (≥35 years), maternal smoking, paternal smoking, maternal stress, maternal anxiety, and prenatal depression. These effects were modest with odds ratios under 1.5 and were based on observational studies that could not control for possible confounds. For example, it is likely that the effect of prenatal depression is in part due to genetic factors influencing both depression in mothers and children.

There is evidence that stresses experienced prenatally by the mother may be related to later internalising problems in children. Nomura et al. (2023) studied the impact on children's behaviour of their mothers having been exposed to a hurricane (Superstorm Sandy) during pregnancy. Those exposed to the stress of the experience of this storm in utero had a substantially elevated risk of depressive, anxiety, and ADHD disorders compared to those not exposed. The elevated risk remained after controlling for concurrent family stress, and demographic and psychosocial confounders, such as maternal age, race, SES, maternal substance use, and normative prenatal stress. Doubts have been expressed over the magnitude of the elevated risks reported by Nomura et al. (2023) because the small sample size may have inflated the estimates (Gilman et al., 2023). Despite this uncertainty Gilman et al. (2023) accept that maternal stress during pregnancy has been shown to be harmful in this study.

Digital Technologies and Social Media Use There are concerns that the use of digital technologies and social media may have adverse influences on the mental health of children and adolescents. Eirich et al. (2022) undertook a meta-analysis of studies on screen time and internalising and externalising behaviour in children under the age of 12 years. They identified 87 eligible studies. In both cases there were only modest correlations between screen time and behaviour – $r = 0.11$ ($CI_{.95}$ 0.10 to 0.12) (externalising) and $r = 0.07$ ($CI_{.95}$ 0.05 to 0.08) (internalising).

An analysis of three data sets, one from the United Kingdom and two from the United States, with a combined $n = 430{,}561$ found that the relationship between use of digital technology and mental health was slight; marginally greater for conduct problems than for emotional problems and depression (Vuorre et al., 2021). This study also showed that over time the small negative association between digital technology use and mental health was not getting stronger. Similar marginal results emerged from a study of time spent on videogame playing and well-being (Vuorre et al., 2022). The evidence base is too weak to permit any conclusions to be drawn about the causal relationships between digital technology use and adolescent mental health. The causal relationship could go in either direction or may indeed be bidirectional.

Using a more general measure of life satisfaction, Orben et al. (2022) applied longitudinal analyses of the relationship between social media use and well-being in a sample of 17,409 adolescents. They found evidence that indicated a direction of effect whereby social media use led to lower life satisfaction ratings but not the reverse. They report that over the period of 10–21 years there are particular ages when this effect was most marked. For females this was at 11–13 and 19 years of age and for males at 14–15 and 19 years of age.

The complexity of this relationship was demonstrated in a longitudinal study of 10,172 Irish children between the ages of 3 and 9 (Neville et al., 2021). At each age caregivers reported the time (hours/day) children spent watching television and using electronic devices and completed the SDQ. The design of the study allowed an analysis using a random intercepts cross-lagged panel model (RI-CLPM) (see Sect. 4.3) which can identify influences on within-child changes over time. The presence of internalising and of externalising problems at age 3 was associated with an increase in screen time at age 5 years. Higher levels of screen time at 3 and 5 years were directionally associated with increased internalising at ages 5 and 7 but not with an increase in externalising. This directional association was reversed between screen time at 7 years and internalising at 9 years, that is, more initial screen time was associated with a later decrease in internalising. These age-related variations in the relationship between screen time and internalising and externalising suggest a possible causal relationship but one that runs in both directions.

A subsequent study of screen time and behaviour and developmental problems in 101,350 children aged between 0 and 17 years living in the United States found an association between screen time and externalising problems especially in boys and preschool children (Qu et al., 2023). The study did not measure internalising and was cross-sectional in design. This means that it cannot attempt to replicate the causal relationships suggested by the Neville et al. (2021) study. The increasing concern over the possible impact of screen time on children's development makes it important that attempts are made to replicate these findings from Neville et al. (2021).

Other Risk Factors There is evidence that depression in children is associated with sleep disturbance (Gregory et al., 2009). This longitudinal study of twins at ages 8 and 10 years showed that sleep at 8 years was directionally associated with depression at 10 years $\beta = 0.10$ ($CI_{.95}$ 0.01 to 0.18) but the effects of early depression on later sleep were not significant $\beta = 0.03$ ($CI_{.95}$ −0.03 to 0.10). This suggests that sleep problems in children may be a risk factor for the development of depression. To test this it is necessary to avoid item overlap between measures of sleep disturbance and depression. In the Gregory et al. (2009) study this was achieved by removing two sleep-related items from the measure of depression – the Child Depression Inventory (Kovacs, 1985).

A systematic review and meta-analysis of 22 studies on the association between sleep and depression was produced by Marino et al. (2021). She concluded that there is a small but statistically significant effect, suggesting an association between sleep disruption and depressive symptoms in children and adolescents and that sleep disruption may be a potentially modifiable risk factor for depression. This conclusion was reinforced by a cross-lagged analysis of sleep and depression in a general population sample of 2802 children and adolescent studied longitudinally between the ages of 5 and 17 years (Marino et al., 2022). The results suggest that disturbed sleep is related to the consolidation of depressive symptoms by age 12 years. This putative role of sleep influencing the development of depressive symptoms led to the recommendation that intervention for sleep problems should be targeted in middle childhood to help prevent depression in adolescence.

Anxiety sensitivity is a trait that is predictive of both anxiety and depression (Muris et al., 2001). It has been distinguished from anxiety per se as follows:

> A distinction is proposed between anxiety (frequency of symptom occurrence) and anxiety sensitivity (beliefs that anxiety experiences have negative implications). (Reiss et al., 1986, p. 1)

Anxiety sensitivity has been found to be relatively stable in twins during the adolescent years with correlation between yearly measures between $r = 0.39$ ($CI_{.95}$ 0.33 to 0.42) and $r = 0.48$ ($CI_{.95}$ 0.44 to 0.52) (Zavos et al., 2012). This continuity results from both stable genetic and non-shared environmental influences.

Features that may create a greater vulnerability to anxiety and depression are biases in attention, threat–safety cue discrimination, and memory. However the extent to which these biases act as proximal mechanisms that mediate other distal risk factors is uncertain (Lau & Waters, 2017). A detailed examination of this issue was undertaken by Booth et al. (2022) in a longitudinal study of 504 adolescents.

They defined resilience (the opposite of vulnerability) as the adolescent showing fewer internalising symptoms than would be predicted from the number of negative life events experienced. They found that memory bias, interpretation bias, worry, rumination, and self-esteem were all related to resilience. Of these memory bias was particularly strongly related to resilience at subsequent time points.

7.5 Genetics and Internalising Problems

Association Between Parent and Child Mental Health There is clear evidence that severe mental disorders, that is, schizophrenia, bipolar disorders, and major depressive disorders, in parents are associated with psychopathology in children (Thorup et al., 2018). Children in such families were 2–4 times more likely to have mental disorder than other children. This familial transmission seems to be general rather than symptom specific. This result is consistent with the p-factor model where a generic genetic risk for psychopathology is transmitted within families. Increased cross-generational risk is also seen with less severe parental mental health problems. For example, higher levels of maternal shyness during the preschool period contribute to increased social wariness in childhood and subsequently to greater social anxiety in mid-adolescence (Zeytinoglu et al., 2022).

The relationship between parent mental health and internalising and externalising problems in children was examined in a meta-analysis of studies on the mental health of mothers (more than 90 studies) and fathers (more than 56 studies) and their children's behaviour (Connell & Goodman, 2002). There were significant associations for both parents for both types of problem. However the size of the association was small. For internalising the effect sizes were $r = 0.18$ (mothers) and $r = 0.14$ (fathers) and for externalising $r = 0.17$ and $r = 0.16$, respectively.

Goodman et al. (2011) reviewed 193 studies on the relationship between maternal depression and child psychopathology. They found slightly greater effect sizes both for internalising ($r = 0.23$, SMD = 0.50) and externalising ($r = 0.21$, SMD = 0.42) than for the broader measure of mental health used by Connell and Goodman (2002). The effect sizes for internalising were significantly higher for girls but there was no difference between the sexes for externalising. The effect size for the relationship with maternal depression was greater for younger children for all child measures.

Lawrence et al. (2019) showed that parent anxiety disorders pose specific risks of anxiety disorders to offspring. In a meta-analysis of 25 studies they found that where parents had an anxiety disorder, their children were significantly more likely to have anxiety RR = 1.76 ($CI_{.95}$ 1.58 to 1.96) and depressive disorders RR = 1.31 (CI_{95} 1.13 to 1.52) than offspring of parents without anxiety disorders. The family design of the studies in this meta-analysis could not differentiate between environmental and genetic factors contributing to these parent–child associations.

The relationship between parental mental health and child behaviours identified in the above meta-analyses could arise either via a social mechanism resulting from exposure of the child to parental mental health problems or via a genetic mechanism. To disentangle which of these might be operating requires the use of genetically informative research designs.

Adoption Studies Using data from the Colorado adoption project, Daniels and Plomin (1985) showed that from an early age, 24 months, adopted children's shyness was related to their biological mothers' shyness and low sociability; this suggests a genetic influence. Also the adopted way child's shyness was related to the adoptive mothers' low sociability: this suggests an additional environmental effect.

A study on a number of different types of adoptive families allowed Kendler et al. (2018) to estimate the relative role of genetics and rearing experiences within the family in the transmission of major depression. They found that both forms of cross-generational transmission act additively on the risk for major depression in the offspring.

Ahmadzadeh et al. (2019) examined within-family processes by using data from an adoptive parent/adopted child study where there is no genetic-mediated association between parent and child. They found that prospectively between the ages of 6 and 8 years that child anxiety predicted maternal anxiety but not the other way round. In addition they found an association between paternal anxiety and later child anxiety. These results suggest environmentally mediated associations between parent and child anxiety symptoms and support models emphasising the impact of the child on caregivers.

Twin Studies on Internalising Problems in General There is some variation in the findings of genetic and environmental influences on internalising problems in preschool children. Examining a range of internalising problems Eley et al. (2003) found moderate genetic influences in a study of 4564 four-year-old twin pair-olds. The proportion of the variance explained by genetic and environmental factors was as follows: general distress (worries, unhappy, somatic complaints, and cries easily), genetic (h^2) = 0.43, shared environment (c^2) 0.14, non-shared environment (e^2) = 0.43; separation anxiety $h^2 = 0.39$, $c^2 = 0.36$, $e^2 = 0.25$; and fears $h^2 = 0.44$, $c^2 = 0.18$, $e^2 = 0.37$. Schmitz et al. (1995) conducted a study on two samples of twins aged 3 and 8 years, and their findings suggest that genetic factors may become more important with age. At 3 years of age internalising problems were influenced by the following components: $h^2 = 0.17$, $c^2 = 0.45$, $e^2 = 0.38$, and at 8 years $h^2 = 0.37$, $c^2 = 0.26$, $e^2 = 0.37$. By contrast van den Oord et al. (1996) found a larger heritability in a twin study of 3-year-olds with estimates of $h^2 = 0.77$, $c^2 = 0.00$, and $e^2 = 0.23$ for internalising. It is not clear why the effects of genes should be so much larger in these Dutch twins. However using the combination of observational and parent report measures of behavioural inhibition and shyness, Smith et al. (2012) found that up to age 3 years substantial estimates of heritability were obtained for a latent variable underlying these combined measures (h^2 range from 0.53 to 0.91, c^2 from 0.00 to 0.37, and e^2 from 0.02 to 0.19).

Longitudinal studies on twins have shown how the genetics of internalising disorders changes with age (Lubke et al., 2016). The symptoms of anxiety and depression show marked fluctuations over time. By studying repeated measures of these symptoms between the ages of 7 and 18 years in a large sample of twins, Lubke et al. (2016) were able to analyse the role of genetic and environmental factors on these overtime changes. They found that the fluctuations in symptom severity were largely idiosyncratic and were not explained by these factors. However the average of the measures was highly heritable (h^2 = 0.60 to 0.84). The authors suggest that quantitative genetics and GWAS of anxiety and depression should adopt the average scores in the changing overtime patterns of symptomatology these problems show. This suggestion was supported by the results of Cheesman et al. (2018). They found that single-nucleotide polymorphism heritabilities (h^2_{SNP}) were low for emotional problems (5%) but can be increased to 14% by examining stable emotional problems in children from 7 to 16 years of age. Twin heritability also increased from 45% on average for individual measures to 76% by focusing on stable trait variance.

A quantitative genetic analysis of data on depression and anxiety from a sample of 2619 twins studied prospectively from mid-adolescence to young adulthood was conducted by Waszczuk et al. (2016). They found evidence that stable and later emerging genes contribute to the comorbidity between depression and anxiety across adolescence and young adulthood. Environmental influences are largely limited to specific time periods and produce changes in symptoms from adolescence into adulthood. These results were supported by a finding based on PRS data from the ALSPAC study (Kwong et al., 2021). They tested genetic effects on depression, anxiety, and neuroticism in adolescence and into young adulthood. They found evidence that genetic factors had a marked effect on the occurrence and maintenance of depression in adolescence.

Twin Studies on Anxiety The complexity of the transmission of anxiety in families was shown by Eley et al. (2015). By studying the children of MZ and DZ twins sets of correlations can be obtained that allow estimates to be derived which can, for example, provide indicators of environmental transmission that is not confounded by genetic factors. This Children of Twins study (CoT; see Sect. 3.1) produced a result that suggested that transmission of anxiety within families was independent of genetic influences. This is unexpected given the previously demonstrated heritability of anxiety in children (Lau et al., 2006; Waszczuk et al., 2014) and adults (Kendler et al., 1986). Three explanations for this seeming disparity were put forward by Eley et al. (2015). The first is that different genes influence adult and adolescent anxiety. The second is that the heritability estimate for anxiety phenotypes obtained from child/adolescent twin studies includes interactions between genetic factors and the shared environment. Third, it is possible that measurement error reduced the association between the generations. They suggest that the third explanation is unlikely given that at least adequate reliability of the measures is used. They considered both age-related changes in genetic influence and gene–environment interactions as the most plausible reasons for this unexpected finding.

Twin Studies on Depression There is well-established evidence that genetics makes a substantial contribution to the risk of major depression (Kendall et al., 2021). Both environmental and genetic factors have been found to be involved in the transmission of mental health problems in families with a depressed parent. Using a CoT design, Silberg et al. (2010) also showed that parental depression could be transmitted to the child via direct environmental exposure. In addition conduct problems in the children in these families were linked by both genetic and environmental risks to depression in the parents. These results suggest that conduct problem may be an early indicator of a risk for depression in adulthood for children with a depressed parent.

Twin Studies on Fears Genetic differences and environmental risk factors have been shown to contribute to individual differences in common fears in children and adolescence. Twin studies on self-reports from adolescents (Kendler et al., 2008) and parent reports (Stevenson et al., 1992) have shown a complex pattern of changes in heritability both between specific types of fears and with age. It has been suggested that the structure of influences on fears and anxiety in children is less clearly differentiated than that found in adults (Sawyers et al., 2019). A twin study in early adulthood, using an experimental technique of fear conditioning, showed that genetics has pervasive effects on individual differences in multiple aspects of fears (Purves et al., 2023). There are significant genetic influences on fear acquisition and the consolation and extinction of fear. These findings may have implications for understanding the variation in the response to treatments for anxiety such as exposure-based cognitive behaviour therapy.

Molecular Genetic Studies Initial studies suggested that h^2_{SNP} was extremely low, if not non-existent, for behaviour problems in children (Trzaskowski et al., 2013). Pappa et al. (2015) also found a low h^2_{SNP} for internalising and externalising scores on the CBCL.

Subsequently, Jami et al. (2022) have produced a meta-analysis of GWAS data on internalising from 22 cohorts comprising 64,561 children aged between 3 and 18 years. They found an overall very modest h^2_{SNP} of 0.02 and no specific locus was significantly associated with internalising. A striking feature of the results was the high genetic correlation with other childhood disorders, such as ADHD and ASD, and with adult disorders, such as anxiety and depression. These high genetic correlations may explain the stability of internalising symptoms over time and the high level of comorbidity with other problems in childhood. Molecular genetic studies of internalising problems in preschool children have suggested that they are influenced by polymorphisms in many genes. Each of these genes has a very minor effect, but many of these polymorphisms are the same as those that influence disorders in childhood and adulthood (Benke et al., 2014).

The genetics of nurture approach of Kong et al. (2018) (see Sect. 3.2) was applied to the transmission of anxiety and depression in families to 8-year-old children (Cheesman et al., 2020). This was based on genotyping 11,598 parent–offspring trios. They found that depressive symptoms were influenced by both genetic nurture and direct genetic effects. They found that direct genetic effects accounted for 19% of the variance in child depression scores and 5% of the variance in anxiety. The effects of genetic nurture were 14% for depression and 0 for anxiety. The genetic nurture effect was partially mediated via an observed measure of maternal anxiety and depression, which explained 64% of the original genetic nurture effect.

7.6 Interventions for Internalising Problems

Cognitive Behaviour Therapy (CBT) The treatment of internalising problems with cognitive behaviour therapy has been supported in efficacy studies, that is, randomised controlled trials (RCTs) where treatment is delivered in specialist research setting. A systematic review and meta-analysis by James et al. (2015) found that the odds ratio of remission from anxiety in response to CBT compared to that for waiting list controls was OR = 7.85 ($CI_{.95}$ 5.31 to 11.60) (this converts to SMD = 0.48). They concluded that CBT is an effective treatment for childhood and adolescent anxiety disorders but it may not be more helpful than other active therapies such as self-help books. Oud et al. (2019) reached similar conclusions for depression. They found that CBT reduced depressive symptoms immediately after the end of treatment (SMD = −0.41) and at follow-up (17–39 weeks; SMD = −0.20). There is some limited evidence that CBT can be an effective treatment for anxiety and post-traumatic stress disorder in children who have experienced sexual abuse (Macdonald et al., 2012).

Wergeland et al. (2021) undertook a meta-analysis of CBT treatment in routine clinical care (effectiveness studies) as well as efficacy studies. When the studies were limited to RCTs the effect size at post-treatment for effectiveness studies, SMD = 1.36 ($CI_{.95}$ 1.17 to 1.55), was similar to that for efficacy studies, SMD = 1.55 ($CI_{.95}$ 1.41 to 1.68). Parallel findings were found for the outcomes measured at follow-up. In a meta-analysis of 87 studies concerning the efficacy of CBT for anxiety in children and adolescents, James et al. (2020) suggested that the quality of evidence was "moderate" or "low". They concluded that CBT is more effective than a waiting list or no treatment in reducing anxiety in children and young people. However there was no clear evidence that CBT is more effective than other treatments including treatment as usual.

This raises the question of how well anxiety and depression in children and adolescents respond to the routine treatment provided by clinical services. This question was addressed in a meta-analysis of 38 publications of treatment as usual by Bear et al. (2020). They found that the improvement from baseline to an average of 13 weeks later was SMD = −0.73 ($CI_{.95}$ −0.88 to −0.59) and to 26 weeks later SMD = −0.87 ($CI_{.95}$ −1.01 to −0.74). The design of these studies was such that these improvements could not be differentiated from spontaneous changes in depression which have been shown to be pervasive in childhood and adolescence (Kovacs et al., 2016).

These improvements in internalising problems under treatment are not uniform. In a systematic review of CBT treatments for anxiety in adults, Loerinc et al. (2015) concluded that although significant gains are made under treatment, approximately 50% of the participants do not respond positively. Given the major role of genetics in influencing anxiety, attention has turned to whether genetic factors are influencing the response to treatment. This includes studies on both drug treatments (Ask et al., 2021) and psychological therapies (Lester & Eley, 2013). However to date there has been little success in identifying genetic effects on the response to psychological therapies using molecular genetics estimates of h^2_{SNP} and PRS (Coleman et al., 2016; Rayner et al., 2019).

Psychological Treatments Weisz et al. (2017) undertook a major meta-analysis of RCTs of psychological treatments synthesising 50 years of findings from 447 studies on 30,431 participants aged between 4 and 18 years. The treatments evaluated were placed into four groups: (a) youth-focused behavioural interventions including CBT, modelling, psychoeducation, operant or respondent conditioning, social skills training, biofeedback, and behavioural activation; (b) youth-focused non-behavioural interventions, including client-centred, psychodynamic, and gestalt therapies; (c) caregiver and family-focused behavioural treatment, including behavioural parent training, behavioural parent–youth/family interventions, such as functional family therapy; and (d) caregiver and family-focused non-behavioural treatment, including non-behavioural parent, parent–youth, or family interventions, such as attachment-based family therapy and multisystem treatments.

For all studies pooled together immediate post-treatment effect size was SMD = 0.46 ($CI_{.95}$ 0.41 to 0.51). At a follow-up an average of 44 weeks after treatment ended found an SMD = 0.36 ($CI_{.95}$ 0.27 to 0.44). There were significant differences between the effect sizes for different conditions. The post-treatment and follow-up results were respectively for ADHD SMD = 0.34 ($CI_{.95}$ 0.23 to 0.45) and SMD = 0.22 ($CI_{.95}$ 0.04 to 0.40); for conduct disorder SMD = 0.46 ($CI_{.95}$ 0.38 to 0.54) and SMD = 0.44 ($CI_{.95}$ 0.29 to 0.58); for anxiety SMD = 0.61 ($CI_{.95}$ 0.53 to 0.70) and SMD = 0.55 ($CI_{.95}$ 0.38 to 0.72); and for depression SMD = 0.29 ($CI_{.95}$ 0.14 to 0.43) and SMD = 0.22 ($CI_{.95}$ 0.04 to 0.40). By way of putting these results into context they calculate that an SMD of 0.46 indicated that

> the probability that a randomly selected youth in the treatment condition would be better off after treatment than a randomly selected youth in the control condition was 63% – only moderately better than chance at 50%. This suggests that, although youth therapies have produced beneficial effects over the years, there is much room for improvement. (Weisz et al., 2017, p. 96)

An intriguing question addressed by Weisz et al. (2019) is whether treatment effectiveness is changing over time. They used a database of 453 RCTs of treatments for anxiety, depression, ADHD, and conduct problems for participants aged 4–18 years and published between 1960 and 2017. They found that the mean effect size increased non-significantly for anxiety, decreased non-significantly for ADHD, and decreased significantly for depression and conduct problems. By itself this analysis could not determine what might have produced the decline in the effectiveness of treatments for depression and conduct problems. They suggest that some radical changes may be needed in the design of treatment, particularly to become more relevant to contemporary youth. To this end "skeuomorph-free ideas" are needed for interventions; this (to me unfamiliar!) term refers to forms of treatment that do not nostalgically reflect former approaches and that are truly innovative.

It has become recognised that children as young as 3 years can show depression in a form equivalent to that found in older children (Whalen et al., 2017). The outcome of depression in this preschool age group is an increased risk of depression in adolescence (Whalen et al., 2016). The approaches to the treatment of early childhood depression have been little studied. Luby et al. (2018) undertook an RCT of parent–child psychotherapy for depression in children aged 3–7 years. It was found that the early identification and intervention were effective with effect sizes of SMD >1.0 on depression measures.

A review of group-based parent training programmes for young children with emotional (internalising) or behaviour problems (externalising) was undertaken by Barlow et al. (2016). They identified 24 clinical trials, of which 22 were RCTs. There was a significantly greater improvement post-intervention in the treatment group compared to controls, SMD = −0.81 ($CI_{.95}$ −1.37 to 0.25). Although the quality of the evidence was graded as low, Barlow et al. (2016) concluded that there was tentative evidence that the use of group-based parenting programmes can improve the overall emotional and behavioural adjustment of young children in the short term.

Ng et al. (2020) conducted a systematic review of studies on mediators of treatment effectiveness for evidence-based psychotherapies for depression in young people. They suggest that there were wasted opportunities to test for mediators. Although significant mediators were identified, findings "are sparse, conflicting, and clouded by methodological issues". They suggest that studying mediators might provide insights into how to improve treatment, and the examination of moderated mediators would perhaps identify who might benefit most from interventions.

Given the increasing prevalence of mental health problems in children and adolescents (Collishaw, 2015; Ford, 2020) and the present unmet needs (Patel et al., 2018) there is an onus to produce interventions that are both effective and economic. The situation identified by Patel et al. in 2018, that on a global scale "access to mental health services remains very poor and fragmented for most people in the world", has been exacerbated by the impact of COVID-19 on the mental health of children and adolescents (Pierce et al., 2020; Zhang-James et al., 2023).

One approach to affordability is to make treatments less expensive in terms of professional time and brief therapies can provide such economies. Weersing et al. (2017) developed a brief behaviour therapy (BBT) programme consisted of 8–12 weekly 45-minute sessions delivered in paediatric clinics by master's-level therapists. The participants were children and adolescents aged 8–16 years with anxiety and/or depression diagnoses. Families were randomised either BBT or to a form of treatment as usual which consisted of personalised referrals to mental health care and telephone calls to support access to care. At the end of treatment there were significant gains compared to the control group with an SMD = 0.58 ($CI_{.95}$ 0.26 to 0.90). The effects remained significant at follow-up 32 weeks later (Brent et al., 2020). An important aim of BBT is to counter a tendency for avoidance of threatening situations which is seen as maladaptive, for those with anxiety and depression. Baca et al. (2023) examined whether changing behavioural avoidance might mediate the impact of BBT. They found that this was the case for anxiety but not for depression. The BBT treatment programme was subjected to a health economic analysis by Lynch et al. (2021). The total cost of BBT was less than treatment as usual, and the greater gains in well-being under BTT indicated that it was a cost-effective approach to service provision.

Prevention A distinction has been made between different types of preventive intervention, which are interventions occurring before the onset of a disorder (Munoz et al., 1996). These types are *universal* (targeted at the population as a whole), *selective* (targeted at those who on the basis of biological or social factors are at a higher-than-average risk of a disorder), and *indicated* prevention (targeted at those who are showing detectable signs of the onset of disorder that fall short of a diagnosis). These types of preventive intervention are distinct from treatment interventions which are directed at those meeting the diagnostic criteria for a disorder.

A prerequisite for selective prevention is the availability of tools that can identify children and adolescents at risk of developing depression. There is evidence that progress is being made to put such measures in place for children without current or previous depression. Rocha et al. (2021) demonstrated that a predictive tool developed with Brazilian children can be successfully applied in other cultural contexts, namely New Zealand and the United Kingdom. However they conclude that additional refinements are needed to improve the predictive validity of the tool in other culture to address the heterogeneity between samples.

There have been a number of meta-analyses of studies on the prevention of depression in children and adolescents following the initial review produced by Horowitz and Garber (2006). A systematic review of these meta-analyses was produced by Bellón et al. (2015). They found that for studies aimed at preventing depression in children there was only evidence for modest short-term effects and that longer-term effectiveness was questionable. A meta-analysis of CBT-based approaches to the prevention of depression was produced by Hetrick et al. (2016). They found a small but statistically significant beneficial effect of CBT across 70 trials (SMD = −0.21 ($CI_{.95}$ −0.27 to −0.15)) in the short term, but this effect was attenuated after a 12-month or longer period. Similar conclusions about the short-term benefits of universal, selective, and indicated prevention interventions for internalising problems were reached by Stockings et al. (2016).

Studies of using school-based prevention programmes to reduce the risk of anxiety and depression were the subject of a systematic review and meta-analysis by Werner-Seidler et al. (2017). Based on the findings of 81 studies they found relatively small effect sizes for both depression, SMD = 0.23 ($CI_{.95}$ 0.19 to 0.28), and anxiety, SMD = 0.20 ($CI_{.95}$ 0.14 to 0.25). Targeted interventions were more effective than universal interventions for depression, but for anxiety these interventions were equally effective. A subsequent network meta-analysis suggested that there were overestimates of effect sizes in previous reviews (such as that by Werner-Seidler et al. (2017)) that arose from the conflation of heterogeneous control conditions (Caldwell et al., 2019). When this conflation was taken into account Caldwell et al. (2019) concluded that there is little evidence that educational setting-based interventions focused solely on the prevention of depression or anxiety are effective.

Pilling et al. (2020) conducted a meta-analysis of the long-term efficacy of psychosocial interventions of child and adolescent mental health for studies that provided medium-term outcomes at 12 months after intervention. The 138 trials identified included both selective and indicated interventions. The latter included studies of treatment. The effects identified at the end of intervention for all studies were SMD = 0.39 ($CI_{.95}$ 0.30 to 0.47). The effect size was only reduced slightly at 12-month follow-up, SMD = 0.31 ($CI_{.95}$ 0.25 to 0.37). At both ends of intervention and at 12-month follow-up the SMDs for selective interventions were lower than for the indicated interventions. A particular value of the findings presented in the Pilling et al. (2020) paper is that there was a large range of disorders analysed in parallel. In terms of improvement maintained to 12-month follow-up they found the following effect sizes: for anxiety SMD = 0.51 ($CI_{.95}$ 0.31 to 0.68), for depression SMD = 0.21 ($CI_{.95}$ 0.10 to 0.32), and for conduct disorder SMD = 0.23 ($CI_{.95}$ 0.14 to 0.33). However the results are not presented for indicated and selective interventions by type of disorder.

Drug Treatments There have been concerns that the use of antidepressants by children and adolescents led to an increased risk of suicidal thoughts or behaviours. A meta-analysis of studies on this question by Bridge et al. (2007) concluded that the increased risk was very small and the benefits of such treatment for children and adolescents with depression and anxiety far outweighed these risks. They also noted that in none of the 27 trials in their review were completed suicides reported. A more recent umbrella review of studies on this issue also failed to find an absolute contraindication for the use of antidepressants by young people (Dragioti et al., 2019).

The British Association of Psychopharmacology recommends that tricyclic antidepressants (TCAs) should not be given to children and adolescents. Rather for these age groups they say only selective serotonin reuptake inhibitors (SSRIs) should be used (Cleare et al., 2015). The safety and efficacy of SSRIs and serotonin-norepinephrine reuptake inhibitors (SNRIs) for the treatment of children and adolescents was the subject of a systematic review and meta-analysis by Locher et al. (2017). They identified 36 placebo-controlled trials which in aggregate showed a small benefit for SSRIs and SNRIs compared to placebo. The effects for children with anxiety disorders were greater than those for other internalising conditions.

It is suggested that SSRI combined with CBT is the most effective treatment for anxiety (Walkup et al., 2008). Locher et al. (2017) noted that the extent of adverse events whilst on the SSRI and SNRI treatments requires that careful monitoring of the benefits during these treatments be conducted for each individual. These conclusions were endorsed in a subsequent systematic review and meta-analysis by Stefánsdóttir et al. (2023). One reason for the relatively small effect sizes for antidepressants for children with depression may be these children's tendency to show a strong placebo response (Feeney et al., 2022).

Zhou et al. (2020) undertook a network meta-analysis of 71 trials of the treatment of acute depression in children and adolescents. They concluded that despite the scarcity of high-quality evidence, the SSRI fluoxetine (alone or in combination with CBT) seems to be the best choice for the acute treatment of moderate-to-severe depressive disorder in children and adolescents, SMD = −0.73 ($CI_{.95}$ −1.39 to −0.07). It is clear that antidepressant treatments are more effective in adults (Cipriani et al., 2018) than in children and adolescents (Cipriani et al., 2016). Indeed this latter network meta-analysis suggested that fluoxetine was the best, and only, drug treatment for depression in children and adolescents that could be recommended for routine clinical practice.

Doubt has been cast on the significance of low levels of serotonin as a cause of depression in a systematic umbrella review (Moncrieff et al., 2022). The evidence reviewed explicitly excluded studies on serotonin in depressed children. Nevertheless it seems likely that their conclusion that there was no support for the hypothesis that depression is caused by lowered serotonin activity or concentrations applies to children and adolescents too. The implications of this review for the use of SSRIs to treat depression are not clear. It should be noted that others have suggested that the evidence against the serotonin hypothesis is not as strong as claimed in this umbrella review (Jauhar et al., 2023; Kendrick & Collinson, 2022). As Moncrieff et al. (2022) point out, there are a number of explanations for the effects of antidepressants other than via an increase in serotonin level. These include an amplified placebo effect or through the restriction or blunting of emotions in general. As it currently stands it appears that fluoxetine is the drug of choice for the treatment of depression in children and adolescents, but its therapeutic mode of action is uncertain.

7.7 Final Thoughts on Internalising Problems

It has long been recognised that mental health problems represent a major source of burden for young people (Patel et al., 2007). Internalising problems, such as anxiety and depression, form a substantial proportion of these mental health problems. There is a huge gap between the mental healthcare needs of young people and the services currently available. Patel et al. (2007) emphasise the need for "affordable and feasible" interventions to be developed. They suggest that this might most helpfully be achieved by integrating a focus on mental health across services directed at families, schools, primary health settings, and those provided in specialist mental health care. This recommendation is reinforced by evidence that social support from a variety of sources, including families, teachers, and peers, can be beneficial in reducing depression symptoms (Rueger et al., 2016). This meta-analysis found an effect size of $r = 0.26$ (SMD = 0.56) between the support received and depression. This effect was similar for boys and girls and indicates that efforts to enhance social support for children and adolescents are likely to be an "affordable and feasible" approach to mitigating the risk of depression in young people.

There are concerns that recent threats arising from events such as global heating and the COVID-19 pandemic have exacerbated the mental health problems of young people. There are suggestions from a meta-analysis of studies that examined changes in mental health in general population cohorts followed from before the COVID-19 pandemic that during the pandemic there was a small increase in mental health symptoms soon after the outbreak (Robinson et al., 2022). There was subsequent decrease and symptoms returned to their pre-pandemic levels within a 6-month period. This pattern held for samples of adults and for children/adolescents. Newlove-Delgado et al. (2023) also reviewed studies on this topic. They were stringent in their appraisal of the evidence and concluded that only 4 out of 51 eligible studies were of high quality. They tentatively suggested that negative effects on mental health of young people had occurred and, though these effects were small and were not found in all studies, they should not be ignored. For children and adolescents these findings are not unexpected given the association between periods of social isolation and loneliness and an increased risk of depression, and possibly anxiety, at the time at which loneliness was experienced, and up to 9 years later (Loades et al., 2020).

A separate meta-analysis examined the effects of the pandemic specifically on symptoms of depression in children and adolescents (Ludwig-Walz et al., 2022). This found a significant increase in mean depression symptom score over the time of the pandemic of SMD = 0.21 ($CI_{.95}$ 0.12 to 0.30) in the better conducted studies with a "low-risk-of-bias". This increase was most marked when more stringent pandemic-related restrictions, such as school closures, had been imposed. These findings were replicated in a meta-analysis by Harrison et al. (2022). This identified a pandemic-related increase in both anxiety and depression in children and adolescents. They place particular emphasis on the role of schools to support children in these periods of crisis and consequently conclude that school closure should be considered only as a last resort. Similar conclusions were reached by Panchal et al. (2023), who undertook analyses to establish whether there were particular subgroups who were vulnerable to the adverse effects of the pandemic. In this meta-analysis children with special educational needs and prior mental health problems were identified as being most at risk.

These considerations suggest that the experience of internalising problems in the lives of young people is only going to become more common and makes more urgent the need for effective systems to support children and adolescents to mitigate the adverse effect on their quality of life.

This concern is powerfully expressed by Tamsin Ford as follows:

> If 'Children are the living messages we send to a time we will not see.' (John F. Kennedy, 35th President of the United States), then recent epidemiological studies suggest that we should be worried about what we are conveying. We should respond by working harder to effect change in policy, practice and research to promote mental health, prevent mental ill-health and to intervene effectively for those who have poor mental health or are vulnerable. Given the strong data on the impact of poor parental mental health on child development, we need to act quickly to support the current cohort of young people, who are battling higher rates of anxiety, depression and self-harm as they become parents, to minimise intergenerational transfer of their parents' difficulties (Patel et al., 2018). (Ford, 2020, p. 1276)

References

Achenbach, T. M. (1966). The classification of children's psychiatric symptoms: A factor-analytic study. *Psychological Monographs, 80*(7), 1–37. https://doi.org/10.1037/h0093906

Ahmadzadeh, Y. I., Eley, T. C., Leve, L. D., Shaw, D. S., Natsuaki, M. N., Reiss, D., et al. (2019). Anxiety in the family: A genetically informed analysis of transactional associations between mother, father and child anxiety symptoms. *Journal of Child Psychology and Psychiatry, 60*(12), 1269–1277. https://doi.org/10.1111/jcpp.13068

Ahmadzadeh, Y. I., Schoeler, T., Han, M., Pingault, J.-B., Creswell, C., & McAdams, T. A. (2021). Systematic review and meta-analysis of genetically informed research: Associations between parent anxiety and offspring internalizing problems. *Journal of the American Academy of Child and Adolescent Psychiatry, 60*(7), 823–840. https://doi.org/10.1016/j.jaac.2020.12.037

Ahmadzadeh, Y. I., Eley, T. C., Hannigan, L., Creswell, C., Lichtenstein, P., Spotts, E., et al. (2022). Parental criticism and adolescent internalising symptoms: Using a Children-of-Twins design with power calculations to account for genetic influence. *Journal of Child Psychology and Psychiatry, 63*(5), 599–607. https://doi.org/10.1111/jcpp.13498

Allmann, A. E. S., Klein, D. N., & Kopala-Sibley, D. C. (2022). Bidirectional and transactional relationships between parenting styles and child symptoms of ADHD, ODD, depression, and anxiety over 6 years. *Development and Psychopathology, 34*, 1400–1411. https://doi.org/10.1017/s0954579421000201

Anda, R. F., Felitti, V. J., Bremner, J. D., Walker, J. D., Whitfield, C., Perry, B. D., et al. (2006). The enduring effects of abuse and related adverse experiences in childhood – A convergence of evidence from neurobiology and epidemiology. *European Archives of Psychiatry and Clinical Neuroscience, 256*(3), 174–186. https://doi.org/10.1007/s00406-005-0624-4

Anda, R. F., Porter, L. E., & Brown, D. W. (2020). Inside the adverse childhood experience score: Strengths, limitations, and misapplications. *American Journal of Preventive Medicine, 59*(2), 293–295. https://doi.org/10.1016/j.amepre.2020.01.009

Ask, H., Cheesman, R., Jami, E. S., Levey, D. F., Purves, K. L., & Weber, H. (2021). Genetic contributions to anxiety disorders: Where we are and where we are heading. *Psychological Medicine, 51*(13), 2231–2246. https://doi.org/10.1017/s0033291720005486

Baca, S. A., Goger, P., Glaser, D., Rozenman, M., Gonzalez, A., Dickerson, J. F., et al. (2023). Reduction in avoidance mediates effects of brief behavioral therapy for pediatric anxiety and depression. *Behaviour Research and Therapy, 164*, 104290. https://doi.org/10.1016/j.brat.2023.104290

Barlow, J., Bergman, H., Kornør, H., Wei, Y., & Bennett, C. (2016). Group-based parent training programmes for improving emotional and behavioural adjustment in young children. *Cochrane Database of Systematic Reviews, 2016*(8), CD003680. https://doi.org/10.1002/14651858.CD003680.pub3

Bayer, J. K., Ukoumunne, O. C., Mathers, M., Wake, M., Abdi, N., & Hiscock, H. (2012). Development of children's internalising and externalising problems from infancy to five years of age. *Australian and New Zealand Journal of Psychiatry, 46*(7), 659–668. https://doi.org/10.1177/0004867412450076

Bear, H. A., Edbrooke-Childs, J., Norton, S., Krause, K. R., & Wolpert, M. (2020). Systematic review and meta-analysis: Outcomes of routine specialist mental health care for young people with depression and/or anxiety. *Journal of the American Academy of Child and Adolescent Psychiatry, 59*(7), 810–841. https://doi.org/10.1016/j.jaac.2019.12.002

Bellón, J. A., Moreno-Peral, P., Motrico, E., Rodriguez-Morejon, A., Fernandez, A., Serrano-Blanco, A., et al. (2015). Effectiveness of psychological and/or educational interventions to prevent the onset of episodes of depression: A systematic review of systematic reviews and meta-analyses. *Preventive Medicine, 76*, S22–S32. https://doi.org/10.1016/j.ypmed.2014.11.003

Benke, K. S., Nivard, M. G., Velders, F. P., Walters, R. K., Pappa, I., Scheet, P. A., et al. (2014). A genome-wide association meta-analysis of preschool internalizing problems. *Journal of the American Academy of Child and Adolescent Psychiatry, 53*(6), 667–676. https://doi.org/10.1016/j.jaac.2013.12.028

Bevilacqua, L., Kelly, Y., Heilmann, A., Priest, N., & Lacey, R. E. (2021). Adverse childhood experiences and trajectories of internalizing, externalizing, and prosocial behaviors from childhood to adolescence. *Child Abuse and Neglect, 112*, 104890. https://doi.org/10.1016/j.chiabu.2020.104890

Bhutta, A. T., Cleves, M. A., Casey, P. H., Cradock, M. M., & Anand, K. J. S. (2002). Cognitive and behavioral outcomes of school-aged children who were born preterm – A meta-analysis. *JAMA-Journal of the American Medical Association, 288*(6), 728–737. https://doi.org/10.1001/jama.288.6.728

Boardman, J. D., Alexander, K. B., & Stallings, M. C. (2011). Stressful life events and depression among adolescent twin pairs. *Biodemography and Social Biology, 57*(1), 53–66. https://doi.org/10.1080/19485565.2011.574565

Bokhorst, C. L., Westenberg, P. M., Oosterlaan, J., & Heyne, D. A. (2008). Changes in social fears across childhood and adolescence: Age-related differences in the factor structure of the Fear Survey Schedule for Children-Revised. *Journal of Anxiety Disorders, 22*(1), 135–142. https://doi.org/10.1016/j.janxdis.2007.01.014

Booth, C., Songco, A., Parsons, S., & Fox, E. (2022). Cognitive mechanisms predicting resilient functioning in adolescence: Evidence from the CogBIAS longitudinal study. *Development and Psychopathology, 34*(1), 345–353. https://doi.org/10.1017/s0954579420000668

Bradley, R. H., Corwyn, R. F., McAdoo, H. P., & Garcıa Coll, C. (2001). The home environments of children in the United States part I: Variations by age, ethnicity, and poverty status. *Child Development, 72*, 1844–1867. https://doi.org/10.1111/1467-8624.t01-1-00382

Brent, D. A., Porta, G., Rozenman, M. S., Gonzalez, A., Schwartz, K. T. G., Lynch, F. L., et al. (2020). Brief behavioral therapy for pediatric anxiety and depression in primary care: A follow-up. *Journal of the American Academy of Child and Adolescent Psychiatry, 59*(7), 856–867. https://doi.org/10.1016/j.jaac.2019.06.009

Bridge, J. A., Iyengar, S., Salary, C. B., Barbe, R. P., Birmaher, B., Pincus, H. A., et al. (2007). Clinical response and risk for reported suicidal ideation and suicide attempts in pediatric antidepressant treatment – A meta-analysis of randomized controlled trials. *JAMA-Journal of the American Medical Association, 297*(15), 1683–1696. https://doi.org/10.1001/jama.297.15.1683

Briggs, E. C., Amaya-Jackson, L., Putnam, K. T., & Putnam, F. W. (2021). All adverse childhood experiences are not equal: The contribution of synergy to adverse childhood experience scores. *American Psychologist, 76*(2), 243–252. https://doi.org/10.1037/amp0000768

Broeren, S., Muris, P., Diamantopoulou, S., & Baker, J. R. (2013). The course of childhood anxiety symptoms: Developmental trajectories and child-related factors in normal children. *Journal of Abnormal Child Psychology, 41*(1), 81–95. https://doi.org/10.1007/s10802-012-9669-9

Brown, G. W., & Harris, T. O. (1978). *Social origins of depression: A study of psychiatric disorder in women*. Tavistock.

Brown, G. W., Sklair, F., Harris, T. O., & Birley, J. L. T. (1973). Life-events and psychiatric disorders 1. Some methodological issues. *Psychological Medicine, 3*(1), 74–87. https://doi.org/10.1017/s0033291700046365

Buss, K. A. (2011). Which fearful toddlers should we worry about? Context, fear regulation, and anxiety risk. *Developmental Psychology, 47*(3), 804–819. https://doi.org/10.1037/a0023227

Caldwell, D. M., Davies, S. R., Hetrick, S. E., Palmer, J. C., Caro, P., Lopez-Lopez, J. A., et al. (2019). School-based interventions to prevent anxiety and depression in children and young people: A systematic review and network meta-analysis. *Lancet Psychiatry, 6*(12), 1011–1020. https://doi.org/10.1016/s2215-0366(19)30403-1

Cheesman, R., Purves, K. L., Pingault, J.-B., Breen, G., Rijsdij, F. K., Plomin, R., et al. (2018). Extracting stability increases the SNP heritability of emotional problems in young people. *Translational Psychiatry, 8*, 223. https://doi.org/10.1038/s41398-018-0269-5

Cheesman, R., Eilertsen, E. M., Ahmadzadeh, Y. I., Gjerde, L. C., Hannigan, L. J., Havdahl, A., et al. (2020). How important are parents in the development of child anxiety and depression? A genomic analysis of parent-offspring trios in the Norwegian Mother Father and Child Cohort Study (MoBa). *BMC Medicine, 18*(1), 284. https://doi.org/10.1186/s12916-020-01760-1

Cipriani, A., Zhou, X. Y., Del Giovane, C., Hetrick, S. E., Qin, B., Whittington, C., et al. (2016). Comparative efficacy and tolerability of antidepressants for major depressive disorder in children and adolescents: A network meta-analysis. *Lancet, 388*(10047), 881–890. https://doi.org/10.1016/s0140-6736(16)30385-3

Cipriani, A., Furukawa, T. A., Salanti, G., Chaimani, A., Atkinson, L. Z., Ogawa, Y., et al. (2018). Comparative efficacy and acceptability of 21 antidepressant drugs for the acute treatment of adults with major depressive disorder: A systematic review and network meta-analysis. *Lancet, 391*(10128), 1357–1366. https://doi.org/10.1016/s0140-6736(17)32802-7

Cleare, A., Pariante, C. M., Young, A. H., Anderson, I. M., Christmas, D., Cowen, P. J., et al. (2015). Evidence-based guidelines for treating depressive disorders with antidepressants: A revision of the 2008 British Association for Psychopharmacology guidelines. *Journal of Psychopharmacology, 29*(5), 459–525. https://doi.org/10.1177/0269881115581093

Coleman, J. R. I., Lester, K. J., Keers, R., Roberts, S., Curtis, C., Arendt, K., et al. (2016). Genome-wide association study of response to cognitive-behavioural therapy in children with anxiety disorders. *British Journal of Psychiatry, 209*(3), 236–243. https://doi.org/10.1192/bjp.bp.115.168229

Collishaw, S. (2015). Annual research review: Secular trends in child and adolescent mental health. *Journal of Child Psychology and Psychiatry, 56*(3), 370–393. https://doi.org/10.1111/jcpp.12372

Collishaw, S., Maughan, B., Natarajan, L., & Pickles, A. (2010). Trends in adolescent emotional problems in England: A comparison of two national cohorts twenty years apart. *Journal of Child Psychology and Psychiatry, 51*(8), 885–894. https://doi.org/10.1111/j.1469-7610.2010.02252.x

Connell, A. M., & Goodman, S. H. (2002). The association between psychopathology in fathers versus mothers and children's internalizing and externalizing behavior problems: A meta-analysis. *Psychological Bulletin, 128*(5), 746–773. https://doi.org/10.1037//0033-2909.128.5.746

Copeland, W. E., Angold, A., Shanahan, L., & Costello, E. J. (2014). Longitudinal patterns of anxiety from childhood to adulthood: The Great Smoky Mountains Study. *Journal of the American Academy of Child and Adolescent Psychiatry, 53*(1), 21–33. https://doi.org/10.1016/j.jaac.2013.09.017

Croft, S., Stride, C., Maughan, B., & Rowe, R. (2015). Validity of the strengths and difficulties questionnaire in preschool-aged children. *Pediatrics, 135*(5), E1210–E1219. https://doi.org/10.1542/peds.2014-2920

Cummings, C. M., Caporino, N. E., & Kendall, P. C. (2014). Comorbidity of anxiety and depression in children and adolescents: 20 years after. *Psychological Bulletin, 140*(3), 816–845. https://doi.org/10.1037/a0034733

Dahlberg, A., Ghaderi, A., Sarkadi, A., & Salari, R. (2019). SDQ in the hands of fathers and preschool teachers. Psychometric properties in a non-clinical sample of 3-5-year-olds. *Child Psychiatry & Human Development, 50*(1), 132–141. https://doi.org/10.1007/s10578-018-0826-4

Daniels, D., & Plomin, R. (1985). Origins of individual differences in infant shyness. *Developmental Psychology, 21*(1), 118–121. https://doi.org/10.1037/0012-1649.21.1.118

Digman, J. (1963). Principal dimensions of child personality as inferred from teachers' judgments. *Child Development, 34*, 43–60.

Doering, S., Larsson, H., Halldner, L., Gillberg, C., Kuja-Halkola, R., & Lundstrom, S. (2022). Internalizing symptoms in adolescence are modestly affected by symptoms of anxiety, depression, and neurodevelopmental disorders in childhood. *BMC Psychiatry, 22*(1), 233. https://doi.org/10.1186/s12888-022-03875-6

Donolato, E., Cardillo, R., Mammarella, I. C., & Melby-Lervag, M. (2022). Research review: Language and specific learning disorders in children and their co-occurrence with internalizing and externalizing problems: A systematic review and meta-analysis. *Journal of Child Psychology and Psychiatry, 63*, 507–518. https://doi.org/10.1111/jcpp.13536

Dragioti, E., Solmi, M., Favaro, A., Fusar-Poli, P., Dazzan, P., Thompson, T., et al. (2019). Association of antidepressant use with adverse health outcomes: A systematic umbrella eview. *JAMA Psychiatry, 76*(12), 1241–1255. https://doi.org/10.1001/jamapsychiatry.2019.2859

Dreger, R. M., Lewis, P. M., Rich, T. A., Miller, K. S., Reid, M. P., Overlade, D. C., et al. (1964). Behavioral classification project. *Journal of Consulting Psychology, 28*(1), 1–13. https://doi.org/10.1037/h0046180

Egger, H. L., & Angold, A. (2006). Common emotional and behavioral disorders in preschool children: Presentation, nosology, and epidemiology. *Journal of Child Psychology and Psychiatry, 47*(3–4), 313–337. https://doi.org/10.1111/j.1469-7610.2006.01618.x

Eirich, R., McArthur, B. A., Anhorn, C., McGuinness, C., Christakis, D. A., & Madigan, S. (2022). Association of screen time with internalizing and externalizing behavior problems in children 12 years or younger: A systematic review and meta-analysis. *JAMA Psychiatry, 79*(5), 393–405. https://doi.org/10.1001/jamapsychiatry.2022.0155

El Rafihi-Ferreira, R., Silvares, E. F. M., Asbahr, F. R., & Ollendick, T. H. (2018). Brief treatment for nighttime fears and co-sleeping problems: A randomized clinical trial. *Journal of Anxiety Disorders, 58*, 51–60. https://doi.org/10.1016/j.janxdis.2018.06.008

Eley, T. C., & Stevenson, J. (2000). Specific life events and chronic experiences differentially associated with depression and anxiety in young twins. *Journal of Abnormal Child Psychology, 28*(4), 383–394. https://doi.org/10.1023/a:1005173127117

Eley, T. C., Bolton, D., O'Connor, T. G., Perrin, S., Smith, P., & Plomin, R. (2003). A twin study of anxiety-related behaviours in pre-school children. *Journal of Child Psychology and Psychiatry, 44*(7), 945–960. https://doi.org/10.1111/1469-7610.00179

Eley, T. C., McAdams, T. A., Rijsdijk, F. V., Lichtenstein, P., Narusyte, J., Reiss, D., et al. (2015). The intergenerational transmission of anxiety: A Children-of-Twins Study. *American Journal of Psychiatry, 172*(7), 630–637. https://doi.org/10.1176/appi.ajp.2015.14070818

Evans, G. W., Li, D. P., & Whipple, S. S. (2013). Cumulative risk and child development. *Psychological Bulletin, 139*(6), 1342–1396. https://doi.org/10.1037/a0031808

Ezpeleta, L., Granero, R., de la Osa, N., Penelo, E., & Domenech, J. M. (2013). Psychometric properties of the Strengths and Difficulties Questionnaire(3-4) in 3-year-old preschoolers. *Comprehensive Psychiatry, 54*(3), 282–291. https://doi.org/10.1016/j.comppsych.2012.07.009

Feeney, A., Hock, R. S., Fava, M., Ortiz, J. M. H., Iovieno, N., & Papakostas, G. I. (2022). Antidepressants in children and adolescents with major depressive disorder and the influence of placebo response: A meta-analysis. *Journal of Affective Disorders, 305*, 55–64. https://doi.org/10.1016/j.jad.2022.02.074

Finkelhor, D. (2018). Screening for adverse childhood experiences (ACEs): Cautions and suggestions. *Child Abuse and Neglect, 85*, 174–179. https://doi.org/10.1016/j.chiabu.2017.07.016

Finlay-Jones, R., & Brown, G. W. (1981). Types of stressful life event and the onset of anxiety and depressive disorders. *Psychological Medicine, 11*(4), 803–815. https://doi.org/10.1017/s0033291700041301

Fombonne, E., Wostear, G., Cooper, V., Harrington, R., & Rutter, M. (2001). The Maudsley long-term follow-up of child and adolescent depression 1. Psychiatric outcomes in adulthood. *British Journal of Psychiatry, 179*, 210–217. https://doi.org/10.1192/bjp.179.3.210

Ford, T. (2020). Editorial perspective: Why I am now convinced that emotional disorders are increasingly common among young people in many countries. *Journal of Child Psychology and Psychiatry, 61*(11), 1275–1276. https://doi.org/10.1111/jcpp.13211

Fowler, P. J., Tompsett, C. J., Braciszewski, J. M., Jacques-Tiura, A. J., & Baltes, B. B. (2009). Community violence: A meta-analysis on the effect of exposure and mental health outcomes of children and adolescents. *Development and Psychopathology, 21*(1), 227–259. https://doi.org/10.1017/s0954579409000145

Fryers, T., & Brugha, T. (2013). Childhood determinants of adult psychiatric disorder. *Clinical Practice and Epidemiology in Mental Health, 9*, 1–50. https://doi.org/10.2174/1745017901309010001

Funkhouser, C. J., Chacko, A. A., Correa, K. A., Kaiser, A. J. E., & Shankman, S. A. (2021). Unique longitudinal relationships between symptoms of psychopathology in youth: A cross-lagged panel network analysis in the ABCD study. *Journal of Child Psychology and Psychiatry, 62*(2), 184–194. https://doi.org/10.1111/jcpp.13256

Gaffrey, M. S., Tillman, R., Barch, D. M., & Luby, J. L. (2018). Continuity and stability of preschool depression from childhood through adolescence and following the onset of puberty. *Comprehensive Psychiatry, 86*, 39–46. https://doi.org/10.1016/j.comppsych.2018.07.010

Gardner, F., & Shaw, D. (2008). Behavioral problems of infancy and preschool children (0-5). In M. Rutter, D. Bishop, D. Pine, S. Scott, J. Stevenson, E. Taylor, & A. Thapar (Eds.), *Rutter's child and adolescent psychiatry* (5th ed.). Blackwell Publishing.

Ghandour, R. M., Sherman, L. J., Vladutiu, C. J., Ali, M. M., Lynch, S. E., Bitsko, R. H., & Blumberg, S. J. (2019). Prevalence and treatment of depression, anxiety, and conduct problems in US children. *Journal of Pediatrics, 206*, 256–267.e3. https://doi.org/10.1016/j.jpeds.2018.09.021

Gilman, S. E., Govender, T., Augustin, D., & Yu, J. (2023). Uncertainty in developmental origins of health and disease research: Commentary on Nomura et al. (2022). *Journal of Child Psychology and Psychiatry, 64*(9), 1396–1398. https://doi.org/10.1111/jcpp.13842

Goh, S. K. Y., Griffiths, S., Norbury, C. F., & SCALES Team. (2021). Sources of variability in the prospective relation of language to social, emotional, and behavior problem symptoms: Implications for developmental language disorder. *Journal of Abnormal Psychology, 130*(6), 676–689. https://doi.org/10.1037/abn0000691

Goodman, R. (2001). Psychometric properties of the strengths and difficulties questionnaire. *Journal of the American Academy of Child and Adolescent Psychiatry, 40*(11), 1337–1345. https://doi.org/10.1097/00004583-200111000-00015

Goodman, R., & Scott, S. (1999). Comparing the strengths and difficulties questionnaire and the child behavior checklist: Is small beautiful? *Journal of Abnormal Child Psychology, 27*(1), 17–24. https://doi.org/10.1023/a:1022658222914

Goodman, A., Lamping, D. L., & Ploubidis, G. B. (2010). When to use broader internalising and externalising subscales instead of the hypothesised five subscales on the strengths and difficulties questionnaire (SDQ): Data from British parents, teachers and children. *Journal of Abnormal Child Psychology, 38*(8), 1179–1191. https://doi.org/10.1007/s10802-010-9434-x

Goodman, S. H., Rouse, M. H., Connell, A. M., Broth, M. R., Hall, C. M., & Heyward, D. (2011). Maternal depression and child psychopathology: A meta-analytic review. *Clinical Child and Family Psychology Review, 14*(1), 1–27. https://doi.org/10.1007/s10567-010-0080-1

Gregory, A. M., Rijsdijk, F. V., Lau, J. Y. F., Dahl, R. E., & Eley, T. C. (2009). The direction of longitudinal associations between sleep problems and depression symptoms: A study of twins aged 8 and 10 years. *Sleep, 32*(2), 189–199. https://doi.org/10.5665/sleep/32.2.189

Gullone, E. (2000). The development of normal fear: A century of research. *Clinical Psychology Review, 20*(4), 429–451. https://doi.org/10.1016/s0272-7358(99)00034-3

Gutman, L. M., & McMaster, N. C. (2020). Gendered pathways of internalizing problems from early childhood to adolescence and associated adolescent outcomes. *Journal of Abnormal Child Psychology, 48*, 703–718. https://doi.org/10.1007/s10802-020-00623-w

Guzman-Holst, C., Zaneva, M., Chessell, C., Creswell, C., & Bowes, L. (2022). Research review: Do antibullying interventions reduce internalizing symptoms? A systematic review, meta-analysis, and meta-regression exploring intervention components, moderators, and mechanisms. *Journal of Child Psychology and Psychiatry, 63*, 1454–1465. https://doi.org/10.1111/jcpp.13620

Haahr-Pedersen, I., Hyland, P., Hansen, M., Perera, C., Spitz, P., Bramsen, R. H., & Vallieres, F. (2021). Patterns of childhood adversity and their associations with internalizing and externalizing problems among at-risk boys and girls. *Child Abuse and Neglect, 121*, 105272. https://doi.org/10.1016/j.chiabu.2021.105272

Hannigan, L. J., Walaker, N., Waszczuk, M. A., McAdams, T. A., & Eley, T. C. (2017). Aetiological influences on stability and change in emotional and behavioural problems across development: A systematic review. *Psychopathology Review, 4*(1), 52–108. https://doi.org/10.5127/pr.038315

Harrison, L., Carducci, B., Klein, J. D., & Bhutta, Z. A. (2022). Indirect effects of COVID-19 on child and adolescent mental health: An overview of systematic reviews. *BMJ Global Health, 7*(12), e010713. https://doi.org/10.1136/bmjgh-2022-010713

Hawker, D. S. J., & Boulton, M. J. (2000). Twenty years' research on peer victimization and psychosocial maladjustment: A meta-analytic review of cross-sectional studies. *Journal of Child Psychology and Psychiatry, 41*(4), 441–455. https://doi.org/10.1111/1469-7610.00629

Hawton, K., & van Heeringen, K. (2009). Suicide. *Lancet, 373*(9672), 1372–1381. https://doi.org/10.1016/s0140-6736(09)60372-x

Hentges, R. F., Devereux, C., Graham, S. A., & Madigan, S. (2021). Child language difficulties and internalizing and externalizing symptoms: A meta-analysis. *Child Development, 92*, e691–e715. https://doi.org/10.1111/cdev.13540

Herrman, H., Patel, V., Kieling, C., Berk, M., Buchweitz, C., Cuijpers, P., et al. (2022). Time for united action on depression: A Lancet-World Psychiatric Association Commission. *Lancet, 399*(10328), 957–1022. https://doi.org/10.1016/s0140-6736(21)02141-3

Hetrick, S. E., Cox, G. R., Witt, K. G., Bir, J. J., & Merry, S. N. (2016). Cognitive behavioural therapy (CBT), third-wave CBT and interpersonal therapy (IPT) based interventions for preventing depression in children and adolescents. *Cochrane Database of Systematic Reviews, 2016*(8), CD003380. https://doi.org/10.1002/14651858.CD003380.pub4

Horowitz, J. L., & Garber, J. (2006). The prevention of depressive symptoms in children and adolescents: A meta-analytic review. *Journal of Consulting and Clinical Psychology, 74*(3), 401–415. https://doi.org/10.1037/0022-006x.74.3.401

Hu, L. T., & Bentler, P. M. (1999). Cutoff criteria for fit indexes in covariance structure analysis: Conventional criteria versus new alternatives. *Structural Equation Modeling: A Multidisciplinary Journal, 6*(1), 1–55. https://doi.org/10.1080/10705519909540118

Hudson, J. L., Murayama, K., Meteyard, L., Morris, T., & Dodd, H. F. (2019). Early childhood predictors of anxiety in early adolescence. *Journal of Abnormal Child Psychology, 47*(7), 1121–1133. https://doi.org/10.1007/s10802-018-0495-6

Hughes, K., Bellis, M. A., Hardcastle, K. A., Sethi, D., Butchart, A., Mikton, C., et al. (2017). The effect of multiple adverse childhood experiences on health: A systematic review and meta-analysis. *The Lancet Public Health, 2*(8), E356–E366. https://doi.org/10.1016/S2468-2667(17)30118-4

Hyde, J. S., & Mezulis, A. H. (2020). Gender differences in depression: Biological, affective, cognitive, and sociocultural factors. *Harvard Review of Psychiatry, 28*(1), 4–13. https://doi.org/10.1097/hrp.0000000000000230

Hyde, J. S., Mezulis, A. H., & Abramson, L. Y. (2008). The ABCs of depression: Integrating affective, biological, and cognitive models to explain the emergence of the gender difference in depression. *Psychological Review, 115*(2), 291–313. https://doi.org/10.1037/0033-295x.115.2.291

James, A. C., James, G., Cowdrey, F. A., Soler, A., & Choke, A. (2015). Cognitive behavioural therapy for anxiety disorders in children and adolescents. *Cochrane Database of Systematic Reviews, 2015*(2), CD004690. https://doi.org/10.1002/14651858.CD004690.pub4

James, T. D., Choi, H. J., Wiebe, S. A., & Espy, K. A. (2016). II. The preschool problem solving study: Sample, data and statistical methods. *Monographs of the Society for Research in Child Development, 81*(4), 30–46. https://doi.org/10.1111/mono.12269

James, A. C., Reardon, T., Soler, A., James, G., & Creswell, C. (2020). Cognitive behavioural therapy for anxiety disorders in children and adolescents. *Cochrane Database of Systematic Reviews, 11*(11), CD013162. https://doi.org/10.1002/14651858.CD013162.pub2

Jami, E. S., Hammerschlag, A. R., Ip, H. F., Allegrini, A. G., Benyamin, B., Border, R., et al. (2022). Genome-wide association meta-analysis of childhood and adolescent internalizing symptoms. *Journal of the American Academy of Child and Adolescent Psychiatry, 61*(7), 934–945. https://doi.org/10.1016/j.jaac.2021.11.035

Jauhar, S., Cowen, P. J., & Browning, M. (2023). Fifty years on: Serotonin and depression. *Journal of Psychopharmacology, 37*(3), 237–241. https://doi.org/10.1177/02698811231161813

Jenkins, R., & Hewitt, L. (1944). Types of personality structure encountered in child guidance clinics. *American Journal of Orthopsychiatry, 14*, 84–94. https://doi.org/10.1111/j.1939-0025.1944.tb04853.x

Johnson, D., Dupuis, G., Piche, J., Clayborne, Z., & Colman, I. (2018). Adult mental health outcomes of adolescent depression: A systematic review. *Depression and Anxiety, 35*(8), 700–716. https://doi.org/10.1002/da.22777

Kendall, K. M., Van Assche, E., Andlauer, T. F. M., Choi, K. W., Luykx, J. J., Schulte, E. C., & Lu, Y. (2021). The genetic basis of major depression. *Psychological Medicine, 51*(13), 2217–2230. https://doi.org/10.1017/s0033291721000441

Kendler, K. S., Heath, A., Martin, N. G., & Eaves, L. J. (1986). Symptoms of anxiety and depression in a volunteer twin population – The etiologic role of genetic and environmental-factors. *Archives of General Psychiatry, 43*(3), 213–221. https://doi.org/10.1001/archpsyc.1986.01800030023002

Kendler, K. S., Karkowski, L. M., & Prescott, C. A. (1999). The assessment of dependence in the study of stressful life events: Validation using a twin design. *Psychological Medicine, 29*(6), 1455–1460. https://doi.org/10.1017/s0033291798008198

Kendler, K. S., Gardner, C. O., Annas, P., & Lichtenstein, P. (2008). The development of fears from early adolescence to young adulthood: A multivariate study. *Psychological Medicine, 38*(12), 1759–1769. https://doi.org/10.1017/s0033291708002936

Kendler, K. S., Ohlsson, H., Sundquist, K., & Sundquist, J. (2018). Sources of parent-offspring resemblance for major depression in a national Swedish extended adoption study. *JAMA Psychiatry, 75*(2), 194–200. https://doi.org/10.1001/jamapsychiatry.2017.3828

Kendrick, T., & Collinson, S. (2022). Antidepressants and the serotonin hypothesis of depression. *BMJ-British Medical Journal, 378*, o1993. https://doi.org/10.1136/bmj.o1993

Kessler, R. C., Avenevoli, S., & Merikangas, K. R. (2001). Mood disorders in children and adolescents: An epidemiologic perspective. *Biological Psychiatry, 49*(12), 1002–1014. https://doi.org/10.1016/s0006-3223(01)01129-5

Kim, S., Thibodeau, R., & Jorgensen, R. S. (2011). Shame, guilt, and depressive symptoms: A meta-analytic review. *Psychological Bulletin, 137*(1), 68–96. https://doi.org/10.1037/a0021466

Kok, R., Linting, M., Bakermans-Kranenburg, M. J., van Ijzendoorn, M. H., Jaddoe, V. W. V., Hofman, A., et al. (2013). Maternal sensitivity and internalizing problems: Evidence from two longitudinal studies in early childhood. *Child Psychiatry & Human Development, 44*(6), 751–765. https://doi.org/10.1007/s10578-013-0369-7

Kong, A., Thorleifsson, G., Frigge, M. L., Vilhjalmsson, B. J., Young, A. I., Thorgeirsson, T. E., et al. (2018). The nature of nurture: Effects of parental genotypes. *Science, 359*(6374), 424–428. https://doi.org/10.1126/science.aan6877

Kovacs, M. (1985). The Children's Depression Inventory (CDI). *Psychopharmacology Bulletin, 21*(4), 995–998. https://doi.org/10.1037/t00788-000

Kovacs, M., Obrosky, S., & George, C. (2016). The course of major depressive disorder from childhood to young adulthood: Recovery and recurrence in a longitudinal observational study. *Journal of Affective Disorders, 203*, 374–381. https://doi.org/10.1016/j.jad.2016.05.042

Kuehner, C. (2017). Why is depression more common among women than among men? *Lancet Psychiatry, 4*(2), 146–158. https://doi.org/10.1016/s2215-0366(16)30263-2

Kwong, A. S. F., Morris, T. T., Pearson, R. M., Timpson, N. J., Rice, F., Stergiakouli, E., & Tilling, K. (2021). Polygenic risk for depression, anxiety and neuroticism are associated with the severity and rate of change in depressive symptoms across adolescence. *Journal of Child Psychology and Psychiatry, 62*, 1462–1474. https://doi.org/10.1111/jcpp.13422

Lacey, R. E., Howe, L. D., Kelly-Irving, M., Bartley, M., & Kelly, Y. (2022). The clustering of adverse childhood experiences in the Avon longitudinal study of parents and children: Are gender and poverty important? *Journal of Interpersonal Violence, 37*(5–6), 2218–2241. https://doi.org/10.1177/0886260520935096

Lahey, B. B., Rathouz, P. J., Keenan, K., Stepp, S. D., Loeber, R., & Hipwell, A. E. (2015). Criterion validity of the general factor of psychopathology in a prospective study of girls. *Journal of Child Psychology and Psychiatry, 56*(4), 415–422. https://doi.org/10.1111/jcpp.12300

Lau, J. Y. F., & Eley, T. C. (2008). Disentangling gene-environment correlations and interactions on adolescent depressive symptoms. *Journal of Child Psychology and Psychiatry, 49*(2), 142–150. https://doi.org/10.1111/j.1469-7610.2007.01803.x

Lau, J. Y. F., & Waters, A. M. (2017). Annual research review: An expanded account of information-processing mechanisms in risk for child and adolescent anxiety and depression. *Journal of Child Psychology and Psychiatry, 58*(4), 387–407. https://doi.org/10.1111/jcpp.12653

Lau, J. Y. F., Eley, T. C., & Stevenson, J. (2006). Examining the state-trait anxiety relationship: A behavioural genetic approach. *Journal of Abnormal Child Psychology, 34*(1), 19–27. https://doi.org/10.1007/s10802-005-9006-7

Lavigne, J. V., Hopkins, J., Gouze, K. R., & Bryant, F. B. (2015). Bidirectional influences of anxiety and depression in young children. *Journal of Abnormal Child Psychology, 43*(1), 163–176. https://doi.org/10.1007/s10802-014-9884-7

Lawrence, P. J., Murayama, K., & Creswell, C. (2019). Systematic review and meta-analysis: Anxiety and depressive disorders in offspring of parents with anxiety disorders. *Journal of the American Academy of Child and Adolescent Psychiatry, 58*(1), 46–60. https://doi.org/10.1016/j.jaac.2018.07.898

Lester, K. J., & Eley, T. C. (2013). Therapygenetics: Using genetic markers to predict response to psychological treatment for mood and anxiety disorders. *Biology of Mood & Anxiety Disorders, 3*(1), 4. https://doi.org/10.1186/2045-5380-3-4

Lewinsohn, P. M., Gotlib, I. H., Lewinsohn, M., Seeley, J. R., & Allen, N. B. (1998). Gender differences in anxiety disorders and anxiety symptoms in adolescents. *Journal of Abnormal Psychology, 107*(1), 109–117. https://doi.org/10.1037/0021-843x.107.1.109

Lewis, K. M., Amatya, K., Coffman, M. F., & Ollendick, T. H. (2015). Treating nighttime fears in young children with bibliotherapy: Evaluating anxiety symptoms and monitoring behavior change. *Journal of Anxiety Disorders, 30*, 103–112. https://doi.org/10.1016/j.janxdis.2014.12.004

Lewis, K. M., Rafihi-Ferreira, R. E., Freitag, G. F., Coffman, M., & Ollendick, T. H. (2021). A 25-year review of nighttime fears in children: Past, present, and future. *Clinical Child and Family Psychology Review, 24*(3), 391–413. https://doi.org/10.1007/s10567-021-00354-4

Loades, M. E., Chatburn, E., Higson-Sweeney, N., Reynolds, S., Shafran, R., Brigden, A., et al. (2020). Rapid systematic review: The impact of social isolation and loneliness on the mental health of children and adolescents in the context of COVID-19. *Journal of the American Academy of Child and Adolescent Psychiatry, 59*(11), 1218–1239. https://doi.org/10.1016/j.jaac.2020.05.009

Locher, C., Koechlin, H., Zion, S. R., Werner, C., Pine, D. S., Kirsch, I., et al. (2017). Efficacy and safety of selective serotonin reuptake inhibitors, serotonin-norepinephrine reuptake inhibitors, and placebo for common psychiatric disorders among children and adolescents: A systematic review and meta-analysis. *JAMA Psychiatry, 74*(10), 1011–1020. https://doi.org/10.1001/jamapsychiatry.2017.2432

Loerinc, A. G., Meuret, A. E., Twohig, M. P., Rosenfield, D., Bluett, E. J., & Craske, M. G. (2015). Response rates for CBT for anxiety disorders: Need for standardized criteria. *Clinical Psychology Review, 42*, 72–82. https://doi.org/10.1016/j.cpr.2015.08.004

Lubke, G. H., Miller, P. J., Verhulst, B., Bartels, M., van Beijsterveldt, T., Willemsen, G., et al. (2016). A powerful phenotype for gene-finding studies derived from trajectory analyses of symptoms of anxiety and depression between age seven and 18. *American Journal of Medical Genetics Part B-Neuropsychiatric Genetics, 171*(7), 948–957. https://doi.org/10.1002/ajmg.b.32375

Luby, J. L., Barch, D. M., Whalen, D., Tillman, R., & Freedland, K. E. (2018). A randomized controlled trial of parent-child psychotherapy targeting emotion development for early childhood depression. *American Journal of Psychiatry, 175*(11), 1102–1110. https://doi.org/10.1176/appi.ajp.2018.18030321

Ludwig-Walz, H., Dannheim, I., Pfadenhauer, L. M., Fegert, J. M., & Bujard, M. (2022). Increase of depression among children and adolescents after the onset of the COVID-19 pandemic in Europe: A systematic review and meta-analysis. *Child and Adolescent Psychiatry and Mental Health, 16*(1), 109. https://doi.org/10.1186/s13034-022-00546-y

Lussier, A. A., Hawrilenko, M., Wang, M. J., Choi, K. W., Cerutti, J., Zhu, Y. W., et al. (2021). Genetic susceptibility for major depressive disorder associates with trajectories of depressive symptoms across childhood and adolescence. *Journal of Child Psychology and Psychiatry, 62*, 895–904. https://doi.org/10.1111/jcpp.13342

Lynch, F. L., Dickerson, J. F., Rozenman, M. S., Gonzalez, A., Schwartz, K. T. G., Porta, G., et al. (2021). Cost-effectiveness of brief behavioral therapy for pediatric anxiety and depression in primary aare. *JAMA Network Open, 4*(3), e211778. https://doi.org/10.1001/jamanetworkopen.2021.1778

Macdonald, G., Higgins, J. P. T., Ramchandani, P., Valentine, J. C., Bronger, L. P., Klein, P., et al. (2012). Cognitive-behavioural interventions for children who have been sexually abused. *Cochrane Database of Systematic Reviews, 2012*(5), CD001930. https://doi.org/10.1002/14651858.CD001930.pub3

Marino, C., Andrade, B., Campisi, S. C., Wong, M., Zhao, H., Jing, X., et al. (2021). Association between disturbed sleep and depression in children and youths: A systematic review and meta-analysis of cohort studies. *JAMA Network Open, 4*(3), e212373. https://doi.org/10.1001/jamanetworkopen.2021.2373

Marino, C., Andrade, B., Montplaisir, J., Petit, D., Touchette, E., Paradis, H., et al. (2022). Testing bidirectional, longitudinal associations between disturbed sleep and depressive symptoms in children and adolescents using cross-lagged models. *JAMA Network Open, 5*(8), e2227119. https://doi.org/10.1001/jamanetworkopen.2022.27119

McLaughlin, K. A., Green, J. G., Gruber, M. J., Sampson, N. A., Zaslavsky, A. M., & Kessler, R. C. (2012). Childhood adversities and first onset of psychiatric disorders in a national sample of US adolescents. *Archives of General Psychiatry, 69*(11), 1151–1160. https://doi.org/10.1001/archgenpsychiatry.2011.2277

McLean, C. P., & Anderson, E. R. (2009). Brave men and timid women? A review of the gender differences in fear and anxiety. *Clinical Psychology Review, 29*(6), 496–505. https://doi.org/10.1016/j.cpr.2009.05.003

McLeod, B. D., Weisz, J. R., & Wood, J. J. (2007a). Examining the association between parenting and childhood depression: A meta-analysis. *Clinical Psychology Review, 27*(8), 986–1003. https://doi.org/10.1016/j.cpr.2007.03.001

McLeod, B. D., Wood, J. J., & Weisz, J. R. (2007b). Examining the association between parenting and childhood anxiety: A meta-analysis. *Clinical Psychology Review, 27*(2), 155–172. https://doi.org/10.1016/j.cpr.2006.09.002

Merikangas, K. R., He, J. P., Burstein, M., Swanson, S. A., Avenevoli, S., Cui, L. H., et al. (2010). Lifetime prevalence of mental disorders in U.S. adolescents: Results from the National Comorbidity Survey Replication-Adolescent Supplement (NCS-A). *Journal of the American Academy of Child and Adolescent Psychiatry, 49*(10), 980–989. https://doi.org/10.1016/j.jaac.2010.05.017

Messer, S. C., Angold, A., Costello, E. J., Loeber, R., VanKammen, W., & StouthamerLoeber, M. (1995). Development of a short questionnaire for use in epidemiological studies of depression in children and adolescents: Factor composition and structure across development. *International Journal of Methods in Psychiatric Research, 5*(4), 251–262.

Miller, A. B., Machlin, L., Mclaughlin, K. A., & Sheridan, M. A. (2021). Deprivation and psychopathology in the fragile families study: A 15-year longitudinal investigation. *Journal of Child Psychology and Psychiatry, 62*, 382–391. https://doi.org/10.1111/jcpp.13260

Moncrieff, J., Cooper, R. E., Stockmann, T., Amendola, S., Hengartner, M. P., & Horowitz, M. A. (2022). The serotonin theory of depression: A systematic umbrella review of the evidence. *Molecular Psychiatry*. https://doi.org/10.1038/s41380-022-01661-0

Morneau-Vaillancourt, G., Oginni, O., Assary, E., Krebs, G., Thompson, E. J., Palaiologou, E., et al. (2023). A cross-lagged twin study of emotional symptoms, social isolation and peer victimisation from early adolescence to emerging adulthood. *Journal of Child Psychology and Psychiatry*. https://doi.org/10.1111/jcpp.13847

Munoz, R. F., Mrazek, P. J., & Haggerty, R. J. (1996). Institute of medicine report on prevention of mental disorders – Summary and commentary. *American Psychologist, 51*(11), 1116–1122. https://doi.org/10.1037/0003-066x.51.11.1116

Muris, P., Schmidt, H., Merckelbach, H., & Schouten, E. (2001). Anxiety sensitivity in adolescents: Factor structure and relationships to trait anxiety and symptoms of anxiety disorders and depression. *Behaviour Research and Therapy, 39*, 89–100. https://doi.org/10.1016/S0005-7967(99)00179-5

Muris, P., Ollendick, T. H., Roelofs, J., & Austin, K. (2014). The short form of the fear survey schedule for children-revised (FSSC-R-SF): An efficient, reliable, and valid scale for measuring fear in children and adolescents. *Journal of Anxiety Disorders, 28*(8), 957–965. https://doi.org/10.1016/j.janxdis.2014.09.020

Neville, R. D., McArthur, B. A., Eirich, R., Lakes, K. D., & Madigan, S. (2021). Bidirectional associations between screen time and children's externalizing and internalizing behaviors. *Journal of Child Psychology and Psychiatry, 62*(12), 1475–1484. https://doi.org/10.1111/jcpp.13425

Newlove-Delgado, T., Russell, A. E., Mathews, F., Cross, L., Bryant, E., Gudka, R., et al. (2023). Annual research review: The impact of Covid-19 on psychopathology in children and young people worldwide: Systematic review of studies with pre- and within-pandemic data. *Journal of Child Psychology and Psychiatry, 64*(4), 611–640. https://doi.org/10.1111/jcpp.13716

Ng, M. Y., DiVasto, K. A., Cootner, S., Gonzalez, N. A. R., & Weisz, J. R. (2020). What do 30 years of randomized trials tell us about how psychotherapy improves youth depression? A systematic review of candidate mediators. *Clinical Psychology-Science and Practice*, e12367. https://doi.org/10.1111/cpsp.12367

Nikolic, M., Hannigan, L. J., Krebs, G., Sterne, A., Gregory, A. M., & Eley, T. C. (2022). Aetiology of shame and its association with adolescent depression and anxiety: Results from a prospective twin and sibling study. *Journal of Child Psychology and Psychiatry, 63*(1), 99–108. https://doi.org/10.1111/jcpp.13465

Nivard, M. G., Dolan, C. V., Kendler, K. S., Kan, K. J., Willemsen, G., van Beijsterveldt, C. E. M., et al. (2015). Stability in symptoms of anxiety and depression as a function of genotype and environment: A longitudinal twin study from ages 3 to 63 years. *Psychological Medicine, 45*(5), 1039–1049. https://doi.org/10.1017/s003329171400213x

Nomura, Y., Newcorn, J. H., Ginalis, C., Heitz, C., Zaki, J., Khan, F., et al. (2023). Prenatal exposure to a natural disaster and early development of psychiatric disorders during the preschool years: Stress in pregnancy study. *Journal of Child Psychology and Psychiatry, 64*(7), 1080–1091. https://doi.org/10.1111/jcpp.13698

Olino, T. M., Dougherty, L. R., Bufferd, S. J., Carlson, G. A., & Klein, D. N. (2014). Testing models of psychopathology in preschool-aged children using a structured interview-based assessment. *Journal of Abnormal Child Psychology, 42*(7), 1201–1211. https://doi.org/10.1007/s10802-014-9865-x

Ollendick, T. H. (1983). Reliability and validity of the revised fear survey schedule for children (FSSC-R). *Behaviour Research and Therapy, 21*(6), 685–692. https://doi.org/10.1016/0005-7967(83)90087-6

Orben, A., Przybylski, A. K., Blakemore, S.-J., & Kievit, R. A. (2022). Windows of developmental sensitivity to social media. *Nature Communications, 13*(1), 1649. https://doi.org/10.1038/s41467-022-29296-3

Oud, M., de Winter, L., Vermeulen-Smit, E., Bodden, D., Nauta, M., Stone, L., et al. (2019). Effectiveness of CBT for children and adolescents with depression: A systematic review and meta-regression analysis. *European Psychiatry, 57*, 33–45. https://doi.org/10.1016/j.eurpsy.2018.12.008

Panchal, U., de Pablo, G. S., Franco, M., Moreno, C., Parellada, M., Arango, C., & Fusar-Poli, P. (2023). The impact of COVID-19 lockdown on child and adolescent mental health: Systematic review. *European Child and Adolescent Psychiatry, 32*(7), 1151–1177. https://doi.org/10.1007/s00787-021-01856-w

Pappa, I., Fedko, I. O., Mileva-Seitz, V. R., Hottenga, J.-J., Bakermans-Kranenburg, M. J., Bartels, M., et al. (2015). Single nucleotide polymorphism heritabiliiy of behavior problems in childhood: Genome-wide complex trait analysis. *Journal of the American Academy of Child and Adolescent Psychiatry, 54*(9), 737–744. https://doi.org/10.1016/j.jaac.2015.06.004

Patel, V., Flisher, A. J., Hetrick, S., & McGorry, P. (2007). Adolescent Health 3 – Mental health of young people: A global public-health challenge. *Lancet, 369*(9569), 1302–1313. https://doi.org/10.1016/s0140-6736(07)60368-7

Patel, V., Saxena, S., Lund, C., Thornicroft, G., Baingana, F., Bolton, P., et al. (2018). The Lancet Commission on global mental health and sustainable development. *Lancet, 392*(10157), 1553–1598. https://doi.org/10.1016/s0140-6736(18)31612-x

Peterson, D. R. (1961). Behavior problems of middle childhood. *Journal of Consulting Psychology, 25*, 205–209. https://doi.org/10.1037/h0038994

Peverill, M., Dirks, M. A., Narvaja, T., Herts, K. L., Comer, J. S., & McLaughlin, K. A. (2021). Socioeconomic status and child psychopathology in the United States: A meta-analysis of population-based studies. *Clinical Psychology Review, 83*, 101933. https://doi.org/10.1016/j.cpr.2020.101933

Phillips, E. M., Brock, R. L., James, T. D., Nelson, J. M., Mason, W. A., Espy, K. A., & Nelson, T. D. (2023). Does preschool executive control mediate the impact of early environmental unpredictability and deprivation on the general factor of psychopathology a decade later? *Journal of Child Psychology and Psychiatry, 64*(10), 1505–1516. https://doi.org/10.1111/jcpp.13775

Pierce, M., Hope, H., Ford, T., Hatch, S., Hotopf, M., John, A., et al. (2020). Mental health before and during the COVID-19 pandemic: A longitudinal probability sample survey of the UK population. *Lancet Psychiatry, 7*(10), 883–892. https://doi.org/10.1016/s2215-0366(20)30308-4

Pilling, S., Fonagy, P., Allison, E., Barnett, P., Campbell, C., Constantinou, M., et al. (2020). Long-term outcomes of psychological interventions on children and young people's mental health: A systematic review and meta-analysis. *PLoS One, 15*(11), e0236525. https://doi.org/10.1371/journal.pone.0236525

Purves, K. L., Krebs, G., McGregor, T., Constantinou, E., Lester, K. J., Barry, T. J., et al. (2023). Evidence for distinct genetic and environmental influences on fear acquisition and extinction. *Psychological Medicine, 53*(3), 1106–1114. https://doi.org/10.1017/s0033291721002580

Qu, G. B., Hu, W. J., Meng, J., Wang, X. Y., Su, W. Q., Liu, H. X., et al. (2023). Association between screen time and developmental and behavioral problems among children in the United States: Evidence from 2018 to 2020 NSCH. *Journal of Psychiatric Research, 161*, 140–149. https://doi.org/10.1016/j.jpsychires.2023.03.014

Rayner, C., Coleman, J. R. I., Purves, K. L., Hodsoll, J., Goldsmith, K., Alpers, G. W., et al. (2019). A genome-wide association meta-analysis of prognostic outcomes following cognitive behavioural therapy in individuals with anxiety and depressive disorders. *Translational Psychiatry, 9*, 150. https://doi.org/10.1038/s41398-019-0481-y

Reijntjes, A., Kamphuis, J. H., Prinzie, P., & Telch, M. J. (2010). Peer victimization and internalizing problems in children: A meta-analysis of longitudinal studies. *Child Abuse and Neglect, 34*(4), 244–252. https://doi.org/10.1016/j.chiabu.2009.07.009

Reiss, S., Peterson, R. A., Gursky, D. M., & McNally, R. J. (1986). Anxiety sensitivity, anxiety frequency and the prediction of fearfulness. *Behaviour Research and Therapy, 24*(1), 1–8. https://doi.org/10.1016/0005-7967(86)90143-9

Rice, F., Riglin, L., Thapar, A. K., Heron, J., Anney, R., O'Donovan, M. C., & Thapar, A. (2019). Characterizing developmental trajectories and the role of neuropsychiatric genetic risk variants in early-onset depression. *JAMA Psychiatry, 76*(3), 306–313. https://doi.org/10.1001/jamapsychiatry.2018.3338

Robinson, E., Sutin, A. R., Daly, M., & Jones, A. (2022). A systematic review and meta-analysis of longitudinal cohort studies comparing mental health before versus during the COVID-19 pandemic in 2020. *Journal of Affective Disorders, 296*, 567–576. https://doi.org/10.1016/j.jad.2021.09.098

Rocha, T. B. M., Fisher, H. L., Caye, A., Anselmi, L., Arseneault, L., Barros, F. C., et al. (2021). Identifying adolescents at risk for depression: A prediction score performance in cohorts based in 3 different continents. *Journal of the American Academy of Child and Adolescent Psychiatry, 60*(2), 262–273. https://doi.org/10.1016/j.jaac.2019.12.004

Rodrigues, M., Sokolovic, N., Madigan, S., Luo, Y. Q., Silva, V., Misra, S., & Jenkins, J. (2021). Paternal sensitivity and children's cognitive and socioemotional outcomes: A meta-analytic review. *Child Development, 92*(2), 554–577. https://doi.org/10.1111/cdev.13545

Rueger, S. Y., Malecki, C. K., Pyun, Y., Aycock, C., & Coyle, S. (2016). A meta-analytic review of the association between perceived social support and depression in childhood and adolescence. *Psychological Bulletin, 142*(10), 1017–1067. https://doi.org/10.1037/bul0000058

Rutter, M. (1967). A children's behaviour questionnaire for completion by teachers: Preliminary findings. *Journal of Child Psychology and Psychiatry, 8*(1), 1–11. https://doi.org/10.1111/j.1469-7610.1967.tb02175.x

Rutter, M., & Sandberg, S. (1992). Psychosocial stressors: Concepts, causes and effects. *European Child and Adolescent Psychiatry, 1*(1), 3–13. https://doi.org/10.1007/BF02084429

Salk, R. H., Hyde, J. S., & Abramson, L. Y. (2017). Gender differences in depression in representative national samples: Meta-analyses of diagnoses and symptoms. *Psychological Bulletin, 143*(8), 783–822. https://doi.org/10.1037/bul0000102

Salmon, K., O'Kearney, R., Reese, E., & Fortune, C. A. (2016). The role of language skill in child psychopathology: Implications for intervention in the early years. *Clinical Child and Family Psychology Review, 19*(4), 352–367. https://doi.org/10.1007/s10567-016-0214-1

Sandberg, S., Rutter, M., Giles, S., Owen, A., Champion, L., Nicholls, J., et al. (1993). Assessment of psychosocial experiences in childhood: Methodological issues and some illustrative findings. *Journal of Child Psychology and Psychiatry, 34*(6), 879–897. https://doi.org/10.1111/j.1469-7610.1993.tb01096.x

Sands, A., van Dijk, M. T., Abraham, E., Yangchen, T., Talati, A., & Weissman, M. M. (2022). The long-term outcomes of prepubertal depression and internalizing problems: A scoping review. *Harvard Review of Psychiatry, 30*(3), 163–180. https://doi.org/10.1097/hrp.0000000000000337

Sawyers, C., Ollendick, T., Brotman, M. A., Pine, D. S., Leibenluft, E., Carney, D. M., et al. (2019). The genetic and environmental structure of fear and anxiety in juvenile twins. *American Journal of Medical Genetics Part B-Neuropsychiatric Genetics, 180*(3), 204–212. https://doi.org/10.1002/ajmg.b.32714

Schlechter, P., Wilkinson, P. O., Ford, T. J., & Neufeld, S. A. S. (2023). The Short Mood and Feelings Questionnaire from adolescence to emerging adulthood: Measurement invariance across time and sex. *Psychological Assessment, 35*(5), 405–418. https://doi.org/10.1037/pas0001222

Schmitz, S., Fulker, D. W., & Mrazek, D. A. (1995). Problem behavior in early and middle childhood: An initial behavior genetic analysis. *Journal of Child Psychology and Psychiatry, 36*(8), 1443–1458. https://doi.org/10.1111/j.1469-7610.1995.tb01674.x

Silberg, J. L., Maes, H., & Eaves, L. J. (2010). Genetic and environmental influences on the transmission of parental depression to children's depression and conduct disturbance: An extended Children of Twins study. *Journal of Child Psychology and Psychiatry, 51*(6), 734–744. https://doi.org/10.1111/j.1469-7610.2010.02205.x

Silverman, W. K., Kurtines, W. M., Jaccard, J., & Pina, A. A. (2009). Directionality of change in youth anxiety treatment involving parents: An initial examination. *Journal of Consulting and Clinical Psychology, 77*(3), 474–485. https://doi.org/10.1037/a0015761

Silverman, W. K., Marin, C. E., Rey, Y., Jaccard, J., & Pettit, J. W. (2021). Directional effects of parent and child anxiety 1 year following treatment of child anxiety, and the mediational role of parent psychological control. *Depression and Anxiety, 38*(12), 1289–1297. https://doi.org/10.1002/da.23210

Singham, T., Viding, E., Schoeler, T., Arseneault, L., Ronald, A., Cecil, C. M., et al. (2017). Concurrent and longitudinal contribution of exposure to bullying in childhood to mental health: The role of vulnerability and resilience. *JAMA Psychiatry, 74*(11), 1112–1119. https://doi.org/10.1001/jamapsychiatry.2017.2678

Smith, A. K., Rhee, S. H., Corley, R. P., Friedman, N. P., Hewitt, J. K., & Robinson, J. L. (2012). The magnitude of genetic and environmental influences on parental and observational measures of behavioral inhibition and shyness in toddlerhood. *Behavior Genetics, 42*(5), 764–777. https://doi.org/10.1007/s10519-012-9551-0

Spence, S. H. (1998). A measure of anxiety symptoms among children. *Behaviour Research and Therapy, 36*(5), 545–566. https://doi.org/10.1016/s0005-7967(98)00034-5

Spence, S. H., Rapee, R., McDonald, C., & Ingram, M. (2001). The structure of anxiety symptoms among preschoolers. *Behaviour Research and Therapy, 39*(11), 1293–1316. https://doi.org/10.1016/s0005-7967(00)00098-x

Stefánsdóttir, I. H., Ivarsson, T., & Skarphedinsson, G. (2023). Efficacy and safety of serotonin reuptake inhibitors (SSRI) and serotonin noradrenaline reuptake inhibitors (SNRI) for children and adolescents with anxiety disorders: A systematic review and meta-analysis. *Nordic Journal of Psychiatry, 77*(2), 137–146. https://doi.org/10.1080/08039488.2022.2075460

Steinsbekk, S., Ranum, B., & Wichstrom, L. (2022). Prevalence and course of anxiety disorders and symptoms from preschool to adolescence: A 6-wave community study. *Journal of Child Psychology and Psychiatry, 63*, 527–534. https://doi.org/10.1111/jcpp.13487

Stevenson, J., Richman, N., & Graham, P. (1985). Behaviour problems and language abilities at 3 years and behavioural-deviance at 8 years. *Journal of Child Psychology and Psychiatry, 26*(2), 215–230. https://doi.org/10.1111/j.1469-7610.1985.tb02261.x

Stevenson, J., Batten, N., & Cherner, M. (1992). Fears and fearfulness in children and adolescents – A genetic-analysis of twin data. *Journal of Child Psychology and Psychiatry, 33*(6), 977–985. https://doi.org/10.1111/j.1469-7610.1992.tb00919.x

Stockings, E. A., Degenhardt, L., Dobbins, T., Lee, Y. Y., Erskine, H. E., Whiteford, H. A., & Patton, G. (2016). Preventing depression and anxiety in young people: A review of the joint efficacy of universal, selective and indicated prevention. *Psychological Medicine, 46*(1), 11–26. https://doi.org/10.1017/s0033291715001725

Su, Y. Y., D'Arcy, C., & Meng, X. F. (2021). Research review: Developmental origins of depression – A systematic review and meta-analysis. *Journal of Child Psychology and Psychiatry, 62*(9), 1050–1066. https://doi.org/10.1111/jcpp.13358

Sullivan, A. D. W., Forehand, R., Vreeland, A., & Compas, B. E. (2022). Does parenting explain the link between cumulative SES risk and child problems in the context of parental depression? *Child Psychiatry & Human Development, 53*, 330–341. https://doi.org/10.1007/s10578-021-01130-9

Tackett, J. L., Lahey, B. B., van Hulle, C., Waldman, I., Krueger, R. F., & Rathouz, P. J. (2013). Common genetic influences on negative emotionality and a general psychopathology factor in childhood and adolescence. *Journal of Abnormal Psychology, 122*(4), 1142–1153. https://doi.org/10.1037/a0034151

Tanguay-Garneau, L., Boivin, M., Feng, B., Matte-Landry, A., Brendgen, M., Vitaro, F., & Dionne, G. (2020). A genetic cross-lagged study of the longitudinal association between anxiety and depressive symptoms during childhood. *Behavior Genetics, 50*(2), 105–118. https://doi.org/10.1007/s10519-019-09988-1

Thapar, A., Collishaw, S., Pine, D. S., & Thapar, A. K. (2012). Depression in adolescence. *Lancet, 379*(9820), 1056–1067. https://doi.org/10.1016/s0140-6736(11)60871-4

Thorup, A. A. E., Laursen, T. M., Munk-Olsen, T., Ranning, A., Mortensen, P. B., Plessen, K. J., & Nordentoft, M. (2018). Incidence of child and adolescent mental disorders in children aged 0-17 with familial high risk for severe mental illness – A Danish register study. *Schizophrenia Research, 197*, 298–304. https://doi.org/10.1016/j.schres.2017.11.009

Trzaskowski, M., Zavos, H. M. S., Haworth, C. M. A., Plomin, R., & Eley, T. C. (2012). Stable genetic influence on anxiety-related behaviours across middle childhood. *Journal of Abnormal Child Psychology, 40*(1), 85–94. https://doi.org/10.1007/s10802-011-9545-z

Trzaskowski, M., Dale, P. S., & Plomin, R. (2013). No genetic influence for childhood behavior problems from DNA analysis. *Journal of the American Academy of Child and Adolescent Psychiatry, 52*(10), 1048–1056. https://doi.org/10.1016/j.jaac.2013.07.016

van den Oord, E., Verhulst, F. C., & Boomsma, D. I. (1996). A genetic study of maternal and paternal ratings of problem behaviors in 3-year-old twins. *Journal of Abnormal Psychology, 105*(3), 349–357. https://doi.org/10.1037/0021-843x.105.3.349

Vos, T., Allen, C., Arora, M., Barber, R. M., Bhutta, Z. A., Brown, A., et al. (2016). Global, regional, and national incidence, prevalence, and years lived with disability for 310 diseases and injuries, 1990-2015: A systematic analysis for the Global Burden of Disease Study 2015. *Lancet, 388*(10053), 1545–1602. https://doi.org/10.1016/s0140-6736(16)31678-6

Vuorre, M., Orben, A., & Przybylski, A. K. (2021). There is no evidence that associations between adolescents' digital technology engagement and mental health problems have increased. *Clinical Psychological Science, 9*(5), 823–835. https://doi.org/10.1177/2167702621994549

Vuorre, M., Johannes, N., Magnusson, K., & Przybylski, A. K. (2022). Time spent playing video games is unlikely to impact wellbeing. *Royal Society Open Science, 9*, 220411. https://doi.org/10.1098/rsos.220411

Walkup, J. T., Albano, A. M., Piacentini, J., Birmaher, B., Compton, S. N., Sherrill, J. T., et al. (2008). Cognitive behavioral therapy, sertraline, or a combination in childhood anxiety. *New England Journal of Medicine, 359*(26), 2753–2766. https://doi.org/10.1056/NEJMoa0804633

Waszczuk, M. A., Zavos, H. M. S., Gregory, A. M., & Eley, T. C. (2014). The phenotypic and genetic structure of depression and anxiety disorder symptoms in childhood, adolescence, and young adulthood. *JAMA Psychiatry, 71*(8), 905–916. https://doi.org/10.1001/jamapsychiatry.2014.655

Waszczuk, M. A., Zavos, H. M. S., Gregory, A. M., & Eley, T. C. (2016). The stability and change of etiological influences on depression, anxiety symptoms and their co-occurrence across adolescence and young adulthood. *Psychological Medicine, 46*(1), 161–175. https://doi.org/10.1017/s0033291715001634

Weersing, V. R., Brent, D. A., Rozenman, M. S., Gonzalez, A., Jeffreys, M., Dickerson, J. F., et al. (2017). Brief behavioral therapy for pediatric anxiety and depression in primary care: A randomized clinical trial. *JAMA Psychiatry, 74*(6), 571–578. https://doi.org/10.1001/jamapsychiatry.2017.0429

Weisz, J. R., Kuppens, S., Ng, M. Y., Eckshtain, D., Ugueto, A. M., Vaughn-Coaxum, R., et al. (2017). What five decades of research tells us about the effects of youth psychological therapy: A multilevel meta-analysis and implications for science and practice. *American Psychologist, 72*(2), 79–117. https://doi.org/10.1037/a0040360

Weisz, J. R., Kuppens, S., Ng, M. Y., Vaughn-Coaxum, R. A., Ugueto, A. M., Eckshtain, D., & Corteselli, K. A. (2019). Are psychotherapies for young people growing stronger? Tracking trends over time for youth anxiety, depression, attention-deficit/hyperactivity disorder, and conduct problems. *Perspectives on Psychological Science, 14*(2), 216–237. https://doi.org/10.1177/1745691618805436

Wergeland, G. J. H., Riise, E. N., & Ost, L. G. (2021). Cognitive behavior therapy for internalizing disorders in children and adolescents in routine clinical care: A systematic review and meta-analysis. *Clinical Psychology Review, 83*, 101918. https://doi.org/10.1016/j.cpr.2020.101918

Werner-Seidler, A., Perry, Y., Calear, A. L., Newby, J. M., & Christensen, H. (2017). School-based depression and anxiety prevention programs for young people: A systematic review and meta-analysis. *Clinical Psychology Review, 51*, 30–47. https://doi.org/10.1016/j.cpr.2016.10.005

Whalen, D. J., Luby, J. L., Tilman, R., Mike, A., Barch, D., & Belden, A. C. (2016). Latent class profiles of depressive symptoms from early to middle childhood: Predictors, outcomes, and gender effects. *Journal of Child Psychology and Psychiatry, 57*(7), 794–804. https://doi.org/10.1111/jcpp.12518

Whalen, D. J., Sylvester, C. M., & Luby, J. L. (2017). Depression and anxiety in preschoolers: A review of the past 7 years. *Child and Adolescent Psychiatry Clinics of North America, 26*(3), 503–522. https://doi.org/10.1016/j.chc.2017.02.006

Williamson, D. E., Birmaher, B., Dahl, R. E., & Ryan, N. D. (2005). Stressful life events in anxious and depressed children. *Journal of Child and Adolescent Psychopharmacology, 15*(4), 571–580. https://doi.org/10.1089/cap.2005.15.571

Yew, S. G. K., & O'Kearney, R. (2013). Emotional and behavioural outcomes later in childhood and adolescence for children with specific language impairments: Meta-analyses of controlled prospective studies. *Journal of Child Psychology and Psychiatry, 54*(5), 516–524. https://doi.org/10.1111/jcpp.12009

Zahn-Waxler, C., Klimes-Dougan, B., & Slattery, M. J. (2000). Internalizing problems of childhood and adolescence: Prospects, pitfalls, and progress in understanding the development of anxiety and depression. *Development and Psychopathology, 12*(3), 443–466. https://doi.org/10.1017/s0954579400003102

Zahn-Waxler, C., Shirtcliff, E. A., & Marceau, K. (2008). Disorders of childhood and adolescence: Gender and psychopathology. *Annual Review of Clinical Psychology, 4*, 275–303. https://doi.org/10.1146/annurev.clinpsy.3.022806.091358

Zalsman, G., Hawton, K., Wasserman, D., van Heeringen, K., Arensman, E., Sarchiapone, M., et al. (2016). Suicide prevention strategies revisited: 10-year systematic review. *Lancet Psychiatry, 3*(7), 646–659. https://doi.org/10.1016/s2215-0366(16)30030-x

Zavos, H. M. S., Gregory, A. M., & Eley, T. C. (2012). Longitudinal genetic analysis of anxiety sensitivity. *Developmental Psychology, 48*(1), 204–212. https://doi.org/10.1037/a0024996

Zeytinoglu, S., Neuman, K. J., Degnan, K. A., Almas, A. N., Henderson, H., Chronis-Tuscano, A., et al. (2022). Pathways from maternal shyness to adolescent social anxiety. *Journal of Child Psychology and Psychiatry, 63*(3), 342–349. https://doi.org/10.1111/jcpp.13477

Zhang-James, Y., Clay, J. W. S., Aber, R. B., Gamble, H. M., & Faraone, S. V. (2023). *Mental health crisis in children and adolescents with COVID-19: A retrospective cohort study of over seven million youth from electronic health records*. Available at https://doi.org/10.2139/ssrn.4410789

Zhou, A. M., & Buss, K. A. (2021). Trajectories of internalizing symptoms in early childhood: Associations with maternal internalizing symptoms and child physiology. *Developmental Psychobiology, 63*, 1295–1308. https://doi.org/10.1002/dev.22104

Zhou, X. Y., Teng, T., Zhang, Y. Q., Del Giovane, C., Furukawa, T. A., Weisz, J. R., et al. (2020). Comparative efficacy and acceptability of antidepressants, psychotherapies, and their combination for acute treatment of children and adolescents with depressive disorder: A systematic review and network meta-analysis. *Lancet Psychiatry, 7*(7), 581–601. https://doi.org/10.1016/S2215-0366(20)30137-1

Chapter 8
Externalising Problems

8.1 Structure of Externalising Problems

There is a wide range of terms that are used to refer to externalising behaviour problems. These include the diagnostic categories of conduct disorder (CD) and oppositional-defiant disorder (ODD). ODD is defined as a recurrent pattern of negativistic, defiant, disobedient, and hostile behaviours. CD is the repetitive and persistent violation of the basic rights of others and societal norms. These two diagnoses are clearly related, with the earlier developing ODD often leading to subsequent CD. A broad umbrella term of antisocial behaviour (AB) refers to this constellation of aggressive and disruptive behaviour. The HiTOP framework, developed to account for behavioural disorders in adults, includes an externalising superspectrum of behaviours (Krueger et al., 2021). This framework identifies a common set of underlying features of behaviours related to broad subsets of externalising – disinhibition and antagonism.

There is good evidence for the distinction between two components of externalising behaviour in children and adolescents – rule-breaking behaviour and aggressive behaviour. These two dimensions emerged as distinct in confirmatory factor analyses (CFAs) of items from parents' ratings on the CBCL for 58,051 6 to 18-year-olds across 30 disparate societies (Ivanova et al., 2007). Rule-breaking is indicated by delinquent or antisocial behaviours such as "lying or cheating", "stealing at home", and "setting fire". Aggressive behaviour includes conduct disorder behaviours such as "fights", "cruelty, bullying, or meanness to others", and "destroys his/her own things". These two patterns of behaviour are aggregated under the heading of externalising behaviour but have somewhat distinct characteristics.

Cheong and Raudenbush (2000) showed that, although these two subscales were highly associated, they had distinct correlates. For example rule-breaking or delinquency was shown to increase with age between 9 and 15 years but aggression did not. Rule-breaking/delinquency was significantly greater in boys but no sex

J. Stevenson, *Developmental Psychopathology*,
https://doi.org/10.1007/978-3-031-45787-6_8

difference was seen for aggressive behaviour. This suggests that although the subscales can be combined to indicate a child's overall level of externalising behaviour, it would be prudent to keep them apart in studies investigating the origins and consequences of rule-breaking and aggression.

Kliem et al. (2018) produced indicators of core elements of disruptive behaviour in 2–6-year-old children based on scores from the Eyberg Child Behavior Inventory (ECBI) (Eyberg & Ross, 1978) and the Strengths and Difficulties Questionnaire (SDQ) (Goodman, 1997). These elements were temper loss, aggression, noncompliance, and low concern for others. They applied taxometric methods to test whether the scores on these elements could be construed as categories. These included comparison curve fit indices (CCFI) which can differentiate between categorical and dimensional latent structures (see Sect. 5.3). They found that the latent structure of disruptive behaviours in these preschool children was essentially dimensional without sub-groups or classes. They argue that intervention efforts should be organised by tailoring treatment intensity to the position of the child on this dimension of severity.

Psychopathy Psychopathy is a specific form of externalising behaviour which can be conceptualised either as a category or as a dimension. There is not a consensus definition of psychopathy but it is generally accepted that psychopathy comprises three components: interpersonal traits (e.g. grandiose-manipulative), affective traits (e.g. callous-unemotional), and behaviour traits (e.g. impulsive-irresponsible and daring-impulse) (da Silva et al., 2020). A triarchic formulation using slightly different labels was suggested by Patrick et al. (2009). This comprises disinhibition, meanness, and boldness. An early difficult temperament and low fear are thought to play an important role in initiating the development of these psychopathy traits. In children and adolescents the formulation of psychopathy places an emphasis on callous-unemotional (CU) traits such as a lack of empathy, lack of guilt, and shallow emotions and antisocial behaviour.

It has been argued that it is more appropriate to consider psychopathy as a behaviour that demonstrates marked individual differences but is not a distinct taxonomic category (Edens et al., 2006). This has been concluded most forcibly by Sellbom and Drislane (2021), who stated that

> the research to date is largely unequivocal in that there is no support for psychopathy as a categorical construct ... (Sellbom and Drislane (2021), p. 2)

Psychopathy and Criminality There has been a debate concerning the place of criminal behaviour in the formulation of psychopathy. It has been argued that criminal behaviour is a correlate or a consequence and not a core component of psychopathy (Skeem & Cooke, 2010). One related issue is the separation of psychopathy from antisocial behaviour (AB). On the basis of the analysis of twin data Viding et al. (2005) showed that CU was a trait with a high heritability. Moreover those children demonstrating high callous-unemotional traits (CU) had AB with a very high heritability. By contrast those with high AB but low CU were subject to a less strong genetic influence on AB but to a moderate influence of the shared environment. This suggests that high levels of AB in general may be influenced by a range of social and genetic influences. However when high AB is found associated with high levels of CU, as in psychopathy, both AB and CU are strongly influenced by genetic factors.

Parenting and Psychopathy There is evidence from a study of differences in CU trait scores in monozygotic twins that these are related to aspects of parenting such as harshness and warmth (Waller et al., 2018). They concluded that parenting is related to child CU traits and aggression, over and above genetically mediated effects, with low parental warmth being a unique environmental correlate of CU traits. Although such a study can control for genetic influences it cannot differentiate the direction of effects: does such parenting lead to CU or does CU foster these behaviours from parents? However this group of authors also conducted an adoption study that suggested that positive reinforcement by mothers could reduce the risk of CU traits that might arise from a child having biological mother who showed antisocial behaviour (Hyde et al., 2016). There is some preliminary evidence that early intervention in parenting can modify amygdala-prefrontal cortex connectivity and via this change enhance the development of emotion regulation (Valadez et al., 2023). These changes were seen in a randomised controlled trial of nurturance training for parents and provide preliminary evidence that adverse parenting can have a causal effect on brain development.

A related set of analyses was undertaken by Perlstein et al. (2022). They showed that low social affiliation (measured by variables, including social engagement, positive effect, enthusiasm and interest in the surroundings), at age 2 years was predictive of callous-unemotional behaviours 1 year later at age 3 years. However this association was only seen for children who experience low levels of parental positivity. This suggests that parental positivity, as index by parents reporting, for example, warm feeling when thinking about their child, may act in concert with the effects of early low social affiliation to influence the emergence of callous-unemotional behaviours. Parenting quality has also been found to moderate the risk of CU traits in older children. In a study of 600 twin pairs aged 6–11 years, Tomlinson et al. (2021) found that the heritability of CU traits decreased with increasing parental warmth and decreasing harshness.

Genetics and Psychopathy There is good evidence that CU traits are heritable with heritability (h^2) between 0.36 and 0.67, and there is some evidence to suggest that the serotonin and oxytocin systems may play a role in CU traits (Moore et al., 2019). However molecular genetic studies have yet to identify specific genetic loci that are significantly associated with CU traits. One of the difficulties in establishing such association may lie in the variability of CU traits. A longitudinal study of 8958 twin pairs found that the risk of a high CU trait was highly heritable ($h^2 = 0.76$) but a different set of genes with a lower heritability ($h^2 = 0.44$) were responsible, with non-shared environmental factors, for subsequent changes in the level of CU with age (Takahashi et al., 2021).

The need for such a developmental perspective on psychopathy was elaborated by Blair et al. (2006). They argued that genetic factors are primarily responsible for the development of the core emotional dysfunction in psychopathy, that is, CU traits. They suggest that the effects of these genetic risk factors are mediated via atypical functional development of the amygdala and orbital/ventrolateral frontal cortex. This view has been supported by more recent imaging studies (Blair & Zhang, 2020). The developmental perspective also underpins an understanding of early emerging psychopathy traits being linked with psychopathy in adulthood. This link has been demonstrated in longitudinal studies. For example, Lynam et al. (2007) found a correlation of $r = 0.31$ between psychopathy measured at age 13 years and 24 years.

8.2 Stability of Externalising Problems

The starting point for consideration of continuities in antisocial behaviour has to be the studies conducted by Lee Robins (e.g. Robins, 1966). These are landmark studies in psychiatric epidemiology and laid the foundations for the investigation of links between disorders in childhood and adulthood. Robins (1978) summarised the longitudinal findings on antisocial behaviour in four cohorts of males in the United States and concluded that

> … (1) adult antisocial behaviour virtually requires childhood antisocial behaviour; (2) most antisocial children do not become antisocial adults; (3) the variety of antisocial behaviour in childhood is a better predictor of adult antisocial behaviour than is any particular behaviour; (4) adult antisocial behaviour is better predicted by childhood behaviour than by family background or social class of rearing; (5) social class makes little contribution to the prediction of serious adult antisocial behaviour. (Robins (1978), p. 611)

The pattern of changes within childhood and adolescence in internalising and externalising behaviours was studied longitudinally in a representative sample of 2076 children by Bongers et al. (2003). They found that the trajectories were linearly increasing for internalising but decreasing for externalising between the ages of 4 and 18 years. Girls had a higher level of internalising, and this difference became more marked as the children aged. Boys had higher externalising scores, but in this case the difference between the mean scores for the sexes declined with age. Gustafsson et al. (2018) showed in a longitudinal study of a general population sample from Sweden that children's conduct problems decrease over the ages of 3–5 years. However children with higher levels of hyperactivity at age 3 have less of a reduction in conduct problems over time.

The development and course of conduct problems in children were studied between the ages of 3 and 11 years in a large nationally representative sample by Gutman et al. (2018). They identified four distinct trajectories of these behaviours that were present in both boys and girls. These trajectories were "low", "early-onset, desisting", "early-onset persistent", and "school onset". They found socio-economic deprivation to be associated with both early-onset groups in both boys and girls. The risk factors for early onset in boys, but not for girls, were being raised by a single parent, maternal detachment, and a neglectful attitude among parents. A subsequent report on this sample extended the analysis up to age 14 and an adolescent onset group emerged. It was striking that all the trajectories where conduct problems were present were associated with maternal smoking during pregnancy (Gutman et al., 2019).

The importance of considering genetic and environmental risk factors as acting in concert has been shown in relation to the stability of externalising behaviours (Womack et al., 2021). They found that genetic factors moderated the link between familiar instability and the course of aggressive behaviour. Using a PRS it was seen that children with lower levels of family instability and lower polygenic risk demonstrated a more rapid decline in aggression between the ages 7 and 14 years. Plomin et al. (2022) also used PRS to test whether genes are moderating the impact of environmental risks on behaviour problems. Using a sample of 6687 twins for whom behaviour measures were available at ages 7, 9, and 12, they found evidence for effects from genes, environmental risks, and GxE. Although the effects were small, GxE effects were often found to contribute to the development of hyperactivity/inattention and conduct problems across these ages.

Longitudinal studies have shown that there is a group of children with early-onset conduct problems that can be distinguished from those with consistently low-conduct problem scores. The factors contributing to this risk are male sex, poor inhibitory control, maternal depression, harsh parenting, and limited parental education (Shaw et al., 2019).

Adolescence-Limited and Life-Course-Persistent Antisocial Behaviour In 1993 Moffitt produced a landmark paper that drew the distinction between adolescence-limited (AL) and life-course-persistent (LCP) antisocial behaviour. These two groups of children are distinguished by the duration of their antisocial behaviour. A small group of almost exclusively boys, perhaps 5% of the population, showed LCP and for whom antisocial behaviour is evident in early child and is shown persistently through adolescence into adulthood. By contrast a larger group of AL children show antisocial behaviour only during their adolescent years.

Moffitt (1993) suggested that the LCP group has a history of difficulties whose origins lie in disrupted neural development early in life. These are associated with two neuropsychological deficits. The first are difficulties in processing verbal material such receptive listening and reading, expressive speech, and memory. The second are deficits in executive functions and self-control. A major feature of this framework is that children with these neuropsychological deficits are likely to live in families that are less able to provide the support they may need to avoid developing antisocial behaviour. Indeed such families may provide an environment that fosters the development of such behaviours – an example of a correlation between biological and environmental risks.

Children who show AL antisocial behaviour represent a group with more "normative" development. They constitute a larger section of the population and for whom antisocial behaviour is restricted to a limited period of their adolescent years.

The antisocial behaviours shown by the AL group are primarily nonaggressive. This group experiences a "maturity gap", where, in many societies, they are excluded from being entitled to engage in the social activities and responsibilities of adulthood but at the same time are undergoing the biological transition to adulthood associated with puberty. An important aspect of Moffitt's theorising is that at this same time these adolescents are developing contacts with older adolescents who have adopted antisocial behaviours as a way of coping with the alienation created by the "maturity gap". These older adolescents provide a role model and will include those in the LCP group. There is an incentive to mimic the behaviour of the LCP adolescents, and this behaviour is reinforced by their demonstration of independence from childhood constraints. In addition there are gains from the negative consequences of crime imposed by society but which are valued by the adolescent's peer group.

This theoretical formulation by Moffitt (1993) was largely based on findings from the Dunedin study (Poulton et al., 2023). It has been supported by subsequent research on LCP antisocial behaviour (Assink et al., 2015; Eme, 2020). However there are suggestions that the AL group may be prone to antisocial behaviours that persist into adulthood and that these behaviours are also associated with biologically based deficits in cognition and emotion processing (Fairchild et al., 2013). The primacy of temperament and neuropsychological functioning in influencing LCP antisocial behaviour has been questioned by Aguilar et al. (2000). They suggest that the children's early psychosocial history as measured by maternal depression, life stress, and the quality of care in the home was of greater importance in distinguishing the LCP and AL groups.

In Odgers et al. (2008) the framework of trajectories of antisocial behaviour, based on the Dunedin study data, was extended to four groups: life-course-persistent (LCP) [sometimes referred to as early-onset persistent (EOP)], adolescent onset (AO), childhood-limited (CL), and low antisocial (LA). A systematic review and meta-analysis of studies examining the psychosocial outcome of these groups in early adulthood was undertaken by Bevilacqua et al. (2018). They identified 13 studies that met their inclusion criteria. The LA group had the lowest risk of an adverse outcome. The groups showing antisocial behaviour at some stage all are at high risk compared to the LA group in the following order from highest risk to lower: EOP, AO, and then CL.

8.3 Risk Factors for Externalising Problems

Gender One of the strongest risk factors for externalising problems is gender. The prevalence of conduct disorder is approximately 2–3 times higher in boys than in girls (Moffitt et al., 2008). Bayer et al. (2012) showed that this higher rate in boys is evident from an early age. They investigated the risk factors for externalising in a general population sample of 733 Australian children during the preschool period.

The strongest predictors of externalising behaviours at 5 years of age were male sex, harsh discipline, and maternal stress.

There is evidence that there are sex differences in the presentation of externalising problems. For example, in conduct disorder the frequency of comorbid conditions is greater in girls. These girls show greater functional impairments, and the age of onset is later in girls than boys, often not being shown until adolescence (Konrad et al., 2021). There is some evidence that the origins of antisocial behaviour are different in boys and girls (Burt et al., 2018). When measured by teacher reports genetic factors were more important for girls and environmental factors more important for boys. However this difference was not detected in ratings of behaviour obtained from mothers.

Adverse Childhood Experiences The background to the term adverse childhood experiences (ACE) is given in Chap. 7. Appleyard et al. (2005) investigated the cumulative nature of risk factors associated with early experience of violent and unstable homes. This used measures of child maltreatment, inter-parental violence, family disruption, low socio-economic status, and high parental stress. The cumulative ACE score from these risk factors in early childhood was significantly linearly related to externalising problems at age 16 years. The prediction of internalising scores in adolescence fell just short of statistical significance. The presence of multiple risks in early childhood continued to have a significant effect even after considering the effect of middle childhood risk. Evans et al. (2008) reviewed the evidence specifically on exposure to domestic violence and behaviour in children from 60 studies. The effect size of such exposure was similar for internalising and externalising: SMD = 0.48 and 0.47, respectively. These effects were stronger on boys than on girls.

Dodge et al. (1990) used a prospective study of 4-year-old children to examine the specific association between the experience of physical abuse and later aggressive behaviour. There was a threefold increase in the risk of a high score on teacher-rated aggression in children who had been "harmed' compared to those who were not. The measure of being "harmed' was based on an interview with the mother and referred physical abuse of the child in the time period before the age of 4. This category represented 15% of this general population sample. This elevated risk was not due to low socio-economic status, single parenthood, marital dissolution, and marital violence or child health problems and temperament. Dodge et al. (1990) conclude that physical abuse per se leads to a cycle of violence.

The number of children and adolescents experiencing abuse or victimisation in the United Kingdom was estimated by Radford et al. (2013). In the under 11-year-olds 2.5% had had experience of some kind of abuse from a parent in the past year – the figure was 6% for those aged 11–17 years old. Abuse is not only associated with later aggressive behaviour and criminal offending (Malvaso et al., 2018); it can have a lifelong impact on a range of aspects of well-being and social functioning (Stevenson, 1999). Sexualised behaviour is particularly associated with a history of sexual abuse. The risk of developing persistent sexualised behaviour during childhood is increased if the child also develops externalising problems, but it is not exacerbated by the presence of internalising problems (Ensink et al., 2018).

Currie and Widom (2010) found the level of unemployment in those individuals with histories of abuse/neglect to be 14% higher compared to controls controlling for background characteristics. They found the effects of abuse to be greater on women than on men. However many children appear to be resilient in the face of early physical abuse (Rutter, 2013). In a follow-up study of the Isle of Wight sample (Rutter et al., 1970), Collishaw et al. (2007) found that 45% of abused children showed no psychiatric disorder in adulthood. But what is unclear is just how psychological characteristics of the child interact with broader social influences to facilitate a more optimal outcome for those experiencing adversity and maltreatment (Cicchetti, 2013).

Bullying and Victimisation Attempts are being made to develop methods for assembling data that could be used to predict which of those experiencing abuse or bullying might be more vulnerable to develop later psychopathology. Meehan et al. (2020) used 22 indicators based on the child's own characteristics and those of family and community to predict psychopathology at age 18 years amongst those victimised before the age of 12 years. Only 40% of these children did not demonstrate either an internalising or externalising disorder at age 18 years. The risk calculator showed a promising accuracy of prediction for the individual child. Potentially this could be used to detect vulnerable children but further developmental testing is needed.

Schaefer et al. (2018) addressed directly the question of whether there was a causal relationship between adolescent victimisation and later psychopathology. Victimisation was measured as exposure to domestic violence between the mother and her partner, frequent bullying by peers, physical maltreatment by an adult, sexual abuse, emotional abuse and neglect, and physical neglect. Using design features from their longitudinal twin study they were able to rule out a number of non-causal reasons for the association between victimisation and psychopathology. They concluded that very different types of victimisation appear to predict similarly poor mental health above that expected from baseline measures in childhood. This risk related to the generalised liability to psychiatric disorder (the "p factor"), and this was independent of family background and genetic risk.

Bevilaqua et al. (2021) showed how a range of adverse childhood experiences (ACE) before the age of 3 years are associated with continuing internalising and externalising problems through childhood and into adolescence. This association is shown both when aggregated into an overall ACE score and for individual ACEs. Some ACEs were most strongly associated with internalising, for example, parental depression and parental discord, and others with externalising, for example, harsh parenting and physical punishment. As the authors recognise, the results presented in this paper cannot identify the causal relationships between the ACEs and outcome. For example, the association between parental characteristics and internalising might not represent a causal relationship but rather arises from genetic factors shared between both.

There is strong evidence that criminality in parents is linked to criminality in the child. Besemer et al. (2017) undertook a systematic review and meta-analysis of studies relating to intergenerational transmission of criminal behaviour. They found that, based on 21 samples, children of parents with a history of criminal behaviour were at a substantially greater risk of criminal behaviour themselves, OR = 2.38 ($CI_{.95}$ 2.18 to 2.60). This review could not differentiate between social and biological mechanisms that might contribute to the transmission of risk.

Parenting A meta-analysis of studies on less extreme variations in parental care found that parenting accounted for less than 6% of the variance in child externalising problems and disorders (Rothbaum & Weisz, 1994). Barnes et al. (2013) made clear the complexities of the relationship between aspects of parenting and the development of externalising problems in preschool children. They showed that both passive and evocative gene–environment correlations were involved.

The possibility that abuse experienced by mothers in their own childhood might increase the risk of problems in their children was examined in a meta-analysis by Loheide-Niesmann et al. (2022). They found that data from 39 studies indicated a small but significant effect of maternal childhood maltreatment and externalising problems in their children. These cross-generational effects were shown to be mediated by maternal depression and their offspring's exposure to maltreatment.

Impulsivity Bell et al. (2021) tested a "trait impulsivity" theory of externalising behaviours. This theory postulates that early emerging features of hyperactivity and impulsivity represent markers of an underlying deficit in the mesolimbic dopamine system. This system includes neural projections from the ventral tegmental area to the nucleus accumbens and ventral regions of the caudate nucleus and putamen (Beauchaine et al., 2017). These impulsivity behaviours are predictive of later emerging oppositional-defiant behaviour and subsequent conduct problems. Bell et al. (2021) found this progression of externalising behaviours in the 685 children they followed longitudinally. Support for the impulsivity theory was found by Ahmad and Hinshaw (2017) in a longitudinal study of 228 girls in young adulthood. In this group hyperactive/impulsive behaviours in middle childhood were predictive of externalising behaviours in adolescence and early adulthood. Inattentive symptoms were not predictive.

Prenatal and Perinatal Risks There is evidence that experiences before birth can influence the development of later behaviour in the child. It has been suggested that prenatal caffeine exposure has been found to have an effect on externalising behaviour as strong as that of prenatal alcohol and cannabis exposure (Zhang et al., 2022). This same study showed altered brain structures arising from prenatal caffeine exposure. Factors such as maternal smoking, alcohol, toxins/drugs, nutrition, and infection during pregnancy can have an effect often mediated by restriction on foetal growth (Schlotz & Phillips, 2009). The interpretation of the putative causal relationship between these antenatal risks and later behaviour needs to be treated with caution, not least as some of the effects may arise through common genetic effects (Thapar & Rutter, 2009). However an analysis of data pooled from a number of twin studies on over 60,000 children has suggested that maternal smoking in pregnancy has a small impact on aggression in childhood and adolescence (Malanchini et al.,

2019). The effect, explaining less than 1% of the variance, remains when other potential confounding factors were controlled including maternal stress during pregnancy, gestation age, length of breastfeeding, and socio-demographic factors, such as parental education and occupation.

The development of polygenic risk scores (PRS) (see Sect. 3.4) has provided a method to control possible genetic confounds in studies of prenatal effects. Luo et al. (2022) used PRS scores for aggressive behaviour in an analysis of the relationship between maternal anxiety, depression, and hostility during pregnancy and child externalising problems at age 6 years. Self-regulated compliance was measured at age 3 years and was considered as a possible mediator of the effect of maternal mental state in pregnancy and later externalising problems. The analysis showed that self-regulated compliance mediated between maternal prenatal mental health and externalising problems at 6 years and was significant even after genetic factors had been controlled using the PRS scores.

Social and Biological Changes During Adolescence There are marked changes in brain structural and brain function associated with puberty (Vijayakumar et al., 2018). Some of these changes have a significant impact on aspects of cognition and social functioning (Blakemore & Choudhury, 2006). For example, there is evidence from an fMRI study that there are puberty-related changes in brain regions involved in risky decision-making (Goddings et al., 2023). This study did not establish the link with self-reported risky behaviour in this sample of boys.

It is unclear just what significance these changes in brain development associated with puberty have for behaviour (Vijayakumar et al., 2018).

Indeed it has been argued that behavioural change in adolescence arises from social causes such as family disharmony, examination stress, and exposure to social media (Graham, 2019) rather than brain changes. These social influences are exacerbated by the "maturity gap" (Moffitt, 1993) (see above). This gap has arisen as a result of improved health and nutrition producing earlier puberty onset and concomitant social changes that have resulted in deferred entry to the adult workforce and its associated responsibilities. This has led adolescents to experience what Moffitt labels a "5- to 10-year role vacuum". However the notion that adolescence is a period of extreme behavioural change has been called into question (Rutter et al., 1976). Although feelings of misery and self-deprecation are common at this age, the increase in psychiatric conditions is not marked. Furthermore, those disorders arising in adolescence have a similar prognosis to those arising in younger children.

Poor Educational Attainment The association of externalising problems and poor academic attainment and reading retardation was identified in the early epidemiological studies in the Isle of Wight and Inner London (Rutter et al., 1970, 1975). It is now possible to examine the possible causes of this association in large samples of twins. Vuoksimaa et al. (2021) used data from 27,000 twin children and found a robust negative association between aggression and academic performance. The association was explained in part by shared genetic effects and in part by shared environmental effects. Over and above these genetic and environmental influences, there was evidence of a negative association between aggression and academic performance which suggests that these characteristics influence one another. However it was not possible within this study to determine the direction of effects, that is, does poor attainment produce aggressive behaviour or vice versa? There is an indication that attention problems may lead to underachievement in a longitudinal study of 1577 Dutch children (Schuurmans et al., 2022). Attention problems at 6 years were associated with academic underachievement (in relation to that expected from IQ) at age 12 years when concurrent mental health problems were controlled.

8.4 Genetics and Externalising Problems

Twin Studies There have been a number of studies on twins to identify the role of genetic and environmental influences on externalising problems. A twin study of 3-year-old children found the following estimates for externalising from quantitative genetic analyses genetic – $h^2 = 0.60$, shared environment – $c^2 = 0.20$, non-shared environment $e^2 = 0.20$ (van den Oord et al., 1996). These results were supported by a later study of a larger sample of Dutch twins (Derks et al., 2004). Schmitz et al. (1995) also conducted a twin study on two samples of young twins aged 3 years and 8 years. At 3 years of age externalising problems were influenced by the following components: $h^2 = 0.34$, $c^2 = 0.45$, $e^2 = 0.36$; and at 8 years $h^2 = 0.57$, $c^2 = 0.38$, $e^2 = 0.24$. A meta-analysis of 51 twin and adoption studies estimated the role of genetic and environmental influences on antisocial behaviour across the life span (Rhee & Waldman, 2002). The best-fitting model found the following proportions of variance due to additive genetic influences (0.32), non-additive genetic influences (0.09), shared environmental influences (0.16), and non-shared environmental influences (0.43).

A twin study has shown that genetics plays a role in the persistence of delinquent rule-breaking behaviour, with $h^2 = 0.67$ (Isen et al., 2022). The heritability of aggression was estimated on a very large sample of 42,468 twins obtained by pooling data from five large European twin cohorts (Luningham et al., 2020). They obtained an overall heritability of 0.60, with slightly higher values in boys (0.64) than in girls (0.58). There is also evidence from two large longitudinally studied cohorts, one from Australia and the other from the Netherlands, that the genetic influences on aggressive behaviour that are expressed in childhood continue to be influential into middle adulthood and beyond (van der Laan et al., 2021).

Adoption Studies Sellers et al. (2020) conducted a longitudinal study of adoptive parents and adopted children that also included information on the biological mother. Such design can identify family-based environmental influences on the child independent of shared parental genetic factors. They found that genetic liability influences early child temperamental attributes (e.g. impulsivity), and these temperament features evoked maternal hostility that contributed to the development of both ADHD and aggression.

Molecular Genetic Studies Molecular genetic studies have attempted to identify specific genes linked to aggressive behaviour. It is suggested that polymorphisms (rs7632287 and rs4564970) in the oxytocin receptor gene may independently influence antisocial behaviour in adolescent boys (Hovey et al., 2016). This finding was replicated in two independent samples. In a subsequent review of studies on the oxytocin receptor gene, Kohlhoff et al. (2022) concluded that, although there was some inconsistency in the results, oxytocin receptor gene polymorphism showed both direct effect on conduct disorder and that gene–environment interactions were also found. Pappa et al. (2016) applied GWAS to aggressive behaviour using a pooled sample of 18,988 children and found that common variants at a specific site on chromosome 2 (2p12) are associated with childhood aggression. To date this association has not been replicated.

There is evidence from a GWAS meta-analysis of data from over 85,000 individuals that implicates the FOXP2 gene in the development of antisocial behaviour (ASB) (Tielbeek et al., 2022). It is of interest that this same gene has been found to be associated with ADHD (Demontis et al., 2019). Initially FOXP2 was shown to be associated with language disorders (Lai et al., 2001; Vernes et al., 2008). A wide range of laboratory studies on the biology of FOXP2 have shown it to play a crucial role in brain development and function (den Hoed et al., 2021). Although this evidence from a number of independent studies suggests that FOXP2 variation is implicated in disorders of cognition and behaviour, Tielbeek et al. (2022) are cautious about its significance. They say:

> … it is premature to over-interpret the FOXP2 findings here. SNPs at this locus have been associated, through GWAS, with a range of externalizing traits, including ADHD, cannabis use disorder, and generalized risk tolerance. Given the involvement of SNPS at this locus in different behavioral traits and diagnoses, and considering the small effect sizes, it is clear the association of FOXP2 variation with ASB has limited explanatory value on its own. That said, nothing yet precludes the possibility that this SNP may help to yield deeper insights once placed in broader context by future research. (Tielbeek et al. (2022), p. 4458)

Grotzinger et al. (2019) developed a powerful multivariate GWAS technique for the identification of genes influencing traits that vary on continua. They labelled this technique genomic structural equation modelling (genomic SEM). Genomic SEM was used by Linnér et al. (2021) to explore the association between gene variants and externalising behaviour. They calculated a PRS based on a weighted sum of the genes identified as being associated with externalising in a GWAS of over 1.5 million people. This PRS was able to explain 10% of the variance in a common factor measure underlying seven measures of externalising behaviour. This study identified over 500 genetic variants associated with externalising behaviour. Linnér et al. (2021) suggest that the implicated genes have early neurodevelopmental effects, which are then associated with behavioural patterns that have repercussions across the life span. They hypothesise that deficits in self-regulation carry this neurodevelopmental risk for a wide range of adverse social and health outcomes.

Gene–Environment Interactions There is evidence that monoamine oxidase A (MAOA) may play a role in increasing the risk of antisocial behaviour, specifically aggression. MAOA is involved in regulating the action of neurotransmitters in the brain. One version of the MAOA gene is associated with a low level of MAOA activity. Caspi et al. (2002) found that children with the low-activity MAOA gene were more likely to respond to the experience of maltreatment in childhood by developing antisocial problems in early adulthood. It was the interaction between this gene and adverse early experiences that produced the risk of later violent behaviour. They reported that only 12% of the males in the group they were studying had the combination of a low MAOA genotype and the experience of maltreatment. However they accounted for 44% of the violent convictions in this cohort.

A meta-analysis of 20 studies on the moderation of the effects maltreatment on later violent behaviour by the MAOA genotype in males was undertaken by Byrd and Manuck (2014). They concluded that

> MAOA variation moderates effects of early life adversity on male subjects' aggressive and antisocial behaviors, and this interaction is attributable to studies that, like the initial report, delimit adversity to experiences of maltreatment, such as physical and sexual abuse, harsh discipline, neglect, assault, or other ill treatment. (Byrd and Manuck (2014), p. 16)

A number of other candidate genes have been tested to examine whether interactions between genetic polymorphisms and adverse experiences can be detected as influencing externalising behaviour. A review of 53 such studies was produced by Weeland et al. (2015). They found that the MAOA polymorphism had the most consistent pattern of significant effects. There was greater heterogeneity in the results from the other genes studied, that is, DRD4, DRD2, DAT1, 5-HTTLPR, and COMT.

It appears that a wide variety of genes may play a role in increasing the vulnerability to the adverse effects of early maltreatment. It has been shown that a number gene–environment interaction effects can be detected in relation to antisocial behaviour (Ruisch et al., 2019). Polygenic scores based on dopamine genes have been found to interact with adverse life events to increase callous and unemotional traits in children; a precursor to development of psychopathy (Ruisch et al., 2020). This is an indication of possible mechanisms mediating the effect of these gene–environment interactions. In studies where this GxE interaction has not been found this may be due to the interaction being only shown when maltreatment is more severe (Ouellet-Morin et al., 2016).

Familial Transmission of Risk Using data on SNPs in mother/father/offspring trios Eilertsen et al. (2021) developed a method for estimating the size of direct genetic effects (from parent to child genotype) and indirect effects, including those transmitted by the effects of parental genes on the child's environment. Applying this method to a large Norwegian sample they showed that for conduct problems measured at 8 years direct genetic effects explained 24% of the variance and indirect genetic effects a further 16% (Eilertsen et al., 2022). They also found that these effects were associated, indicating the action of a gene–environment correlation. They suggest that their results show that parents contribute substantially to externalising problems in their children via both direct genetic transmission and influences on the environment experienced by the child.

Rather different conclusions were reached from the results of a study following externalising behaviour in 2734 children from the age of 11–29 years (Kretschmer et al., 2022). They constructed PRS for mothers, fathers, and their offspring. For externalising behaviour in early adulthood they found no evidence of genetic nurture effects (see Sect. 3.2) and only a very small evocative gene–environment correlation. There was a strong continuity in externalising behaviour from childhood to adulthood, and they suggest that this might militate against detecting indirect effects on adult externalising behaviour mediated by the family environment in their analysis of longitudinal data. This would explain why Eilertsen et al. (2022) did find such indirect family effects at the earlier age of 8 years but Kretschmer et al. (2022) did not.

Overview of Genetics The full range of quantitative and molecular genetic studies on antisocial behaviour was reviewed by Gard et al. (2019). They observe that most candidate gene studies have concentrated on genes related to dopaminergic and serotonergic neurotransmission. Although some associations have been reported with polymorphism in genes related to dopamine, they suggest that the role of these genes needs to be considered in terms of gene–environment interactions. It has been shown that antisocial behaviour is highly polygenic and there are further complications in that there may be sex differences in these genetic effects (Tielbeek et al., 2017). Whilst powerful methods for detecting gene associations with externalising behaviour have been applied, an understanding of the significance of development of this plethora of associations is lacking. This is reflected in Linnér et al. (2021) reaching the following conclusion from their study of the genetics of self-regulation and externalising behaviour based on the DNA of 1.5 million people:

> future work will be needed to tease apart the pathways by which biological and social risks unfold within and across generations ... (Linnér et al. (2021), p. 1374)

8.5 Interventions for Externalising Problems

Conduct problems in children make a considerable demand for educational, social, and judicial services into adulthood. Rissanen et al. (2022) followed up 5011 Finish children into adulthood to look at the subsequent costs of services of those with the lowest and the highest conduct problem scores at 8 years of age. The former accumulated €10,547 of service costs and the latter a sum roughly four times high (€44, 348). Similar high later costs have been found for conduct problems in the preschool period. Goulter et al. (2023) examined the cost to services into the early adult years of children showing conduct problems at around 5 years of age. The children had taken part in one of two longitudinal studies in the United States. A 1 standard deviation increase in the conduct problem score of the CBCL was associated with an increased cost to the criminal system, government, and medical services of

$146,279. Therefore there is a need for effective early interventions not only to benefit the child and the family but also to produce large net savings to social and other services.

Parenting Programmes There is good evidence that parenting programmes can be effective (Scott & Gardner, 2015). They can also be cost-effective in relation to long-term demands of services (Bachmann et al., 2022). There is some evidence that programmes that combine interventions addressing behaviour and reading attainment may be particularly efficacious for children with early-onset antisocial behaviour (Scott et al., 2010).

Psychosocial treatments of disruptive behaviour have been reviewed periodically (Eyberg et al., 2008; Kaminski & Claussen, 2017). These reviews concluded that two treatment approaches had well-established efficacy, that is, group parent behaviour therapy and individual parent behaviour therapy with child participation. A less positive systematic review and meta-analysis was produced by Bakker et al. (2017). They suggested that psychological treatments have a small effect in reducing conduct problems in children and adolescents with a clinical diagnosis. Depending on the source of reports of behaviour changes the effect sizes ranged from SMD = 0.26 to 0.36. In addition the quality and number of the available studies did not allow conclusions to be drawn on the relative efficacy of different types of psychological treatment.

It has been consistently reported that those with conduct problems and CU traits are particularly resistant to good treatment outcomes (Hawes et al., 2014). A more optimistic subsequent meta-analysis has suggested that children with conduct problems plus CU traits do show significant improvements under treatment although their level of disruptive behaviours remains high (Perlstein et al., 2023). In addition this analysis found that interventions that included a parenting component appeared effective in directly reducing CU traits.

The issue of the effectiveness of parenting programmes for children's externalising problems was addressed in a meta-analysis of 154 trials by Leijten et al. (2019). They found that effects on disruptive behaviour gradually increased across the levels of prevention (universal SMD = −0.21, selective SMD = −0.27, indicated SMD= −0.55) and treatment (SMD= −0.69). Of 26 parenting techniques, 3 were associated with stronger programme effects: positive reinforcement, praise in particular, and reacting to disruptive child behaviour with natural and/or logical consequences (e.g. take a toy away when the child plays too roughly with it).

Although only modest, these effect sizes are in line with those found for psychological and pharmacological treatments for mental health conditions across all ages and conditions. Leichsenring et al. (2019) suggest that most treatments only achieve an effect size of an SMD of 0.30 or below against placebo or treatment as usual. They make the rather pessimistic conclusion that

> …. recent evidence across multiple meta-analyses on key mental disorders provides an overarching picture of limited benefits for both psychotherapy and pharmacotherapy. Some differences for specific disorders are not strong enough to weaken the overall impression that a dead end has been reached in the treatment of mental disorders. (Leichsenring et al. (2019), p. 2112)

These conclusions were supported by a subsequent umbrella review (Leichsenring et al., 2022). This review was based on RCTs on psychotherapies and pharmacotherapies for mental disorders in adults. However it is likely that the same broad conclusions can be applied to treatments of mental disorders in children and adolescents.

Multisystemic Therapy In a narrative overview of treatments for the mental health of children and adolescents, Kazdin and Weisz (1998) identified a number of promising approaches for treating anxiety, depression, oppositional, aggressive, and antisocial behaviour. A number of these treatments have been shown to produce significant effects in RCTs; however, evidence for clinical significance (Jacobson & Truax, 1991) is often lacking. One of the therapeutic approaches deemed promising by Kazdin and Weisz (1998) is multisystemic therapy (MST). This is a family systems-based approach that has been used successfully with serious juvenile offenders (Henggeler et al., 1992). Riedinger et al. (2017) suggest that

> systemic therapy is defined by the inclusion of other relevant persons into the process of therapy, with the goal to change interpersonal communication and interactions, and hence lower personal suffering. (Riedinger et al. (2017), p. 880)

The RCTs where the MST approach has been applied to delinquency have been subject to a meta-analysis (van der Stouwe et al., 2014). Based on findings from 22 studies they found small but significant treatment effects on delinquency (SMD = 0.20), the primary outcome, and also on psychopathology (SMD= 0.27). Rather different conclusions have recently been reached by Littell et al. (2021). They show that the review by Kazdin and Weisz (1998) overlooked studies undertaken by investigators from outside the United States which tend to produce results less favourable to MST. They suggest that the differences in their conclusions from those of van der Stouwe et al. (2014) stem from the inclusion of different studies and the use of different analytic methods. Based on the more stringent methods they employ, Littell et al. (2021) conclude that

> the quality of evidence for MST is mixed and effects are inconsistent across studies. Reductions in out-of-home placements and arrest/conviction were observed in the USA, but not in other high-income countries. Studies that compared MST to more active treatments showed fewer benefits, and there is evidence that MST may have had some negative effects on youth outside of the USA. Based on moderate to low quality evidence, MST may reduce self-reported delinquency and improve parent and family outcomes, but there is no overall evidence of effects on youth symptoms, substance abuse, peer relations, or school outcomes. (Littell et al. (2021), p. 3)

Carr (2019) produced an extensive narrative review of studies on the efficacy of systemic therapies (defined more broadly than just MST) on a wide range of problems in childhood. This overview by Carr (2019) includes a valuable listing of resources for access to details about systemic treatments.

Externalising behaviours may subsequently lead to criminality and to be associated with a range of social disadvantages. A meta-analysis has shown that conduct disorders before the age of 18 years are strongly associated with later crimes of violence, OR = 3.52 ($CI_{.95}$ 2.34 to 5.31) (Erskine et al., 2016). There are a number of social and genetic factors that influence the transmission of criminal behaviour across generations in families (Kendler et al., 2014). The transmission of risk for criminality both within and between generations is therefore a major concern for children showing externalising behaviours. Andersen et al. (2021) have shown in a multigenerational study in Denmark that remaining in education can offset the transmission of such disadvantages particularly for those in a small group of families who show multiple health and social disadvantages. The encouragement to remain within the education system may therefore be a very effective intervention of such children.

Prevention Hendricks et al. (2018) produced a systemic review of published meta-analyses of interventions for prevention and treatment of aggressive behaviour and externalising problems in children. The majority of meta-analyses on prevention found small effect sizes – SMD less than 0.49. This held for universal, selective and indicative prevention interventions (see Sect. 7.6 for an account of this distinction between types of prevention based on Munoz et al. (1996)). Treatment produced somewhat greater effect sizes. Neither age nor gender was found to moderate these effect sizes but interventions were more effective if the pre-intervention levels of aggression were higher and if there was parental involvement in the intervention.

There is evidence that school-based interventions to reduce bullying can be effective. Ttofi and Farrington (2011) reported on a meta-analysis that identified 44 evaluations of such interventions. They found that bullying decreased by 20–23% and victimisation decreased by 17–20% compared to controls. The characteristics of the more effective programmes were greater intensity of intervention, the inclusion of parent meetings, firm disciplinary methods, and improved playground supervision. It has been shown that being a victim of bullying and being a perpetrator has long-term consequences both for the individual and for the society at large (Olweus, 2013). Reviews such as that of Ttofi and Farrington (2011) have shown that school-based interventions can reduce the number of perpetrators and victims of bullying, it has proved more problematic to show longer term and broader benefits for school performance and crime reduction at the population level (Borgen et al., 2021).

Drug Treatments There is scant evidence indicating that a pharmacological approach to the treatment of externalising behaviours can be effective. The only drug to receive endorsement, albeit qualified, for use in the treatment of aggressive and disruptive behaviour is the atypical antipsychotic risperidone (Gorman et al., 2015; Khan et al., 2019). The endorsement is qualified over concerns about major side effects of this treatment including weight gain and adverse metabolic changes. For this reason risperidone should only be considered for use with children and adolescents with severely disruptive and aggressive behaviour. This cautious recognition of possible clinical benefit of risperidone in treating aggression and conduct problems in children over the age of 5 years was echoed in a systematic review by Loy et al. (2017). Given that aspects of externalising behaviour, such as rule-breaking and aggression, are often a feature of the behaviour shown by children with ADHD, Gorman et al. (2015) strongly recommend that psychostimulants, such as methylphenidate and amphetamine, should first be used in children with aggressive or disruptive behaviour plus ADHD. In these recommendations there is a proviso that they should only be used if non-pharmacological therapies have been found not to be beneficial.

8.6 Co-occurrence of Internalising and Externalising Problems

The question of the co-occurrence of internalising and externalising problems can be addressed either as the relationship between categories (diagnoses), between dimensions or between symptoms. The co-occurrence of categories is referred to as comorbidity. The analysis of the association between dimensions underlies the hierarchal models of behavioural differences that was extensively discussed in Chap. 6. An alternative is to adopt a network analysis framework where co-occurrence arises from behavioural symptoms having a direct effect on each other and not arising from a shared underlying influence (Cramer et al., 2010). Examples of the application of this network approach to morbidity are a study of the co-occurrence anxiety and depression in girls (Rouquette e al., 2018) and the association between internalising, externalising, and attention symptoms in middle childhood (Funkhouser et al., 2021).

Comorbidity The development of systematic classification schemes raised the question of how to deal with individuals that showed the characteristics of more than one diagnostic category (Feinstein, 1970). The consequences of comorbidity for studies of child psychopathology were reviewed by Caron and Rutter (1991). They show how comorbidity can produce bias in epidemiology studies that are based on clinical samples. They present a number of routes whereby comorbidity can occur, including shared risk factors, overlapping risk factors, comorbid patterns constituting a meaningful syndrome, and one disorder creating an increased risk for the other.

A major review and meta-analysis of studies on general population samples of psychopathology comorbidity children and adolescents was produced by Angold et al. (1999). They show that comorbidity occurs frequently and that it is found between conditions that cross the internalising/externalising boundary. For example, depression is almost as strongly related to conduct problems as it is to anxiety. They also conclude that comorbidity in children and adolescents does not arise as a result of methodological artefacts such as halo effects, that is, the identification of one diagnosis in a child lowering the bar for a clinician to make a second diagnosis. It has also been shown to be pervasive as comorbidity is similar in magnitude and type in large epidemiological studies of adults from four different countries (Merikangas et al., 1996). This leads to the conclusion that comorbidity is a real phenomenon and raises questions about the factors that might be a cause.

Comorbidity Case–Control Approach Weiss et al. (1998) investigated which characteristics differentiate levels of common and specific features of child psychopathology: common features, which differentiate psychopathology from normality; broadband-specific features, which differentiate internalising problems (e.g. anxiety, somatisation) from externalising problems (e.g. aggression, hyperactivity); and narrowband- specific features, which differentiate different narrowband syndromes (e.g. anxiety from somatisation, hyperactivity from aggression) within each of the broadband syndromes. They found that common features are related to severity of psychopathology, whereas specific features may be more related to differentiation of psychopathology. Common features included low self-worth. Broadband features that differentiated internalising from externalising problems included a relatively greater sense of academic and social incompetence. Findings along these lines were reported by Brunnekreef et al. (2007), who investigated cognitive processing in 10–12-year-old children with internalising and externalising problems. They found that cognitive processing deficits are more strongly related to the degree than to the type of maladaptive behaviour.

The approach to analysis adopted by Weiss et al. (1998) was that of profile analysis (see Tabachnik & Fidell, 2013, Chap. 10) which is based on the comparison of the characteristics of groups with contrasting profiles of symptoms and is an extension of the case/control design, the weaknesses of which are discussed below.

In Sect. 6.4 it was shown that a general psychopathology factor (GPF) could be identified that can create a susceptibility to develop a wide range of behaviour problems. Consequently in all age groups GPF could act to produce the association between internalising problems and externalising problems. Therefore there is a need to take into account the influences on the GPF if factors acting on a specific type of behaviour problem are to be identified.

This raises the question of how to select groups in case–control studies that can identify specificity. Specificity refers to causal factors that make a unique contribution to a specific disorder (Garber & Hollon, 1991). In the present situation this is complex. Both the factors influencing the GPF, and those with more specific effects, need to be differentiated. This means that in terms of research design it is not sufficient simply to compare a group with a specific behaviour problem to a group with no behaviour problems. As argued by Lilienfeld (2018):

> The problem is that without inclusion of well-validated indices of other disorders, ascertaining the specificity of one's results to a given disorder becomes extremely challenging. (Lilienfeld (2018), p. 82)

To identify a factor that shows a specific association in this case–control framework it is necessary to study at least three groups – for example, those with internalising problems, those externalising problems, and a typically developing comparison group (TDCG). This latter term is preferred to "normal" or "control" group because the implication of the first of these alternatives is that the children with behaviour problem are "abnormal" in a more general sense. "Comparison group" is preferred to the use of the term "control" group as the latter is really only appropriate in an experimental study in which extraneous factors can be attempted to be "controlled" by random allocation.

Using these three groups it may be possible to differentiate between factors related to both internalising and externalising but not to the TDCG, that is, influences on the GPF. Specific factors will be related to just one of the problem groups but not to the other or to the GPF. However such case/control studies are almost inevitably observational correlational studies. In the absence of experimental interventions these studies lack the potential to differentiate a cause of a problem from a consequence of a problem (Garber & Hollon, 1991). This situation can be partially addressed using longitudinal data. As Kraemer et al. (2001) suggest the ambiguity of the directionality of causal is remedied by temporal precedence. Longitudinal data can be used to identify which factors precede the onset of a problem. This is necessary but not sufficient to establish causality as the possibility of a third factor confound remains.

The above discussion of the issues raised by Garber and Hollon (1991) is couched in terms of the selection of groups in an analysis of between group research designs, for example, what distinguishes children with externalising problems, children with internalising problems, and children in the TDCG. The limitations of such a case–control design have been summarised by Ofrat and Krueger (2012) – see also Schwartz and Susser (2011). They emphasise that the identification of "pure" diagnostic cases often excludes children with comorbidities and thereby limits the external validity of the findings. They endorse the transdiagnostic or dimensional approach to the identification of general and specific risk factors.

Challenges to the Categorical Diagnostic Approach The strengths and potential of this transdiagnostic modelling of mental health have been reviewed by Dalgleish et al. (2020). They identify the following as "challenges" to the diagnostic framework approach to mental health. The first is that unlike physical illness mental health problems do not arise from a small number of discrete causes. Instead they are influenced by a wide range biological and psychosocial factors that interact with one another. Second, in mental health symptoms do not present as a binary present or absent. Instead they are distributed along a continuum in the general population. Third, mental health problems do not present in isolation. Comorbidity is the rule rather than the exception, so that they are not discrete but rather are positioned in a complex multidimensional framework. Fourth, there is rarely a clear profile of symptoms but rather there is extensive heterogeneity in the symptom profile of disorders. The categorical approach cannot produce a system of discrete homogeneous disorders. Fifth, associated with the problem of heterogeneity is the failure of categorical diagnoses to identify a cardinal set of symptoms for any specific condition and consequently when applied the "diagnosis" is unlikely to capture the range of symptoms shown by the individual. Sixth, mental health problems show marked changes over time. The binary present/absent approach is not framed to reflect these dynamic changes in symptoms and fluctuations in severity. Seventh, the diagnostic framework leads to a search for treatments that map on to single disorders. This fails to deal with the complexities arising from comorbidities and is not consistent with the findings that many treatments, both pharmacological and behavioural, are effective across a broad range of symptoms.

Comorbidity Dimensional Approach Within a transdiagnostic/dimensional framework, the issue of comorbidity becomes that of identifying the specificity of associations between risk factors and continuous measures of behaviour (Krueger & Markon, 2006). This paper by Krueger and Markon provides a detailed history of the notion and study of comorbidity. In the multilevel hierarchical models outlined in Chap. 6 the dimensions in this framework are the latent variables of internalising, externalising, and the general psychopathology factor (GPF).

Lynch et al. (2021) used this framework to produce a systematic review of studies of transdiagnostic risks, that is, those related to the GPF, and specific risks, that is, those related to the group factors of internalising and externalising. They suggested that there were a number of biological (executive functioning deficits, earlier pubertal timing, genetic risk for ADHD and schizophrenia, reduced grey matter volume), socio-environmental (stressful life events, maternal depression), and psychological (low effortful control, high neuroticism, negative affectivity) that constituted transdiagnostic risk factors. The risk factors for internalising, for which there was replicated evidence, were three biological factors (being female, earlier pubertal timing, and executive functioning deficits), one socio-environmental factor (maternal depression), and three psychological factors (high neuroticism, low extroversion, high behavioural inhibition). The risk factors, with replicated evidence, for externalising were three biological factors (executive functioning deficits, earlier pubertal timing, being male), one socio-environmental factor (stressful life events), two psychological factors (high neuroticism, low effortful control). The importance of these findings on specific risk factors is that they were obtained from studies where the modelling had allowed control for pervasive general risks on behaviour.

Comorbidity as Severity and Directionality An alternative framework for considering the emergence of co-occurring behaviours was developed by Essex et al. (2003). This framework has two component scores – severity and directionality. In the case of internalising and externalising these two scores are obtained for each person by first standardising the internalising and externalising measures to obtain z-scores. Severity is then calculated as the mean of these two z-scores. Directionality is derived by halving the difference of the two z-scores. Severity is therefore an indication of the degree of shared psychopathology shown by the individual. Directionality is an indication of how much the scores are directed towards either internalising or externalising. Importantly the severity and directionality indicators are uncorrelated with one another.

The analysis can then address the question of to what extent external risk factors are increasing the level of psychopathology shown and whether these same risk factors are influencing the type of psychopathology shown. A study by Ekblad et al. (2020) on the effects of mothers smoking during pregnancy on their child's behaviour will be used to illustrate the severity/directionality approach. An additional component of this study was the use of discordant sibling pairs where mothers smoked when pregnant with one child but not when pregnant with the other child in the family. This provides a control for a number of possible within-family confounds. They found that the severity score was not related to maternal smoking during pregnancy. However the directionally score was significantly related to the direction of smoking increasing the risk of externalising behaviour. It is surprising that this simple and elegant approach to identifying the effects of risk factors on behaviour is not more widely applied.

Comorbidity Over Time Willner et al. (2016) used latent profile analysis (see Sect. 2.5) to examine the developmental course of comorbidity in a longitudinal study of 336 children from an urban low-income community. They found a high degree of stability of comorbidity between internalising and externalising problems suggesting a common vulnerability was acting. In addition those children who were initially high on just externalising symptoms were at risk for accumulating internalising symptoms over time. Ip et al. (2019) undertook a longitudinal study of 238 children between the ages of 3 and 10 years. They were interested in the change over time in relationship between emotional and disruptive problems. They found that few children developed "pure" internalising or externalising problems – co-occurrence was the norm.

There are some distinguishing features of internalising and externalising problems that are identifiable during the preschool period. Bayer et al. (2012) followed a group of 733 Australian children with repeated measurements up to age 3 years and then again at 5 years of age. The factors that predicted internalising behaviours at 5 years of age were harsh discipline, maternal stress, having no older siblings, single parenthood, and maternal substance misuse. For externalising behaviours at 5 years of age the strongest predictors were male sex, harsh discipline, and maternal stress. These predictors explained 22% of the variation in internalising behaviours and 24% of the variation in externalising behaviours. Although there are distinct predictors of internalising and externalising as discussed above these problems do co -occur. What factors might account for this association between these two types of psychological problems in children? The evidence for a number of these factors will now be considered.

Co-occurrence and Stressful Life Events McMahon et al. (2003) undertook a systematic review of studies investigating the impact of particular life stresses on internalising and externalising problems in children. They identified 16 studies concerned with exposure to violence, 33 on abuse, and 8 on divorce/marital conflict plus 8 others on various stresses. Their interest was in whether there was a specific association between particular stresses and types of outcome. What they found was consistent not with specificity but with both equifinality (i.e. multiple stresses leading to the same outcome) and multifinality (i.e. multiple outcomes from any one stress). The only stress with a specific outcome was sexual abuse was specifically associated with internalising problems.

This same group of researchers tested a model of the mediation and moderation of the effects of risk on psychopathology in children (Grant et al., 2003). They present the results of the effects of poverty on internalising and externalising using meta-analytic path analysis synthesising the findings from up to 30 studies. The

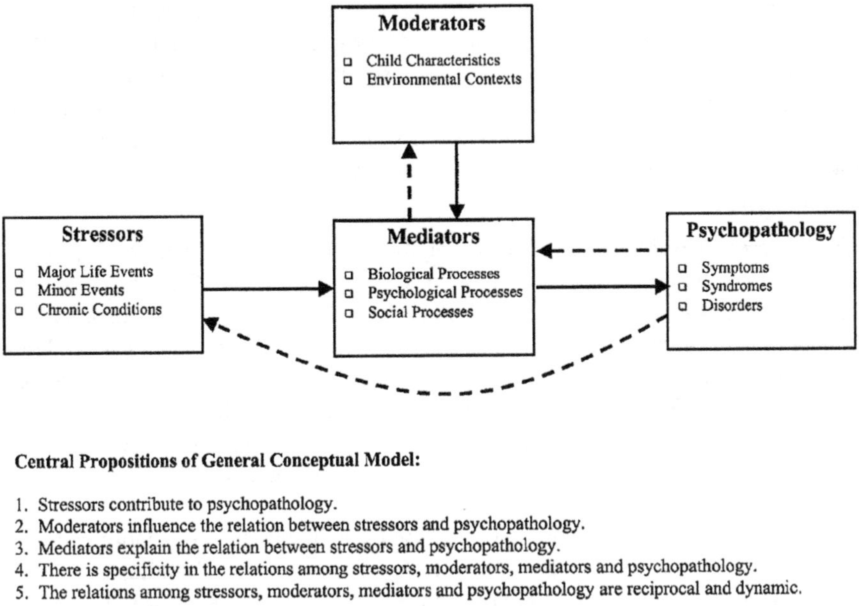

Fig. 8.1 Conceptual model of the role of stressors in the aetiology of child psychopathology. (Reproduced with the permission of the American Psychological Association from Fig. 1 Grant et al. (2003); permission conveyed through Copyright Clearance Center, Inc.)

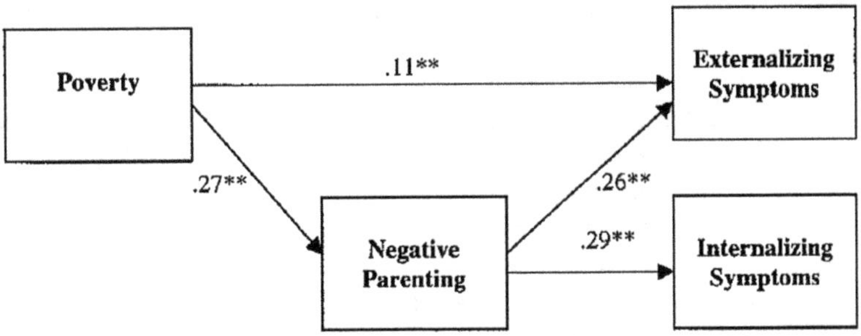

Fig. 8.2 Mediation model of the effect of poverty on child psychopathology [** $p < 0.01$]. (Reproduced with the permission of the American Psychological Association from Fig. 3 Grant et al. (2003); permission conveyed through Copyright Clearance Center, Inc.)

model they tested is presented in Fig. 8.1 using negative parenting as a mediator. This showed that there was no evidence of specificity in outcome. Poverty was linked both directly to externalising and indirectly via negative parenting to internalising and externalising problems (see Fig. 8.2). They found some evidence for moderation of these effects by sex, with negative parenting having a slightly larger effect on internalising for girls compared to boys.

The pattern of results reported by McMahon et al. (2003) and Grant et al. (2003) was replicated in a study by Shanahan et al. (2008). However Shanahan et al. (2008) undertook additional analyses that did not just consider the bivariate link between risk factors and psychopathology. They took into account comorbidity and the effects of other risk factors. In this analysis some risks such as parental unemployment and parent depression still showed nonspecific links to both internalising and externalising problems.

Co-occurrence and Genetics It has been found that depression and conduct disorders are associated in childhood and adolescence. The origin of this association is uncertain. Does depression lead to conduct disorders? Does conduct disorder lead to depression? Do both arise from a common cause? Or perhaps there is a combination of these processes operating? One candidate for a common cause is genetics. Caserini et al. (2023) undertook a systematic review of studies on shared genetic influences between depression and conduct disorder. They found that across 10 relevant studies there was consistent evidence for genetic factors making a strong contribution to the association.

The Caserini et al. (2023) review addressed specifically the association between depression and conduct disorder. There have been a number of studies examining the role of genetic and environmental factors to the co-occurrence of more general internalising and externalising problems. Gjone and Stevenson (1997) used the internalising and externalising problem scales of the CBCL with a sample of 915 same-sex Norwegian twin pairs aged 5–15 years. They found that the covariance between these measures ($r = 0.51$ to 0.56) was largely accounted for by the common environment, though genetic factors were important too. Similar findings came from a study of 398 same-sex Italian twins by Pesenti-Gritti et al. (2008).

Other studies have found a stronger genetic influence on the association between internalising and externalising. O'Connor et al. (1998) tested for influences on this association in a sample of twins and siblings aged between 10 and 18 years. Depression and antisocial behaviour were the measures used of internalising and externalising, respectively. The co-occurrence of depressive and antisocial symptoms was explained by genetic (45%) and shared (30%) and non-shared (25%) environmental influences. Cosgrove et al. (2011) found no evidence of shared environmental influences on the internalising/externalising latent variables correlation. The correlation between latent internalising and externalising factors ($r = 0.72$) was due to both common genetic (62%) and non-shared environmental (38%) influences. Mikolajewski et al. (2013) found common shared environmental and genetic influences on internalising and externalising, and these were also influencing negative affectivity. Cosgrove et al. (2011) suggest that the difference between studies may arise from differences in the measurement of behaviour. For example, Gjone and Stevenson (1997) used parent ratings which might inflate shared environment estimates. Whereas Cosgrove et al. (2011) used behaviour measures based on self-report interviews which are likely to be more prone to identify non-shared environment effects.

The notion of generalist genes was introduced by Eley (1997). She provided evidence that both within externalising and within internalising there are genes that acted on more than one subset of a set of symptoms, that is, the same genes influence both aggressive and nonaggressive antisocial behaviour and depression and anxiety have genes in common. A complement to generalist genes are specialist environments, and a model of "generalist genes, specialist environments" was proposed for cognitive abilities by Kovas and Plomin (2007) and was subsequently applied to psychopathology (Lahey et al., 2011). This model proposes that genes are primarily responsible for the correlation between characteristics and environments for their differentiation. Using the terminology of Essex et al. (2003) genes drive severity and environments drive directionality.

Marceau et al. (2022) have examined whether the "generalist genes, specialist environment" notion applies between internalising and externalising using the severity/directionality framework. The participants were adolescent twins, and so Marceau et al. (2022) were able to test the effects of genes and environments on the indices of severity and directionality. They found that severity was mainly influenced by genes. However directionality was influenced not only by the non-shared environment but also by genes. They conclude:

> Overall, the generalist genes specialist environments model (although originally developed for the intersection of anxiety and depression symptoms) is a nice heuristic for thinking about comorbid internalizing and externalizing problems. However, the present data generally show that comorbidity is more nuanced, and that specialist genes and generalist environments are also important for understanding the commonalities and differentiation of internalizing and externalizing problems during adolescence. (Marceau et al. (2022), p. 385)

Under hierarchical factor models influences on the GPF will contribute to the co-occurrence of internalising and externalising problems. As discussed in Sect. 6.7 genetic influences on the GPF have been demonstrated by Waldman et al. (2016). They found that genes accounted for a substantial proportion of the variance in the general factor (43%). The contributions of the shared environment and non-shared environment were 25% and 32%, respectively. Substantial genetic influences were also found for externalising (65%) with a less marked contribution from the shared (16%) and non-shared environments (19%). The reverse pattern was found for internalising where the shared (44%) and non-shared environment (37%) had larger effects than genes (19%). The findings in relation to genetic and shared environment effects on the general factor were broadly replicated in a separate twin study by Allegrini et al. (2020). However they found less of a contribution from the non-shared environment. Gjerde et al. (2023) have found an even larger genetic influence ($h^2 = 0.75$) on the p-factor in an analysis of psychopathology in a wider set of family members (twins, siblings, cousins, and half-siblings) in a total population cohort of Norwegian children ($N > 114{,}500$).

An important development in the understanding of general genetic influences on psychopathology was the study of the co-development of conduct and emotional problems by Hannigan et al. (2018). They showed that there were a number of joint symptom trajectories for emotional and conduct problems in twin children over the ages of 4–16 years, for example, jointly stable and jointly increasing. The heritability of the trajectory groups was substantial ($h^2 = 0.41$ to 0.78). Additionally PRS based on depression symptom-associated alleles were predictive of membership of the most symptomatic trajectory class. They summarise their findings as follows:

> Overall, our results demonstrate that, in childhood and adolescence, comorbidity is as much about *co-development* as co-occurrence. We found that, while many individuals showed normative levels of conduct and emotional problems across development, those that had elevated or developmentally-increasing levels of one trait were also more likely to be on similar trajectories for the other. Beyond this, we show that joint symptom trajectories of conduct and emotional problems are associated with genetic factors – both as inferred by known genetic relationships *and* as measured directly from genotype data. This highlights the potential informativeness and utility of joint trajectories for aetiological studies of developing psychopathology. (Hannigan et al. (2018))

There is evidence that there is a continuing association between internalising and externalising behaviour in middle age (Gustavson et al., 2020). This longitudinal twin study found that there are shared genetic factors accounting for the association. These influences contributed to the considerable stability of internalising and externalising psychopathology symptoms across middle age.

Passive gene–environment correlations have been identified that are related to both internalising and externalising behaviour in children at ages 5–6 and 11–12 years (Ensink et al., 2020). They found that PRS for psychiatric disorders were correlated with pre- and postnatal features of the early environment, specifically aspects of maternal well-being, behaviour, and lifestyle. These environmental risk factors were related to both internalising and externalising behaviour in the children. In this study the origins of the association between internalising and externalising were via shared passive gene–environment correlations rather than by a direct effect of shared genes.

Co-occurrence and Parental Mental Health There is long-standing evidence that links mental health in parents and children (e.g. Rutter, 1966). This association may arise through genetic mechanisms or through social interactions within families. An examination of these relations was undertaken by Speyer et al. (2022) in a longitudinal study of ages 3–17 years of 10,746 families. Parental mental health was measured by a widely adopted brief questionnaire that focuses on symptoms of depression and anxiety (Kessler et al., 2003). Child mental health was assessed by the SDQ (Goodman, 1997). Speyer et al. (2022) found that maternal psychological distress was positively associated with subsequent internalising and externalising problems for girls but only with internalising problems for boys. Paternal psychological distress was associated with boys' later internalising and externalising problems during early adolescence. Bidirectional effects were also present whereby child mental health was associated with later parental psychological distress. In this study the effects were not large. Xerxa et al. (2021) found similar modest overtime associations in a study of 5536 children and their parents in a cohort of younger children from the Netherlands. Child externalising and internalising problems were both predicted by earlier parental psychopathology. The findings from these two studies indicate that parental psychopathology may be a contributing factor to the co-occurrence of internalising and externalising problems in children.

Speyer et al. (2022) and Xerxa et al. (2021) both used an autoregressive latent trajectory modelling with structured residuals (ALT-SR) (see Sect. 4.3). This method of analysis takes into account within- and between-person effects. That is, it can detect how changes from a usual level of psychopathology in the parent can affect changes in child problems at subsequent time points, and, in addition, how child problems can affect changes in parent psychopathology. Although these two studies suggest that there may be small but robust reciprocal effects between child and parent psychopathology, in themselves they cannot identify what mechanisms, for example, social or genetic, may account for these associations.

Co-occurrence and Emotion Regulation Emotion regulation is the process by which people modify the intensity and/or duration of their emotions in response to contextual demands and has been posited as influential in the emergence of both internalising and externalising behaviour and in their co-occurrence. In an extensive meta-analysis of 212 studies, Compas et al. (2017) examined the association of emotion regulation and coping strategies with internalising and externalising symptoms. They found that maladaptive coping was associated with higher levels of internalising and adaptive coping was associated with lower levels of externalising. The greater use of emotion regulation was linked to lower levels of both internalising and externalising. The effect sizes in these analyses were modest with correlations with internalising and externalising being no greater than $r = 0.27$. However modest effect sizes are the norm – see the discussion of Götz et al. (2022) in Sect. 2.9.

Aldao et al. (2016) undertook a narrative review of this possible role of emotional dysregulation. One component of emotional dysregulation is depressive rumination which is defined as repetitively dwelling upon one's past mistakes, regrets, and/or shortcomings. Aldao et al. (2016) found that depressive rumination is associated with the development of internalising, and to a lesser extent, externalising, symptoms over time and therefore plays a role in their co-occurrence.

Temperament It has been proposed that irritability, defined as excessive reactivity to negative emotional stimuli, is an early developing risk factor for a number of internalising and externalising disorders (Beauchaine & Tackett, 2020). Irritability is expressed as impatience, annoyance, anger, and sometimes aggression, and it is a risk factor for the development of impulsivity, negative affectivity, and poor inhibitory control – features of the hyperactive-impulsive symptoms of ADHD. Irritability has been found to be the component of oppositional-defiant behaviours that are most closely related to the development of depression and that this reflects shared genetic factors (Waldman et al., 2021).

Mesman and Koot (2000) examined the temperament characteristics that differentiated children with internalising and externalising psychopathology in a sample of children followed for 9 years from the age of 2.5 years. The characteristics that were found in those with internalising problems in boys and girls were temperamental withdrawal in the preschool period and parental internalising psychopathology.

Early temperamental high general activity level was identified as specific to externalising. Parenting stress, poor school results (only for boys), and stressful life events (only for girls) were found to be common correlates of both types of psychopathology.

Co-occurrence and IQ There is well-replicated evidence that IQ is related to psychopathology. This holds for variation in IQ across the normal range and for those with low IQ. For example Pettersson et al. (2021) found a correlation of $r = -0.17$ between IQ and a general psychopathology factor in a prospective general population study of 899,398 Swedish men.

This correlation is similar to that found for behaviour problems rated by parents and IQ in a general population sample of 13-year-old twins ($r = -0.15$) – the correlation was somewhat higher for teacher-rated behaviour ($r = -0.33$) (Goodman et al., 1995). This study found that IQ was related to both internalising (emotional symptoms) and externalising (conduct problems) and will therefore contribute to their co-occurrence. Goodman et al. (1995) appraised the evidence for various mechanisms that might result in this association between internalising, externalising, and IQ. They suggest that either lower IQ is a cause or that there is a biological third factor acting on IQ and behaviour.

The association between intellectual disability and psychopathology was demonstrated by Emerson and Hatton (2007) in a systematically identified sample of children with learning disabilities in the United Kingdom aged 5–16 years. The rate of disorders was substantially higher among those with intellectual disability (36%) compared to those without intellectual disability (8%). Emerson and Hatton (2007) showed that in part this increased prevalence was a result of an increase in exposure to social disadvantage.

Co-occurrence and Specific Learning Disabilities A factor that contributes to the co-occurrence of internalising and externalising problems is the presence of specific learning disabilities, especially those related to language. Donolato et al. (2022) undertook a meta-analysis of studies that have examined the relationship between language and learning disorders (LLD) and internalising and externalising problems. They found that both internalising and externalising problems were more common in those with LLD than in TD children. The effect sizes for internalising were larger for those with language disorders, SMD= 0.49 ($CI_{.95}$ 0.38 to 0.61), than for other LLDs. Externalising problems were also more frequent in this group than in TD children, SMD= 0.45 ($CI_{.95}$ 0.32 to 0.59).

Prospective studies on the relationship between language impairment, emotional, and behavioural problems were reviewed in a meta-analysis by Yew and O'Kearney (2013). They identified 19 studies of children aged between 3 and 9 years who had been followed up from between 2 and 12 years later. Children with language impairments were found to have double the rate of later emotional and behavioural disorders. This finding held for both internalising and externalising problems. Although there is a relationship between language and emotional and behaviour problems across the normal range of language ability, it has been shown that the effect is most marked for those with very low language abilities (Goh et al., 2021).

Co-occurrence and Network Analysis Using the ALSPAC data set McElroy et al. (2018) adopted a network analysis (see Sect. 2.6) to address the question of the co-occurrence of internalising and externalising problems. The pattern of behavioural associations was consistent across the age points 7.5, 10.5, and 14 years. Generalised anxiety disorders and oppositional-defiant disorders were identified as having the greatest influence in the networks, and they concluded that these disorders may play the strongest role in either producing and/or maintaining the association between internalising and externalising.

8.7 Final Thoughts on Internalising and Externalising Problems

In Chaps. 7 and 8 findings on the origins and consequences of internalising and externalising problems have been reviewed. It is a sign of the maturity of this field of research that reference can now be made to a study that integrates an analysis of the relationship between measures of experience and of the genetic make-up of individuals to predict a substantial proportion of the variance in internalising and externalising behaviour. This paper by Choi et al. (2022) uses an integrated index based on 133 measures of both proximal and more distal environmental circumstances and life events; this is a measure of the exposome (Miller, 2021) (see Sect. 10.9). It is augmented by genomic data in a large sample of American youth ($N = 4314$) from the Adolescent Brain and Cognitive Development study (see Sect. 3.1). The methods employed allowed the estimation of the effects of the genome (G), the exposome (E), GxE interactions, and ExE interactions on internalising and externalising behaviours. These estimates for internalising and externalising are summarised in Fig. 8.3.

The genomic assessment of genome-wide similarity and differences between individuals that was adopted represents an improvement in the prediction of behaviour from genomic measures based on PRS. The state-of-the-art modelling methods employed were able to explain 35% of the variance in internalising and 63% of the variance in externalising. It was striking that there was a substantial contribution from GxE in externalising (33% of the variance) but less so for internalising (13%).

When components of the exposome were examined, life events were a key influence on internalising but the broader contexts of family, school, and peer group were more influential for externalising. The contribution of G, apart from GxE, was modest for both behavioural measures – 7% or less. This paper represents a step change in the ability of genetic and environmental measures to predict behaviour. The methods employed are bound to become more widely adopted. The key finding for externalising behaviours is that future research could profit from a focus on gene–environment interactions as these were found to represent the single largest influence. For depression and anxiety the examination of loss and threat events in triggering problems should be a priority.

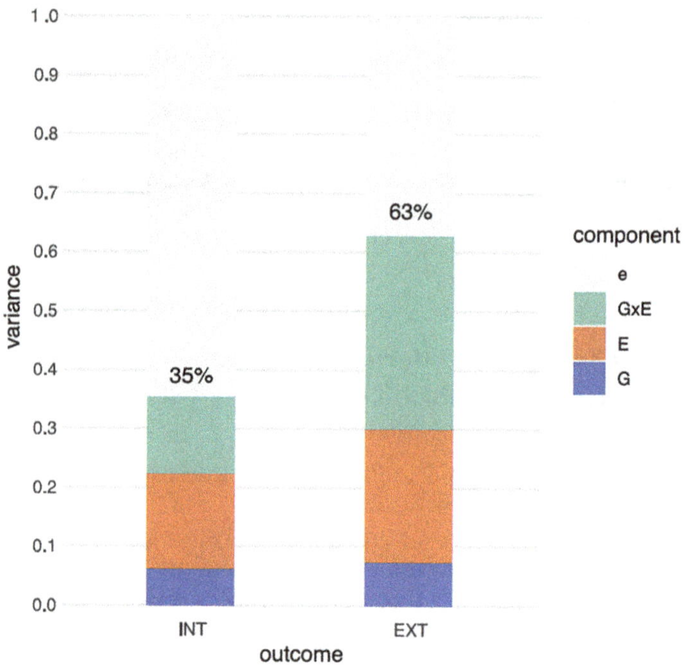

Fig. 8.3 Estimated total proportion of variance in INT and EXT symptoms explained by G, E, and GxE components. e, residual variance; E, modelled exposome effects based on 133 exposure variables; G, genomic effects; GxE, genome-by-exposome effects. (Reproduced with the permission of John Wiley and Sons from Fig. 1 Choi et al. (2022); permission conveyed through Copyright Clearance Center, Inc.)

Despite these advances there are enduring concerns. For example, there is continuing uncertainty over the long-term benefit of treatments for common childhood behavioural and emotional disorders. Roest et al. (2022) suggest that although there is good evidence for the effectiveness of such treatments in the short term (2 years), there is a paucity of evidence on longer outcomes. Under these circumstances they propose that "watchful waiting may be the best choice, especially if symptoms are mild". Dekkers et al. (2022) disagree. They suggest that the review by Roest et al. (2022) was compromised by a lack of methodological rigour and that important evidence for long-term effectiveness for treatments of both internalising and externalising problems was overlooked. In addition, they say it would be unjust to withhold treatments that are known to be effective in the short term on the basis that longer-term benefits were uncertain.

What is clear is that the burden of internalising and externalising problems on children and adolescent is substantial. A review of this burden globally concluded that

> mental and substance use disorders are the leading cause of disability in children and youth worldwide. (Erskine et al. (2015), p. 1558)

This review also showed that mental and substance use disorders are also the sixth leading cause of disability-adjusted life-years (DALYs) – the number of years of healthy life lost. These findings are made even more concerning as there is evidence that, over a 40-year period bridging the 2000 millennium, child mental health problems have become more strongly associated with negative social, educational, and mental health outcomes (Sellers et al., 2019).

There are treatments for internalising and externalising behaviours that are effective at least in the short term. However there is a drastic shortfall in the number of affected young people getting access to treatment. For example, in a survey of the general population in the Netherlands, Vanheusden et al. (2008) found:

> Among young adults with internalizing and externalizing psychopathology ($n = 367$), only 34.6% ($n = 126$) had used any mental health services; 16.2% ($n = 59$) had used only primary mental health care and 18.4% ($n = 67$) had used specialty mental health care (with or without primary care). (Vanheusden et al. (2008), p. 811)

At about the same time a study of 5–15-year-olds in the United Kingdom found that of those children with psychiatric disorders, 58% had been in contact with one of a range of social services for help with emotional, behavioural, or concentration difficulties, including 23% who had been in contact with mental health services (Ford et al., 2005). A similar level of access to service for those with mental health disorders was found in the United States in the early 2000s (Merikangas et al., 2011). Indeed it has been demonstrated that this is a global issue:

> Irrespective of increased prevalence across adolescence, evidence suggests that most adolescents and young adults with mental health problems do not receive treatment from health professionals. (Patton et al. (2016), p. 28)

This shortfall is in large part due to the lack of provision but is also influenced by social factors including teachers' and parents' perception of the nature of children's psychological problems and of the potential value of referral and treatment (Ford et al., 2008). A range of issues surround the structure of service provision and attitudes towards and knowledge about services and treatment have been shown to be key influencing parents gaining access to mental health services for children (Reardon et al., 2017).

It is, of course, preferable to prevent these mental health problems from occurring in the first place. In relation both to internalising (e.g. Herrman et al., 2022) and externalising (e.g. Fairchild et al., 2019) it has been concluded that prevention should be a priority.

The focus of these comments on service provision in this chapter has been problems of internalising and externalising. The same concerns over the lack of treatment and support hold for children with neurodevelopmental disorders such as attention-deficit hyperactivity disorder and autism spectrum disorders which are the focus of the final two chapters.

References

Aguilar, B., Sroufe, L. A., Egeland, B., & Carlson, E. (2000). Distinguishing the early-onset/persistent and adolescence-onset antisocial behavior types: From birth to 16 years. *Development and Psychopathology, 12*(2), 109–132. https://doi.org/10.1017/s0954579400002017

Ahmad, S. I., & Hinshaw, S. P. (2017). Attention-deficit/hyperactivity disorder, trait impulsivity, and externalizing behavior in a longitudinal sample. *Journal of Abnormal Child Psychology, 45*(6), 1077–1089. https://doi.org/10.1007/s10802-016-0226-9

Aldao, A., Gee, D. G., De Los Reyes, A., & Seager, I. (2016). Emotion regulation as a transdiagnostic factor in the development of internalizing and externalizing psychopathology: Current and future directions. *Development and Psychopathology, 28*(4), 927–946. https://doi.org/10.1017/s0954579416000638

Allegrini, A. G., Cheesman, R., Rimfeld, K., Selzam, S., Pingault, J. B., Eley, T. C., & Plomin, R. (2020). The p factor: Genetic analyses support a general dimension of psychopathology in childhood and adolescence. *Journal of Child Psychology and Psychiatry, 61*(1), 30–39. https://doi.org/10.1111/jcpp.13113

Andersen, S. H., Richmond-Rakerd, L. S., Moffitt, T. E., & Caspi, A. (2021). Nationwide evidence that education disrupts the intergenerational transmission of disadvantage. *Proceedings of the National Academy of Sciences of the United States of America, 118*(31). https://doi.org/10.1073/pnas.2103896118

Angold, A., Costello, E. J., & Erkanli, A. (1999). Comorbidity. *Journal of Child Psychology and Psychiatry, 40*(1), 57–87. https://doi.org/10.1111/1469-7610.00424

Appleyard, K., Egeland, B., van Dulmen, M. H. M., & Sroufe, L. A. (2005). When more is not better: The role of cumulative risk in child behavior outcomes. *Journal of Child Psychology and Psychiatry, 46*(3), 235–245. https://doi.org/10.1111/j.1469-7610.2004.00351.x

Assink, M., van der Put, C. E., Hoeve, M., de Vries, S. L. A., Stams, G., & Oort, F. J. (2015). Risk factors for persistent delinquent behavior among juveniles: A meta-analytic review. *Clinical Psychology Review, 42*, 47–61. https://doi.org/10.1016/j.cpr.2015.08.002

Bachmann, C. J., Beecham, J., O'Connor, T. G., Briskman, J., & Scott, S. (2022). A good investment: Longer-term cost savings of sensitive parenting in childhood. *Journal of Child Psychology and Psychiatry, 63*(1), 78–87. https://doi.org/10.1111/jcpp.13461

Bakker, M. J., Greven, C. U., Buitelaar, J. K., & Glennon, J. C. (2017). Practitioner review: Psychological treatments for children and adolescents with conduct disorder problems – a systematic review and meta-analysis. *Journal of Child Psychology and Psychiatry, 58*(1), 4–18. https://doi.org/10.1111/jcpp.12590

Barnes, J. C., Boutwell, B. B., Beaver, K. M., & Gibson, C. L. (2013). Analyzing the origins of childhood externalizing behavioral problems. *Developmental Psychology, 49*(12), 2272–2284. https://doi.org/10.1037/a0032061

Bayer, J. K., Ukoumunne, O. C., Mathers, M., Wake, M., Abdi, N., & Hiscock, H. (2012). Development of children's internalising and externalising problems from infancy to five years of age. *Australian and New Zealand Journal of Psychiatry, 46*(7), 659–668. https://doi.org/10.1177/0004867412450076

Beauchaine, T. P., & Tackett, J. L. (2020). Irritability as a transdiagnostic vulnerability trait: Current issues and future directions. *Behavior Therapy, 51*(2), 350–364. https://doi.org/10.1016/j.beth.2019.10.009

Beauchaine, T. P., Zisner, A. R., & Sauder, C. L. (2017). Trait impulsivity and the externalizing spectrum. In T. Widiger & T. D. Cannon (Eds.), *Annual review of clinical psychology* (Vol. 13, pp. 343–368).

Bell, Z. E., Fristad, M. A., Youngstrom, E. A., Arnold, L. E., Beauchaine, T. P., & Consortium, L. (2021). Attention-deficit/hyperactivity disorder symptoms and externalizing progression in the LAMS study: A test of trait impulsivity theory. *Journal of the American Academy of Child and Adolescent Psychiatry*. https://doi.org/10.1016/j.jaac.2021.05.018

Besemer, S., Ahmad, S. I., Hinshaw, S. P., & Farrington, D. P. (2017). A systematic review and meta-analysis of the intergenerational transmission of criminal behavior. *Aggression and Violent Behavior, 37*, 161–178. https://doi.org/10.1016/j.avb.2017.10.004

Bevilacqua, L., Hale, D., Barker, E. D., & Viner, R. (2018). Conduct problems trajectories and psychosocial outcomes: A systematic review and meta-analysis. *European Child and Adolescent Psychiatry, 27*(10), 1239–1260. https://doi.org/10.1007/s00787-017-1053-4

Bevilacqua, L., Kelly, Y., Heilmann, A., Priest, N., & Lacey, R. E. (2021). Adverse childhood experiences and trajectories of internalizing, externalizing, and prosocial behaviors from childhood to adolescence. *Child Abuse and Neglect, 112*. https://doi.org/10.1016/j.chiabu.2020.104890

Blair, R. J. R., Peschardt, K. S., Budhani, S., Mitchell, D. G. V., & Pine, D. S. (2006). The development of psychopathy. *Journal of Child Psychology and Psychiatry, 47*(3–4), 262–275. https://doi.org/10.1111/j.1469-7610.2006.01596.x

Blair, R. J. R., & Zhang, R. (2020). Recent neuro-imaging findings with respect to conduct disorder, callous-unemotional traits and psychopathy. *Current Opinion in Psychiatry, 33*(1), 45–50. https://doi.org/10.1097/yco.0000000000000559

Blakemore, S. J., & Choudhury, S. (2006). Development of the adolescent brain: Implications for executive function and social cognition. *Journal of Child Psychology and Psychiatry, 47*(3–4), 296–312. https://doi.org/10.1111/j.1469-7610.2006.01611.x

Bongers, I. L., Koot, H. M., van der Ende, J., & Verhulst, F. C. (2003). The normative development of child and adolescent problem behavior. *Journal of Abnormal Psychology, 112*(2), 179–192. https://doi.org/10.1037/0021-843x.112.2.179

Borgen, N. T., Olweus, D., Kirkeboen, L. J., Breivik, K., Solberg, M. E., Frones, I., et al. (2021). The potential of anti-bullying efforts to prevent academic failure and youth crime. A case using the Olweus Bullying Prevention Program (OBPP). *Prevention Science, 22*(8), 1147–1158. https://doi.org/10.1007/s11121-021-01254-3

Brunnekreef, J. A., De Sonneville, L. M. J., Althaus, M., Minderaa, R. B., Oldehinkel, A. J., Verhulst, F. C., & Ormel, J. (2007). Information processing profiles of internalizing and externalizing behavior problems: Evidence from a population-based sample of preadolescents. *Journal of Child Psychology and Psychiatry, 48*(2), 185–193. https://doi.org/10.1111/j.1469-7610.2006.01695.x

Burt, S. A., Slawinski, B. L., & Klump, K. L. (2018). Are there sex differences in the etiology of youth antisocial behavior? *Journal of Abnormal Psychology, 127*(1), 66–78. https://doi.org/10.1037/abn0000324

Byrd, A. L., & Manuck, S. B. (2014). MAOA, childhood maltreatment, and antisocial behavior: Meta analysis of a gene-environment interaction. *Biological Psychiatry, 75*(1), 9–17. https://doi.org/10.1016/j.biopsych.2013.05.004

Caron, C., & Rutter, M. (1991). Comorbidity in child psychopathology - concepts, issues and research strategies. *Journal of Child Psychology and Psychiatry, 32*(7), 1063–1080. https://doi.org/10.1111/j.1469-7610.1991.tb00350.x

Carr, A. (2019). Family therapy and systemic interventions for child-focused problems: The current evidence base. *Journal of Family Therapy, 41*(2), 153–213. https://doi.org/10.1111/1467-6427.12226

Caserini, C., Ferro, M., Nobile, M., Scaini, S., & Michelini, G. (2023). Shared genetic influences between depression and conduct disorder in children and adolescents: A systematic review. *Journal of Affective Disorders, 322*, 31–38. https://doi.org/10.1016/j.jad.2022.11.001

Caspi, A., McClay, J., Moffitt, T. E., Mill, J., Martin, J., Craig, I. W., et al. (2002). Role of genotype in the cycle of violence in maltreated children. *Science, 297*(5582), 851–854. https://doi.org/10.1126/science.1072290

Cheong, Y. F., & Raudenbush, S. W. (2000). Measurement and structural models for children's problem behaviors. *Psychological Methods, 5*(4), 477–495. https://doi.org/10.1037/1082-989x.5.4.477

Choi, K. W., Wilson, M., Ge, T., Kandola, A., Patel, C. J., Lee, S. H., & Smoller, J. W. (2022). Integrative analysis of genomic and exposomic influences on youth mental health. *Journal of Child Psychology and Psychiatry, 63*(10), 1196–1205. https://doi.org/10.1111/jcpp.13664

Cicchetti, D. (2013). Annual research review: Resilient functioning in maltreated children - past, present, and future perspectives. *Journal of Child Psychology and Psychiatry, 54*(4), 402–422. https://doi.org/10.1111/j.1469-7610.2012.02608.x

Collishaw, S., Pickles, A., Messer, J., Rutter, M., Shearer, C., & Maughan, B. (2007). Resilience to adult psychopathology following childhood maltreatment: Evidence from a community sample. *Child Abuse and Neglect, 31*(3), 211–229. https://doi.org/10.1016/j.chiabu.2007.02.004

Compas, B. E., Jaser, S. S., Bettis, A. H., Watson, K. H., Gruhn, M. A., Dunbar, J. P., et al. (2017). Coping, emotion regulation, and psychopathology in childhood and adolescence: A meta-analysis and narrative review. *Psychological Bulletin, 143*(9), 939–991. https://doi.org/10.1037/bul0000110

Cosgrove, V. E., Rhee, S. H., Gelhorn, H. L., Boeldt, D., Corley, R. C., Ehringer, M. A., et al. (2011). Structure and etiology of co-occurring internalizing and externalizing disorders in adolescents. *Journal of Abnormal Child Psychology, 39*(1), 109–123. https://doi.org/10.1007/s10802-010-9444-8

Cramer, A. O. J., Waldorp, L. J., van der Maas, H. L. J., & Borsboom, D. (2010). Comorbidity: A network perspective. *Behavioral and Brain Sciences, 33*(2–3), 137-+. https://doi.org/10.1017/s0140525x09991567

Currie, J., & Widom, C. S. (2010). Long-term consequences of child abuse and neglect on adult economic well-being. *Child Maltreatment, 15*(2), 111–120. https://doi.org/10.1177/1077559509355316

da Silva, D. R., Rijo, D., & Salekin, R. T. (2020). Psychopathic traits in children and youth: The state-of-the-art after 30 years of research. *Aggression and Violent Behavior, 55*. https://doi.org/10.1016/j.avb.2020.101454

Dalgleish, T., Black, M., Johnston, D., & Bevan, A. (2020). Transdiagnostic approaches to mental health problems: Current status and future directions. *Journal of Consulting and Clinical Psychology, 88*(3), 179–195. https://doi.org/10.1037/ccp0000482

Dekkers, T. J., Groenman, A. P., Cuijpers, P., Hoekstra, P. J., Luman, M., de Castro, B. O., et al. (2022). Commentary: Why treatment is the best choice for childhood mental disorders - a commentary on Roest et al. *Journal of Child Psychology and Psychiatry*. https://doi.org/10.1111/jcpp.13715

Demontis, D., Walters, R. K., Martin, J., Mattheisen, M., Als, T. D., Agerbo, E., & Wilson, C. H. (2019). Discovery of the first genome-wide significant risk loci for attention deficit/hyperactivity disorder. *Nature Genetics, 51*(1), 63-+. https://doi.org/10.1038/s41588-018-0269-7

den Hoed, J., Devaraju, K., & Fisher, S. E. (2021). Molecular networks of the FOXP2 transcription factor in the brain. *EMBO Reports, 22*(8). https://doi.org/10.15252/embr.202152803

Derks, E. M., Hudziak, J. J., van Beijsterveldt, C. E. M., Dolan, C. V., & Boomsma, D. I. (2004). A study of genetic and environmental influences on maternal and paternal CBCL syndrome scores in a large sample of 3-year-old Dutch twins. *Behavior Genetics, 34*(6), 571–583. https://doi.org/10.1007/s10519-004-5585-2

Dodge, K. A., Bates, J. E., & Pettit, G. S. (1990). Mechanisms in the cycle of violence. *Science, 250*(4988), 1678–1683. https://doi.org/10.1126/science.2270481

Donolato, E., Cardillo, R., Mammarella, I. C., & Melby-Lervag, M. (2022). Research review: Language and specific learning disorders in children and their co-occurrence with internalizing and externalizing problems: A systematic review and meta-analysis. *Journal of Child Psychology and Psychiatry, 63*, 507–518. https://doi.org/10.1111/jcpp.13536

Edens, J. F., Marcus, D. K., Lilienfeld, S. O., & Poythress, N. G. (2006). Psychopathic, not psychopath: Taxometric evidence for the dimensional structure of psychopathy. *Journal of Abnormal Psychology, 115*(1), 131–144. https://doi.org/10.1037/0021-843x.115.1.131

Eilertsen, E. M., Cheesman, R., Ayorech, Z., Roysamb, E., Pingault, J.-B., Njolstad, P. R., et al. (2022). On the importance of parenting in externalizing disorders: An evaluation of indi-

rect genetic effects in families. *Journal of Child Psychology and Psychiatry*. https://doi.org/10.1111/jcpp.13654
Eilertsen, E. M., Jami, E. S., McAdams, T. A., Hannigan, L. J., Havdahl, A. S., Magnus, P., et al. (2021). Direct and indirect effects of maternal, paternal, and offspring genotypes: Trio-GCTA. *Behavior Genetics, 51*(2), 154–161. https://doi.org/10.1007/s10519-020-10036-6
Ekblad, M. O., Marceau, K., Rolan, E., Palmer, R. H. C., Todorov, A., Heath, A. C., & Knopik, V. S. (2020). The effect of smoking during pregnancy on severity and directionality of externalizing and internalizing symptoms: A genetically informed approach. *International Journal of Environmental Research and Public Health, 17*(21). https://doi.org/10.3390/ijerph17217921
Eley, T. C. (1997). General genes: A new theme in developmental psychopathology. *Current Directions in Psychological Science, 6*(4), 90–95. https://doi.org/10.1111/1467-8721.ep11512831
Eme, R. (2020). Life course persistent antisocial behavior silver anniversary. *Aggression and Violent Behavior, 50*. https://doi.org/10.1016/j.avb.2019.101344
Emerson, E., & Hatton, C. (2007). Mental health of children and adolescents with intellectual disabilities in Britain. *British Journal of Psychiatry, 191*, 493–499. https://doi.org/10.1192/bjp.bp.107.038729
Ensink, J. B. M., de Moor, M. H. M., Zafarmand, M. H., de Laat, S., Uitterlinden, A., Vrijkotte, T. G. M., et al. (2020). Maternal environmental risk factors and the development of internalizing and externalizing problems in childhood: The complex role of genetic factors. *American Journal of Medical Genetics Part B-Neuropsychiatric Genetics, 183*(1), 17–25. https://doi.org/10.1002/ajmg.b.32755
Ensink, K., Godbout, N., Bigras, N., Lampron, J., Sabourin, S., & Normandin, L. (2018). Persistent and transitory sexualized behavior problems in children. *Child Psychiatry & Human Development, 49*(4), 621–631. https://doi.org/10.1007/s10578-017-0778-0
Erskine, H. E., Moffitt, T. E., Copeland, W. E., Costello, E. J., Ferrari, A. J., Patton, G., et al. (2015). A heavy burden on young minds: The global burden of mental and substance use disorders in children and youth. *Psychological Medicine, 45*(7), 1551–1563. https://doi.org/10.1017/s0033291714002888
Erskine, H. E., Norman, R. E., Ferrari, A. J., Chan, G. C. K., Copeland, W. E., Whiteford, H. A., & Scott, J. G. (2016). Long-term outcomes of attention-deficit/hyperactivity disorder and conduct disorder: A systematic review and meta-analysis. *Journalof the American Academy of Child and Adolescent Psychiatry, 55*(10), 841–850. https://doi.org/10.1016/j.jaac.2016.06.016
Essex, M. J., Klein, M. H., Cho, E., & Kraemer, H. C. (2003). Exposure to maternal depression and marital conflict: Gender differences in children's later mental health symptoms. *Journal of the American Academy of Child and Adolescent Psychiatry, 42*(6), 728–737. https://doi.org/10.1097/01.Chi.0000046849.56865.1d
Evans, S. E., Davies, C., & DiLillo, D. (2008). Exposure to domestic violence: A meta-analysis of child and adolescent outcomes. *Aggression and Violent Behavior, 13*(2), 131–140. https://doi.org/10.1016/j.avb.2008.02.005
Eyberg, S. M., Nelson, M. M., & Boggs, S. R. (2008). Evidence-based psychosocial treatments for children and adolescents with disruptive behavior. *Journal of Clinical Child and Adolescent Psychology, 37*(1), 215–237. https://doi.org/10.1080/15374410701820117
Eyberg, S. M., & Ross, A. W. (1978). Assessment of child-behavior problems - validation of a new inventory. *Journlal of Clinical Child Psychology, 7*(2), 113–116. https://doi.org/10.1080/15374417809532835
Fairchild, G., Hawes, D. J., Frick, P. J., Copeland, W. E., Odgers, C. L., Franke, B., et al. (2019). Conduct disorder. *Nature Reviews Disease Primers, 5*. https://doi.org/10.1038/s41572-019-0095-y
Fairchild, G., van Goozen, S. H. M., Calder, A. J., & Goodyer, I. M. (2013). Research review: Evaluating and reformulating the developmental taxonomic theory of antisocial behaviour. *Journal of Child Psychology and Psychiatry, 54*(9), 924–940. https://doi.org/10.1111/jcpp.12102

Feinstein, A. R. (1970). Pre-therapeutic classification of co-morbidity in chronic disease. *Journal of Chronic Diseases, 23*(7), 455-+. https://doi.org/10.1016/0021-9681(70)90054-8

Ford, T., Hamilton, H., Goodman, R., & Meltzer, H. (2005). Service contacts among the children participating in the British Child and Adolescent Mental Health Surveys. *Child and Adolescent Mental Health, 10*(1), 2–9. https://doi.org/10.1111/j.1475-3588.2005.00108.x

Ford, T., Hamilton, H., Meltzer, H., & Goodman, R. (2008). Predictors of service use for mental health problems among British schoolchildren. *Child and Adolescent Mental Health, 13*(1), 32–40. https://doi.org/10.1111/j.1475-3588.2007.00449.x

Funkhouser, C. J., Chacko, A. A., Correa, K. A., Kaiser, A. J. E., & Shankman, S. A. (2021). Unique longitudinal relationships between symptoms of psychopathology in youth: A cross-lagged panel network analysis in the ABCD study. *Journal of Child Psychology and Psychiatry, 62*(2), 184–194. https://doi.org/10.1111/jcpp.13256

Garber, J., & Hollon, S. D. (1991). What can specificity designs say about causality in psychopathology research. *Psychological Bulletin, 110*(1), 129–136. https://doi.org/10.1037/0033-2909.110.1.129

Gard, A. M., Dotterer, H. L., & Hyde, L. W. (2019). Genetic influences on antisocial behavior: Recent advances and future directions. *Current Opinion in Psychology, 27*, 46–55. https://doi.org/10.1016/j.copsyc.2018.07.013

Gjerde, L. C., Eilertsen, E. M., McAdams, T. A., Cheesman, R., Moffitt, T. E., Caspi, A., et al. (2023). The p factor of psychopathology and personality in middle childhood: Genetic and gestational risk factors. *Psychological Medicine*, 1–11. https://doi.org/10.1017/s0033291723000077

Gjone, H., & Stevenson, J. (1997). The association between internalizing and externalizing behavior in childhood and early adolescence: Genetic or environmental common influences? *Journal of Abnormal Child Psychology, 25*(4), 277–286. https://doi.org/10.1023/a:1025708318528

Goddings, A. L., Dumontheil, I., Viner, R. M., & Blakemore, S. J. (2023). Puberty and risky decision-making in male adolescents. *Developmental Cognitive Neuroscience, 60*. https://doi.org/10.1016/j.dcn.2023.101230

Goh, S. K. Y., Griffiths, S., Norbury, C. F., & Team, S. (2021). Sources of variability in the prospective relation of language to social, emotional, and behavior problem symptoms: Implications for developmental language disorder. *Journal of Abnormal Psychology, 130*(6), 676–689. https://doi.org/10.1037/abn0000691

Goodman, R. (1997). The strengths and difficulties questionnaire: A research note. *Journal of Child Psychology and Psychiatry, 38*(5), 581–586. https://doi.org/10.1111/j.1469-7610.1997.tb01545.x

Goodman, R., Simonoff, E., & Stevenson, J. (1995). The impact of child IQ, parent IQ and sibling IQ on child behavioural-deviance scores. *Journal of Child Psychology and Psychiatry, 36*(3), 409–425. https://doi.org/10.1111/j.1469-7610.1995.tb01299.x

Gorman, D. A., Gardner, D. M., Murphy, A. L., Feldman, M., Belanger, S. A., Steele, M. M., et al. (2015). Canadian guidelines on pharmacotherapy for disruptive and aggressive behaviour in children and adolescents with attention-deficit hyperactivity disorder, oppositional defiant disorder, or conduct disorder. *Canadian Journal of Psychiatry-Revue Canadienne De Psychiatrie, 60*(2), 62–76. https://doi.org/10.1177/070674371506000204

Gotz, F. M., Gosling, S. D., & Rentfrow, P. J. (2022). Small effects: The indispensable foundation for a cumulative psychological science. *Perspectives on Psychological Science, 17*(1), 205–215. https://doi.org/10.1177/1745691620984483

Goulter, N., Hur, Y. S., Jones, D. E., Godwin, J., McMahon, R. J., Dodge, K. A., et al. (2023). M. Kindergarten conduct problems are associated with monetized outcomes in adolescence and adulthood. *Journal of Child Psychology and Psychiatry*. https://doi.org/10.1111/jcpp.13837

Graham, P. (2019). Against the stream: The teenage brain is not unique. *Bjpsych Bulletin, 43*(6), 287–289. https://doi.org/10.1192/bjb.2019.37

Grant, K. E., Compas, B. E., Stuhlmacher, A. F., Thurm, A. E., McMahon, S. D., & Halpert, J. A. (2003). Stressors and child and adolescent psychopathology: Moving from markers to mechanisms of risk. *Psychological Bulletin, 129*(3), 447–466. https://doi.org/10.1037/0033-2909.129.3.447

Grotzinger, A. D., Rhemtulla, M., de Vlaming, R., Ritchie, S. J., Mallard, T. T., Hill, W. D., et al. (2019). Genomic structural equation modelling provides insights into the multivariate genetic architecture of complex traits. *Nature Human Behaviour, 3*(5), 513–525. https://doi.org/10.1038/s41562-019-0566-x

Gustafsson, B. M., Danielsson, H., Granlund, M., Gustafsson, P. A., & Proczkowska, M. (2018). Hyperactivity precedes conduct problems in preschool children: A longitudinal study. *Bjpsych Open, 4*(4), 186–191. https://doi.org/10.1192/bjo.2018.20

Gustavson, D. E., Franz, C. E., Panizzon, M. S., Lyons, M. J., & Kremen, W. S. (2020). Internalizing and externalizing psychopathology in middle age: Genetic and environmental architecture and stability of symptoms over 15 to 20 years. *Psychological Medicine, 50*(9), 1530–1538. https://doi.org/10.1017/s0033291719001533

Gutman, L. M., Joshi, H., Parsonage, M., & Schoon, I. (2018). Gender-specific trajectories of conduct problems from ages 3 to 11. *Journal of Abnormal Child Psychology, 46*(7), 1467–1480. https://doi.org/10.1007/s10802-017-0379-1

Gutman, L. M., Joshi, H., & Schoon, I. (2019). Developmental trajectories of conduct problems and cumulative risk from early childhood to adolescence. *Journal of Youth and Adolescence, 48*(2), 181–198. https://doi.org/10.1007/s10964-018-0971-x

Hannigan, L. J., Pingault, J.-B., Krapohl, E., McAdams, T. A., Rijsdijk, F. V., & Eley, T. C. (2018). Genetics of co-developing conduct and emotional problems during childhood and adolescence. *Nature Human Behaviour, 2*(7), 514+. https://doi.org/10.1038/s41562-018-0373-9

Hawes, D. J., Price, M. J., & Dadds, M. R. (2014). Callous-unemotional traits and the treatment of conduct problems in childhood and adolescence: A comprehensive review. *Clinical Child and Family Psychology Review, 17*(3), 248–267. https://doi.org/10.1007/s10567-014-0167-1

Hendriks, A. M., Bartels, M., Colins, O. F., & Finkenauer, C. (2018). Childhood aggression: A synthesis of reviews and meta-analyses to reveal patterns and opportunities for prevention and intervention strategies. *Neuroscience and Biobehavioral Reviews, 91*, 278–291. https://doi.org/10.1016/j.neubiorev.2018.03.021

Henggeler, S. W., Melton, G. B., & Smith, L. A. (1992). Family preservation using multisystemic therapy – an effective alternative to incarcerating serious juvenile-offenders. *Journal of Consulting and Clinical Psychology, 60*(6), 953–961. https://doi.org/10.1037/0022-006x.60.6.953

Herrman, H., Patel, V., Kieling, C., Berk, M., Buchweitz, C., Cuijpers, P., et al. (2022). Time for united action on depression: A lancet-world psychiatric association commission. *Lancet, 399*(10328), 957–1022. https://doi.org/10.1016/s0140-6736(21)02141-3

Hovey, D., Lindstedt, M., Zettergren, A., Jonsson, L., Johansson, A., Melke, J., et al. (2016). Antisocial behavior and polymorphisms in the oxytocin receptor gene: Findings in two independent samples. *Molecular Psychiatry, 21*(7), 983–988. https://doi.org/10.1038/mp.2015.144

Hyde, L. W., Waller, R., Trentacosta, C. J., Shaw, D. S., Neiderhiser, J. M., Ganiban, J. M., et al. (2016). Heritable and nonheritable pathways to early callous-unemotional behaviors. *American Journal of Psychiatry, 173*(9), 903–910. https://doi.org/10.1176/appi.ajp.2016.15111381

Ip, K. I., Jester, J. M., Sameroff, A., & Olson, S. L. (2019). Linking Research Domain Criteria (RDoC) constructs to developmental psychopathology: The role of self-regulation and emotion knowledge in the development of internalizing and externalizing growth trajectories from ages 3 to 10. *Development and Psychopathology, 31*(4), 1557–1574. https://doi.org/10.1017/s0954579418001323

Isen, J., Tuvblad, C., Younan, D., Ericson, M., Raine, A., & Baker, L. A. (2022). Developmental trajectories of delinquent and aggressive behavior: Evidence for differential heritability. *Child Psychiatry & Human Development, 53*, 199–211. https://doi.org/10.1007/s10578-020-01119-w

Ivanova, M. Y., Achenbach, T. M., Dumenci, L., Almqvist, F., Weintraub, S., Bilenberg, N., et al. (2007). Testing the 8-syndrome structure of the child behavior checklist in 30 societies. *Journal of Clinical Child and Adolescent Psychology, 36*(3), 405–417. https://doi.org/10.1080/15374410701444363

Jacobson, N. S., & Truax, P. (1991). Clinical-significance – a statistical approach to defining meaningful change in psychotherapy-research. *Journal of Consulting and Clinical Psychology, 59*(1), 12–19. https://doi.org/10.1037/0022-006x.59.1.12

Kaminski, J. W., & Claussen, A. H. (2017). Evidence base update for psychosocial treatments for disruptive behaviors in children. *Journal of Clinical Child and Adolescent Psychology, 46*(4), 477–499. https://doi.org/10.1080/15374416.2017.1310044

Kazdin, A. E., & Weisz, J. R. (1998). Identifying and developing empirically supported child and adolescent treatments. *Journal of Consulting and Clinical Psychology, 66*(1), 19–36. https://doi.org/10.1037/0022-006x.66.1.19

Kendler, K. S., Lonn, S. L., Morris, N. A., Sundquist, J., Langstrom, N., & Sundquist, K. (2014). A Swedish national adoption study of criminality. *Psychological Medicine, 44*(9), 1913–1925. https://doi.org/10.1017/s0033291713002638

Kessler, R. C., Barker, P. R., Colpe, L. J., Epstein, J. F., Gfroerer, J. C., Hiripi, E., et al. (2003). Screening for serious mental illness in the general population. *Archives of General Psychiatry, 60*(2), 184–189. https://doi.org/10.1001/archpsyc.60.2.184

Khan, S., Down, J., Aouira, N., Bor, W., Haywood, A., Littlewood, R., et al. (2019). Current pharmacotherapy options for conduct disorders in adolescents and children. *Expert Opinion on Pharmacotherapy, 20*(5), 571–583. https://doi.org/10.1080/14656566.2018.1561862

Kliem, S., Heinrichs, N., Lohmann, A., Bussing, R., Schwarzer, G., & Briegel, W. (2018). Dimensional latent structure of early disruptive behavior disorders: A taxometric analysis in preschoolers. *Journal of Abnormal Child Psychology, 46*(7), 1385–1394. https://doi.org/10.1007/s10802-017-0383-5

Kohlhoff, J., Cibralic, S., Hawes, D. J., & Eapen, V. (2022). Oxytocin receptor gene (OXTR) polymorphisms and social, emotional and behavioral functioning in children and adolescents: A systematic narrative review. *Neuroscience and Biobehavioral Reviews, 135*. https://doi.org/10.1016/j.neubiorev.2022.104573

Konrad, K., Kohls, G., Baumann, S., Bernhard, A., Martinelli, A., Ackermann, K., et al. (2021). Sex differences in psychiatric comorbidity and clinical presentation in youths with conduct disorder. *Journal of Child Psychology and Psychiatry*. https://doi.org/10.1111/jcpp.13428

Kovas, Y., & Plomin, R. (2007). Learning abilities and disabilities: Generalist genes, specialist environments. *Current Directions in Psychological Science, 16*(5), 284–288. https://doi.org/10.1111/j.1467-8721.2007.00521.x

Kraemer, H. C., Stice, E., Kazdin, A., Offord, D., & Kupfer, D. (2001). How do risk factors work together? Mediators, moderators, and independent, overlapping, and proxy risk factors. *American Journal of Psychiatry, 158*(6), 848–856. https://doi.org/10.1176/appi.ajp.158.6.848

Kretschmer, T., Vrijen, C., Nolte, I. M., Wertz, J., & Hartman, C. A. (2022). Gene-environment interplay in externalizing behavior from childhood through adulthood. *Journal of Child Psychology and Psychiatry, 63*(10), 1206–1213. https://doi.org/10.1111/jcpp.13652

Krueger, R. F., Hobbs, K. A., Conway, C. C., Dick, D. M., Dretsch, M. N., Eaton, N. R., et al. (2021). Validity and utility of hierarchical taxonomy of psychopathology (HiTOP): II.Externalizing superspectrum. *World Psychiatry, 20*(2), 171–193. https://doi.org/10.1002/wps.20844

Krueger, R. E., & Markon, K. E. (2006). Reinterpreting comorbidity: A model-based approach to understanding and classifying psychopathology. *Annual Review of Clinical Psychology, 2*, 111–133. https://doi.org/10.1146/annurev.clinpsy.2.022305.095213

Lahey, B. B., Van Hulle, C. A., Singh, A. L., Waldman, I. D., & Rathouz, P. J. (2011). Higher-order genetic and environmental structure of prevalent forms of child and adolescent psychopathology. *Archives of General Psychiatry, 68*(2), 181–189. https://doi.org/10.1001/archgenpsychiatry.2010.192

Lai, C. S. L., Fisher, S. E., Hurst, J. A., Vargha-Khadem, F., & Monaco, A. P. (2001). A forkhead-domain gene is mutated in a severe speech and language disorder. *Nature, 413*(6855), 519–523. https://doi.org/10.1038/35097076

Leichsenring, F., Steinert, C., & Ioannidis, J. P. A. (2019). Toward a paradigm shift in treatment and research of mental disorders. *Psychological Medicine, 49*(13), 2111–2117. https://doi.org/10.1017/s0033291719002265

Leichsenring, F., Steinert, C., Rabung, S., & Ioannidis, J. P. A. (2022). The efficacy of psychotherapies and pharmacotherapies for mental disorders in adults: An umbrella review and meta-analytic evaluation of recent meta-analyses. *World Psychiatry, 21*(1), 133–145. https://doi.org/10.1002/wps.20941

Leijten, P., Gardner, F., Melendez-Torres, G. J., van Aar, J., Hutchings, J., Schulz, S., et al. (2019). Meta-analyses: Key parenting program components for disruptive child behavior. *Journal of the American Academy of Child and Adolescent Psychiatry, 58*(2), 180–190. https://doi.org/10.1016/j.jaac.2018.07.900

Lilienfeld, S. O. (2018). The multidimensional nature of psychopathy: Five recommendations for research. *Journal of Psychopathology and Behavioral Assessment, 40*(1), 79–85. https://doi.org/10.1007/s10862-018-9657-7

Linnér, R. K., Mallard, T. T., Barr, P. B., Sanchez-Roige, S., Madole, J. W., Driver, M. N., et al. (2021). Multivariate analysis of 1.5 million people identifies genetic associations with traits related to self-regulation and addiction. *Nature Neuroscience, 24*(10), 1367–1376. https://doi.org/10.1038/s41593-021-00908-3

Littell, J. H., Pigott, T. D., Nilsen, K. H., Green, S. J., & Montgomery, O. L. K. (2021). Multisystemic therapy® for social, emotional, and behavioural problems in youth age 10 to 17: An updated systematic review and meta-analysis. *Campbell Systematic Reviews, 17*(4). https://doi.org/10.1002/cl2.1158

Loheide-Niesmann, L., Riem, M. M. E., & Cima, M. (2022). The impact of maternal childhood maltreatment on child externalizing behaviour and the mediating factors underlying this association: A three-level meta-analysis and systematic review. *European Child and Adolescent Psychiatry*. https://doi.org/10.1007/s00787-022-02117-0

Loy, J. H., Merry, S. N., Hetrick, S. E., & Stasiak, K. (2017). Atypical antipsychotics for disruptive behaviour disorders in children and youths (review). *Cochrane Database of Systematic Reviews, 8*. https://doi.org/10.1002/14651858.CD008559.pub3

Luningham, J. M., Hendriks, A. M., Krapohl, E., Ip, H. F., van Beijsterveldt, C. E. M., Lundstrom, S., et al. (2020). Harmonizing behavioral outcomes across studies, raters, and countries: Application to the genetic analysis of aggression in the ACTION Consortium. *Journal of Child Psychology and Psychiatry, 61*(7), 807–817. https://doi.org/10.1111/jcpp.13188

Luo, M., Pappa, I., Cecil, C. A. M., Jansen, P., van Ijzendoorn, M. H., & Kok, R. (2022). Maternal psychological problems during pregnancy and child externalizing problems: Moderated mediation model with child self-regulated compliance and polygenic risk scores for aggression. *Child Psychiatry & Human Development, 53*, 654–666. https://doi.org/10.1007/s10578-021-01154-1

Lynam, D. R., Caspi, A., Moffitt, T. E., Loeber, R., & Stouthamer-Loeber, M. (2007). Longitudinal evidence that psychopathy scores in early adolescence predict adult psychopathy. *Journal of Abnormal Psychology, 116*(1), 155–165. https://doi.org/10.1037/0021-843x.116.1.155

Lynch, S. J., Sunderland, M., Newton, N. C., & Chapman, C. (2021). A systematic review of transdiagnostic risk and protective factors for general and specific psychopathology in young people. *Clinical Psychology Review, 87*. https://doi.org/10.1016/j.cpr.2021.102036

Malanchini, M., Smith-Woolley, E., Ayorech, Z., Rimfeld, K., Krapohl, E., Vuoksimaa, E., et al. (2019). Aggressive behaviour in childhood and adolescence: The role of smoking during pregnancy, evidence from four twin cohorts in the EU-ACTION consortium. *Psychological Medicine, 49*(4), 646–654. https://doi.org/10.1017/s0033291718001344

Malvaso, C. G., Delfabbro, P., & Day, A. (2018). The maltreatment-offending association: A systematic review of the methodological features of prospective and longitudinal studies. *Trauma Violence & Abuse, 19*(1), 20–34. https://doi.org/10.1177/1524838015620820

Marceau, K., Yu, L., Knopik, V. S., Ganiban, J. M., & Neiderhiser, J. M. (2022). Intergenerational transmission of psychopathology: An examination of symptom severity and directionality. *Development and Psychopathology, 34*(5), 1767–1780. https://doi.org/10.1017/s0954579422000852

McElroy, E., Shevlin, M., Murphy, J., & McBride, O. (2018). Co-occurring internalizing and externalizing psychopathology in childhood and adolescence: A network approach. *European Child and Adolescent Psychiatry, 27*(11), 1449–1457. https://doi.org/10.1007/s00787-018-1128-x

McMahon, S. D., Grant, K. E., Compas, B. E., Thurm, A. E., & Ey, S. (2003). Stress and psychopathology in children and adolescents: Is there evidence of specificity? *Journal of Child Psychology and Psychiatry, 44*(1), 107–133. https://doi.org/10.1111/1469-7610.00105

Meehan, A. J., Latham, R. M., Arseneault, L., Stahl, D., Fisher, H. L., & Danese, A. (2020). Developing an individualized risk calculator for psychopathology among young people victimized during childhood: A population-representative cohort study. *Journal of Affective Disorders, 262*, 90–98. https://doi.org/10.1016/j.jad.2019.10.034

Merikangas, K. R., Angst, J., Eaton, W., Canino, G., RubioStipec, M., Wacker, H., et al. (1996). Comorbidity and boundaries of affective disorders with anxiety disorders and substance misuse: Results of an international task force. *British Journal of Psychiatry, 168*, 58–67. https://doi.org/10.1192/s0007125000298425

Merikangas, K. R., He, J. P., Burstein, M., Swendsen, J., Avenevoli, S., Case, B., et al. (2011). Service utilization for lifetime mental disorders in U.S. adolescents: Results of the National Comorbidity Survey-Adolescent Supplement (NCS-A). *Journal of the American Academy of Child and Adolescent Psychiatry, 50*(1), 32–45. https://doi.org/10.1016/j.jaac.2010.10.006

Mesman, J., & Koot, H. M. (2000). Common and specific correlates of preadolescent internalizing and externalizing psychopathology. *Journal of Abnormal Psychology, 109*(3), 428–437. https://doi.org/10.1037//0021-843x.109.3.428

Mikolajewski, A. J., Allan, N. P., Hart, S. A., Lonigan, C. J., & Taylor, J. (2013). Negative affect shares genetic and environmental influences with symptoms of childhood internalizing and externalizing disorders. *Journal of Abnormal Child Psychology, 41*(3), 411–423. https://doi.org/10.1007/s10802-012-9681-0

Miller, G. W. (2021). Exposome: A new field, a new journal. *Exposome, 1*, 1–2.

Moffitt, T. E. (1993). Adolescence-limited and life-course-persistent antisocial-behavior – a developmental taxonomy. *Psychological Review, 100*(4), 674–701. https://doi.org/10.1037/0033-295x.100.4.674

Moffitt, T. E., Arseneault, L., Jaffee, S. R., Kim-Cohen, J., Koenen, K. C., Odgers, C. L., et al. (2008). Research review: DSM-V conduct disorder: Research needs for an evidence base. *Journal of Child Psychology and Psychiatry, 49*(1), 3–33. https://doi.org/10.1111/j.1469-7610.2007.01823.x

Moore, A. A., Blair, R. J., Hettema, J. M., & Roberson-Nay, R. (2019). The genetic underpinnings of callous-unemotional traits: A systematic research review. *Neuroscience and Biobehavioral Reviews, 100*, 85–97. https://doi.org/10.1016/j.neubiorev.2019.02.018

Munoz, R. F., Mrazek, P. J., & Haggerty, R. J. (1996). Institute of medicine report on prevention of mental disorders – summary and commentary. *American Psychologist, 51*(11), 1116–1122. https://doi.org/10.1037/0003-066x.51.11.1116

O'Connor, T. G., McGuire, S., Reiss, D., Hetherington, E. M., & Plomin, R. (1998). Co-occurrence of depressive symptoms and antisocial behavior in adolescence: A common genetic liability. *Journal of Abnormal Psychology, 107*(1), 27–37. https://doi.org/10.1037/0021-843x.107.1.27

Odgers, C. L., Moffitt, T. E., Broadbent, J. M., Dickson, N., Hancox, R. J., Harrington, H., et al. (2008). Female and male antisocial trajectories: From childhood origins to adult outcomes. *Development and Psychopathology, 20*(2), 673–716. https://doi.org/10.1017/s0954579408000333

Ofrat, S., & Krueger, R. F. (2012). How research on the meta-structure of psychopathology aids in understanding biological correlates of mood and anxiety disorders. *Biology of Mood & Anxiety Disorders, 2*(1). https://doi.org/10.1186/2045-5380-2-13

Olweus, D. (2013). School bullying: Development and some important challenges. In S. NolenHoeksema (Ed.), *Annual review of clinical psychology* (Vol. 9, pp. 751–780).

Ouellet-Morin, I., Cote, S. M., Vitaro, F., Hebert, M., Carbonneau, R., Lacourse, E., et al. (2016). Effects of the MAOA gene and levels of exposure to violence on antisocial outcomes. *British Journal of Psychiatry, 208*(1), 42–48. https://doi.org/10.1192/bjp.bp.114.162081

Pappa, I., St Pourcain, B., Benke, K., Cavadino, A., Hakulinen, C., Nivard, M. G., et al. (2016). A genome-wide approach to children's aggressive behavior: The EAGLE consortium. *American Journal of Medical Genetics Part B-Neuropsychiatric Genetics, 171*(5), 562–572. https://doi.org/10.1002/ajmg.b.32333

Patrick, C. J., Fowles, D. C., & Krueger, R. F. (2009). Triarchic conceptualization of psychopathy: Developmental origins of disinhibition, boldness, and meanness. *Development and Psychopathology, 21*(3), 913–938. https://doi.org/10.1017/s0954579409000492

Patton, G. C., Sawyer, S. M., Santelli, J. S., Ross, D. A., Afifi, R., Allen, N. B., et al. (2016). Our future: A Lancet commission on adolescent health and wellbeing. *Lancet, 387*(10036), 2423–2478. https://doi.org/10.1016/s0140-6736(16)00579-1

Perlstein, S., Fair, M., Hong, E. M. Y., & Waller, R. (2023). Treatment of childhood disruptive behavior disorders and callous-unemotional traits: A systematic review and two multilevel meta-analyses. *Journal of Child Psychology and Psychiatry*. https://doi.org/10.1111/jcpp.13774

Perlstein, S., Waller, R., Wagner, N. J., & Saudino, K. J. (2022). Low social affiliation predicts increases in callous-unemotional behaviors in early childhood. *Journal of Child Psychology and Psychiatry, 63*(1), 109–117. https://doi.org/10.1111/jcpp.13466

Pesenti-Gritti, P., Spatola, C. A. M., Fagnani, C., Ogliari, A., Patriarca, V., Stazi, M. A., & Battaglia, M. (2008). The co-occurrence between internalizing and externalizing behaviors. *European Child and Adolescent Psychiatry, 17*(2), 82–92. https://doi.org/10.1007/s00787-007-0639-7

Pettersson, E., Lichtenstein, P., Larsson, H., D'Onofrio, B. M., Lahey, B. B., & Latvala, A. (2021). Associations of resting heart rate and intelligence with general and specific psychopathology: A prospective population study of 899,398 Swedish men. *Clinical Psychological Science, 9*(3), 524–532. https://doi.org/10.1177/2167702620961081

Plomin, R., Gidziela, A., Malanchini, M., & von Stumm, S. (2022). Gene-environment interaction using polygenic scores: Do polygenic scores for psychopathology moderate predictions from environmental risk to behavior problems? *Development and Psychopathology, 34*(5), 1816–1826. https://doi.org/10.1017/s0954579422000931

Poulton, R., Guiney, H., Ramrakha, S., & Moffitt, T. E. (2023). The Dunedin study after half a century: Reflections on the past, and course for the future. *Journal of the Royal Society of New Zealand, 53*, 446–465. https://doi.org/10.1080/03036758.2022.2114508

Radford, L., Corral, S., Bradley, C., & Fisher, H. L. (2013). The prevalence and impact of child maltreatment and other types of victimization in the UK: Findings from a population survey of caregivers, children and young people and young adults. *Child Abuse and Neglect, 37*(10), 801–813. https://doi.org/10.1016/j.chiabu.2013.02.004

Reardon, T., Harvey, K., Baranowska, M., O'Brien, D., Smith, L., & Creswell, C. (2017). What do parents perceive are the barriers and facilitators to accessing psychological treatment for mental health problems in children and adolescents? A systematic review of qualitative and quantitative studies. *European Child and Adolescent Psychiatry, 26*(6), 623–647. https://doi.org/10.1007/s00787-016-0930-6

Rhee, S. H., & Waldman, I. D. (2002). Genetic and environmental influences on antisocial behavior: A meta-analysis of twin and adoption studies. *Psychological Bulletin, 128*(3), 490–529. https://doi.org/10.1037//0033-2909.128.3.490

Riedinger, V., Pinquart, M., & Teubert, D. (2017). Effects of systemic therapy on mental health of children and adolescents: A meta-analysis. *Journal of Clinical Child and Adolescent Psychology, 46*(6), 880–894. https://doi.org/10.1080/15374416.2015.1063427

Rissanen, E., Kuvaja-Kollner, V., Elonheimo, H., Sillanmaki, L., Sourander, A., & Kankaanpaa, E. (2022). The long-term cost of childhood conduct problems: Finnish Nationwide 1981 Birth Cohort Study. *Journal of Child Psychology and Psychiatry, 63*(6), 683–692. https://doi.org/10.1111/jcpp.13506

Robins, L. (1966). *Deviant children grown up*. Williams & Wilkins.

Robins, L. N. (1978). Sturdy childhood predictors of adult antisocial behavior - replications from longitudinal-studies. *Psychological Medicine, 8*(4), 611–622. https://doi.org/10.1017/s0033291700018821

Roest, A. M., de Vries, Y. A., Wienen, A. W., & de Jonge, P. (2022). Editorial perspective: Are treatments for childhood mental disorders helpful in the long run? An overview of systematic reviews. *Journal of Child Psychology and Psychiatry*. https://doi.org/10.1111/jcpp.13677

Rothbaum, F., & Weisz, J. R. (1994). Parental caregiving and child externalizing behavior in nonclinical samples – a meta-analysis. *Psychological Bulletin, 116*(1), 55–74. https://doi.org/10.1037/0033-2909.116.1.55

Rouquette, A., Pingault, J. B., Fried, E. I., Orri, M., Falissard, B., Kossakowski, J. J., et al. (2018). Emotional and behavioral symptom network structure in elementary school girls and association with anxiety disorders and depression in adolescence and early adulthood: A network analysis. *JAMA Psychiatry, 75*(11), 1173–1181. https://doi.org/10.1001/jamapsychiatry.2018.2119

Ruisch, I. H., Dietrich, A., Glennon, J. C., Buitelaar, J. K., & Hoekstra, P. J. (2019). Interplay between genome-wide implicated genetic variants and environmental factors related to childhood antisocial behavior in the UK ALSPAC cohort. *European Archives of Psychiatry and Clinical Neuroscience, 269*(6), 741–752. https://doi.org/10.1007/s00406-018-0964-5

Ruisch, I. H., Dietrich, A., Klein, M., Faraone, S. V., Oosterlaan, J., Buitelaar, J. K., & Hoekstra, P. J. (2020). Aggression based genome-wide, glutamatergic, dopaminergic and neuroendocrine polygenic risk scores predict callous-unemotional traits. *Neuropsychopharmacology, 45*(5), 761–769. https://doi.org/10.1038/s41386-020-0608-0

Rutter, M. (1966). *Children of sick parents: An environmental and psychiatric study*. Oxford University Press.

Rutter, M. (2013). Annual research review: Resilience – clinical implications. *Journal of Child Psychology and Psychiatry, 54*(4), 474–487. https://doi.org/10.1111/j.1469-7610.2012.02615.x

Rutter, M., Graham, P., Chadwick, O. F. D., & Yule, W. (1976). Adolescent turmoil – fact or fiction. *Journal of Child Psychology and Psychiatry, 17*(1), 35–56. https://doi.org/10.1111/j.1469-7610.1976.tb00372.x

Rutter, M., Tizard, J., & Whitmore, K. (Eds.). (1970). *Education, health and behaviour*. Longman.

Rutter, M., Yule, B., Quinton, D., Rowlands, O., Yule, W., & Berger, M. (1975). Attainment and adjustment in 2 geographical areas.3. some factors accounting for area differences. *British Journal of Psychiatry, 126*(JUN), 520–533. https://doi.org/10.1192/bjp.126.6.520

Schaefer, J. D., Moffitt, T. E., Arseneault, L., Danese, A., Fisher, H. L., Houts, R., et al. (2018). Adolescent victimization and early-adult psychopathology: Approaching causal inference using a longitudinal twin study to rule out noncausal explanations. *Clinical Psychological Science, 6*(3), 352–371. https://doi.org/10.1177/2167702617741381

Schlotz, W., & Phillips, D. I. W. (2009). Fetal origins of mental health: Evidence and mechanisms. *Brain Behavior and Immunity, 23*(7), 905–916. https://doi.org/10.1016/j.bbi.2009.02.001

Schmitz, S., Fulker, D. W., & Mrazek, D. A. (1995). Problem behavior in early and middle childhood: An initial behavior genetic analysis. *Journal of Child Psychology and Psychiatry, 36*(8), 1443–1458. https://doi.org/10.1111/j.1469-7610.1995.tb01674.x

Schuurmans, I. K., Martinez, N. T., Blok, E., Hillegers, M. H. J., Ikram, M. A., Luik, A. I., & Cecil, C. A. M. (2022). Child mental health problems as a risk factor for academic underachievement: A multi-informant, population-based study. *Acta Psychiatrica Scandinavica, 145*(6), 578–590. https://doi.org/10.1111/acps.13426

Schwartz, S., & Susser, E. (2011). The use of well controls: An unhealthy practice in psychiatric research. *Psychological Medicine, 41*(6), 1127–1131. https://doi.org/10.1017/s0033291710001595

Scott, S., & Gardner, F. (2015). Parenting progams. In A. Thapar, D. Pine, J. Leckman, S. Scott, M. Snowling, & E. Taylor (Eds.), *Rutter's child and adolescent psychiatry* (6th ed.). Wiley Blackwell.

Scott, S., Sylva, K., Doolan, M., Price, J., Jacobs, B., Crook, C., & Landau, S. (2010). Randomised controlled trial of parent groups for child antisocial behaviour targeting multiple risk factors: The SPOKES project. *Journal of Child Psychology and Psychiatry, 51*(1), 48–57. https://doi.org/10.1111/j.1469-7610.2009.02127.x

Sellbom, M., & Drislane, L. E. (2021). The classification of psychopathy. *Aggression and Violent Behavior, 59*. https://doi.org/10.1016/j.avb.2020.101473

Sellers, R., Harold, G. T., Thapar, A., Neiderhiser, J. M., Ganiban, J. M., Reiss, D., et al. (2020). Examining the role of genetic risk and longitudinal transmission processes underlying maternal parenting and psychopathology and children's ADHD symptoms and aggression: Utilizing the advantages of a prospective adoption design. *Behavior Genetics, 50*(4), 247–262. https://doi.org/10.1007/s10519-020-10006-y

Sellers, R., Warne, N., Pickles, A., Maughan, B., Thapar, A., & Collishaw, S. (2019). Cross-cohort change in adolescent outcomes for children with mental health problems. *Journal of Child Psychology and Psychiatry, 60*(7), 813–821. https://doi.org/10.1111/jcpp.13029

Shanahan, L., Copeland, W., Costello, E. J., & Angold, A. (2008). Specificity of putative psychosocial risk factors for psychiatric disorders in children and adolescents. *Journal of Child Psychology and Psychiatry, 49*(1), 34–42. https://doi.org/10.1111/j.1469-7610.2007.01822.x

Shaw, D. S., Galan, C. A., Lemery-Chalfant, K., Dishion, T. J., Elam, K. K., Wilson, M. N., & Gardner, F. (2019). Trajectories and predictors of children's early-starting conduct problems: Child, family, genetic, and intervention effects. *Development and Psychopathology, 31*(5), 1911–1921. https://doi.org/10.1017/s0954579419000828

Skeem, J. L., & Cooke, D. J. (2010). Is criminal behavior a central component of psychopathy? Conceptual directions for resolving the debate. *Psychological Assessment, 22*(2), 433–445. https://doi.org/10.1037/a0008512

Speyer, L. G., Hall, H. A., Hang, Y., Hughes, C., & Murray, A. L. (2022). Within-family relations of mental health problems across childhood and adolescence. *Journal of Child Psychology and Psychiatry*. https://doi.org/10.1111/jcpp.13572

Stevenson, J. (1999). The treatment of the long-term sequelae of child abuse. *Journal of Child Psychology and Psychiatry, 40*(1), 89–111. https://doi.org/10.1017/s0021963098003345

Tabachnick, B. G., & Fidell, L. S. (2013). *Using multivariate statistics* (Sixth ed.). Pearson.

Takahashi, Y., Pease, C. R., Pingault, J. B., & Viding, E. (2021). Genetic and environmental influences on the developmental trajectory of callous-unemotional traits from childhood to adolescence. *Journal of Child Psychology and Psychiatry, 62*(4), 414–423. https://doi.org/10.1111/jcpp.13259

Thapar, A., & Rutter, M. (2009). Do prenatal risk factors cause psychiatric disorder? Be wary of causal claims. *British Journal of Psychiatry, 195*(2), 100–101. https://doi.org/10.1192/bjp.bp.109.062828

Tielbeek, J. J., Johansson, A., Polderman, T. J. C., Rautiainen, M. R., Jansen, P., Taylor, M., et al. (2017). Genome-wide association studies of a broad spectrum of antisocial behavior. *JAMA Psychiatry, 74*(12), 1242–1250. https://doi.org/10.1001/jamapsychiatry.2017.3069

Tielbeek, J. J., Uffelmann, E., Williams, B. S., Colodro-Conde, L., Gagnon, E., Mallard, T. T., et al. (2022). Uncovering the genetic architecture of broad antisocial behavior through a genome-wide association study meta-analysis. *Molecular Psychiatry, 27*(11), 4453–4463. https://doi.org/10.1038/s41380-022-01793-3

Tomlinson, R. C., Hyde, L. W., Dotterer, H. L., Klump, K. L., & Burt, S. A. (2021). Parenting moderates the etiology of callous-unemotional traits in middle childhood. *Journal of Child Psychology and Psychiatry*. https://doi.org/10.1111/jcpp.13542

Ttofi, M. M., & Farrington, D. P. (2011). Effectiveness of school-based programs to reduce bullying: A systematic and meta-analytic review. *Journal of Experimental Criminology, 7*(1), 27–56. https://doi.org/10.1007/s11292-010-9109-1

Valadez, E. A., Tottenham, N., Korom, M., Tabachnick, A. R., Pine, D. S., & Dozier, M. (2023). A randomized controlled trial of a parenting intervention during infancy alters amygdala-prefrontal circuitry in middle childhood. *Journal of the American Academy of Child & Adolescent Psychiatry*. https://doi.org/10.1016/j.jaac.2023.06.015

van den Oord, E., Verhulst, F. C., & Boomsma, D. I. (1996). A genetic study of maternal and paternal ratings of problem behaviors in 3-year-old twins. *Journal of Abnormal Psychology, 105*(3), 349–357. https://doi.org/10.1037/0021-843x.105.3.349

van der Laan, C. M., Morosoli-Garcia, J. J., van de Weijer, S. G. A., Colodro-Conde, L., Lupton, M. K., Mitchell, B. L., et al. (2021). Continuity of genetic risk for aggressive behavior across the life-course. *Behavior Genetics, 51*(5), 592–606. https://doi.org/10.1007/s10519-021-10076-6

van der Stouwe, T., Asscher, J. J., Stams, G., Dekovic, M., & van der Laan, P. H. (2014). The effectiveness of multisystemic therapy (MST): A meta-analysis. *Clinical Psychology Review, 34*(6), 468–481. https://doi.org/10.1016/j.cpr.2014.06.006

Vanheusden, K., van der Ende, J., Mulder, C. L., van Lenthe, F. J., Verhulst, F. C., & Mackenbach, J. P. (2008). The use of mental health services among young adults with emotional and behavioural problems: Equal use for equal needs? *Social Psychiatry and Psychiatric Epidemiology, 43*(10), 808–815. https://doi.org/10.1007/s00127-008-0367-4

Vernes, S. C., Newbury, D. F., Abrahams, B. S., Winchester, L., Nicod, J., Groszer, M., et al. (2008). A functional genetic link between distinct developmental language disorders. *New England Journal of Medicine, 359*(22), 2337–2345. https://doi.org/10.1056/NEJMoa0802828

Viding, E., Blair, R. J. R., Moffitt, T. E., & Plomin, R. (2005). Evidence for substantial genetic risk for psychopathy in 7-year-olds. *Journal of Child Psychology and Psychiatry, 46*(6), 592–597. https://doi.org/10.1111/j.1469-7610.2004.00393.x

Vijayakumar, N., Op de Macks, Z., Shirtcliff, E. A., & Pfeifer, J. H. (2018). Puberty and the human brain: Insights into adolescent development. *Neuroscience and Biobehavioral Reviews, 92*, 417–436. https://doi.org/10.1016/j.neubiorev.2018.06.004

Vuoksimaa, E., Rose, R. J., Pulkkinen, L., Palviainen, T., Rimfeld, K., Lundstrom, S., et al. (2021). Higher aggression is related to poorer academic performance in compulsory education. *Journal of Child Psychology and Psychiatry, 62*, 327–338. https://doi.org/10.1111/jcpp.13273

Waldman, I. D., Poore, H. E., van Hulle, C., Rathouz, P. J., & Lahey, B. B. (2016). External validity of a hierarchical dimensional model of child and adolescent psychopathology: Tests using confirmatory factor analyses and multivariate behavior genetic analyses. *Journal of Abnormal Psychology, 125*(8), 1053–1066. https://doi.org/10.1037/abn0000183

Waldman, I. D., Rowe, R., Boylan, K., & Burke, J. D. (2021). External validation of a bifactor model of oppositional defiant disorder. *Molecular Psychiatry, 26*(2), 682–693. https://doi.org/10.1038/s41380-018-0294-z

Waller, R., Hyde, L. W., Klump, K. L., & Burt, A. (2018). Parenting is an environmental predictor of callous unemotional traits and aggression: A monozygotic twin differences study. *Journal of the American Academy of Child and Adolescent Psychiatry, 57*(12), 955–963. https://doi.org/10.1016/j.jaac.2018.07.882

Weeland, J., Overbeek, G., de Castro, B. O., & Matthys, W. (2015). Underlying mechanisms of gene-environment interactions in externalizing behavior: A systematic review and search for theoretical mechanisms. *Clinical Child and Family Psychology Review, 18*(4), 413–442. https://doi.org/10.1007/s10567-015-0196-4

Weiss, B., Susser, K., & Catron, T. (1998). Common and specific features of childhood psychopathology. *Journal of Abnormal Psychology, 107*(1), 118–127. https://doi.org/10.1037/0021-843x.107.1.118

Willner, C. J., Gatzke-Kopp, L. M., & Bray, B. C. (2016). The dynamics of internalizing and externalizing comorbidity across the early school years. *Development and Psychopathology, 28*(4), 1033–1052. https://doi.org/10.1017/s0954579416000687

Womack, S. R., Clifford, S., Wilson, M. N., Shaw, D. S., & Lemery-Chalfant, K. (2021). Genetic moderation of the association between early family instability and trajectories of aggressive behaviors from middle childhood to adolescence. *Behavior Genetics*. https://doi.org/10.1007/s10519-021-10069-5

Xerxa, Y., Rescorla, L. A., van der Ende, J., Hillegers, M. H. J., Verhulst, F. C., & Tiemeier, H. (2021). From parent to child to carent: Associations between parent and offspring psychopathology. *Child Development, 92*(1), 291–307. https://doi.org/10.1111/cdev.13402

Yew, S. G. K., & O'Kearney, R. (2013). Emotional and behavioural outcomes later in childhood and adolescence for children with specific language impairments: Meta-analyses of controlled prospective studies. *Journal of Child Psychology and Psychiatry, 54*(5), 516–524. https://doi.org/10.1111/jcpp.12009

Zhang, R., Manza, P., & Volkow, N. D. (2022). Prenatal caffeine exposure: Association with neurodevelopmental outcomes in 9-to 11-year-old children. *Journal of Child Psychology and Psychiatry, 63*(5), 563–578. https://doi.org/10.1111/jcpp.134

Chapter 9
Neurodevelopmental Aspects of Behavioural Differences: I. Attention Deficit Hyperactivity Disorder (ADHD)

There are two dimensions of behavioural differences that emerge early in development and that have enduring influences on children's functioning. These dimensions underlie attentional deficit hyperactivity disorder (ADHD) and autism spectrum disorders (ASD). These behavioural dimensions will be covered in this chapter and in Chap. 10. Both ADHD and ASD are recognised as being on continua of behavioural differences that extend through the general population. Historically, this has not been the case and both were previously seen as diagnostic categories that were qualitatively distinct. They are also now seen as being underpinned by neurodevelopmental differences rather than primarily arising from adverse experiences during development. For this reason, they are being considered here separately from internalising and externalising behaviours.

Morris-Rosendahl and Crocq (2020) provide a history of the conditions classified as neurodevelopmental disorders in DSM-5. They review the moves towards a continuum model for these neurodevelopmental disorders and argue the case for a genetic neurodevelopmental continuum with individual genes influencing a range of behaviours. They suggest this is an orientation that may be fruitful in the development of transdiagnostic therapies.

The status of neurodevelopmental disorders was reviewed by Thapar et al. (2017). They endorsed the importance of recognising these as disorders distinct from other groupings such as internalising and externalising behaviours. They also suggested that considering them as traits has been central to the development of research studies but that a categorical framework is needed, not least to assist with decision-making in the clinical context.

A more radical critique of the use of a categorical framework for neurodevelopmental disorders has been be made by Astle et al. (2022). The range of neurodevelopmental disorders they address covers ADHD, ASD, specific reading disorder, specific maths disorder, developmental language disorder, and social pragmatic communication disorder. The reading and language-focussed neurodevelopmental disorders are outside the scope of this book. Astle et al. (2022) identify three

J. Stevenson, *Developmental Psychopathology*,
https://doi.org/10.1007/978-3-031-45787-6_9

problems that arise from a categorical diagnostic approach. The first is that the categorical taxonomies do not capture the needs of all the children that may have poor functioning in learning, behaviour, and social functioning. In particular, this approach fails to identify the significant number of children who show milder difficulties which may nevertheless need support; the use of a diagnostic threshold misses the needs of many children. The second is that the categorical approach is not suited to deal with the high level of symptom variability within diagnostic categories. The third problem is that the categorical approach cannot readily accommodate the overlap between supposedly discrete groups.

The alternative that they endorse is the transdiagnostic approach. This has at its core a set of dimensions on which children with neurodevelopmental problems vary. They propose that these dimensions may include hyperactivity and impulsivity, inattention, social communication, executive functioning, and phonological processing. They suggest that

> ..neurodevelopment can be more usefully understood in terms of multiple continuous dimensions relating to cognition, behaviour, or neurobiology – with graduated levels ranging from typical through to atypical functioning.
>
> … individuals may have elevated levels of difficulty across multiple dimensions, with the particular combination reflecting both the nature and complexity of their difficulties. (Astle et al., 2022, p.5)

They show how a more flexible set of categories can be derived from measures on these dimensions plus additional data, such as neurobiological characteristics, by the use of data-driven cluster analyses. They illustrate this approach by reference to Kushki et al. (2019), who used data on behaviour and on cortical neuroanatomy to examine the relationships between data-derived clusters and existing diagnostic groups (ADHD, ASD, and obsessive compulsive disorder) and found little agreement between the two approaches. Kushki et al. (2019) concluded that this transdiagnostic approach, coupled with cluster analysis, identifies groupings that more closely align with the known features of large between-disorder overlap and of within-disorder variability.

Du Rietz et al. (2021b) undertook a confirmatory factor analysis of diagnoses in the Swedish National Patients Register on a large sample of 774,416 full and maternal half-sibling pairs. They applied latent variables underlying neurodevelopmental, internalising, and externalising behaviours as well as a general psychopathology factor. They found that when the general psychopathology factor was taken into account, ADHD remained highly correlated with the neurodevelopmental factor $r = 0.43$ ($CI_{.95} = 0.42–0.45$) and was almost exclusively influenced by genetic factors. They conclude that the comorbidities found for ADHD with internalising and externalising behaviours largely arise from influences shared with the general psychopathology factor. However, there was some evidence consistent with the notion that ADHD might be a precursor of some later externalising behaviours.

The application of a hierarchical modelling approach to behaviour in children with a variety of neurodevelopmental disorders was undertaken by Holmes et al. (2021). The 403 children in their sample were aged 5 to 18 years and had been referred for support with problems in attention, learning and/or memory. As for other children, there was general psychopathology (p-factor) which accounted for variance across all psychopathology measures. In addition, this factor predicted a wide range of clinical, educational, and social measures. Additional variance in the behaviour measures was explained by latent variables of broad internalising and broad externalising. This again echoes the pattern seen in models derived for children in the general population. There were an additional three lower-order factors of specific internalising, social maladjustment, and neurodevelopment. The latter was the strongest predictor of learning problems in this sample. Holmes et al. (2021) argue that this study demonstrates the value of a hierarchical and multidimensional approach to the description of psychopathology in children with neurodevelopmental problems.

This change from a categorical to dimensional framework presents a potential difficulty in labelling. It has become standard to use the term ASD spectrum to refer to the dimension of behaviour differences related to autism, and that is the term that will be adopted here. With the dimension related to ADHD, there is a less clear consensus. Following Taylor (1998), the term "hyperactivity" has been used for the dimension as distinct from the ADHD category. Under his formulation, hyperactivity is a trait continuously distributed in the population – an enduring disposition to behave in a restless, inattentive, impulsive, and disorganised fashion. Unfortunately, the use of "hyperactivity" for the behavioural dimension underlying ADHD has not been widely adopted. Consequently, here, the dimension will be referred to as ADHD symptoms or score.

For neurodevelopmental conditions such as ADHD and ASD, Morton and Frith (2001) have provided a framework for formulating the relationships between underlying causes. This postulates that biology causes cognition via influences on the brain and cognition causes behaviour. This framework will be used here to summarise studies on ADHD and ASD. All three levels (biology, cognition, and behaviour) can be influenced by environmental factors. Here, cognition represents an essential intermediary explaining the connections between biology and behaviour. In this framework, the role of emotions in influencing behaviour is divided between their biological basis and their cognitive interpretation (for example, see Fava & Morton, 2009).

9.1 Behavioural Aspects of ADHD

Diagnoses of problems with inattention and activity The behaviours comprising ADHD include being unable to sit still, especially in calm or quiet surroundings, constant fidgeting, being unable to concentrate on tasks, excessive physical movement, excessive talking, being unable to wait their turn, acting without thinking and interrupting conversations. The DSM-5 criteria for an ADHD diagnosis require that these behaviours are present before the age of 12 years; that they should be seen in two or more settings, typically home and school; that they produce an impairment in functioning; and that the behaviours cannot be attributed to another mental disorder.

There is clear evidence that internationally ADHD is one of the most common mental disorders in children (Polanczyk et al., 2015). This systematic review and meta-analysis of the worldwide literature indicated a prevalence rate of ADHD of 5.3%, with males more than twice as likely to show ADHD than females (Polanczyk et al., 2007). A later systematic review and meta-analysis produced a slightly higher estimate of prevalence. Based on 175 eligible studies, the prevalence of ADHD was estimated to be 7.2% ($CI_{.95}$ 6.7 to 7.8) (Thomas et al., 2015). The slightly higher estimate of prevalence is partly a result of the inclusion of an additional 83 studies and by not having a restriction on the language in which the studies were published. It may also be that the diagnosis of ADHD is being made more often in clinical settings. A large scale study (N = 11,878) examined the prevalence of ADHD in 9–10-year-olds in the USA using a variety of criteria for ADHD (Cordova et al., 2022). They found a prevalence of about 3.5% using the most stringent criteria of a DSM-5 definition requiring multiple informants.

Hyperkinetic disorder is the diagnostic category used in the World Health Organization's International Classification of Disease and is a sub-group of those with ADHD. The diagnosis is applicable to perhaps 1.5% of the primary school-aged population (Swanson et al., 1998). This sub-group has to conform to more stringent criteria than those receiving an ADHD diagnosis. Inattentiveness, hyperactivity, and impulsiveness have to be present at both home and school for hyperkinetic disorder. Children with hyperkinetic disorder are the sub-group of those with ADHD that are particularly responsive to treatment with stimulants (Santosh et al., 2005).

Taylor (2017) has reviewed both prevalence rates for cases of ADHD identified by research studies and compared these to the administrative prevalence rates. These are the rates at which the diagnosis is made in clinical services. He concludes that ADHD is under diagnosed by clinicians. The UK shows a particularly low level of diagnosis. The administrative prevalence in the UK is around 1% compared to a research-based prevalence in the UK of about 2.5%. This matters as there are interventions that can improve functioning in those with ADHD, although the impact of treatments on core ADHD impairments of inattention and impulsiveness is limited. An additional adverse consequence of not receiving a diagnosis is that "less helpful" labels may be applied, such as "'idle', 'difficult', and 'naughty'" (Taylor, 2017).

There is a suggestion that there may be an increase in the diagnosis of ADHD whilst the frequency of hyperactive/inattentive behaviours is at relatively constant levels over time (Rydell et al., 2018). The frequency of a diagnosis of ADHD was found to increase from 4.6% to 5.6% in two cohorts of Australian children born in 1999/2000 and 2003/2004 (Kazda et al., 2022). These two samples were of about 4500 children in each case. These results from Australia are in line with the increased prevalence found in the meta-analyses by Polanczyk et al. (2007) and Thomas et al. (2015) discussed above. However, a striking feature of these results is that the increase in prevalence was observed in cohorts born only 4 years apart.

It is possible that the increased prevalence is due to changes in exposure to environmental risks, such as air pollution. This possibility was tested by Taylor et al. (2023) based on twin samples in Sweden born between 1992 and 2008. They found no significant changes in the relative contribution of genetic and environmental factors over this time period. They suggest that changes in the underlying aetiology of ADHD over time are unlikely to account for the increase in ADHD prevalence. Instead, it is more likely that ADHD is being more frequently recognised by parents, teacher, and clinicians, resulting in increases in ADHD diagnoses.

Behavioural measures of ADHD The performance of the available screening measures for ADHD was the subject of a systematic review and meta-analysis by Mulraney et al. (2022). They identified 41 different measures that could be used for this purpose. They concluded that most of the instruments have a very good overall diagnostic accuracy. However, they recommend that reliance should not be placed on a single measure completed by a single reporter. Multiple measures are needed to achieve the sensitivity and specificity needed in the clinical setting or for population screening.

The identification of a continuum of ADHD behaviours leads to the consideration of both positive and negative aspects of behaviour. By adopting such a method, it is possible to produce scales that show an approximately normal distribution. This approach was applied in the development of the Strengths and Weaknesses of ADHD symptoms and Normal Behavior (SWAN) scale (Swanson et al., 2012). Other scales, which are based on counts of the number of symptoms, tend to produce J-shaped distributions, with many children scoring zero and only a few at the high-end extreme. It is suggested that this SWAN scale provides a distribution of scores that is more suitable for analysis with parametric statistics and which corrects for a tendency of symptom count measures to over-identify high-end cases.

Sub-types of ADHD There is extensive evidence to support the distinction between behaviours related to inattention and to hyperactive-impulsivity. However, there is not sufficient evidence for sub-types of ADHD based on this distinction. Rather, it is preferable to use a dimensional approach whereby a child with ADHD is characterised at different ages by the degree to which inattention and hyperactive-impulsivity behaviours are shown (Willcutt et al., 2012).

A test of the distinction between inattentive and hyperactive-impulsivity aspects of ADHD was made by Martel et al. (2022). It is known that both polygenic factors and prenatal risk can lead to ADHD. Martel et al. (2022) postulated that these two causal factors influenced different facets of ADHD via separate temperament routes. They tested this model on data from a sample of 849 children studied longitudinally between middle childhood through adolescence. Results showed the mediation pathway from prenatal smoking through surgency to hyperactivity-impulsivity was significant ($\beta = 0.053$, $p < 0.01$). The second route from polygenic risk through effortful control to inattention was also significant ($\beta = 0.084$, $p < 0.01$). These results held when other associations were controlled – for example, with the other risk factor and held across parent- and teacher-report of ADHD symptoms. Based on these findings, ADHD is seen as multifaceted with children varying on at least two behavioural dimensions, each of which may have separate developmental origins in aspects of earlier temperament, and each of which is influenced by distinct genetic and environmental risk factors.

ADHD in young children A meta-analysis by Joseph et al. (2023) found that there were modest associations between temperament, measured in infancy and toddlerhood, and later ADHD symptoms. The correlations were of the order $r = 0.39 - 0.25$. They suggest that infant temperament is an early risk factor for ADHD in childhood and that such measures "could be used for early intervention identification". These correlations are not large and suggest that many children with elevated temperament profiles of raised activity levels, for example, would not go on to show clinically diagnostic severity of ADHD behaviour. Under these circumstances, the adverse effects of elevating parental concerns about their child would outweigh the gains to be made from labelling the child at risk for ADHD.

Wilens et al. (2002) demonstrated that children aged 4 to 6 years diagnosed with ADHD were very similar to older (7–9-year-olds) with the same diagnosis in the quality of the ADHD symptoms, the high level of comorbidity, and impaired functioning. These findings suggest that ADHD was an appropriate formulation to apply to preschool children but left open the question of whether it is best conceptualised as a categorical diagnosis or as an extreme on a continuum.

The debate over whether it was developmentally appropriate to apply an ADHD diagnosis to the behaviour of preschool children or whether this behaviour was better considered as extremes on a dimension was evaluated by Sonuga-Barke et al. (2005). The diagnostic approach they label the "mental disorder framework." The dimensional approach they characterize as a "developmental psychopathology framework". They conclude that findings related to the mental disorder perspective indicate that preschool children can have a pattern of ADHD impairment equivalent to that shown by older children and adolescents. Using the developmental psychopathology approach, Sonuga-Barke et al. (2005) proposed four developmental pathways involving preschool hyperactivity: emergent oppositionality, late-onset ADHD, preschool limited ADHD, and early-onset/chronic ADHD. They suggest that these pathways have distinct developmental courses from infancy to middle childhood. At successive phases, different temperament characteristics interact with features of the parent–child relationship and negative aspects of the child's experience at school to influence the emergence of these types of early hyperactivity. They conclude that if ADHD in preschool children is to be considered as a clinical diagnosis under the mental disorder model, the approach to treatment and intervention needs to be based on an understanding of the developmental psychopathology pathway the child may be following.

Behaviours associated with ADHD Those with ADHD have been shown to be more likely to show aggressive behaviour, particularly reactive or impulsive aggression (Saylor & Amann, 2016). Speyer et al. (2022) studied a sample of 1246 Swiss children between the ages of 7 and 9 to examine the relationship between ADHD behaviours and types of aggressive behaviour. They found evidence that there were many reciprocal relationships between these sets of behaviours. Inattention was seen to be predictive of both proactive and reactive aggression. Saylor and Amann (2016) showed that proactive aggression in those with ADHD did not necessarily remit when ADHD treatments are given. Such behaviours have adverse social consequences for the child with ADHD, for example, for in peer relations.

9.2 Cognitive Aspects of ADHD

There has been an extensive range of neuropsychological deficits that have been shown to be associated with ADHD. Coghill et al. (2014) undertook a study using measures in domains that had been thought to characterise the cognitive deficits of those with ADHD. They used confirmatory factor analysis (CFA) to identify a six-factor model on data obtained from boys with ADHD and typically developing (TD) boys with mean ages of 9 years. The effect sizes (standardised mean differences from the mean of TD boys) on these six factor scores were as follows: working memory 0.95, inhibition 0.61, delay aversion 0.82, decision-making 0.55, timing 0.71, and response variability 0.37. There was a 0.60 correlation between delay aversion and inhibition, but the other factor correlations were only modest. This provides evidence that these six areas of neuropsychological functioning represent relatively discrete areas of cognitive deficits in boys with ADHD.

Self-control Moffitt et al. (2011) assessed children's self-control during their first decade of life using nine measures: observational ratings of children's lack of control (at 3 and 5 years of age) and parent, teacher, and self-reports of impulsive aggression, hyperactivity, lack of persistence, inattention, and impulsivity (at 5, 7, 9, and 11 years). These measures produced a gradient of self-control from low to high. This gradient was shown to be linearly related to a number of outcomes up to age 32 years of age. These include health, wealth and criminality. The effects of the gradient remained even when children with an ADHD diagnosis were removed. These findings suggest that, in the population at large, individual differences in self-control during the first 11 years of life can predict significant adverse outcomes in adulthood. These associations remain when other factors are controlled, such as the children's intelligence, social class, and home lives of their families.

Time perception The studies on the perception of time by those with ADHD was subjected to a meta-analysis by Marx et al. (2022). They found deficits in those with ADHD, especially in discriminating stimuli of very brief durations. ADHD was associated with more variability in estimating the duration of stimuli of longer duration. Deficits in time estimation and time production accuracy were interpreted as indicating an accelerated internal clock. They suggest that these findings indicate the need for improved measures of timing ability to aid the development of interventions for those with ADHD.

Sluggish cognitive tempo A particular cognitive style has come to be known as "sluggish cognitive tempo" (SCT). It is characterised by excessive daydreaming, mental confusion and fogginess, being lost in one's thoughts, and slowed behaviour and thinking. A number of measures of SCT have been developed which show adequate reliability and validity (Becker, 2021). SCT has been examined as a possible pure form of inattentive ADHD. However it has become to be recognised as a distinctive pattern of behaviour that is distinguishable from ADHD (Becker et al., 2016). Unlike ADHD, there is not strong evidence for an excess of males with SCT. Nevertheless, SCT does show a strong correlation with ADHD inattention

($r = 0.63$) and a less strong correlation with hyperactivity-impulsivity ($r = 0.32$). There is no clear profile of neuropsychological deficits in SCT, but there is some evidence of poor processing speed, sustained attention, and metacognition (Becker et al., 2016). There is a suggestion that SCT is also linked to ASD and is particularly common when ASD and ADHD co-occur (Mayes et al., 2020).

Executive function There has been an extensive range of studies examining whether executive function (EF) deficits contribute to ADHD behaviours. EF involves high-level cognitive processes, often associated with the frontal lobes, that control lower level processes in the service of goal-directed behaviour (Friedman & Miyake, 2017). They include abilities such as response inhibition, interference control, working memory updating, and set shifting. A landmark paper by Pennington and Ozonoff (1996) reviewed the history of the concept of executive function and discusses how this relates to loss of ability arising from damage to the prefrontal cortex. The executive functions contribute to the maintenance of an appropriate problem-solving set to attain a later goal.

There is a need for caution in the interpretation of studies of EF that use different types of measures. In particular, it has been shown that performance-based measures (such as the Stop Task: Oosterlaan et al., 1998) and rating measures of executive function (such as the Behavior Rating Inventory of Executive Function – BRIEF: Gioia et al., 2000) assess different aspects of executive function (Toplak et al., 2013). The administration, task demands, and scoring of these domains of measures are different. Toplak et al. (2013) found that the median correlation between these two types of EF measures was only 0.19 in the 20 studies they reviewed.

Structure of executive function Karr et al. (2018) undertook a review of studies that had examined the structure of EF using confirmatory factor analysis (CFA). The first paper to present such findings was that by Miyake et al. (2000) which showed that for young adults the three executive function factors of shifting, updating, and inhibition are separable but not independent; they are moderately correlated. Data from a set of 46 samples were re-analysed by Karr et al. (2018). They found evidence of differentiation with age in the structure of EF from the preschool onward with models involving one or two factors in young children and more complex and nested factor models in adults. The inconsistencies between studies lead the authors to caution that the findings are tentative and do not offer definitive conclusions regarding the true nature of executive functions.

Following Karr et al. (2018) there have been a number of commentaries that have suggested that the use of latent variable approaches, such as CFA, may not be the optimal method to capture the structure of EF. Camerota et al. (2020) show that different measurement models produce different findings about EF. They contrasted a CFA measurement model producing latent variables and composite scores derived from principal component analysis. Indeed it has been suggested that this latent variable approach presenting EF as a set of domain-general components is inappropriate (Doebel, 2020). Instead she suggests that EF should be viewed as developing from specific tasks

> well-established age-related improvements on measures of executive function may in part reflect the acquisition of knowledge, beliefs, values, and more that shape how control is used in the service of particular goals. For example, in this proposal, children do not simply develop an inhibitory process that they then apply across a wide range of situations. Rather, they develop skills in using control in specific ways in the service of specific goals, such as avoiding hitting a playmate who takes one of their toys. (Doebel, 2020, p.946)

Executive function and behaviour The review by Pennington and Ozonoff (1996) found that EF deficits are consistently found in both ADHD and ASD but not in conduct disorder. The nature of the EF deficit is different for ASD and ADHD. EF deficits on complex tasks are more severe in the ASD than in ADHD. In the few studies of more specific EF tasks, there are impairments in motor inhibition in ADHD but not in autism, whereas there are impairments in verbal working memory in autism but not ADHD.

A later review of EF, focussed on studies of inhibition, set shifting, working memory, planning, and fluency, was produced by Sergeant et al. (2002). They concluded that there were EF deficits in children with ADHD but that there was no clear consensus between studies on the precise nature of the deficit. These conclusions were reflected in the results of meta-analysis of 83 studies on EF in children with ADHD (Willcutt et al., 2005). They found effect sizes in the range of 0.46 to 0.69. They suggest that EF weaknesses are neither necessary nor sufficient to cause all cases of ADHD but that they are an important part of the complex neuropsychology of ADHD.

There is a possibility that some of the common comorbidities of ADHD influence the association with EF deficits. For example, Noordermeer et al. (2020) studied adolescents with ADHD only, ADHD plus Oppositional Defiant Disorder (ODD) and controls. They found that it was on the combined ADHD and ODD group that had a wide range of EF abnormalities whereas those with ADHD alone were impaired only in working memory and time production. These results suggest that ODD may be largely responsible for the EF deficits observed in ADHD.

The question of the nature of the relationship between EF, ADHD, and other aspects of child mental health was studied by Halse et al. (2022). They obtained measures repeatedly between the ages of 6 and 14 years on a community sample of Norwegian children (N = 874). They found a reciprocal relationship over time between poor EF and ADHD. A similar two-way association was found between EF and depression, anxiety, oppositional defiant disorder, and conduct disorder. They concluded that poor EF and a wide range of disorders are both a cause and consequence of each other. This suggests that EF may be one of the factors that comprise the general factor of psychopathology (see Sect. 6.7).

Executive function, IQ, and ADHD The well-established relationship between ADHD and low IQ was summarised in a meta-analysis of 137 studies (Frazier et al., 2004). They reported a highly significant effect size (SMD = 0.61 ($CI_{.95}$ 0.57 to 0.65)) for the difference in mean full-scale IQ between those with ADHD and TD children and adolescents. This association between ADHD and IQ was shown by Kuntsi et al. (2004) to arise from shared genetic factors.

Given that ADHD is related to IQ, it is important to establish whether the association between ADHD and EF is simply due to shared variance with IQ. Friedman and Miyake (2017) estimate that a latent EF factor shares on average 25% of its variance with "g" – the latent factor underlying measures of IQ. They argue that the evidence suggests that although EF is related to IQ, it is not the same as IQ. Indeed, EF predicts behaviour even when IQ is controlled.

Models of executive function deficits in ADHD There are alternative models of the way EF may relate to ADHD behaviour. Castellanos et al. (2006) suggested that EF needs to be recast into those functions reflecting "cool" processes, such as those involved in relatively abstract decontextualised problems related to an instructional set, and "hot" processes that relate to a motivational state where there is a greater emotional load. Their model proposes that some children with ADHD will have "cool" EF deficits, some "hot" EF deficits, and some have both. The relationship between the "cool" and "hot" EF systems and brain sMRI and fMRI were reviewed by Rubia (2011). This indicated that those with ADHD exhibited abnormalities in the "cool" EF system. By contrast those with conduct disorder were distinguished by differences in the "hot" EF structures.

Nigg (2017) has drawn attention to the confusion of terminology that surrounds studies on processes variously labelled self-control, executive functioning, effortful control, cognitive control, impulsivity, risk-taking, and inhibition. He suggests that the term self-regulation be used to encompass the intrinsic regulation of action, emotion, and cognition. This is distinct from extrinsic effects on regulation, i.e. direction by others. Self-regulation incorporates both "bottom-up" or automatic processes, which are automatic, stimulus-driven, rapid, and do not require mental capacity, and "top-down" or deliberate processes, which are subjectively deliberate, slow, sequential and require working memory. Nigg (2017) provides a framework for understanding how the breakdown of self-regulation may lead to psychopathology. Abnormalities in the neural systems involved in executive function in the anterior insula/dorsal anterior cingulate-based network have been found to be a common feature in adults with schizophrenia, bipolar disorder, depression, addiction, obsessive-compulsive disorder, and anxiety. These abnormalities may relate to executive function deficits observed across diagnoses.

Executive function in the preschool child The development of EF during the preschool period was studied by Hughes et al. (2010). They used a variety of tasks to measure EF at ages 4 and 6 in a longitudinally studied sample from the general population. They showed that there is single latent EF variable at these two ages and that there was significant improvement in EF ability over the time of the transition to school.

Espy et al. (2011) developed a model of the relationship between elements of executive control and behaviour problems in preschool children (see Fig. 9.1). They found a single latent variable of executive control could be identified for a set of measures derived from laboratory tasks. Using parent ratings of behaviour, four latent variables were derived – hyperactive behaviours, attention problems, disinhibition behaviours, and emotional dysregulation behaviours. The executive control

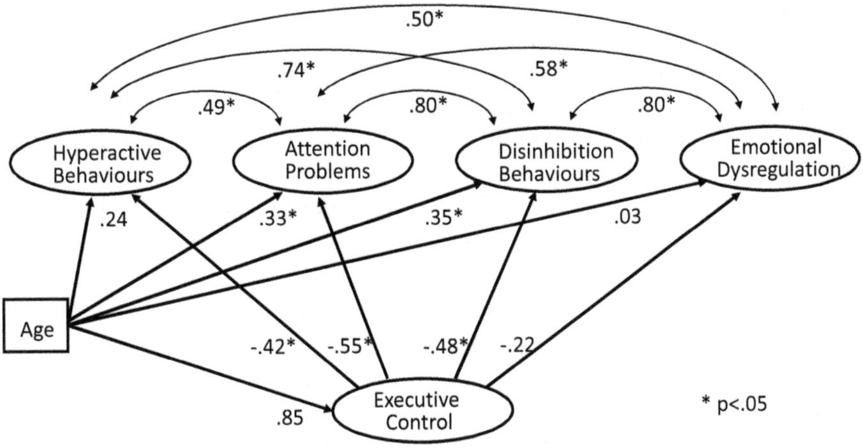

Fig. 9.1 Problem behaviour-executive control model for boys and girls. Only latent variables and age are shown. (Adapted with the permission of John Wiley & Sons from Figure 3 Espy et al. (2011); permission conveyed through Copyright Clearance Center, Inc.)

latent variable was significantly related to the first three of these latent variables with standardised paths coefficients at round 0.50. It was not significantly related to emotional dysregulation (see Fig. 9.1). However Espy et al. (2011) also say that the model fit was not significantly changed when the paths from executive control to the other later variables were set to be equal – this solution gave paths of −0.42 for each. This suggests the most parsimonious interpretation is that executive control is related equally strongly to hyperactive behaviour, attention problems, disinhibition, and emotional dysregulation in these young children.

Genetic influences on executive function Twin studies have shown EF to have a very high heritability. In a study using three latent EF variables, Friedman et al. (2008) showed that inhibiting, updating, and shifting had almost all of their variance explained by genetic differences. The heritabilities were 0.99, 1.00, and 0.81, respectively. However, subsequent molecular genetic studies have failed to identify specific genes that might contribute to variation in EF ability (Ibrahim-Verbaas et al., 2016).

The possibility of epigenetic factors modifying EF was reviewed by Ibrahim et al. (2018). They identified 14 studies on the issue; however, these varied in methodology to an extent that precluded the possibility of a meta-analysis. There was little consistency in the findings that have emerged from these studies and the authors concluded that larger studies are needed to clearly identify the possible role of epigenetic influences on EF.

There have been a number of attempts to relate polygenic scores for ADHD to EF. Benca et al. (2017) did not find an association nor did Schork et al. (2019). However, Chang et al. (2020) did find that EF was associated with PRS scores for ADHD and indeed that EF mediated the association between ADHD PRS and ADHD symptoms. In part, this difference between the studies might arise from the Chang et al. (2020) sample being younger than in the other two studies.

Executive function and Theory of Mind Hughes et al. (1998) studied a group of 4-year-old children from a general population sample. A group of "hard to manage" children were selected on the basis of being above the 90th percentile on the hyperactivity sub-scale of the SDQ. These children were poor compared to TD children on a measure of executive control and a measure of Theory of Mind (see Sect. 10.2). Within the "hard to manage" group, these two poor performances were associated. Hughes et al. (1998) conclude that their results suggest that executive dysfunction may lead to problems of disruptive behaviour both directly and indirectly, via deficit in Theory of Mind.

Reaction time variability There have been a number of studies that suggest that variability in reaction time (RT) is a core feature of ADHD (Tamm et al., 2012). In a twin study, Kuntsi, Oosterlaan, and Stevenson (2001) found that reaction time variability was the major discriminator between those with hyperactivity and TD children. In this same study, reaction time variability was shown to share genetic effects with hyperactivity (Kuntsi & Stevenson, 2001). Castellanos et al. (2005) found that RT variability was greater in boys with ADHD than TD boys. In addition, they found that this RT variability was suppressed by methylphenidate, which is an efficacious treatment for ADHD (Cortese, 2020). It has been shown that the genetic influences shared between mean RT, RT variability and ADHD behaviours are independent of the genetic influences shared between ADHD behaviours and IQ (Wood et al., 2010).This illustrates the multiple routes whereby cognitive factors mediate the influence of genetics on ADHD.

Reaction time variability has also been shown to relate to outcomes in adolescents with ADHD. Over a 6-year period, those with ADHD showing most marked reaction time variability at age 12 years were less likely to show improvements in ADHD measures than remitters, i.e those showing improvement (Michelini et al., 2016). Other neuropsychological measures, such as executive function, did not differentiate between remitters and persisters. The authors of this study suggest that the findings indicate that reaction time variability could be a valuable target for nonpharmacological interventions for those with ADHD.

These findings on reaction time variability in ADHD have been shown to be robust in a meta-analysis of 319 studies (Kofler et al., 2013). The effects size for ADHD compared to TD children was SMD = 0.76 – the effect was smaller for adults (SMD = 0.46). However, when compared to other diagnostic groups, it was found that RT variability was not specific to ADHD. Indeed, Kofler et al. (2013) conclude that RT variability should be considered as general marker or shared risk factor among a broad range of psychopathology. Karalunas et al. (2014) point out that children with ADHD in the Kofler et al. (2013) meta-analysis showed more variable RT than the combined clinical group comparisons (SMD = 0.25). They argue that when more fine-grained measures of RT variability are used, they show some specificity to ADHD, but more comparisons across clinical populations are need.

The potential value of reaction time variability as an endophenotype in genetic studies of ADHD was emphasised by Uebel et al. (2010). Endophenotypes are traits that are associated with the expression of an illness and are believed to represent the genetic liability of the disorder among non-affected subjects. In addition, an endophenotype must occur before the onset of illness and must be heritable (Leboyer et al., 1998). There is now evidence that reaction time variability and a component of executive function, working memory, represent endophenotypes for ADHD. Using data from the large population sample in the Adolescent Brain Cognitive Development study, Moses et al. (2022) found that both reaction time variability and working memory partially mediated the relationship between an ADHD PRS and measured ADHD behaviour.

Delay aversion Delay aversion was proposed as an influence acting on ADHD, in parallel with executive functions, and one that was present from the preschool period onwards (Sonuga-Barke et al., 2003). Delay aversion is a negative emotion arising from having to wait for an anticipated reward or experience, which is shown particularly by children with ADHD. It was suggested that delay aversion and executive function represent independent influences on ADHD (Sonuga-Barke et al., 2005). Evidence for this proposal was found in an appraisal of children with ADHD and controls (Solanto et al., 2001; Marco et al., 2009).

Similar findings were obtained in a study of children with hydrocephalus (Stevenson & Cate, 2004). These children have been shown to have problems with attention and executive function (Burmeister et al., 2005). Children with hydrocephalus and a TD comparison group were assessed on executive functions and delay aversion using computerised tasks (Kuntsi et al., 2001b). A mediation path analysis showed that the risk of hyperactivity in children with hydrocephalus was accounted for by independent paths via executive functions and via delay aversion (see Fig. 9.2).

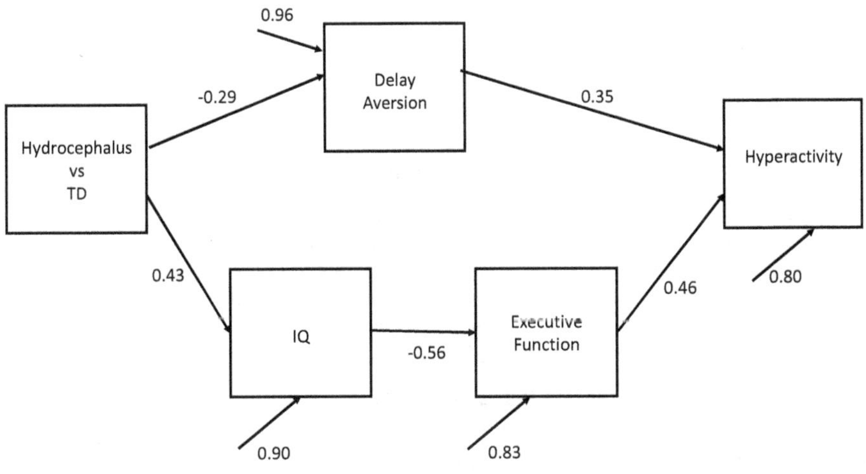

Fig. 9.2 Dual pathway of association between delay aversion, executive function, and hyperactivity. (Adapted with the permission of Hindawi from Figure 1 Stevenson and Cate (2004); permission conveyed through Copyright Clearance Center, Inc.)

The question of the whether neuropsychological deficits associated with ADHD are apparent from an early age was addressed in a meta-analysis of studies on preschool children (Pauli-Pott & Becker, 2011). They found a large effect for delay aversion. The executive function and attention measures showed smaller but significant differences between those with ADHD and TD children. The data indicated that the effect size for delay aversion may decrease with age.

The related issues of impulsive choice-making and delay of gratification deficits associated with ADHD were reviewed in a meta-analysis by Patros et al. (2016). They found an effect size of SMD = 0.47 between those with ADHD and TD children on tasks of impulsive decision-making. A subsequent meta-analysis by Doidge et al. (2021) examined gender differences in performance on delay of gratification tasks. They found a significant gender difference in those with ADHD, with girls preferring a small immediate reward to a larger delayed reward (SMD = −0.23). No such sex difference was found in TD children.

Emotional regulation Delay aversion is related to self-control. This is a feature of self-regulation defined as the capacity to alter unwanted impulses and behaviours in order to bring them into agreement with internal and external standards. The heritability of self-control was estimated in a meta-analysis of 31 twin studies by Willems et al. (2019). The overall MZ correlation was 0.58 and the DZ correlation was 0.28. These values provide a heritability of 0.60, with little evidence for shared environment effects. This suggests that individual differences in self-control arise from genetic differences between people and from experiences unique to the person.

Delay aversion is related to self-control. This is a feature of self-regulation defined as the capacity to alter unwanted impulses and behaviours in order to bring them into agreement with internal and external standards. The heritability of self-control was estimated in a meta-analysis of 31 twin studies by (Willems et al., 2019). The overall MZ correlation was 0.58 and the DZ correlation was 0.28. These values provide a heritability of 0.60, with little evidence for shared environment effects. This suggests that individual differences in self-control arise from genetic differences between people and from experiences unique to the person.

A related feature of behaviour that accompanies ADHD is emotional lability or dysregulation. Emotional regulation is defined as:

> an individual's ability to modify an emotional state so as to promote adaptive, goal oriented behaviors. It encompasses the processes that allow the individual to select, attend to, and appraise emotionally arousing stimuli, and to do so flexibly. These processes trigger behavioral and physiological responses that can be modulated in line with goals. Emotion dysregulation arises when these adaptive processes are impaired, leading to behavior that defeats the individual's interests. (Shaw et al., 2014, p.276)

Shaw et al. go on to explain that emotion dysregulation is a dimensional entity, not a categorical diagnosis, and that there is a full spectrum of emotional dysregulation within ADHD. It does not just occur with extreme ADHD behaviours. A longitudinal study of a UK population cohort of 9619 children between the ages 3 and 7 years found that emotional dysregulation was an important mediator of the association between ADHD symptoms and the development of internalising problems (Antony et al., 2022). There is evidence that the functioning of the right insula brain region may be an important influence on the emotional dysregulation seen in those with ADHD. An analysis of functional MRI data showed that for these children emotion dysregulation was related to increased interconnections in the right insula (Viering et al., 2021).

Banaschewski et al. (2012) examined whether any underlying neuropsychological deficit could account for the association between emotional dysregulation and ADHD. They used measures of working memory, reaction time variability, and delay aversion. They found that, although these were related to emotional dysregulation, this relationship disappeared when ADHD symptoms were controlled. By contrast, these neuropsychological test measures remained significantly related to ADHD symptoms when emotional dysregulation was controlled. In this study, the strongest association between a neuropsychological measure and emotional dysregulation was with mean reaction time and reaction time variability. The same pattern was found by Sjowall et al. (2013) and Van Liefferinge et al. (2021). These results suggest that emotional dysregulation is unlikely to be a causal factor in the development of ADHD.

Concluding comment on cognitive features of ADHD It is clear that there is a rich set of findings related to the neuropsychological basis of ADHD, and many theories have been proposed to account for them, but there is little consensus on which are right or, as Johnson et al. (2009) argue, on how to demonstrate these theories are wrong! It appears that reaction time variability is one of the most robust performance factors consistently related to ADHD (Kuntsi & Klein, 2012). But even in this circumscribed area there is no clear account yet of its biological basis (Killeen, 2019; Bellato et al., 2020).

9.3 Biological Aspects of ADHD

Gender One of the most salient features of ADHD is the increased risk of the condition in males compared to females. Hinshaw et al. (2022) produced a landmark review on the issue of ADHD in girls and women. They concluded that

> (a) Girls meet diagnostic criteria for ADHD at just under half the rates of boys, a ratio that becomes much closer to equal by adulthood. (b) Girls and women with ADHD show a predominance of inattention and associated Internalizing problems; boys and men display greater levels of hyperactive–impulsive symptoms and associated externalizing problems. (c) Sex differences in ADHD symptoms and related outcomes depend heavily on the clinical versus nonreferred nature of the samples under investigation [the higher male prevalence is more marked in clinical samples]. (d) Females with ADHD experience, on average, serious impairments, with a particularly heightened risk for problems in close relationships and engagement in self-harm. (e) Clinicians may overlook symptoms and impairments in females because of less overt (but still impairing) symptom manifestations in girls and women and their frequent adoption of compensatory strategies. (Hinshaw et al., 2022, p.484)

Brain structure, function, and chemistry: Volume There have been a substantial number of studies examining possible differences in brain structure and function in children with ADHD. For example, a meta-analysis by Valera et al. (2007) summarised early studies on brain volumes in ADHD. They found the largest differences between children with ADHD and TD children were in cerebellar regions, the splenium of the corpus callosum, total and right cerebral volume, and right caudate.

There has been a recurrent problem of non-replication in these MRI studies of brain structure. The same is true of studies of functional-MRI (see below). A major subsequent meta-analysis concluded:

> To the best of our knowledge, this study is the largest meta-analysis of structural and functional neuroimaging experiments in children/adolescents with ADHD. We found no significant convergent across structural and functional regional alterations in ADHD, which might be attributable to clinical heterogeneity, experimental and analytical flexibility and positive publication bias, but could also point towards a more distributed, network-based pathology lacking a consistent expression at any particular location. (Samea et al., 2019)

Diffusion-weighted imaging is a method applied to quantify microstructural features in the brain and white matter connections. This approach can provide information on the differences in fine details of brain structure that underpin the possible differences in functional connectivity from the fMRI studies. For example, using diffusion-weighted imaging (Griffiths et al., 2021) found lower local efficiency (i.e. longer distances) in subcortical regions in those with ADHD. However, once again, problems of non-replication have arisen with diffusion-weighted imaging studies of ADHD. A meta-analysis of these studies indicated that there was little consistency in the findings on atypical interhemispheric connections (Aoki et al., 2018). They suggest that in part this inconsistency may be due to artefacts arising from uncorrected group differences in head motion. Head motion during scanning can produce spurious results in diffusion-weighted imaging and the overactive behaviour in children with ADHD will be reflected in increased head motion and thereby is likely to distort any comparisons with TD children.

Brain structure, function, and chemistry: Functional MRI (fMRI) In a review of imaging studies of ADHD, Pereira-Sanchez and Castellanos (2021) suggest:

> Neuroimaging research on ADHD since 2019 has documented that children with ADHD have smaller global and regional brain structural indices than TDCs, in both cortical and subcortical areas, albeit with small effect sizes. Functional imaging results are less clear; some meta-analytic approaches suggest interplay of several key networks is associated with ADHD; this conclusion was not supported by the most comprehensive and unrestricted analyses. Multimodal approaches integrating imaging, genetic, and phenotypic data are emerging, although their replicability has yet to be confirmed. Adoption of open science and best reporting practices are needed to make ADHD neuroimaging research more methodologically sound and relevant to improve the care of patients. (Pereira-Sanchez & Castellanos, 2021, p.109)

Studies on resting-state functional MRI in those with ADHD will be used to illustrate these difficulties. Castellanos and Proal (2012) suggested that ADHD could be associated with differences in a wider range of brain systems, which can be seen when the brain is studied in a resting-state, i.e. using functional imaging when the participant has not been given an explicit task. Norman et al. (2021) undertook a study of a sample of 167 participants enriched with children with high levels of ADHD symptoms, who were followed for 3 years. The found that baseline resting-state functional MRI (R-fMRI) predicted an increase in inattention symptoms over this time period. Specifically, greater connectivity of right inferior frontal gyrus at baseline was associated with fewer inattention symptoms at follow-up. No such effects were found on hyperactivity/impulsivity symptoms.

Meta-analysis of R-fMRI studies have been conducted by Cortese et al. (2021a) and by Sutcubasi et al. (2020). The latter concluded that ADHD is characterised by reduced connectivity both within the core Default Mode Network (DMN) subsystem and between that system and other brain networks involved in cognition and motivation. The DMN is a distributed network of brain regions which are, somewhat paradoxically, more active when the brain is seemingly doing nothing (Whitfield-Gabrieli & Ford, 2012). The Cortese et al. (2021a) review came to a very different conclusion from Sutcubasi et al. (2020)! They adopted a different meta-analytic approach to the fMRI data. They concentrated on identifying "spatial convergence". This reflects the degree to which different fMRI studies agree on the location in the brain where connectivity is higher or lower than in TD comparison children. They concluded that there was no significant agreement on where such brain connectivity difference might be found in those with ADHD. To explain this inconsistency, in addition to methodological differences from the Sutcubasi et al. (2020) review, Cortese et al. (2021a) point out the difficulties in obtaining reproducible findings from fMRI in studies on psychiatric disorders.

In commenting on these disagreements, Pereira-Sanchez and Castellanos (2021) identify disparities in the findings from a third meta-analysis by Gao et al. (2019). They go further to conclude that there is little agree between the results of f-MRI studies on ADHD on just where brain function differences might be found. They suggest that by contrast, structural MRI studies have identified robust replicated differences in brain volume and structure in those with ADHD and TD children but with very small effects sizes (SMD) between 0.10 and 0.30.

However, subsequently, a mega-analysis was produced of resting-state connectivity in patients with ADHD ($N = 1301$) and unaffected controls ($N = 1301$) drawn from several large datasets (Norman et al., 2023). This mega-analysis was based on pooled "raw" data and produced large sample for analysis. The results showed that ADHD was associated with more positive/decreased negative connectivity between the default mode network and attention networks. The effects sizes are small but significant – SMD between 0.14 and 0.17. Norman et al. (2023) conclude that although these results are robust, atypical connectivity for the DMN is neither necessary nor sufficient for the development of ADHD.

One of the reasons for this problem of reproducibility may stem from the low reliability of fMRI and R-fMRI studies. A meta-analysis of 90 experiments with 1008 adult participants found a test–retest reliability of 0.40 for task-functional fMRI measures (Elliott et al., 2020). The test–re-test of R-fMRI by itself was also found to be low (0.54) (Elliott et al., 2019). However, Elliott et al. (2019) suggest that a more reliable measure of connectivity can be derived by combining data from task based fMRI and R-fMRI – they call this general functional connectivity (GFC). With GFC the test–re-test reliability of connectivity measures improved and heritability and power increased. As yet, this approach has not been applied to data from children and adolescents with ADHD.

Castellanos (2021) has provided a bullish but cautious appraisal of brain imaging studies on ADHD. He places particular emphasis on the impact that Big Data/Open Data-sharing may have in future studies. This impact has already been shown by the Norman et al. (2023) mega-analysis on DMN discussed above.

Brain structure, function, and chemistry: EEG An alternative method of investigating brain function is electro-encephalography (EEG). There is a long history of EEG studies on children with ADHD, which has been reviewed by Arns et al. (2013). They concluded that there are group differences in EEG between those with ADHD and TD children. The EEG profile may also be a helpful indicator of the likely response to stimulant medication treatment.

Many of these studies have involved resting state EEG analogous to the R-fMRI approach. Studies have also been based on recording brain activity whilst making a response during an experimental task. Recent studies on the use of these event-related potentials (ERPs) with children with ADHD were the subject of a meta-analysis (Michelini et al., 2022). They found modest differences in ERP between those with and without ADHD in samples of both children and adults. As yet, it is unknown just how specific these ERP differences are to ADHD or whether they will be found in children with other neurodevelopmental disorders.

Brain structure, function, and chemistry: chemistry Perlov et al. (2009) produced a review and meta-analysis of studies using magnetic resonance spectroscopy (MRS) to examine differences in brain chemistry between children with ADHD and TD children. A number of regions of interest (ROI) had been studied. ROI are parts of the brain on which the imaging is concentrated as these regions are thought to be likely to show differences based on previous research. In the Perlov et al. (2009) review, these ROI were the frontal lobes and the prefrontal cortex and basal ganglia. They commented that there were too few studies that had used MRS to establish possible neurochemistry mechanisms in ADHD. The weaknesses in these studies, such as being based on small numbers of participants, were identified in a subsequent review by O'Neill et al. (2013).

Aoki et al. (2013) also undertook a meta-analysis to establish whether there were age-related changes in brain chemistry in those with ADHD. The only ADHD difference from TD children they identified was a significantly higher-than-normal N-acetylaspartate (NAA) in the medial prefrontal cortex (mPFC), but no significant differences in other metabolites in that area. There were no significant differences in metabolite levels in any other region.

A number of the MRS studies have focussed on differentiating ADHD associated with prenatal alcohol exposure (PAE) with familial ADHD. For example, Alger et al. (2021) found that compared to familial ADHD, those with ADHD+PAE had higher glutamate levels, more marked hyperactivity, and distinct white matter pathology. They also identified that children with ADHD without PAE were significantly lower in glutamate levels in white matter than TD children.

Marked age-related changes have been reported for the inhibitory neurotransmitter gamma-aminobutyric acid (GABA) and related metabolites (Bollmann et al., 2015; Spencer et al., 2014). Lower GABA levels were found in children with ADHD compared to TD comparison children but this was not found for adults with ADHD. The opposite pattern was found for glutamine with elevated levels for children with ADHD but not for adults. In a study of adults with ADHD, Bauer et al. (2018) found an increase in glutamate in the anterior cingulate cortex compared to a TD comparison group. In addition, the level of glutamate in those with ADHD was correlated with hyperactivity and impulsivity.

Glutamate and gamma-aminobutyric acid (GABA) are synthesised by the gut microbiome and form part of the "microbiota–gut–brain axis" (Cryan et al., 2019). A model has been proposed that sees a reciprocal relationship between the gut and the brain as playing a role in the development of ADHD (Sandgren & Brummer, 2018). The potential implication of studies on the gut microbiome for the treatment of ADHD have been reviewed (Cenit et al., 2017; Checa-Ros et al., 2021). There is suggestive, but weak, evidence that the use of probiotics early in life may reduce the risk of developing ADHD (Partty et al., 2015). This finding arose from the follow-up of 75 children at 13 years taking part in a randomised trial of the use of probiotics to prevent atopic eczema! There is suggestion that the use of micronutrient supplementation to treat ADHD may result in small, subtle changes to the composition of the microbiome (Stevens et al., 2019). One potential influence on the gut microbiome is exposure to antibiotics. There is evidence that pre-natal (but not post-natal) antibiotic exposure increases the risk of ADHD in the child (Otten et al., 2022).

Reporting on a later meta-analysis, Vidor et al. (2022) point out that the findings in the previous meta-analyses on MRS studies of ADHD were not replicated. Their own analysis of 33 studies identified just one significant difference between those with and without ADHD – glutamate and glutamine were present in higher concentration on the right medial frontal area in those with ADHD. In reflecting on the results of the various meta-analyses of MRS studies on ADHD that raise the following question:

> …how suitable MRS is for the subtle functional changes of psychiatric disorders. Although this is a question for which we have no definitive answer, it is imperative to continuously consider that MRS has eminent limitations as conflicting results consistently emerge. (Vidor et al., 2022, p. 1045)

ENIGMA (Enhancing NeuroImaging Genetics through MetaAnalysis) Consortium Thompson et al. (2020) produced a review of the work of the ENIGMA, which is a global alliance of over 1400 scientists across 43 countries, studying the human brain in health and disease. The key findings of the ENIGMA Consortium ADHD Working Group based on 2246 participants with ADHD were as follows:

> Reduction in bilateral amygdala, striatal, and hippocampal volumes in the ADHD population, especially in children; lower cortical surface area values found in children with ADHD, but not in adolescents or adults; lower surface area associated with ADHD symptoms in the general population in childhood; genetic association studies suggest that genes involved in

> neurite outgrowth play a role in findings of reduced volume in ADHD; gene-expression studies imply that structural brain alterations in ADHD can also be explained in part by the differential vulnerability of these regions to mechanisms mediating apoptosis [or programmed cell death] , oxidative stress, and autophagy. (Thompson et al., 2020, p.3)

There have been sporadic reports of differences between those with ADHD and TD comparison children in asymmetries in a number of brain structures. To obtain a more definitive test, information on brain asymmetries was examined in the ENIGMA Consortium data set (Postema et al., 2021). These data comprise 1933 people with ADHD and 1829 comparison participants. The data set included adults as well as children. Some significant findings were obtained, but the effect sizes were small, with an SMD between −0.18 and 0.18. The authors report that these differences would not survive study-wide correction for multiple testing. The conclusion was reached that brain asymmetries are not likely to prove to be a valuable biomarker for ADHD.

It is striking (and disappointing) that, in reviewing the studies on brain structure, function and chemistry in ADHD, there is such a uniform failure to produce robust findings using the various methods employed. It is even more sobering that these studies have been focused largely on identifying group differences between those with and without ADHD. The application of these assessment methods in the planning of treatment of ADHD for individuals will make the need for reliable measurement even greater.

Genetics ***Family studies*** The transmission of the risk of ADHD across generations has been established (Solberg et al., 2021). This population-based intergenerational study demonstrated a stronger recurrent risk of ADHD from mothers than from fathers, and in both cases, strongest to daughters. A relative risk of 11.7 was found for ADHD in offspring of parents who were both ADHD compared to families where both parents did not have ADHD. This family transmission could be explained by a number of environmental, genetic and interaction mechanisms. To disentangle the effects of these influences, research designs are needed based on twins and adopted children, for example.

Twin studies Faraone and Larsson (2019) summarised the findings from 37 twin studies of children and suggested that the heritability of inattentiveness or hyperactivity is 74% across age groups. Levy et al. (1997) and Gjone et al. (1996) have shown that using twin data that the genetic risk for ADHD was most appropriately considered as a dimension. A similar pattern of results was obtained with hyperactivity ratings in preschool twin children, with heritability at around 0.80 both across the full range of scores and for group heritabilities at the high end of the continuum (Price et al., 2001). Kuntsi et al. (2005), in a longitudinal study of the same sample, showed that genetic factors were largely responsible for the stability of ADHD symptoms from age 2 to 8 years.

Adoption studies There have been fewer studies of ADHD examining genetic and environmental influences using adopted children and their families. However, the findings support the conclusion from twin studies that genetics is a major influence on ADHD. For example, Sprich et al. (2000) found that the rate of ADHD in the adoptive parents of adopted ADHD children was 6% compared with 18% of the biological parents of non-adopted ADHD children and 3% of the biological parents of TD children. This pattern of occurrence of ADHD is consistent with the transmission of ADHD in families via genetics rather than the shared environment.

Molecular genetic studies The SNP-based heritability for ADHD symptom scores indicates a polygenic architecture, with SNP-based heritability ranging from 5% to 34% across studies (Middeldorp et al., 2016). This finding was based on the genotyping of 17,666 children under the age of 13 years from nine population-based cohorts. There were indications in the results that genes involved in neurite outgrowth are possibly involved. In addition, they concluded that continuous and dichotomous measures of ADHD appear to assess a phenotype that was under the influence of the same set of genes.

The investigations into the genetic basis of ADHD have now reached a stage where the first replicated findings of loci from GWAS have been identified (Demontis et al., 2019). This study identified significant loci associated with ADHD in a GWAS meta-analysis of 55,374 individuals from 12 study cohorts. FOXP2 is among the biologically informative genes implicated as important contributors to the aetiology of ADHD. A feature of FOXP2 is its association with language disorders (Lai et al., 2001) and these are the developmental disorders that are most frequently comorbid with ADHD (Jensen & Steinhausen, 2015). This study also suggests a strong overlap with the genetics of ADHD-related traits and is consistent with a dimensional view of ADHD as the extreme end of a continuum of symptoms (Demontis et al., 2019).

A further GWAS was conducted to ascertain which genetic variants are associated with ADHD plus disruptive behaviours disorders (DBD) that included oppositional defiant disorder and conduct disorder (Demontis et al., 2021). This GWAS found three genome-wide significant loci on chromosome 1,7, and 11 associated with ADHD+DBD. The SNP heritability was greater for ADHD+DBD (0.34) than for AHD without DBD (0.20). The results indicate that ADHD plus aggressive behaviours have a higher load of common genetic risk variants than ADHD alone.

There have been a number of subsequent studies that have used the findings from the Demontis et al. (2019) GWAS to create polygenic risk scores (PRS). These have been reviewed by Ronald et al. (2021) and have shown strong association with categorical ADHD and ADHD traits as well as a number of other associated conditions. However, the finding of association between this PRS and ASD is inconclusive.

A range of PRS was used by Martin et al. (2023) to test for the direct genetic transmission of ADHD in families. They produced PRS for ADHD, anxiety, autism, bipolar disorder, depression, obsessive-compulsive disorder, schizophrenia, Tourette syndrome, and cognitive ability. They found that only high scores on the PRS for ADHD and for cognitive ability were transmitted from parent to child in trios of parents and their child with ADHD. Furthermore, from an analysis of non-transmitted alleles, there was no evidence for genetic nurture (see Sect. 3.2) of ADHD. The results suggest a direct transmission of polygenic liability to ADHD from parent to child.

There have been sufficient studies employing PRS to predict aspects of ADHD for a systematic review and meta-analysis to be conducted. Li and He (2021) produced a meta-analysis of studies on PRS for ADHD. This obtained 12 unique effect sizes from ADHD-PRS studies with a pooled N of 40,088 participants. They found that the correlation between the PRS and ADHD status was around 0.20. This is similar to the SNP heritabilities reported by Demontis et al. (2021), which were 0.34 and 0.20 for ADHD plus disruptive behaviour disorder and ADHD alone, respectively, reported above.

These modest values identified for the contribution of common genetic variants to the explanation of ADHD have to be placed in the context of the known heterogeneity of ADHD, the need to take into account comorbidity with other disruptive behaviours, and the requirements to have data available on a very large sample. The latter is especially important to be able to incorporate rare and low-frequency variants that may confer moderate risks. These low-frequency variants are likely to be as polygenic as the common variants (Chatterjee et al., 2016). Clearly, there is a way to go to establish the full power of PRS to predict ADHD and before these scores could be appropriately applied in clinical contexts.

Green et al. (2022) reached a more bullish conclusion about the possible role of ADHD-PRS in clinical practice on the basis of their meta-analysis. They identified 33 relevant studies for inclusion in a systematic review and 16 studies with data on which a meta-analysis could be produced. They found that ADHD-PRS provide important information on the development of ADHD severity, its course, and associated comorbidity. They conclude that by helping to identify these adverse outcomes, ADHD-PRS could be used to provide tools for early identification of children at risk and/or individualised care plans for children suspected of suffering from ADHD. Their results also suggest that a persistent course of ADHD may have genetic underpinnings.

PRS were used by Vainieri et al. (2021) to examine whether genetic variants that contribute to ADHD are also related to individual differences in attention regulation (measured by reaction time variability) and response inhibition (measured by commission errors). The investigation was based on a meta-analysis of results from 5 studies. It provides molecular genetic evidence that attention regulation and ADHD share common genetic factors. This suggests that ADHD common genetic variants not only contribute to the risk of ADHD, but are also an indicator of greater reaction time variability for those with ADHD, which was shown above to be a factor related to the later outcome of ADHD (Michelini et al., 2016).

Gene–environment interactions The role of gene–environment interactions in the development of ADHD was reviewed by Nigg et al. (2010). They suggest that there is emerging evidence that dopaminergic and serotonergic genotypes interact with psychosocial factors to influence the severity of ADHD symptoms in childhood. These initial studies took a candidate gene approach using genotypes related to these neurotransmitter systems. However, subsequent GWAS studies (see Sect. 3.2) have not replicated the association of these genes with ADHD. Using polygenic risk scores (see Sect. 3.4) and measured psychosocial risk factors in a sample of 33,872 individuals with ADHD and a population-based comparison group, Østergaard et al. (2020) were able to identify the main effects of genetic and of psychosocial risk on ADHD but found no evidence for interaction between genes and the environment (GxE) on ADHD. These results were replicated in a study by Mooney et al. (2023). This too used PRS and measures of exposure to environmental risks. The latter included family risks – income and family conflict/negative sentiment, and broader environmental risks – geocoded measures of area deprivation, lead exposure risk, and air pollution exposure (nitrogen dioxide and fine particulate matter). They found significant additive effects for genetic and family environmental risks in two independent samples. The small gene–environment interactions that they found did not replicate across samples and were inconsistent across groups of children with different ethnic/racial backgrounds. What is clear is that at present there is little certainty as to the presence of GxE interactions influencing ADHD or to the mechanisms whereby GxE might arise but it is clear that the size of the GxE effects is small.

Genetic associations between ADHD and other psychopathologies The reason for these association was investigated by Brikell et al. (2020). They used an ADHD PRS derived from a sample of 13,457 children aged 9 to 12 years. They found that the PRS was correlated with the p-factor, externalising, and depression. The results indicate that common genetic variants associated with ADHD contribute to a genetic risk for a wider range of psychopathology symptoms.

Andersson et al. (2020) used meta-analyses to estimate the magnitude of genetic correlations between ADHD and a variety of other disorders in childhood and adulthood based on 31 independent studies. The genetic correlations were around 0.50 for the association between ADHD and both internalising and externalising disorders. These findings suggest that there is shared genetic risk accounting for the presence of internalising, externalising, and neurodevelopmental disorder symptoms in those with ADHD symptoms.

The findings on the role of genes in influencing ADHD with a particular focus on the genetic basis of the relationship between ADHD and a range of psychiatric disorders were reviewed by Ribasés et al. (2023). The studies in this review included those using a number of methodological advances in the Mendelian randomisation (MR) approach (see Sect. 4.6) – namely, Latent Casual Variable (LCV) analysis (O'Connor & Price, 2018) and Causal Analysis Using Summary Effect estimates (CAUSE) (Morrison et al., 2020). These elaborations of the MR analysis have provided firmer evidence of the possible causal effect of ADHD on depression (Artigas et al., 2023).

Mitochondrial DNA Mitochondrial DNA is found outside the nucleus of cells and is inherited solely from the mother. Its potential role in neurodevelopmental disorders may be mediated by the regulation of neuronal functioning (McCormick et al., 2018). There is some suggestive, but only preliminary, evidence that indicates that there may be an association between genetic variants in mitochondrial DNA and ADHD (Giannoulis et al., 2022). However, it is unclear how such mitochondrial DNA variants might play a role in the pathophysiology underlying ADHD.

Integrating information on genetics, cognition, and imaging in ADHD ADHD has been the focus of a number studies that are starting to integrate information on genetic risk, cognition, brain imaging, and behaviour. This integration of complementary methodologies provides valuable insights into the mediation of genetic influences on ADHD. Pinto et al. (2016) provided preliminary findings showing the way genetic polymorphisms in risk alleles for ADHD could be seen to have effects mediated via cognition. For example, an analysis using a SNP in the serotonin receptor gene (HTR2A) showed evidence that it may be related to inattention and that this relationship was explained by its influence on reaction time variability. The authors recognised that the study was under-powered but the findings should encourage future studies to adopt this approach.

Nigg et al. (2018) took this approach a stage further to use a wider set of genetic measures to create a polygenic risk score. The possible role of working memory and vigilance/arousal as mediators of the impact of genetic factors on ADHD was examined. They found a significant mediation effect of 0.10. The effect of the PRS on ADHD that is independent of working memory is 0.13. The mediation therefore represents about 50% of the effects of the polygenic score on ADHD. Similar findings were found of mediation by a vigilance measure of the PRS effect on ADHD. This methodology provides important evidence of the way cumulative common genetic variants influence a behavioural phenotype via a cognitive intermediary.

Sudre et al. (2020) also aimed to investigate the mediation of polygenic scores on aspects of ADHD symptomatology but, as well as measures of cognition as mediators, they also obtained brain imaging data. This allowed them to employ a serial mediation analysis to study the route from polygenic risk, to white matter microstructure of the anterior corona radiata, then cognition (working memory, focused attention), and finally to hyperactivity–impulsivity. The results of this analysis are shown in Fig. 9.3. This study not only replicates the mediation of polygenic risk for

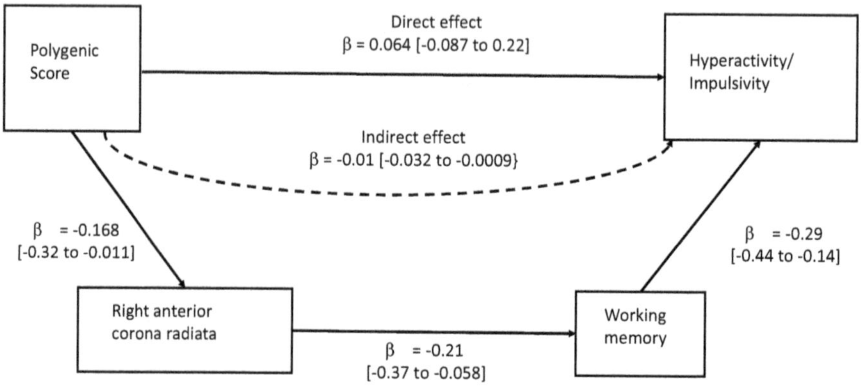

Fig. 9.3 Working memory mediates the association between the polygenic score and hyperactivity/impulsivity showing β and CI_{95}. (Adapted with the permission of Springer Nature from Figure 2 Sudre et al. (2020); permission conveyed through Copyright Clearance Center, Inc.)

ADHD via working memory shown by Nigg et al. (2018), it extends the approach to identify the possible brain systems involved. This is a landmark study.

In a subsequent report, Sudre et al. (2021) go on to use machine learning to address the question of predicting the course of ADHD from a combination of polygenic risk, cognition, and brain structure. They found that polygenic risk and cognitive performance emerged as the most important features in predicting whether ADHD symptoms improved or worsened over time. Brain structure measures made an additional smaller contribution to predicting outcome. For a review of the contribution of machine learning to the study of ADHD (see Cao et al., 2023).

Pre- and peri-natal factors The pre- and perinatal environmental risk factors for ADHD were reviewed by Nigg et al. (2020b). They suggested that although a number of associations with ADHD have been identified, these studies are mainly observational studies that cannot rule out the effects of unmeasured confounders, especially those arising from gene-environment correlations. Where natural experiments have been applied, factors such as maternal smoking and maternal body mass index are not seen as likely to play a causal role. Young maternal age is associated with the risk of later ADHD in the child. However, this seems to be a consequence of the association between young maternal age and socioeconomic disadvantage rather than an effect of young age per se (Baker et al., 2023).

There is evidence that exposure to individual toxins during pregnancy can increase the risk of ADHD in the child (Skogheim et al., 2021). The question of polysubstance use in pregnancy and ADHD was examined in a study of a cohort of 3138 children in the USA (Garrison-Desany et al., 2022). Polysubstance abuse was identified by tobacco smoking, alcohol consumption, and use of cannabis, cocaine, or opioids. It was found that the risk of later ADHD was increased by an interaction between opioids, cannabis and alcohol use and to a lessor extant by an interaction with smoking.

There is well replicated evidence that preterm birth is related to an increased risk of ADHD (Bhutta et al., 2002). El Marroun et al. (2012) have shown that post-term birth is also associated with ADHD both as a dimension and as a category. In a population sample of 5145 children in the Netherlands, they found higher levels of ADHD in children born post-term even after controlling for maternal age, education, ethnicity, psychopathology, smoking and drinking during pregnancy, family income, gender of the child, and age of the child at the assessment. Pre-term birth is closely associated with low birthweight and with sub-optimal neonatal health as indicated by low Apgar scores. There is evidence to suggest that all three of these factors are predictive of later ADHD with the Apgar score having the biggest effect followed by gestational age at birth (Hanc et al., 2018).

It is known that prenatal alcohol exposure (PAE) is associated with higher levels of externalising behaviour, including ADHD related behaviours (Tsang et al., 2016). Although PAE is known to effect the brain of the developing foetus, especially the prefrontal cortex (Moore et al., 2014), it has been uncertain whether the association with ADHD may result from confounds such as a shared genetic risk. However, Wetherill et al. (2018) undertook a meta-analysis of studies on externalising behaviours in children of alcoholics and those with PAE. They were able to show that there was increased risk of ADHD in those with PAE that was greater than that arising from parental alcohol dependence or a genetic liability. They conclude that in children with PAE ADHD arises from direct alcohol exposure during prenatal development.

It has been suggested the quality of maternal diet during pregnancy may influence the neurodevelopment in the child (Borge et al., 2017). However in a meta-analysis of 17 studies there was no consistent evidence that diet in pregnancy is related to the risk of ADHD in children (Li et al., 2019).

Prenatal maternal anxiety may also play a role in the development of ADHD. Maternal anxiety in late pregnancy was associated with hyperactivity/inattention at age 4 in boys and with emotional and behaviour problems in both boys and girls (O'Connor et al., 2002). This association was specific to antenatal anxiety; the association held when postnatal anxiety on mothers was controlled. This suggest that the association was not a result of shared genetic influences. Subsequent studies have indicated how this association might be mediated. Using foetal functional connectivity MRI, De Asis-Cruz et al. (2020) found that maternal anxiety measures when the foetuses were at 33-weeks gestation were associated with differences in foetal brain connectivity.

Risk factors related to maternal health during pregnancy and ADHD have been extensively investigated. A systematic review and meta-analysis of these studies was undertaken by Bitsko et al. (2022). They found a number of prenatal factors (pre-pregnancy weight, preeclampsia, pregnancy complications, elevated testosterone exposure), and postnatal factors (Apgar score, neonatal illness, no breastfeeding) were positively associated with ADHD. Although significant, the effect sizes for these factors were small ranging from SMD = 0.05 to 0.26. Other risk factors arising at the time of birth were not associated. This latter group of risk factors were perinatal asphyxia, labour complications, and mode of delivery. There is a proviso for these putative effects. The meta-analysis could not take into account possible confounds arising from association between the risks and genetic influences (r_{GE}) nor interaction between these risks and genes (GxE). The same limitation holds for a study ante-natal or peri-natal depression in mothers and the risk of ADHD in the child (Nidey et al., 2021). The effect was three-fold increase in ADHD and remained when control for a number of potential confounders was made. However, the design of the study could not rule out a genetic confound between the risk maternal depression and ADHD in the child.

Maternal autoimmune disease and neuroinflammation It has been suggested that a range maternal inflammatory states in pregnancy are associated with common neurodevelopmental disorders in children. A review of meta-analyses on the question was undertaken by Han et al. (2021). They found that those inflammatory states in pregnancy associated with ADHD include obesity, pre-eclampsia, smoking, low socioeconomic status, stress, autoimmune disease, and asthma. These associations are obtained largely from observational studies, which cannot rule out the action of confounds such as gene-environment correlations.

In a cohort of Australian children, Nielsen et al. (2021) identified 12,610 children who had been exposed to maternal autoimmune disease and a propensity score matched (see Sect. 4.8) comparison group of children not exposed in this way. They found that the risk of ADHD in the exposed children was 30% higher than in the comparison group. Maternal type 1 diabetes was the condition with the single highest risk of ADHD (120% higher). The mechanism for the association is uncertain but it is possible that there is a shared genetic vulnerability between autoimmune disease and ADHD or that maternal immune activation impacts directly on neurodevelopment in children. Nielsen et al. (2021) also produced a meta-analysis of five studies (including their own) that replicated this association between maternal autoimmune disease and child ADHD. This risk associated with any maternal autoimmune disease is very similar to the 30% increase in the risk of autism spectrum disorder identified in a meta-analysis of maternal autoimmune disease by Chen et al. (2016).

The evidence that links neuroinflammation to ADHD has been reviewed by Dunn et al. (2019). They identify a number of lines of evidence that suggest a possible role for neuroinflammation in the pathophysiology of ADHD. These include an association between inflammatory and autoimmune disorders and ADHD, an association with increased serum cytokines, possible involvement in ADHD of genes associated with inflammatory pathways, evidence of early life exposure to environmental factors via inflammatory mechanisms, and animal experiment studies. The mechanisms linking these inflammatory factors to ADHD include reductions on grey matter volumes and alterations to neurotransmitter systems (dopaminergic, serotonergic and glutamatergic). They conclude that in sum there is

> substantial indirect and circumstantial evidence supports a hypothesis that neuroinflammation plays an important albeit non-specific role in the pathophysiology of ADHD. (Dunn et al., 2019, p.29)

9.4 Environmental Risk Factors for ADHD

Adverse environmental exposures It is clear that genetic variation does not act alone to influence ADHD behaviours. There are a number of known, or suspected environmental factors, that influence ADHD, e.g. environmental lead exposure (Goodlad et al., 2013), particulate matter air pollution (Myhre et al., 2018; Peterson et al., 2022) and chemical compounds altering the endocrine system (Rivollier et al., 2019). The impact of these exposures on children's brains was made clear in a review by Lanphear (2015). This paper includes a link to an instructive video that explains how cumulative exposure to seemingly low levels of toxins can have a major impact on brain development and behaviour at the level both of the individual and the general population – see https://www.annualreviews.org/do/10.1146/do.multimedia.2015.01.08.351/abs/

In a nationally representative sample of children in the USA, lead exposure was shown to increase the risk of ADHD 2.3 times between the bottom and top third levels of exposure (Froehlich et al., 2009). When experienced along with prenatal tobacco exposure, the effect was to increase the odds of ADHD to 8.1. The causal effect of lead on ADHD in some children was supported by a Mendelian randomization study (Nigg et al., 2016).

There has been uncertainty concerning the possible role of air quality on the risk of ADHD. However, stronger evidence for an effect has been obtained recently from a population-based birth cohort study from Taiwan to investigate the effect on ADHD of exposure to particulate matter in the air of 2.5 microns or less ($PM_{2.5}$) during pregnancy and the preschool period (Chang et al., 2022). The study used satellite data monitoring air quality to determine $PM_{2.5}$ exposure in 425,736 children. They found that the exposure of pregnant women to $PM_{2.5}$ above 16 μg/m^3 from conception to the early life of their children increased the risk of ADHD. This conclusion was supported by the finding of a dose–response relationship between the severity of exposure and the risk of later ADHD.

The role of exposure prenatally to polycyclic aromatic hydrocarbons (PAH), an additional air pollutant, on behaviour was tested by Liu et al. (2022). They found that such PAH exposure combined with maternal stress influences individual differences in socioemotional development. Peterson et al. (2022) have also reported that prenatal $PM_{2.5}$ and PAH exposure disrupts brain development in regions that regulate thought, emotion, and behaviour.

Epigenetics One possible route for the impact of adverse environments on ADHD is via epigenetic mechanisms (Nigg, 2018). These are changes made to the chemistry of DNA (but not the DNA code itself) that may affect gene expression and synaptic transmission – see Sect. 3.3. There is evidence that a wide range of environmental influences that can produce these epigenetic changes, including childhood adversities (Krause et al., 2020). For example, findings from the English Romanian Adoption study suggest that environmental insults of sufficient severity, such as institutional deprivation, may be associated with long-lasting epigenetic changes (Kumsta et al., 2016). These changes may account for some of the risk of the enduring social behavioural deficits, including ADHD, seen in these children adopted into English families (Sonuga-Barke et al., 2017).

The first studies have started to show a possible role of DNA methylation (one type of epigenetic change in DNA) in increasing the risk of ADHD. There is evidence that DNA methylation at birth is associated with later ADHD (Neumann et al., 2020). Mooney et al. (2020) found concurrent associations between DNA methylation and ADHD in children aged 17 to 12 years. It has been suggested in two studies that the severity of symptomology in those with ADHD is related to the degree of DNA methylation (Goodman et al., 2020; Siu et al., 2021). These are as yet initial findings in the study of the epigenetic mechanisms influencing the risk of ADHD. They will require replication but they may provide clues for future avenues to examine the way genes influence the ADHD phenotype. These developments in understanding the possible role of epigenetics in the emergence of ADHD have been reviewed by Cecil and Nigg (2022). They conclude that

> …the field of epigenetics and ADHD is promising but is still in its infancy, and the potential for transformative translational applications remains a distant goal. (Cecil & Nigg, 2022, p.1)

Parenting A review of studies suggested that parenting style may not be a cause of ADHD; instead, children's difficult behaviours induce negative interactions with parents (Modesto-Lowe et al., 2008). However, there is evidence that the absence of maternal sensitivity (as indicated by praise and assisting the child to complete a task), rather than negative interactions, may contribute to ADHD symptoms even when pre-existing problems with attention and executive function are taken into account (Choenni et al., 2019). Whatever its role in the development of ADHD, there is evidence to suggest that interventions to enhance parenting have a role to play in treatment. It would appear that parent training does not change core ADHD symptoms but can reduce oppositional behaviours and noncompliant behaviour in these children (Daley et al., 2018).

An elegant natural experiment design was used by Harold et al. (2013) to investigate the role of variation in parenting and ADHD behaviours. By studying adopted children they were able to identify the effects of parenting that were not confounded with genetic influence – adoptive parents provide care and not genes for the child. As can be seen in Fig. 9.4 genetic effects from the birth mother influence early aspects of behaviour in the child such as impulsivity. In turn the child's behaviour is related to the adoptive mother's hostility, which then has a subsequent impact on ADHD symptomatology. The latter is a pure environmental effect as possible gene-environment correlations have been eliminated.

More extreme negative aspects of parenting are considered as maltreatment and include physical abuse and neglect (including malnutrition), emotional abuse and neglect, sexual abuse, and early deprivation. The link between maltreatment and

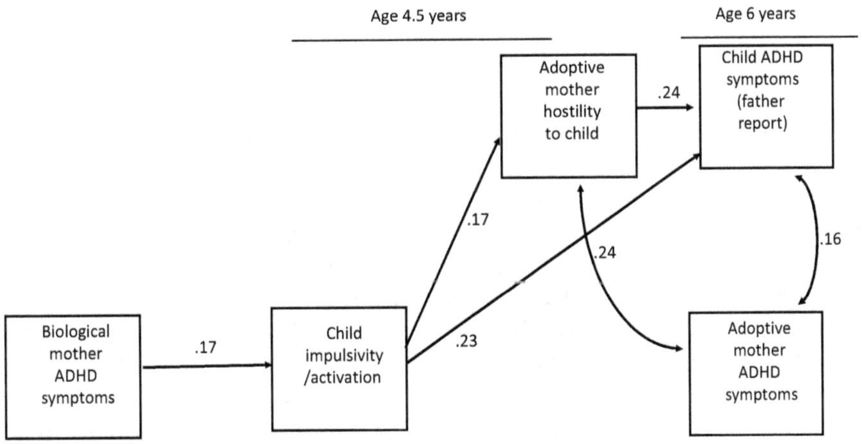

Fig. 9.4 Genetic and social influences on ADHD behaviour in adoptive families. (Adapted with the permission of John Wiley & Sons from Figure 1 Harold et al. (2013); permission conveyed through Copyright Clearance Center, Inc.)

ADHD has been repeatedly demonstrated (e.g. Briscoe-Smith & Hinshaw, 2006). What is unclear is the direction of effects between them. Does ADHD lead to maltreatment via evoking hostile responses from parents and others (Stern et al., 2018)? Does maltreatment lead to ADHD via changes in the child's nervous, endocrine, and immune systems (Danese & McEwen, 2012)?

Bali et al. (2023) produced a systematic review of longitudinal studies that could address this question of the direction of possible causal links between maltreatment and ADHD. They identified 11 relevant prospective studies and used the framework of Hill (1965), described in Sect. 4.2, to examine the evidence for causality. Although they consider the studies to be of high quality and confirm the association between ADHD and maltreatment, there was no consensus between the studies on the direction of effects. In addition, the possibility of a third factor acting as a common influence on ADHD and maltreatment could not be excluded. They concluded that further studies are needed to clearly differentiate between these alternative mechanisms in order to provide guidance on preventive interventions and treatments for children experiencing maltreatment.

Lifestyle Using a composite lifestyle index based on water intake, sweetened beverage intake, supplement use, reading, screen time, physical activity, and sleep, Holton and Nigg (2020) found a robust association of ADHD with a less healthy lifestyle compared to that of controls. These results held even after adjustment for multiple confounding factors, including age, sex, IQ, ADHD medication, comorbid psychiatric conditions, and household income. The findings were replicated when teacher ratings of ADHD symptoms were used, so the effects could not be attributable to shared source variance between the measure of ADHD and the lifestyle index. As the authors recognise, it is unclear from such a cross-sectional study just what is the direction of effects – does an unhealthy lifestyle lead to or exacerbate ADHD or does ADHD lead to an unhealthy lifestyle? In addition, although measured confounds were controlled, it is possible that there may be unmeasured confounds such as gene–environment correlations.

Diet Iv et al. (2022) investigated the association between dietary patterns at age 2 years and the course of hyperactivity-inattention behaviour up to 8 years of age. They identified three dietary profiles at age 2 – a high consumption of processed and fast foods, a healthy diet following "guidelines" and a diet mainly comprising baby foods. The healthy diet was negatively associated with hyperactivity-inattention problems (SMD = −0.16) and the baby food showed the opposite (SMD = 0.19). Similar findings were obtained at an older age where a "Western diet", defined by high levels of total fat, saturated fat, refined sugars, and sodium, was associated with an ADHD diagnosis (SMD = 0.44) (Howard et al., 2011). Both these studies were correlational in design and consequently, the role of possible confounders could not be excluded. However, there is now evidence from an RCT that adopting a healthy diet can improve ADHD symptoms in children at least in the short-term (Huberts-Bosch et al., 2023).

There is evidence that children with ADHD respond to dietary treatments and that therefore dietary factors may be risk factors for ADHD. Both the removal of artificial food colours from the diet and supplementation with free fatty acids show some benefit (Stevenson et al., 2014). The effects sizes for these dietary treatment studies for ADHD are between 0.20 and 0.40. The results for restricted elimination diets are more varied and have been found not to be more effective that the adoption of a healthy diet (Huberts-Bosch et al., 2023)

There is replicated evidence from a meta-analyses that iron deficiency is associated with ADHD (Tseng et al., 2018). Specifically, peripheral serum ferritin level in the children with ADHD is significantly lower than in the children without ADHD (SMD = −0.25 ($CI_{.95}$ −0.44 to −0.05)). Similar findings that ADHD behaviours were related to serum ferritin levels (a protein that stores iron) but not serum iron levels were reported by Wang et al. (2017). However as yet there is no convincing body of evidence that iron supplementation can significantly improve ADHD symptomatology. The same is true for zinc supplementation. There are too few studies with inconsistent findings to warrant conclusions being drawn about possible therapeutic efficacy. The quality of the evidence from these studies was rated as relatively poor (Talebi et al., 2022).

A broader range of micronutrients supplementation has also been tested as a treatment for ADHD in two well conducted RCTs (Rucklidge et al., 2018; Johnstone et al., 2022). There was replicated evidence from these studies that children with ADHD and problems of emotion regulation showed improvement when treated with micronutrients (vitamins, minerals, amino acids, and antioxidants) compared to placebo. Those with problems of emotion regulation children comprise some 40% to 50% of those with ADHD. The risk ratios for responding to treatment compared to placebo are 2.96 and 2.97, respectively, in these two studies (see Stevenson, 2022).

These dietary approaches to intervention are more effective in changing the core symptoms of ADHD than other non-pharmacological treatments (Sonuga-Barke et al., 2013). However the resulting effect sizes are lower than those for stimulant treatment on ADHD itself (Faraone & Buitelaar, 2010). Stimulant medication also produces significant benefits in reducing other functional consequences of ADHD such as mood disorders, accidents and injuries, and educational outcomes (Boland et al., 2020).

Family context It has been postulated that disorganised or chaotic families may contribute to the risk of ADHD, externalising behaviour and cognitive development. There has been repeated demonstrations of these associations (e.g. Pike et al., 2006; Mulligan et al., 2013). However, it is uncertain what mechanisms underly the link. Agnew-Blais et al. (2022) studied household chaos and ADHD in a sample of over 2000 twin pairs between the ages of 7 and 12 years. They identified that children in more chaotic families had higher ADHD scores. However, they also had obtained ADHD PRS scores for the twins and for their mothers. They found that the child's PRS was associated with chaos scores over and above the association of the chaos score with the mothers PRS score. This indicated that the child's ADHD may be creating an evocative gene-environment correlation. These results suggest that household chaos is in part a reflection of the child's genetic risk and this makes it uncertain just what contribution household chaos plays is causing ADHD.

Spencer et al. (2022) examined the relationship between variance in household income and maternal education measures before the age of 5 years and ADHD when the child is 9 to 11 years. The analysis was based on data from seven large cohorts in 6 industrialised countries ($N = 44{,}925$). They found that the prevalence of ADHD was linearly related to both these measures of socioeconomic status (SES) with the rate being higher the lower the SES. These findings replicate those from a meta-analysis by Russell et al. (2016). Based on 42 studies, they found that children in families of low SES are on average 1.85–2.21 times more likely to have ADHD than their peers in high SES families.

The effects of social disadvantaged were tested using an extended family design based on over 800,000 Swedish children (Larsson et al., 2014). This found an increase in ADHD associated with low family income while controlling for covariates, such as gender, parental age, and parental mental health. The study also compared differently exposed cousins and siblings to control for unmeasured familial confounding including genetic influences.

Michaëlsson et al. (2022) used a Mendelian randomisation design (see Sect. 4.5) to investigate the possible direction of effects between SES, intelligence and ADHD. They found that an ADHD diagnosis may be a direct consequence of socio-economic related factors and that this effect was not mediated by low IQ. There were only modest effects in the other direction. Furthermore, low intelligence was neither an independent cause nor a consequence of ADHD. What is not known from this analysis is just what might be the mechanisms leading from low SES and to an ADHD diagnosis. Michaëlsson et al. (2022) discussed a range of possibilities including those with greater resource being able to avoid the ADHD diagnosis for their child by having

> ..greater opportunity to protect, stimulate, and train their children to become physically and mentally competent and thus avoid an ADHD diagnosis. (Michaëlsson et al., 2022, p.8)

Jendreizik et al. (2022) investigated the relationship between various family risk factors and ADHD and ODD behaviours in children aged between 6 and 12 years who had been referred with ADHD. The family adversities included low parental education, marital conflicts, parental delinquency, and crowded housing conditions. They found that there was a cascade of influences with family adversity being associated with more marked parental psychopathology. This in turn being associated with more negative and fewer positive parenting practices. These negative parenting practices were associated with more severe ADHD behaviours (but not ODD behaviours). This pattern of chain of influences indicates that it may be particularly fruitful to focus on negative parenting practices when developing treatments for ADHD. A proviso is that the effectiveness of such parenting interventions may be moderated by genetic risk. Leve et al. (2022) found that parenting interventions were helpful for those children at high genetic risk but may be detrimental for those at low genetic risk. The reason for this detrimental effect is unclear.

9.5 Outcome of ADHD

Associated psychological problems in childhood There are well-replicated findings that ADHD and emotional problems are associated in childhood and later. What has been unclear is whether these conditions effect each other and if so what is the direction of such an effect or whether both arise as a result of a common underlying cause. This question was addressed by Stern et al. (2020) in a longitudinal study of twins. They showed that ADHD symptoms are predictors of later emotional symptoms, and not the other way round. Moreover, that this influence was mediated by shared genes. Emotional dysregulation is a feature often associated with ADHD and has been proposed as mediating the association with later Internalising (Steinberg & Drabick, 2015). It has been shown in a cross-sectional study of children aged 5 to 12 years olds that emotional dysregulation mediates 50% of the association between ADHD and depression.

Antony et al. (2022) investigated the possible role of emotional dysregulation in leading to later Internalising problems using a refined modelling technique. Theirs was a longitudinal study that applied an autoregressive latent trajectory model with structured residuals (ALT-SR). This is a version the class of latent curve modes with structured residuals (LCM-SR) that was developed by Curran et al. (2014) (see Sect. 4.3). They concluded that emotional dysregulation mediates the association between ADHD symptoms and Internalising problems in childhood. As a consequence, it represents an important target for preventive intervention. An examination of broader range sequelae of emotional dysregulation in those with ADHD was made by Faraone et al. (2019). They argued that emotional impulsivity and deficient emotional self-regulation are strong and specific associates of ADHD. Consequently these aspects of emotional dysregulation should be considered as core symptoms of ADHD and could be fruitful targets for treatment.

A longitudinal network analysis was employed by Karalunas et al. (2021) to investigate the transdiagnostic relationship between behaviours related to ADHD and other aspects of psychopathology in a sample of children studied between 9 and 12 years of age. They showed that ADHD symptoms and working memory deficits each had direct and independent links with later depression. The findings indicated that features of ADHD, temperamental irritability, and working memory may be critical transdiagnostic risk factor for psychopathology. This suggests that these may be candidates for underpinning the general psychopathology factor (GPF).

ADHD and somatic health The risk of later adverse health outcomes for those with ADHD was reviewed by Nigg (2013). This was an extensive review of a large number of studies and produced the following main conclusions. The risk of smoking was about 2.5 times higher in those with ADHD. This was not accounted for by an association with conduct disorder but the similar degree of risk of substance use was mainly accounted for by an association with conduct disorder. Night settling may be disrupted in those with ADHD but that was no clear evidence of an association with other sleep disturbances. The risk of injury was nearly doubled but it was unclear if this resulted from ADHD per se or from other associated behaviour problems. The risk of suicide attempts was raised in girls with ADHD and seems to be mediated by mood disorder. There is markedly increased risk of completed suicide in boys with ADHD and this is associated with the increased risk of conduct disturbance and substance use. For a number of other adverse health outcomes, the data were too sparse to make firm conclusions about the risk associated with ADHD, that is, diabetes, hypertension, and risky sexual behaviour.

One health feature that is consistently related to ADHD is obesity (Cortese & Tessari, 2017). A longitudinal study by Kase et al. (2021) found there to be a time invariant relationship, i.e. a consistent association across ages, between hyperactivity and impulsivity (but not inattention) and higher body mass index (BMI) from the age of 11 to 22 years. There was no evidence from the longitudinal analysis that changes in BMI were influenced by ADHD symptoms or that higher BMI was leading to an increase in ADHD severity. The authors suggest that high BMI and ADHD have a shared familial (possible genetic) basis. The establishment of this association at an early age indicates that targeting high BMI in children with ADHD should be implemented early in childhood.

The origins of the association between ADHD and a number of physical conditions in adulthood were investigated by Du Rietz et al. (2021a). They used data from a Swedish population register of nearly 5 million individuals. They could identify family relationships in this data set and so could estimate the role of genetic and environmental factors in the associations that were found. People with ADHD were more at risk for many conditions compared to those without ADHD. The strongest associations were with nervous system conditions such as sleep disorder, epilepsy, and dementia (ORs ranged between 1.50 and 4.62) and with respiratory diseases such as asthma and chronic obstructive pulmonary disorder (ORs 2.42 to 3.24). These associations were found to be largely explained by genetic factors. However, the associations with nervous system disorders arose from non-shared environment factors.

There are now initial findings as to which genes may contribute to the relationship between somatic health and ADHD. Using data on 55,374 participants Garcia-Marin et al. (2021) showed that a wide range of genes influencing somatic disorders were associated with ADHD including iron deficiency anaemia, obesity and type 2 diabetes. The possibility that there is a general risk factor that underlies a propensity to mental as well as physical disease has been raised by Cortese et al. (2021b). This they label a "d" (disease) factor analogous to the p factor for psychopathology (see Sect. 6.2). If this should be the case, the findings from Du Rietz et al. (2021a), and Garcia-Marin et al. (2021) indicate that this propensity may be attributed to genes.

Outcome of preschool ADHD Preschool ADHD is relatively stable into middle childhood. Even when given treatment with medication, the course is generally chronic, with high symptom severity and impairment (Riddle et al., 2013). The extent of in the intractability of preschool ADHD is shown in the conclusion reached by Riddle et al. (2013) that

> almost 90% of clinic-referred preschoolers initially diagnosed with moderate-to-severe ADHD, who mostly received parent training followed by controlled medication treatment, continued to be diagnosed with ADHD into mid-to-late childhood. (Riddle et al., 2013, p.273)

Lavigne et al. (1996) had found that ADHD was present in 2% of children aged between 2 and 5 years in a large sample living in Chicago. It was almost always comorbid with ODD in this sample. It was shown that preschool-age children with ADHD are at significant risk for concurrent behavioural, social, familial, and academic difficulties relative to a typically developing comparison group (DuPaul et al., 2001). A large sample of Norwegian preschoolers were screened for ADHD symptoms at 36 months and a sub-group of participants were assessed for ADHD at age 36 to 44 months on the Preschool Age Psychiatric Assessment (PAPA) (Overgaard et al., 2016). Of those with ADHD symptoms, 33% were reported to have symptoms of anxiety compared to 16% of controls. Children with symptoms of ADHD and anxiety had more severe ADHD symptomatology, in particular more inattentive symptoms compared with children with ADHD symptoms and no anxiety.

A follow-up of children with preschool hyperactivity in a community sample showed them to present a much higher cost to non-mental health services per annum into late adolescence and into early adulthood compared to non-hyperactive controls (£562 vs. £30) (Chorozoglou et al., 2015). This same study showed that for males there were poor adolescent/early adulthood mental health outcomes that were specifically associated with hyperactivity (Smith et al., 2017). For females the smaller effects of hyperactivity on adult outcome were no longer significant when confounds were controlled.

Stability of ADHD Wootton et al. (2022) pooled data from 5 large general population samples from the UK, New Zealand, and Brazil to investigate the pattern of change in ADHD traits across the age range from 3 to 45 years. There was clearly replicated decline with age in ADHD behaviours across all samples. Females consistently had lower scores that males. There were differences between the cohorts in the patterns of decline which may reflect both cultural and measurement variation.

The course of ADHD symptomatology was studied by Vos et al. (2021) over the ages 5 to 28 years. They found the patterns of symptom changes to be very variable and identified 7 sub-groups with distinct trajectories of change. The differentiation between the groups was related to a wide variety of factors including both initial symptom severity and genetic risks measured in a PRS. Agnew-Blais et al. (2021) have also demonstrated that PRS scores were not only related to the presence of ADHD in childhood but also in adulthood. Moreover, these scores were predictive of the course of ADHD.

Outcome in adulthood ADHD is a neurodevelopmental disorder starting early in life but in many cases endures well into adulthood. The life-time consequences of ADHD were reviewed by Franke et al. (2018). They showed that the developmental outcome was very varied. For many, there are long-lasting difficulties in health and well-being. Others with ADHD can live very successful lives. Franke et al. (2018) argue that there is a lack of information on how best to manage and support those with ADHD in adulthood and a particular paucity of studies on ADHD in old age.

ADHD confers a 50% to 300% increased risk for serious secondary mental health problems later in life including substance use disorders, depression, psychosis, and anxiety disorders (Nigg et al., 2020b). The risk for a psychotic disorder or schizophrenia for children and adolescents with ADHD has been summarised in a systematic review and meta-analysis (Nourredine et al., 2021). The odds ratio (OR) for psychotic disorder was 5.04 and for schizophrenia was 4.59.

There is well replicated evidence that those with ADHD are at increased of smoking (Matthies et al., 2013) and of nicotine dependence in adulthood (McClernon & Kollins, 2008). Studies have found a consistent pattern of a genetic association between ADHD and smoking. Using a Mendelian randomisation design, Vink et al. (2021) did not find evidence for a causal relationship from liability for ADHD to nicotine dependence i.e. ADHD does not lead to nicotine dependence. They did find a strong genetic correlation between them (r_g = 0. 53) and suggest that this arises from shared underlying genetic vulnerabilities.

It has been generally assumed that finding an adult with ADHD represented a neurodevelopmental condition that arose in childhood and then was stable into adulthood. An alternative possibility is that it could be a condition with an onset delayed until the adult years. Moffitt et al. (2015) undertook a prospective longitudinal study of a representative birth cohort. In the same group of participants a follow-forward analysis of ADHD cases diagnosed in childhood was compared to a follow-back analysis of ADHD cases diagnosed in adulthood. This was designed to test whether the correlates of adult ADHD are the same as those of childhood ADHD. The vast majority of those with adult ADHD did not have a history of ADHD in childhood. They did not show neuropsychological deficits in either childhood or adulthood nor did they have elevated PRS scores for childhood ADHD. Importantly these results have been largely replicated in an independent sample (Agnew-Blais et al., 2016).

These findings were surprising and raise the unresolved question of just what is causing ADHD in adulthood (Asherson et al., 2016). The distinction between persistent (i.e. starting in childhood) and symptomatic adult ADHD (i.e. onset in adulthood) was made in a study of the global prevalence of ADHD in adults (Song et al., 2021). They estimated the global prevalence of persistent ADHD to be 2.58% and of symptomatic adult ADHD to be (6.76%). These results are consistent with the findings from Moffitt et al. (2015) presented above.

9.6 Treatment of ADHD

Non-pharmacological treatments Sonuga-Barke et al. (2013) reviewed evidence for the efficacy of non-pharmacological treatments for ADHD. There were four key features of this review. First, it included only randomized controlled trials. Second, the participants had to be individuals who were diagnosed with ADHD (or who met a validated cut-off on a recognised rating scale). Third, the outcome of the RCT had to include change in ADHD symptomatology. Fourth, the effect sizes were calculated for outcome measures based on reported by the person closest to the therapeutic setting and separately for measures obtained from the person most likely to be blind as to treatment. These two sets of analyses produced strikingly different results. When the outcome measure was based on ADHD assessments by raters closest to the therapeutic setting, all dietary (SMD = 0.21–0.48) and psychological (SMD = 0.40–0.64) treatments produced statistically significant effects. However, when the best probably blinded assessment was employed, effects remained significant for free fatty acid supplementation (SMD = 0.16) and artificial food colour exclusion (SMD = 0.42) but were substantially attenuated to nonsignificant levels for other treatments.

A subsequent publication based on the behavioural intervention studies from this same team (Daley et al., 2018) suggested that on the basis of current evidence that takes into account whether outcomes are blinded, behavioural intervention cannot be supported as a front-line treatment for core ADHD symptoms. There is, however, evidence from measures that are probably blinded that these interventions benefit parenting practices and improve conduct problems, which commonly co-occur with ADHD, and are often the main reason for referral.

Sonuga-Barke et al. (2013) concluded that free fatty acid supplementation produced small but significant reductions in ADHD symptoms even with probably blinded assessments, although the clinical significance of these effects remains to be determined. Artificial food colour exclusion produced larger effects but often in individuals selected for food sensitivities. Better evidence for efficacy from blinded assessments is required for behavioural interventions, neurofeedback, cognitive training, and restricted elimination diets before they can be supported as treatments for core ADHD symptoms. A similar conclusion concerning the need for more consistent and higher quality evidence of efficacy for nonpharmacological treatments for ADHD was reached in a later systematic review by Sibley et al. (2023).

Behavioural parent training Loe et al. (2021) produced the American Academy of Pediatrics Practice Guidelines for ADHD, which recommends parent training in behaviour management (BPT) as a treatment for young children with ADHD. These recommendations in part draw on a review by Evans et al. (2018) on psychosocial treatment approaches, which updated an earlier review (Evans et al., 2014). These reviews were more positive about the value of BPT interventions than Daley et al. (2018) and Sonuga-Barke et al. (2013). The reasons for this disparity lies primarily in the restriction of the Sonuga-Barke et al. (2013) meta-analysis to measures of ADHD symptom change as the outcome and the inflation of effect sizes in the Evans et al. (2014) review by the inclusion of non-blind assessments.

Evans et al. (2018) conclude that BPT is still well-established for preschool- and elementary-school-age children, but BPT for adolescents is less so. However, the authors suggest that effect size alone cannot be used alone for recommendations for practice:

> we continue to struggle with measures of clinical meaningfulness. The common use of effect sizes is an improvement, but there are still important limitations. For example, depending on the variability of data from a measure within a sample, a relatively small

> difference between groups could be statistically significant and have a moderate to large effect size. Yet the difference may be of a magnitude that parents and teachers could not notice a difference in the child's behavior. (Evans et al., 2018, p.193)

It is interesting to note that Sonuga-Barke et al. (2013) had a similar difficulty appraising the value of free fatty acid supplementation as a treatment for ADHD. This produced statistically significant reductions in ADHD symptoms SMD = 0.16 ($CI_{.95}$ 0.01 to 0.31), but they found the clinical significance of these effects remained to be determined.

Barkley (2016) commented on disagreements about the efficacy of BPT for ADHD. He argues that

1. The evidence does not show BPT to be very effective.
2. BPT was designed to treat behaviour which is linked to parental management methods (such as oppositional defiant behaviour).
3. By contrast, parent skills do not contribute to ADHD.
4. That BPT is not as efficacious as medication even for the preschool child.
5. The BPT is not side-effect free – it can induce an increase in defiant and disruptive behaviour.

He asserts (stridently!) as follows:

> The CDC [Centers for Disease Control and Prevention] should stop pontificating on the value of BPT for ADHD versus medications when it clearly is not well-informed on the facts, theories and etiologies concerning ADHD, nor the evidence of effectiveness for these therapies. (Barkley, 2016, p.6)

Drug treatments It is well-established that psychostimulant drug treatments for ADHD are efficacious (Cortese, 2020). For children, the effect size in RCTs for methylphenidate compared to placebo was around SMD = 0.80 for both teacher and parent ratings (Cortese et al., 2018). A meta-analysis of studies of stimulant treatment for preschool children with ADHD suggested a slightly lower effect size (SMD = 0.59 (CI.95 0.41 to 0.77)) (Sugaya et al., 2023). In the UK, methylphenidate is recommended as a treatment for children aged 5 and older if symptoms persist after a period of support for parents and liaison with school (NICE, 2018). For younger children, NICE recommends that methylphenidate should only be used once parent training has been tried out.

There is now evidence that that both methylphenidate and behavioural parent training are of benefit to preschool children (Sugaya et al., 2022). They conducted a double-blind placebo-controlled trial of combining methylphenidate and behavioural parent training. After 8 weeks of treatment, methylphenidate was effective in reducing ADHD symptoms and improving functionality. Functionality here was measured using the Children's Global Assessment Scale (Shaffer et al., 1983) – a widely used rating scale of children's everyday functioning at home and at school. Behavioural parent training was effective in improving functionality for preschool children with ADHD but not core ADHD behaviours. Sugaya et al. (2022) recommend that

> Preschool children with ADHD should not be left untreated until they reach school age or their impairment becomes severe and they should receive treatments supported by the best available evidence. (Sugaya et al., 2022, p.855)

There are a number of concerns about adverse side effects of such drug treatments for children. These are discussed by Posner et al. (2020) who suggest that growth retardation is the main concern but this can be reduced by the use of "drug holidays", i.e. short breaks from medication. Another potentially serious psychological concern is the risk of medication precipitating psychotic episodes in children, especially those with a history of psychosis. However, a large-scale study in Sweden found no such increased risk for those with or without a psychosis history (Hollis et al., 2019). The potential for α2-adrenergic agonists as a pharmacological treatment for ADHD in preschoolers is discussed by Froehlich (2021). There is evidence that this treatment may be as effective as stimulants and with fewer side effects (Harstad et al., 2021), but there is a need for RCTs to be conducted to confirm the possible benefits of α2-adrenergic agonists for this age group.

Stimulants have been identified as an effective treatment for ADHD but there is a question of just which aspects of cognitive dysfunction in children with ADHD are improved by this treatment. McKenzie et al. (2022) undertook a systematic review of investigations on this issue. They found 10 studies that addressed this question. The results indicated that a number of aspects of attention were improved by the administration of psychostimulants. These included memory, vigilance, divided attention, and focused attention. The benefits for other aspects of cognition, including academic performance and executive function, were inconclusive.

There is an under-investigated issue of when or whether it is safe to discontinue stimulant medication. The treatment recommendations from NICE (2018) are that there should be annual reviews of the medication treatment to consider whether it should be continued. They also recommend the consideration of the use of trial periods when the medication is stopped or the dose reduced in order to assess the overall balance of benefits and harms of discontinuation. There are ethical constraints on using a placebo-controlled study to identify the long-term effectiveness of stimulant treatment, as this would involve denying children in the placebo group access to a treatment of known short-term benefit. Accordingly, Matthijssen et al. (2019) used an alternative discontinuation design that randomly allocated children, aged 8 to 18 years and who had been on methylphenidate for two years or longer, to either continue using methylphenidate for 7 weeks or the gradual withdrawal to placebo over 3 weeks followed by 4 weeks of complete placebo. They found that there were statistically significant benefits from continued medication use, particularly on working memory (Rosenau et al., 2021). However, some children did not show a deterioration after withdrawal. These findings give support to the approach to treatment continuation recommended by NICE (2018).

Combined treatments The Multimodal Treatment Study of Children with ADHD (MTA) was a major investigation of the effectiveness of stimulant medication, behavioural treatment, a combined treatment of the two, and community care for children with ADHD. A group of 579 children aged 7 to 10 years were randomly assigned to one of these four treatments. After 14 months of treatment, it was found that the combined treatment and stimulant medications were equally effective and showed significantly greater improvements than the behavioural and community care treatments (Jensen et al., 1999). However, these initial gains of treatment were lost 6 to 8 years later (Molina et al., 2009). For an appraisal of the significance of the MTA study for the clinical management of ADHD, see Hinshaw et al. (2015). They conclude:

> The paradox is that, despite their proven short-term benefits, no clinically significant and enduring intervention (or intervention combination) exists for this condition, as of yet. (Hinshaw et al., 2015, p.48)

It should be noted that an umbrella review of meta-analyses and network meta-analyses of studies, published up to 2021, on the treatment of mental disorders in children concluded that combining drug treatments with parent training was particularly efficacious for ADHD (Correll et al., 2021) – see also Sugaya et al. (2022) discussed above.

Clinically significant change The question that was raised above of what constitutes a clinically significant effect of treatment is obviously important. Statistical significance in an RCT is a necessary but not sufficient reason for adopting a treatment. Kazdin (2001) produced an overview of not just the statistical issues in identifying clinically significant change but the conceptual issues too. He suggests that although many ways have been developed to quantify such change:

> it is still not entirely clear what any of the ways mean in the lives of clients. (Kazdin, 2001, p.455)

One such way to quantify change is to obtain a reliable change index (RCI) for an individual (Jacobson & Truax, 1991) or for treatment on a group (Abramowitz, 1998). The RCI assesses change in scores in relation to the mean scores of the dysfunctional population and the functional population. This approach addresses the question as to whether, as a result of treatment, the amount of change that has occurred is large enough to be considered meaningful. This is appraised by calculating the difference in scores pre- and post-test in relation to the standard error of the difference between the scores. Reliable change is in this sense real change, that is, it does not simply arise from random fluctuations of measurement. An alternative is the normative comparison approach. This addresses the question as to whether, after treatment, individuals are distinguishable from those in the functional population (Kendall et al., 1999).

Kazdin (2001) takes issue with whether either showing reliable change or improvement on a normative comparison:

> means the client is better in any way that affects daily functioning or that a failure to pass this threshold means otherwise. (Kazdin, 2001, p.461)

These are "comparison methods", that is, judging change in score on measures under treatment against the scores of others. There are two additional approaches to assess clinical significance. The first is "social impact" where change is calibrated on a measure of social functioning such as truancy. The second is "subjective evaluation" where the client, or perhaps their parent, makes their own judgement of improvement in functioning. To meet Kazdin's concerns requires the adoption of an idiographic approach to determining clinical significance, such as this subjective evaluation (see Sect. 5.1).

The issue of clinical significance is unresolved for non-pharmacological treatment. It has been more directly addressed in drug treatment RCTs. Coghill et al. (2017) examined the impact on quality of life and functional outcomes in placebo controlled RCTs of medication treatments for ADHD. They used a 0.5 standard deviation improvement in quality of life as an index of clinically significant improvement – a degree of change that has been repeatedly shown to represent a minimally important difference in quality of life (Norman et al., 2003). They found that the effects sizes for stimulant medication on functional and quality of life measures were large (>0.80). They conclude that these treatments can be used both to improve symptoms and functioning in everyday life.

9.7 Final Thoughts on ADHD

A recurrent theme to emerge from research on ADHD is that it is best conceptualised as being on a continuum with a large number of genetic and environmental factors influencing a child's position on this continuum. In an overarching review of the state of ADHD research, Nigg et al. (2020a) argue that ADHD should not be seen as a discrete category but rather as at the conjunction of dimensions of dysregulation of executive function, attention, and of affect.

A wide range of studies have been reviewed in this chapter, and there are many unresolved questions about the origins, consequences, and treatment of ADHD. However, there is sufficient agreement that in 2021, a World Federation of ADHD International Consensus Statement was produced by over 50 of the leading ADHD researchers worldwide (Faraone et al., 2021). The aim was to provide current and accurate information about ADHD supported by a substantial and rigorous body of evidence. The main conclusions were summarised as follows:

ADHD occurs in 5.9% of youth and 2.5% of adults.
Most cases of ADHD are caused by the combined effects of many genetic and environmental risks.
There are small differences in the brain between people with and without ADHD.
Untreated ADHD can lead to many adverse outcomes.
ADHD costs society hundreds of billions of dollars each year, worldwide.

References

Abramowitz, J. S. (1998). Does cognitive-behavioral therapy cure obsessive-compulsive disorder? A meta-analytic evaluation of clinical significance. *Behavior Therapy, 29*(2), 339–355. https://doi.org/10.1016/s0005-7894(98)80012-9

Agnew-Blais, J. C., Polanczyk, G. V., Danese, A., Wertz, J., Moffitt, T. E., & Arseneault, L. (2016). Evaluation of the persistence, remission, and emergence of Attention-Deficit/Hyperactivity Disorder in young adulthood. *JAMA Psychiatry, 73*(7), 713–720. https://doi.org/10.1001/jamapsychiatry.2016.0465

Agnew-Blais, J. C., Belsky, D. W., Caspi, A., Danese, A., Moffitt, T. E., Polanczyk, G. V., et al. (2021). Polygenic risk and the course of Attention-Deficit/Hyperactivity Disorder from childhood to young adulthood: Findings from a nationally representative cohort. *Journal of the American Academy of Child and Adolescent Psychiatry, 60*(9), 1147–1156. https://doi.org/10.1016/j.jaac.2020.12.033

Agnew-Blais, J. C., Wertz, J., Arseneault, L., Belsky, D. W., Danese, A., Pingault, J.-B., et al. (2022). Mother's and children's ADHD genetic risk, household chaos and children's ADHD symptoms: A gene-environment correlation study. *Journal of Child psychology and Psychiatry*. https://doi.org/10.1111/jcpp.13659

Alger, J. R., O'Neill, J., O'Connor, M. J., Kalender, G., Ly, R., Ng, A., et al. (2021). Neuroimaging of supraventricular frontal white matter in children with familial Attention-Deficit Hyperactivity Disorder and Attention-Deficit Hyperactivity Disorder due to prenatal alcohol exposure. *Neurotoxicity Research, 39*. https://doi.org/10.1007/s12640-021-00342-0

Andersson, A., Tuvblad, C., Chen, Q., Du Rietz, E., Cortese, S., Kuja-Halkola, R., & Larsson, H. (2020). Research Review: The strength of the genetic overlap between ADHD and other psychiatric symptoms - A systematic review and meta-analysis. *Journal of Child Psychology and Psychiatry, 61*(11), 1173–1183. https://doi.org/10.1111/jcpp.13233

Antony, E. M.-A., Pihlajamaki, M., Speyer, L. G., & Murray, A. L. (2022). Does emotion dysregulation mediate the association between ADHD symptoms and internalizing problems? A longitudinal within-person analysis in a large population-representative study. *Journal of Child Psychology and Psychiatry*. https://doi.org/10.1111/jcpp.13624

Aoki, Y., Inokuchi, R., Suwa, H., & Aoki, A. (2013). Age-related change of neurochemical abnormality in attention-deficit hyperactivity disorder: A meta-analysis. *Neuroscience and Biobehavioral Reviews, 37*(8), 1692–1701. https://doi.org/10.1016/j.neubiorev.2013.04.019

Aoki, Y., Cortese, S., & Castellanos, F. X. (2018). Research Review: Diffusion tensor imaging studies of attention-deficit/hyperactivity disorder: Meta-analyses and reflections on head motion. *Journal of Child Psychology and Psychiatry, 59*(3), 193–202. https://doi.org/10.1111/jcpp.12778

Arns, M., Conners, C. K., & Kraemer, H. C. (2013). A decade of EEG Theta/Beta Ratio research in ADHD: A meta-analysis. *Journal of Attention Disorders, 17*(5), 374–383. https://doi.org/10.1177/1087054712460087

Artigas, M. S., Sanchez-Mora, C., Rovira, P., Vilar-Ribo, L., Ramos-Quiroga, J. A., & Ribases, M. (2023). Mendelian randomization analysis for attention deficit/hyperactivity disorder: Studying a broad range of exposures and outcomes. *International Journal of Epidemiology, 52*(2), 386–402. https://doi.org/10.1093/ije/dyac128

Asherson, P., Buitelaar, J., Faraone, S. V., & Rohde, L. A. (2016). Adult attention-deficit hyperactivity disorder: Key conceptual issues. *Lancet Psychiatry, 3*(6), 568–578. https://doi.org/10.1016/s2215-0366(16)30032-3

Astle, D. E., Holmes, J., Kievit, R., & Gathercole, S. E. (2022). Annual Research Review: The transdiagnostic revolution in neurodevelopmental disorders. *Journal of Child Psychology and Psychiatry, 63*(4), 397–417. https://doi.org/10.1111/jcpp.13481

Baker, B. H., Joo, Y. Y., Park, J., Cha, J., Baccarelli, A. A., & Posner, J. (2023). Maternal age at birth and child attention-deficit hyperactivity disorder: Causal association or familial confounding? *Journal of Child Psychology and Psychiatry, 64*(2), 299–310. https://doi.org/10.1111/jcpp.13726

Bali, P., Sonuga-Barke, E., Mohr-Jensen, C., Demontis, D., & Minnis, H. (2023). Is there evidence of a causal link between childhood maltreatment and attention deficit/hyperactivity disorder? A systematic review of prospective longitudinal studies using the Bradford-Hill criteria. *JCPP Advances*, e12169. https://doi.org/10.1002/jcv2.12169

Banaschewski, T., Jennen-Steinmetz, C., Brandeis, D., Buitelaar, J. K., Kuntsi, J., Poustka, L., et al. (2012). Neuropsychological correlates of emotional lability in children with ADHD. *Journal of Child Psychology and Psychiatry, 53*(11), 1139–1148. https://doi.org/10.1111/j.1469-7610.2012.02596.x

Barkley, R. A. (2016). The CDC and behavioral parent training for ADHD. *Mental Health Weekly, 26*, 5–6. https://doi.org/10.1002/mhw.30638

Bauer, J., Werner, A., Kohl, W., Kugel, H., Shushakova, A., Pedersen, A., & Ohrmann, P. (2018). Hyperactivity and impulsivity in adult attention-deficit/hyperactivity disorder is related to glutamatergic dysfunction in the anterior cingulate cortex. *World Journal of Biological Psychiatry, 19*(7), 538–546. https://doi.org/10.1080/15622975.2016.1262060

Becker, S. P. (2021). Systematic review: Assessment of sluggish cognitive tempo over the past decade. *Journal of the American Academy of Child and Adolescent Psychiatry, 60*(6), 690–709. https://doi.org/10.1016/j.jaac.2020.10.016

Becker, S. P., Leopold, D. R., Burns, G. L., Jarrett, M. A., Langberg, J. M., Marshall, S. A., et al. (2016). The internal, external, and diagnostic validity of sluggish cognitive tempo: A meta-analysis and critical review. *Journal of the American Academy of Child and Adolescent Psychiatry, 55*(3), 163–178. https://doi.org/10.1016/j.jaac.2015.12.006

Bellato, A., Arora, I., Hollis, C., & Groom, M. J. (2020). Is autonomic nervous system function atypical in attention deficit hyperactivity disorder (ADHD)? A systematic review of the evidence. *Neuroscience and Biobehavioral Reviews, 108*, 182–206. https://doi.org/10.1016/j.neubiorev.2019.11.001

Benca, C. E., Derringer, J. L., Corley, R. P., Young, S. E., Keller, M. C., Hewitt, J. K., & Friedman, N. P. (2017). Predicting cognitive executive functioning with polygenic risk scores for psychiatric disorders. *Behavior Genetics, 47*(1), 11–24. https://doi.org/10.1007/s10519-016-9814-2

Bhutta, A. T., Cleves, M. A., Casey, P. H., Cradock, M. M., & Anand, K. J. S. (2002). Cognitive and behavioral outcomes of school-aged children who were born preterm - A meta-analysis. *JAMA-Journal of the American Medical Association, 288*(6), 728–737. https://doi.org/10.1001/jama.288.6.728

Bitsko, R. H., Holbrook, J. R., O'Masta, B., Maher, B., Cerles, A., Saadeh, K., et al. (2022). A systematic review and meta-analysis of prenatal, birth, and postnatal factors associated with Attention-Deficit/Hyperactivity Disorder in children. *Prevention Science*. https://doi.org/10.1007/s11121-022-01359-3

Boland, H., DiSalvo, M., Fried, R., Woodworth, K. Y., Wilens, T., Faraone, S. V., & Biederman, J. (2020). A literature review and meta-analysis on the effects of ADHD medications on functional outcomes. *Journal of Psychiatric Research, 123*, 21–30. https://doi.org/10.1016/j.jpsychires.2020.01.006

Bollmann, S., Ghisleni, C., Poil, S. S., Martin, E., Ball, J., Eich-Hochli, D., et al. (2015). Developmental changes in gamma-aminobutyric acid levels in attention-deficit/hyperactivity disorder. *Translational Psychiatry, 5*. https://doi.org/10.1038/tp.2015.79

Borge, T. C., Aase, H., Brantster, A. L., & Biele, G. (2017). The importance of maternal diet quality during pregnancy on cognitive and behavioural outcomes in children: A systematic review and meta-analysis. *BMJ Open, 7*(9). https://doi.org/10.1136/bmjopen-2017-016777

Brikell, I., Larsson, H., Lu, Y., Pettersson, E., Chen, Q., Kuja-Halkola, R., et al. (2020). The contribution of common genetic risk variants for ADHD to a general factor of childhood psychopathology. *Molecular Psychiatry, 25*(8), 1809–1821. https://doi.org/10.1038/s41380-018-0109-2

Briscoe-Smith, A. M., & Hinshaw, S. P. (2006). Linkages between child abuse and attention-deficit/hyperactivity disorder in girls: Behavioral and social correlates. *Child Abuse and Neglect, 30*(11), 1239–1255. https://doi.org/10.1016/j.chiabu.2006.04.008

Burmeister, R., Hannay, H. J., Copeland, K., Fletcher, J. M., Boudousquie, A., & Dennis, M. (2005). Attention problems and executive functions in children with spina bifida and hydrocephalus. *Child Neuropsychology, 11*(3), 265–283. https://doi.org/10.1080/092970490911324

Camerota, M., Willoughby, M. T., & Blair, C. B. (2020). Measurement models for studying child executive functioning: Questioning the status quo. *Developmental Psychology, 56*(12), 2236–2245. https://doi.org/10.1037/dev0001127

Cao, M., Martin, E., & Li, X. (2023). Machine learning in attention-deficit/hyperactivity disorder: New approaches toward understanding the neural mechanisms. *Translational Psychiatry, 13*(1), 236. https://doi.org/10.1038/s41398-023-02536-w

Castellanos, F. X. (2021). A biased perspective on brain imaging of ADHD. *American Journal of Psychiatry, 178*(8), 694–700. https://doi.org/10.1176/appi.ajp.2021.21060609

Castellanos, F. X., & Proal, E. (2012). Large-scale brain systems in ADHD: Beyond the prefrontal-striatal model. *Trends in Cognitive Sciences, 16*(1), 17–26. https://doi.org/10.1016/j.tics.2011.11.007

Castellanos, F. X., Sonuga-Barke, E. J. S., Scheres, A., Di Martino, A., Hyde, C., & Walters, J. R. (2005). Varieties of attention-deficit/hyperactivity disorder-related intra-individual variability. *Developmental Psychology, 57*(11), 1416–1423. https://doi.org/10.1016/j.biopsych.2004.12.005

Castellanos, F. X., Sonuga-Barke, E. J. S., Milham, M. P., & Tannock, R. (2006). Characterizing cognition in ADHD: Beyond executive dysfunction. *Trends in Cognitive Sciences, 10*(3), 117–123. https://doi.org/10.1016/j.tics.2006.01.011

Cecil, C. A. M., & Nigg, J. T. (2022). Epigenetics and ADHD: Reflections on current knowledge, research priorities and translational potential. *Molecular Diagnosis & Therapy, 26*, 581–606. https://doi.org/10.1007/s40291-022-00609-y

Cenit, M. C., Nuevo, I. C., Codoner-Franch, P., Dinan, T. G., & Sanz, Y. (2017). Gut microbiota and attention deficit hyperactivity disorder: New perspectives for a challenging condition. *European Child and Adolescent Psychiatry, 26*(9), 1081–1092. https://doi.org/10.1007/s00787-017-0969-z

Chang, S. H., Yang, L., Wang, Y. F., & Faraone, S. V. (2020). Shared polygenic risk for ADHD, executive dysfunction and other psychiatric disorders. *Translational Psychiatry, 10*(1). https://doi.org/10.1038/s41398-020-00872-9

Chang, Y.-C., Chen, W.-T., Su, S.-H., Jung, C.-R., & Hwang, B.-F. (2022). PM2.5 exposure and incident attention-deficit/hyperactivity disorder during the prenatal and postnatal periods: A birth cohort study. *Environmental Research, 214*(Pt 1), 113769–113769. https://doi.org/10.1016/j.envres.2022.113769

Chatterjee, N., Shi, J., & Garcia-Closas, M. (2016). Developing and evaluating polygenic risk prediction models for stratified disease prevention. *Nature Reviews Genetics, 17*(7), 392–406. https://doi.org/10.1038/nrg.2016.27

Checa-Ros, A., Jerez-Calero, A., Molina-Carballo, A., Campoy, C., & Munoz-Hoyos, A. (2021). Current evidence on the role of the gut microbiome in ADHD pathophysiology and therapeutic Implications. *Nutrients, 13*(1). https://doi.org/10.3390/nu13010249

Chen, S. W., Zhong, X. S., Jiang, L. N., Zheng, X. Y., Xiong, Y. Q., Ma, S. J., et al. (2016). Maternal autoimmune diseases and the risk of autism spectrum disorders in offspring: A systematic review and meta-analysis. *Behavioural Brain Research, 296*, 61–69. https://doi.org/10.1016/j.bbr.2015.08.035

Choenni, V., Lambregtse-van den Berg, M. P., Verhulst, F. C., Tiemeier, H., & Kok, R. (2019). The longitudinal relation between observed maternal parenting in the preschool period and the occurrence of child ADHD symptoms in middle childhood. *Journal of Abnormal Child Psychology, 47*(5), 755–764. https://doi.org/10.1007/s10802-018-0492-9

Chorozoglou, M., Smith, E., Koerting, J., Thompson, M. J., Sayal, K., & Sonuga-Barke, E. J. S. (2015). Preschool hyperactivity is associated with long-term economic burden: Evidence from a longitudinal health economic analysis of costs incurred across childhood, ado-

lescence and young adulthood. *Journal of Child Psychology and Psychiatry, 56*(9), 966–975. https://doi.org/10.1111/jcpp.12437
Coghill, D. R., Seth, S., & Matthews, K. (2014). A comprehensive assessment of memory, delay aversion, timing, inhibition, decision making and variability in attention deficit hyperactivity disorder: Advancing beyond the three-pathway models. *Psychological Medicine, 44*(9), 1989–2001. https://doi.org/10.1017/s0033291713002547
Coghill, D. R., Banaschewski, T., Soutullo, C., Cottingham, M. G., & Zuddas, A. (2017). Systematic review of quality of life and functional outcomes in randomized placebo-controlled studies of medications for attention-deficit/hyperactivity disorder. *European Child and Adolescent Psychiatry, 26*(11), 1283–1307. https://doi.org/10.1007/s00787-017-0986-y
Cordova, M. M., Antovich, D. M., Ryabinin, P., Neighbor, C., Mooney, M. A., Dieckmann, N. F., et al. (2022). Attention-Deficit/Hyperactivity Disorder: Restricted phenotypes prevalence, comorbidity, and polygenic risk sensitivity in the ABCD baseline cohort. *Journal of the American Academy of Child and Adolescent Psychiatry.* https://doi.org/10.1016/j.jaac.2022.03.030
Correll, C. U., Cortese, S., Croatto, G., Monaco, F., Krinitski, D., Arrondo, G., et al. (2021). Efficacy and acceptability of pharmacological, psychosocial, and brain stimulation interventions in children and adolescents with mental disorders: An umbrella review. *World Psychiatry, 20*(2), 244–275. https://doi.org/10.1002/wps.20881
Cortese, S. (2020). Pharmacologic treatment of Attention Deficit-Hyperactivity Disorder. *New England Journal of Medicine, 383*(11), 1050–1056. https://doi.org/10.1056/NEJMra1917069
Cortese, S., & Tessari, L. (2017). Attention-Deficit/Hyperactivity Disorder (ADHD) and obesity: Update 2016. *Current Psychiatry Reports, 19*(1). https://doi.org/10.1007/s11920-017-0754-1
Cortese, S., Adamo, N., Del Giovane, C., Mohr-Jensen, C., Hayes, A. J., Carucci, S., et al. (2018). Comparative efficacy and tolerability of medications for attention-deficit hyperactivity disorder in children, adolescents, and adults: A systematic review and network meta-analysis. *Lancet Psychiatry, 5*(9), 727–738. https://doi.org/10.1016/s2215-0366(18)30269-4
Cortese, S., Aoki, Y. Y., Itahashi, T., Castellanos, F. X., & Eickhoff, S. B. (2021a). Systematic review and meta-analysis: Resting-state functional magnetic resonance imaging studies of Attention-Deficit/Hyperactivity Disorder. *Journal of the American Academy of Child and Adolescent Psychiatry, 60*(1), 61–75. https://doi.org/10.1016/j.jaac.2020.08.014
Cortese, S., Arrondo, G., Correll, C. U., & Solmi, M. (2021b). Beyond the p factor: Is there a d factor? *JCPP Advances*. https://doi.org/10.1002/jcv2.12051
Curran, P. J., Howard, A. L., Bainter, S. A., Lane, S. T., & McGinley, J. S. (2014). The separation of between-person and within-person components of individual change over time: A latent curve model with structured residuals. *Journal of Consulting and Clinical Psychology, 82*(5), 879–894. https://doi.org/10.1037/a0035297
Daley, D., Van Der Oord, S., Ferrin, M., Cortese, S., Danckaerts, M., Doepfner, M., et al. (2018). Practitioner Review: Current best practice in the use of parent training and other behavioural interventions in the treatment of children and adolescents with attention deficit hyperactivity disorder. *Journal of Child Psychology and Psychiatry, 59*(9), 932–947. https://doi.org/10.1111/jcpp.12825
Danese, A., & McEwen, B. S. (2012). Adverse childhood experiences, allostasis, allostatic load, and age-related disease. *Physiology & Behavior, 106*(1), 29–39. https://doi.org/10.1016/j.physbeh.2011.08.019
De Asis-Cruz, J., Krishnamurthy, D., Zhao, L., Kapse, K., Vezina, G., Andescavage, N., et al. (2020). Association of prenatal maternal anxiety with fetal regional brain connectivity. *Jama Network Open, 3*(12). https://doi.org/10.1001/jamanetworkopen.2020.22349
Demontis, D., Walters, R. K., Martin, J., Mattheisen, M., Als, T. D., Agerbo, E., . Wilson, C.H. (2019). Discovery of the first genome-wide significant risk loci for attention deficit/hyperactivity disorder. *Nature Genetics, 51*(1), 63-+. doi:https://doi.org/10.1038/s41588-018-0269-7
Demontis, D., Walters, R. K., Rajagopal, V. M., Waldman, I. D., Grove, J., Als, T. D., et al. (2021). Risk variants and polygenic architecture of disruptive behavior disorders in the context of

attention-deficit/hyperactivity disorder. *Nature Communications, 12*(1), 576–576. https://doi.org/10.1038/s41467-020-20443-2

Doebel, S. (2020). Rethinking executive function and its development. *Perspectives on Psychological Science, 15*(4), 942–956. https://doi.org/10.1177/1745691620904771

Doidge, J. L., Flora, D. B., & Toplak, M. E. (2021). A meta-analytic review of sex differences on delay of gratification and temporal discounting tasks in ADHD and typically developing samples. *Journal of Attention Disorders, 25*(4), 540–561. https://doi.org/10.1177/1087054718815588

Du Rietz, E., Brikell, I., Butwicka, A., Leone, M., Chang, Z., Cortese, S., et al. (2021a). ADHD and physical conditions in adulthood in Sweden: A genetically informed register study. *Lancet Psychiatry, 8*(9), 774–783. https://doi.org/10.1016/S2215-0366(21)00171-1

Du Rietz, E., Pettersson, E., Brikell, I., Ghirardi, L., Chen, Q., Hartman, C., et al. (2021b). Overlap between attention-deficit hyperactivity disorder and neurodevelopmental, externalising and internalising disorders: Separating unique from general psychopathology effects. *British Journal of Psychiatry, 218*(1), 35–42. https://doi.org/10.1192/bjp.2020.152

Dunn, G. A., Nigg, J. T., & Sullivan, E. L. (2019). Neuroinflammation as a risk factor for attention deficit hyperactivity disorder. *Pharmacology Biochemistry and Behavior, 182*, 22–34. https://doi.org/10.1016/j.pbb.2019.05.005

DuPaul, G. J., McGoey, K. E., Eckert, T. L., & VanBrakle, J. (2001). Preschool children with attention-deficit/hyperactivity disorder: Impairments in behavioral, social, and school functioning. *Journal of the American Academy of Child and Adolescent Psychiatry, 40*(5), 508–515. https://doi.org/10.1097/00004583-200105000-00009

El Marroun, H., Zeegers, M., Steegers, E. A. P., van der Ende, J., Schenk, J. J., Hofman, A., et al. (2012). Post-term birth and the risk of behavioural and emotional problems in early childhood. *International Journal of Epidemiology, 41*(3), 773–781. https://doi.org/10.1093/ije/dys043

Elliott, M. L., Knodt, A. R., Cooke, M., Kim, M. J., Melzer, T. R., Keenan, R., et al. (2019). General functional connectivity: Shared features of resting-state and task fMRI drive reliable and heritable individual differences in functional brain networks. *Neuroimage, 189*, 516–532. https://doi.org/10.1016/j.neuroimage.2019.01.068

Elliott, M. L., Knodt, A. R., Ireland, D., Morris, M. L., Poulton, R., Ramrakha, S., et al. (2020). What Is the test-retest reliability of common task-functional MRI measures? New empirical evidence and a meta-analysis. *Psychological Science, 31*(7), 792–806. https://doi.org/10.1177/0956797620916786

Espy, K. A., Sheffield, T. D., Wiebe, S. A., Clark, C. A. C., & Moehr, M. J. (2011). Executive control and dimensions of problem behaviors in preschool children. *Journal of Child Psychology and Psychiatry, 52*(1), 33–46. https://doi.org/10.1111/j.1469-7610.2010.02265.x

Evans, S. W., Owens, J. S., & Bunford, N. (2014). Evidence-based psychosocial treatments for children and adolescents with Attention-Deficit/Hyperactivity Disorder. *Journal of Clinical Child and Adolescent Psychology, 43*(4), 527–551. https://doi.org/10.1080/15374416.2013.850700

Evans, S. W., Owens, J. S., Wymbs, B. T., & Ray, A. R. (2018). Evidence-based psychosocial treatments for children and adolescents with Attention Deficit/Hyperactivity Disorder. *Journal of Clinical Child and Adolescent Psychology, 47*(2), 157–198. https://doi.org/10.1080/15374416.2017.1390757

Faraone, S. V., & Buitelaar, J. (2010). Comparing the efficacy of stimulants for ADHD in children and adolescents using meta-analysis. *European Child and Adolescent Psychiatry, 19*(4), 353–364. https://doi.org/10.1007/s00787-009-0054-3

Faraone, S. V., & Larsson, H. (2019). Genetics of attention deficit hyperactivity disorder. *Molecular Psychiatry, 24*(4), 562–575. https://doi.org/10.1038/s41380-018-0070-0

Faraone, S. V., Rostain, A. L., Blader, J., Busch, B., Childress, A. C., Connor, D. F., & Newcorn, J. H. (2019). Practitioner Review: Emotional dysregulation in attention-deficit/hyperactivity disorder - implications for clinical recognition and intervention. *Journal of Child Psychology and Psychiatry, 60*(2), 133–150. https://doi.org/10.1111/jcpp.12899

Faraone, S. V., Banaschewski, T., Coghill, D., Zheng, Y., Biederman, J., Bellgrove, M. A., et al. (2021). The World Federation of ADHD International Consensus Statement: 208 Evidence-based conclusions about the disorder. *Neuroscience and Biobehavioral Reviews, 128*, 789–818. https://doi.org/10.1016/j.neubiorev.2021.01.022

Fava, L., & Morton, J. (2009). Causal modeling of panic disorder theories. *Clinical Psychology Review, 29*(7), 623–637. https://doi.org/10.1016/j.cpr.2009.08.002

Franke, B., Michelini, G., Asherson, P., Banaschewski, T., Bilbow, A., Buitelaar, J. K., et al. (2018). Live fast, die young? A review on the developmental trajectories of ADHD across the lifespan. *European Neuropsychopharmacology, 28*(10), 1059–1088. https://doi.org/10.1016/j.euroneuro.2018.08.001

Frazier, T. W., Demaree, H. A., & Youngstrom, E. A. (2004). Meta-analysis of intellectual and neuropsychological test performance in attention-deficit/hyperactivity disorder. *Neuropsychology, 18*(3), 543–555. https://doi.org/10.1037/0894-4105.18.3.543

Friedman, N. P., & Miyake, A. (2017). Unity and diversity of executive functions: Individual differences as a window on cognitive structure. *Cortex, 86*, 186–204. https://doi.org/10.1016/j.cortex.2016.04.023

Friedman, N. P., Miyake, A., Young, S. E., DeFries, J. C., Corley, R. P., & Hewitt, J. K. (2008). Individual differences in executive functions are almost entirely genetic in origin. *Journal of Experimental Psychology-General, 137*(2), 201–225. https://doi.org/10.1037/0096-3445.137.2.201

Froehlich, T. E. (2021). Comparison of medication treatments for preschool children with ADHD A first step toward addressing a critical gap. *Jama-Journal of the American Medical Association, 325*(20), 2049–2050. https://doi.org/10.1001/jama.2021.5603

Froehlich, T. E., Lanphear, B. P., Auinger, P., Hornung, R., Epstein, J. N., Braun, J., & Kahn, R. S. (2009). Association of tobacco and lead exposures with Attention-Deficit/Hyperactivity Disorder. *Pediatrics, 124*(6), E1054–E1063. https://doi.org/10.1542/peds.2009-0738

Gao, Y. X., Shuai, D. D., Bu, X., Hu, X. Y., Tang, S., Zhang, L. Q., et al. (2019). Impairments of large-scale functional networks in attention-deficit/hyperactivity disorder: A meta-analysis of resting-state functional connectivity. *Psychological Medicine, 49*(15), 2475–2485. https://doi.org/10.1017/s003329171900237x

Garcia-Marin, L. M., Campos, A. I., Cuellar-Partida, G., Medland, S. E., Kollins, S. H., & Renteria, M. E. (2021). Large-scale genetic investigation reveals genetic liability to multiple complex traits influencing a higher risk of ADHD. *Scientific Reports, 11*(1). https://doi.org/10.1038/s41598-021-01517-7

Garrison-Desany, H. M., Hong, X., Maher, B. S., Beaty, T. H., Wang, G., Pearson, C., et al. (2022). Individual and combined association between prenatal polysubstance exposure and childhood risk of Attention-Deficit/Hyperactivity Disorder. *Jama Network Open, 5*(3). https://doi.org/10.1001/jamanetworkopen.2022.1957

Giannoulis, S. V., Mueller, D., Kennedy, J. L., & Goncalves, V. (2022). Systematic review of mitochondrial genetic variation in attention-deficit/hyperactivity disorder. *European Child and Adolescent Psychiatry*. https://doi.org/10.1007/s00787-022-02030-6

Gioia, G. A., Isquith, P. K., Guy, S. C., & Kenworthy, L. (2000). Behavior rating inventory of executive function. In Odessa: Psychological Assessment Resources.

Gjone, H., Stevenson, J., & Sundet, J. M. (1996). Genetic influence on parent-reported attention-related problems in a Norwegian general population twin sample. *Journal of the American Academy of Child and Adolescent Psychiatry, 35*(5), 588–596. https://doi.org/10.1097/00004583-199605000-00013

Goodlad, J. K., Marcus, D. K., & Fulton, J. J. (2013). Lead and Attention-Deficit/Hyperactivity Disorder (ADHD) symptoms: A meta-analysis. *Clinical Psychology Review, 33*(3), 417–425. https://doi.org/10.1016/j.cpr.2013.01.009

Goodman, S. J., Burton, C. L., Butcher, D. T., Siu, M. T., Lemire, M., Chater-Diehl, E., et al. (2020). Obsessive-compulsive disorder and attention-deficit/hyperactivity disorder: Distinct associations with DNA methylation and genetic variation. *Journal of Neurodevelopmental Disorders, 12*(1). https://doi.org/10.1186/s11689-020-09324-3

Green, A., Baroud, E., DiSalvo, M., Faraone, S. V., & Biederman, J. (2022). Examining the impact of ADHD polygenic risk scores on ADHD and associated outcomes: A systematic review and meta-analysis. *Journal of Psychiatric Research.* https://doi.org/10.1016/j.jpsychires.2022.07.032

Griffiths, K. R., Braund, T. A., Kohn, M. R., Clarke, S., Williams, L. M., & Korgaonkar, M. S. (2021). Structural brain network topology underpinning ADHD and response to methylphenidate treatment. *Translational Psychiatry, 11*(1). https://doi.org/10.1038/s41398-021-01278-x

Halse, M., Steinsbekk, S., Hammar, A., & Wichstrom, L. (2022). Longitudinal relations between impaired executive function and symptoms of psychiatric disorders in childhood. *Journal of Child Psychology and Psychiatry.* https://doi.org/10.1111/jcpp.13622

Han, V. X., Patel, S., Jones, H. F., Nielsen, T. C., Mohammad, S. S., Hofer, M. J., et al. (2021). Maternal acute and chronic inflammation in pregnancy is associated with common neurodevelopmental disorders: A systematic review. *Translational Psychiatry, 11*(1). https://doi.org/10.1038/s41398-021-01198-w

Harold, G. T., Leve, L. D., Barrett, D., Elam, K., Neiderhiser, J. M., Natsuaki, M. N., et al. (2013). Biological and rearing mother influences on child ADHD symptoms: Revisiting the developmental interface between nature and nurture. *Journal of Child Psychology and Psychiatry, 54*(10), 1038–1046. https://doi.org/10.1111/jcpp.12100

Harstad, E., Shults, J., Barbaresi, W., Bax, A., Cacia, J., Deavenport-Saman, A., et al. (2021). alpha(2)-Adrenergic agonists or stimulants for preschool-age children with Attention-Deficit/Hyperactivity Disorder. *Jama-Journal of the American Medical Association, 325*(20), 2067–2075. https://doi.org/10.1001/jama.2021.6118

Hill, A. B. (1965). The environment and disease: Association or causation? *Journal of the Royal Society of Medicine, 58*, 295–300. https://doi.org/10.1177/003591576505800503

Hinshaw, S. P., Arnold, L. E., & MTA Cooperative Group. (2015). Attention-deficit hyperactivity disorder, multimodal treatment, and longitudinal outcome: Evidence, paradox, and challenge. *Wiley Interdisciplinary Reviews-Cognitive Science, 6*(1), 39–52. https://doi.org/10.1002/wcs.1324

Hinshaw, S. P., Nguyen, P. T., O'Grady, S. M., & Rosenthal, E. A. (2022). Annual Research Review: Attention-deficit/hyperactivity disorder in girls and women: Underrepresentation, longitudinal processes, and key directions. *Journal of Child Psychology and Psychiatry, 63*(4), 484–496. https://doi.org/10.1111/jcpp.13480

Hollis, C., Chen, Q., Chang, Z., Quinn, P. D., Viktorin, A., Lichtenstein, P., et al. (2019). Methylphenidate and the risk of psychosis in adolescents and young adults: A population-based cohort study. *Lancet Psychiatry, 6*(8), 651–658. https://doi.org/10.1016/s2215-0366(19)30189-0

Holmes, J., Mareva, S., Bennett, M. P., Black, M. J., & Guy, J. (2021). Higher-Order dimensions of psychopathology in a neurodevelopmental transdiagnostic sample. *Journal of Abnormal Psychology, 130*(8), 909–922. https://doi.org/10.1037/abn0000710

Holton, K. F., & Nigg, J. T. (2020). The association of lifestyle factors and ADHD in children. *Journal of Attention Disorders, 24*(11), 1511–1520. https://doi.org/10.1177/1087054716646452

Howard, A. L., Robinson, M., Smith, G. J., Ambrosini, G. L., Piek, J. P., & Oddy, W. H. (2011). ADHD Is associated with a "Western" dietary pattern in adolescents. *Journal of Attention Disorders, 15*(5), 403–411. https://doi.org/10.1177/1087054710365990

Huberts-Bosch, A., Bierens, M., Ly, V., van der Velde, J., de Boer, H., van Beek, G., et al. (2023). Short-term effects of an elimination diet and healthy diet in children with attention-deficit/hyperactivity disorder: A randomized-controlled trial. *European Child and Adolescent Psychiatry.* https://doi.org/10.1007/s00787-023-02256-y

Hughes, C., Dunn, J., & White, A. (1998). Trick or treat?: Uneven understanding of mind and emotion and executive dysfunction in "hard-to-manage" preschoolers. *Journal of Child Psychology and Psychiatry, 39*(7), 981–994. https://doi.org/10.1111/1469-7610.00401

Hughes, C., Ensor, R., Wilson, A., & Graham, A. (2010). Tracking executive function across the transition to school: A latent variable approach. *Developmental Neurosychology, 35*(1), 20–36. https://doi.org/10.1080/87565640903325691

Ibrahim, O., Sutherland, H. G., Haupt, L. M., & Griffiths, L. R. (2018). An emerging role for epigenetic factors in relation to executive function. *Briefings in Functional Genomics, 17*(3), 170–180. https://doi.org/10.1093/bfgp/elx032

Ibrahim-Verbaas, C. A., Bressler, J., Debette, S., Schuur, M., Smith, A. V., Bis, J. C., et al. (2016). GWAS for executive function and processing speed suggests involvement of the CADM2 gene. *Molecular Psychiatry, 21*(2), 189–197. https://doi.org/10.1038/mp.2015.37

Iv, N., Herbein, M., Heude, B., van der Waerden, J., Melchior, M., Feart, C., et al. (2022). Children's diet at 2 years and trajectories of hyperactivity-inattention symptoms and conduct problems between 3 and 8 years: The EDEN cohort. *Journal of Nutrition, 152*(2), 484–491. https://doi.org/10.1093/jn/nxab398

Jacobson, N. S., & Truax, P. (1991). Clinical-significance - A statistical approach to defining meaningful change in psychotherapy-research. *Journal of Consulting and Clinical Psychology, 59*(1), 12–19. https://doi.org/10.1037/0022-006x.59.1.12

Jendreizik, L. T., Hautmann, C., von Wirth, E., Dose, C., Thoene, A.-K., Treier, A.-K., et al. (2022). The importance of familial risk factors in children with ADHD: Direct and indirect effects of family adversity, parental psychopathology and parenting practices on externalizing symptoms. *Child and Adolescent Psychiatry and Mental Health, 16*(1). https://doi.org/10.1186/s13034-022-00529-z

Jensen, C. M., & Steinhausen, H. C. (2015). Comorbid mental disorders in children and adolescents with attention-deficit/hyperactivity disorder in a large nationwide study. *Adhd-Attention Deficit and Hyperactivity Disorders, 7*(1), 27–38. https://doi.org/10.1007/s12402-014-0142-1

Jensen, P. S., Arnold, L. E., Richters, J. E., Severe, J. B., Vereen, D., Vitiello, B., et al. (1999). A 14-month randomized clinical trial of treatment strategies for attention-deficit/hyperactivity disorder. *Archives of General Psychiatry, 56*(12), 1073–1086. https://doi.org/10.1001/archpsyc.56.12.1073

Johnson, K. A., Wiersema, J. R., & Kuntsi, J. (2009). What would Karl Popper say? Are current psychological theories of ADHD falsifiable? *Behavioral and Brain Functions, 5*. https://doi.org/10.1186/1744-9081-5-15

Johnstone, J. M., Hatsu, I., Tost, G., Srikanth, P., Eiterman, L. P., Bruton, A. M., et al. (2022). Micronutrients for attention-deficit/hyperactivity disorder in youths: A placebo-controlled randomized clinical trial. *Journal of the American Academy of Child and Adolescent Psychiatry, 61*(5), 647–661. https://doi.org/10.1016/j.jaac.2021.07.005

Joseph, H. M., Lorenzo, N. E., Fisher, N., Novick, D. R., Gibson, C., Rothenberger, S. D., et al. (2023). Research Review: A systematic review and meta-analysis of infant and toddler temperament as predictors of childhood attention-deficit/hyperactivity disorder. *Journal of Child Psychology and Psychiatry, 64*(5), 715–735. https://doi.org/10.1111/jcpp.13753

Karalunas, S. L., Geurts, H. M., Konrad, K., Bender, S., & Nigg, J. T. (2014). Annual Research Review: Reaction time variability in ADHD and autism spectrum disorders: measurement and mechanisms of a proposed trans-diagnostic phenotype. *Journal of Child Psychology and Psychiatry, 55*(6), 685–710. https://doi.org/10.1111/jcpp.12217

Karalunas, S. L., Antovich, D., Goh, P. K., Martel, M. M., Tipsord, J., Nousen, E. K., & Nigg, J. T. (2021). Longitudinal network model of the co-development of temperament, executive functioning, and psychopathology symptoms in youth with and without ADHD. *Developmental Psychopathology, 33*(5), 1803–1820. https://doi.org/10.1017/s0954579421000900

Karr, J. E., Areshenkoff, C. N., Rast, P., Hofer, S. M., Iverson, G. L., & Garcia-Barrera, M. A. (2018). The unity and diversity of executive functions: A systematic review and re-analysis of latent variable studies. *Psychological Bulletin, 144*(11), 1147–1185. https://doi.org/10.1037/bul0000160

Kase, B. E., Rommelse, N., Chen, Q., Li, L., Andersson, A., Du Rietz, E., et al. (2021). Longitudinal associations between symptoms of ADHD and BMI from late childhood to early adulthood. *Pediatrics, 147*(6). https://doi.org/10.1542/peds.2020-036657

Kazda, L., McGeechan, K., Bell, K., Thomas, R., & Barratt, A. (2022). Increased diagnosis of attention-deficit hyperactivity disorder despite stable hyperactive/inattentive behaviours:

Evidence from two birth cohorts of Australian children. *Journal of Child Psychology and Psychiatry, 64*(8), 1140–1148. https://doi.org/10.1111/jcpp.13700

Kazdin, A. E. (2001). Almost clinically significant (p < .10): Current measures may only approach clinical significance. *Clinical Psychology-Science and Practice, 8*(4), 455–462. https://doi.org/10.1093/clipsy/8.4.455

Kendall, P. C., Marrs-Garcia, A., Nath, S. R., & Sheldrick, R. C. (1999). Normative comparisons for the evaluation of clinical significance. *Journal of Consulting and Clinical Psychology, 67*(3), 285–299. https://doi.org/10.1037/0022-006x.67.3.285

Killeen, P. R. (2019). Models of attention-deficit hyperactivity disorder. *Behavioural Processes, 162*, 205–214. https://doi.org/10.1016/j.beproc.2019.01.001

Kofler, M. J., Rapport, M. D., Sarver, D. E., Raiker, J. S., Orban, S. A., Friedman, L. M., & Kolomeyer, E. G. (2013). Reaction time variability in ADHD: A meta-analytic review of 319 studies. *Clinical Psychology Review, 33*(6), 795–811. https://doi.org/10.1016/j.cpr.2013.06.001

Krause, B. J., Artigas, R., Sciolla, A. F., & Hamilton, J. (2020). Epigenetic mechanisms activated by childhood adversity. *Epigenomics, 12*(14), 18. https://doi.org/10.2217/epi-2020-0042

Kumsta, R., Marzi, S. J., Viana, J., Dempster, E. L., Crawford, B., Rutter, M., et al. (2016). Severe psychosocial deprivation in early childhood is associated with increased DNA methylation across a region spanning the transcription start site of CYP2E1. *Translational Psychiatry, 6*. https://doi.org/10.1038/tp.2016.95

Kuntsi, J., & Klein, C. (2012). Intraindividual variability in ADHD and its implications for research of causal links. *Current Topics in Behavioral Neurosciences, 9*, 67–91. https://doi.org/10.1007/7854_2011_145

Kuntsi, J., & Stevenson, J. (2001). Psychological mechanisms in hyperactivity: II The role of genetic factors. *Journal of Child Psychology and Psychiatry, 42*(2), 211–219. https://doi.org/10.1111/1469-7610.00712

Kuntsi, J., Oosterlaan, J., & Stevenson, J. (2001a). Psychological mechanisms in hyperactivity: I response inhibition deficit, working memory impairment, delay aversion, or something else? *Journal of Child Psychology and Psychiatry, 42*(2), 199–210. https://doi.org/10.1017/s0021963001006709

Kuntsi, J., Stevenson, J., Oosterlaan, J., & Sonuga-Barke, E. J. S. (2001b). Test-retest reliability of a new delay aversion task and executive function measures. *British Journal of Developmental Psychology, 19*, 339–348. https://doi.org/10.1348/026151001166137

Kuntsi, J., Eley, T. C., Taylor, A., Hughes, C., Asherson, P., Caspi, A., & Moffitt, T. E. (2004). Co-occurrence of ADHD and low IQ has genetic origins. *American Journal of Medical Genetics Part B-Neuropsychiatric Genetics, 124B*(1), 41–47. https://doi.org/10.1002/ajmg.b.20076

Kuntsi, J., Rijsdijk, F., Ronald, A., Asherson, P., & Plomin, R. (2005). Genetic influences on the stability of attention-deficit/hyperactivity disorder symptoms from early to middle childhood. *Developmental Psychology, 57*(6), 647–654. https://doi.org/10.1016/j.biopsych.2004.12.032

Kushki, A., Anagnostou, E., Hammill, C., Duez, P., Brian, J., Iaboni, A., et al. (2019). Examining overlap and homogeneity in ASD, ADHD, and OCD: A data-driven, diagnosis-agnostic approach. *Translational Psychiatry, 9*. https://doi.org/10.1038/s41398-019-0631-2

Lai, C. S. L., Fisher, S. E., Hurst, J. A., Vargha-Khadem, F., & Monaco, A. P. (2001). A forkhead-domain gene is mutated in a severe speech and language disorder. *Nature, 413*(6855), 519–523. https://doi.org/10.1038/35097076

Lanphear, B. P. (2015). The impact of toxins on the developing brain. In J. E. Fielding (Ed.), *Annual Review of Public Health, Vol 36* (Vol. 36, pp. 211–230). https://doi.org/10.1146/annurev-publhealth-031912-114413

Larsson, H., Sariaslan, A., Langstrom, N., D'Onofrio, B., & Lichtenstein, P. (2014). Family income in early childhood and subsequent attention deficit/hyperactivity disorder: A quasi-experimental study. *Journal of Child Psychology and Psychiatry, 55*(5), 428–435. https://doi.org/10.1111/jcpp.12140

Lavigne, J. V., Gibbons, R. D., Christoffel, K. K., Arend, R., Rosenbaum, D., Binns, H., et al. (1996). Prevalence rates and correlates of psychiatric disorders among preschool children. *Journal of the American Academy of Child and Adolescent Psychiatry, 35*(2), 204–214. https://doi.org/10.1097/00004583-199602000-00014

Leboyer, M., Bellivier, F., Nosten-Bertrand, M., Jouvent, R., Pauls, D., & Mallet, J. (1998). Psychiatric genetics: Search for phenotypes. *Trends in Neurosciences, 21*(3), 102–105. https://doi.org/10.1016/s0166-2236(97)01187-9

Leve, L. D., Anderson, D., Harold, G. T., Neiderhiser, J. M., Natsuaki, M. N., Shaw, D. S., et al. (2022). Developmental profiles of child behavior problems from 18 months to 8 years: The protective effects of structured parenting vary by genetic risk. *Development and Psychopathology, 34*(5), 1716–1730. https://doi.org/10.1017/s0954579422000839

Levy, F., Hay, D. A., McStephen, M., Wood, C., & Waldman, I. (1997). Attention-deficit hyperactivity disorder: A category or a continuum? Genetic analysis of a large-scale twin study. *Journal of the American Academy of Child and Adolescent Psychiatry, 36*(6), 737–744. https://doi.org/10.1097/00004583-199706000-00009

Li, J. J., & He, Q. F. (2021). Polygenic scores for ADHD: A meta-Analysis. *Research on Child and Adolescent Psychopathology, 49*(3), 297–310. https://doi.org/10.1007/s10802-021-00774-4

Li, M. Y., Francis, E., Hinkle, S. N., Ajjarapu, A. S., & Zhang, C. L. (2019). Preconception and prenatal nutrition and neurodevelopmental disorders: A systematic review and meta-analysis. *Nutrients, 11*(7). https://doi.org/10.3390/nu11071628

Liu, R., DeSerisy, M., Fox, N. A., Herbstman, J. B., Rauh, V. A., Beebe, B., & Margolis, A. E. (2022). Prenatal exposure to air pollution and maternal stress predict infant individual differences in reactivity and regulation and socioemotional development. *Journal of Child Psychology and Psychiatry, 63*(11), 1359–1367. https://doi.org/10.1111/jcpp.13581

Loe, I. M., Kakar, P. A., & Sanders, L. M. (2021). Diagnosis, evaluation, and treatment of Attention-Deficit/Hyperactivity Disorder. *JAMA Pediatrics, 175*(2), 191–192. https://doi.org/10.1001/jamapediatrics.2020.2218

Marco, R., Miranda, A., Schlotz, W., Melia, A., Mulligan, A., Mueller, U., et al. (2009). Delay and reward choice in ADHD: An experimental test of the role of delay aversion. *Neuropsychology, 23*(3), 367–380. https://doi.org/10.1037/a0014914

Martel, M. M., Elkins, A. R., Eng, A. G., Goh, P. K., Bansal, P. S., Smith-Thomas, T. E., et al. (2022). Longitudinal temperament pathways to ADHD between childhood and adolescence. *Research on Child and Adolescent Psychopathology, 50*, 1055–1066. https://doi.org/10.1007/s10802-022-00902-8

Martin, J., Wray, M., Agha, S. S., Lewis, K. J. S., Anney, R. J. L., O'Donovan, M. C., et al. (2023). Investigating direct and indirect genetic effects in Attention Deficit/Hyperactivity Disorder using parent-offspring trios. *Biol Psychiatry, 93*(1), 37–44. https://doi.org/10.1016/j.biopsych.2022.06.008

Marx, I., Cortese, S., Koelch, M. G., & Hacker, T. (2022). Meta-analysis: Altered perceptual timing abilities in Attention-Deficit/Hyperactivity Disorder. *Journal of the American Academy of Child and Adolescent Psychiatry, 61*(7), 866–880. https://doi.org/10.1016/j.jaac.2021.12.004

Matthies, S., Holzner, S., Feige, B., Scheel, C., Perlov, E., Ebert, D., et al. (2013). ADHD as a serious risk factor for early smoking and nicotine dependence in adulthood. *Journal of Attention Disorders, 17*(3), 176–186. https://doi.org/10.1177/1087054711428739

Matthijssen, A. F. M., Dietrich, A., Bierens, M., Deters, R. K., van de Loo-Neus, G. H. H., van den Hoofdakker, B. J., et al. (2019). Continued benefits of methylphenidate in ADHD after 2 years in clinical practice: A randomized placebo-controlled discontinuation study. *American Journal of Psychiatry, 176*(9), 754–762. https://doi.org/10.1176/appi.ajp.2019.18111296

Mayes, S. D., Calhoun, S. L., & Waschbusch, D. A. (2020). Sluggish cognitive tempo in autism, ADHD, and neurotypical child samples. *Research in Autism Spectrum Disorders, 79*. https://doi.org/10.1016/j.rasd.2020.101678

McClernon, F. J., & Kollins, S. H. (2008). ADHD and smoking from genes to brain to behavior. *Addiction Reviews, 2008(1141)*, 131–147. https://doi.org/10.1196/annals.1441.016

McCormick, E. M., Muraresku, C. C., & Falk, M. J. (2018). Mitochondrial genomics: A complex field now coming of age. *Current Genetic Medicine Reports, 6*(2), 52–61. https://doi.org/10.1007/s40142-018-0137-x

McKenzie, A., Meshkat, S., Lui, L. M. W., Ho, R., Vincenzo, J. D. D., Ceban, F., et al. (2022). The effects of psychostimulants on cognitive functions in individuals with attention-deficit hyperactivity disorder: A systematic review. *Journal of Psychiatry Research, 149*, 252–259. https://doi.org/10.1016/j.jpsychires.2022.03.018

Michaëlsson, M., Yuan, S., Melhus, H., Baron, J. A., Byberg, L., Larsson, S. C., & Michaelsson, K. (2022). The impact and causal directions for the associations between diagnosis of ADHD, socioeconomic status, and intelligence by use of a bi-directional two-sample Mendelian randomization design. *BMC Medicine, 20*(1). https://doi.org/10.1186/s12916-022-02314-3

Michelini, G., Kitsune, G. L., Cheung, C. H. M., Brandeis, D., Banaschewski, T., Asherson, P., et al. (2016). Attention-Deficit/Hyperactivity Disorder remission Is linked to better neurophysiological error detection and attention-vigilance processes. *Biological Psychiatry, 80*(12), 923–932. https://doi.org/10.1016/j.biopsych.2016.06.021

Michelini, G., Salmastyan, G., Vera, J. D., & Lenartowicz, A. (2022). Event-related brain oscillations in attention-deficit/hyperactivity disorder (ADHD): A systematic review and meta-analysis. *International Journal of Psychophysiology, 174*, 29–42. https://doi.org/10.1016/j.ijpsycho.2022.01.014

Middeldorp, C. M., Hammerschlag, A. R., Ouwens, K. G., Groen-Blokhuis, M. M., St Pourcain, B., Greven, C. U., et al. (2016). A genome-wide association meta-analysis of Attention-Deficit/Hyperactivity Disorder symptoms in population-based pediatric cohorts. *Journal of the American Academy of Child and Adolescent Psychiatry, 55*(10), 896–905. https://doi.org/10.1016/j.jaac.2016.05.025

Miyake, A., Friedman, N. P., Emerson, M. J., Witzki, A. H., Howerter, A., & Wager, T. D. (2000). The unity and diversity of executive functions and their contributions to complex "frontal lobe" tasks: A latent variable analysis. *Cognitive Psychology, 41*(1), 49–100. https://doi.org/10.1006/cogp.1999.0734

Modesto-Lowe, V., Danforth, J. S., & Brooks, D. (2008). ADHD: Does parenting style matter? *Clinical Pediatrics, 47*(9), 865–872. https://doi.org/10.1177/0009922808319963

Moffitt, T. E., Arseneault, L., Belsky, D., Dickson, N., Hancox, R. J., Harrington, H., et al. (2011). A gradient of childhood self-control predicts health, wealth, and public safety. *Proceedings of the National Academy of Sciences of the United States of America, 108*(7), 2693–2698. https://doi.org/10.1073/pnas.1010076108

Moffitt, T. E., Houts, R., Asherson, P., Belsky, D. W., Corcoran, D. L., Hammerle, M., et al. (2015). Is adult ADHD a childhood-onset neurodevelopmental disorder? Evidence from a four-decade longitudinal cohort study. *American Journal of Psychiatry, 172*(10), 967–977. https://doi.org/10.1176/appi.ajp.2015.14101266

Molina, B. S. G., Hinshaw, S. P., Swanson, J. M., Arnold, L. E., Vitiello, B., Jensen, P. S., et al. (2009). The MTA at 8 Years: Prospective follow-up of children treated for combined-type ADHD in a multisite study. *Journal of the American Academy of Child and Adolescent Psychiatry, 48*(5), 484–500. https://doi.org/10.1097/CHI.0b013e31819c23d0

Mooney, M. A., Ryabinin, P., Wilmot, B., Bhatt, P., Mill, J., & Nigg, J. T. (2020). Large epigenome-wide association study of childhood ADHD identifies peripheral DNA methylation associated with disease and polygenic risk burden. *Translational Psychiatry, 10*(1). https://doi.org/10.1038/s41398-020-0710-4

Mooney, M. A., Ryabinin, P., Morton, H., Selah, K., Gonoud, R., Kozlowski, M., et al. (2023). Joint polygenic and environmental risks for childhood attention-deficit/hyperactivity disorder (ADHD) and ADHD symptom dimensions. *JCPP Advances, 3*(2), e12152. https://doi.org/10.1002/jcv2.12152

Moore, E., Migliorini, R., Infante, M., & Riley, E. (2014). Fetal alcohol spectrum disorders: Recent neuroimaging findings. *Current Developmental Disorders Reports, 1*, 161–172. https://doi.org/10.1007/s40474-014-0020-8

Morrison, J., Knoblauch, N., Marcus, J. H., Stephens, M., & He, X. (2020). Mendelian randomization accounting for correlated and uncorrelated pleiotropic effects using genome-wide summary statistics. *Nature Genetics, 52*(7), 740-+. https://doi.org/10.1038/s41588-020-0631-4

Morris-Rosendahl, D. J., & Crocq, M. A. (2020). Neurodevelopmental disorders-the history and future of a diagnostic concept. *Dialogues in Clinical Neuroscience, 22*(1), 65–72. https://doi.org/10.31887/DCNS.2020.22.1/macrocq

Morton, J., & Frith, U. (2001). Why we need cognition: Cause and developmental disorder. In E. Dupoux (Ed.), *Language, brain, and cognitive development, Festschrift for Jacques Mehler* (pp. 263–278). MIT Press.

Moses, M., Tiego, J., Demontis, D., Walters, G. B., Stefansson, H., Stefansson, K., et al. (2022). Working memory and reaction time variability mediate the relationship between polygenic risk and ADHD traits in a general population sample. *Molecular Psychiatry, 27*(12), 5028–5037. https://doi.org/10.1038/s41380-022-01775-5

Mulligan, A., Anney, R., Butler, L., O'Regan, M., Richardson, T., Tulewicz, E. M., et al. (2013). Home environment: Association with hyperactivity/impulsivity in children with ADHD and their non-ADHD siblings. *Child Care Health and Development, 39*(2), 202–212. https://doi.org/10.1111/j.1365-2214.2011.01345.x

Mulraney, M., Arrondo, G., Musullulu, H., Iturmendi-Sabater, I., Cortese, S., Westwood, S. J., et al. (2022). Systematic review and meta-analysis: Screening tools for Attention-Deficit/Hyperactivity Disorder in children and adolescents. *Journal of the American Academy of Child and Adolescent Psychiatry, 61*(8), 982–996. https://doi.org/10.1016/j.jaac.2021.11.031

Myhre, O., Lag, M., Villanger, G. D., Oftedal, B., Ovrevik, J., Holme, J. A., et al. (2018). Early life exposure to air pollution particulate matter (PM) as risk factor for attention deficit/hyperactivity disorder (ADHD): Need for novel strategies Check for updates for mechanisms and causalities. *Toxicology and Applied Pharmacology, 354*, 196–214. https://doi.org/10.1016/j.taap.2018.03.015

Neumann, A., Walton, E., Alemany, S., Cecil, C., Gonzalez, J. R., Jima, D. D., et al. (2020). Association between DNA methylation and ADHD symptoms from birth to school age: A prospective meta-analysis. *Translational Psychiatry, 10*(1). https://doi.org/10.1038/s41398-020-01058-z

NICE. (2018, March). *Attention deficit hyperactivity disorder: Diagnosis and management.* Retrieved from https://www.nice.org.uk/guidance/ng87

Nidey, N. L., Momany, A. M., Strathearn, L., Carter, K. D., Wehby, G. L., Bao, W., et al. (2021). Association between perinatal depression and risk of attention deficit hyperactivity disorder among children: A retrospective cohort study. *Annals of Epidemiology, 63*, 1–6. https://doi.org/10.1016/j.annepidem.2021.06.005

Nielsen, T. C., Nassar, N., Shand, A. W., Jones, H., Guastella, A. J., Dale, R. C., & Lain, S. J. (2021). Association of maternal autoimmune disease with Attention-Deficit/Hyperactivity Disorder in children. *JAMA Pediatrics, 175*(3). https://doi.org/10.1001/jamapediatrics.2020.5487

Nigg, J. T. (2013). Attention-deficit/hyperactivity disorder and adverse health outcomes. *Clinical Psychology Review, 33*(2), 215–228. https://doi.org/10.1016/j.cpr.2012.11.005

Nigg, J. T. (2017). Annual Research Review: On the relations among self-regulation, self-control, executive functioning, effortful control, cognitive control, impulsivity, risk-taking, and inhibition for developmental psychopathology. *Journal of Child Psychology and Psychiatry, 58*(4), 361–383. https://doi.org/10.1111/jcpp.12675

Nigg, J. T. (2018). Toward an emerging paradigm for understanding Attention-Deficit/Hyperactivity Disorder and other neurodevelopmental, mental, and behavioral disorders environmental risks and epigenetic associations. *JAMA Pediatrics, 172*(7), 619–621. https://doi.org/10.1001/jamapediatrics.2018.0920

Nigg, J., Nikolas, M., & Burt, S. A. (2010). Measured gene-by-environment interaction in relation to Attention-Deficit/Hyperactivity Disorder. *Journal of the American Academy of Child and Adolescent Psychiatry, 49*(9), 863–873. https://doi.org/10.1016/j.jaac.2010.01.025

Nigg, J. T., Elmore, A. L., Natarajan, N., Friderici, K. H., & Nikolas, M. A. (2016). Variation in an iron metabolism gene moderates the association between blood lead levels and Attention-Deficit/Hyperactivity Disorder in children. *Psychological Science, 27*(2), 257–269. https://doi.org/10.1177/0956797615618365

Nigg, J. T., Gustafsson, H. C., Karalunas, S. L., Ryabinin, P., McWeeney, S. K., Faraone, S. V., et al. (2018). Working memory and vigilance as multivariate endophenotypes related to common genetic risk for Attention-Deficit/Hyperactivity Disorder. *Journal of the American Academy of Child and Adolescent Psychiatry, 57*(3), 175–182. https://doi.org/10.1016/j.jaac.2017.12.013

Nigg, J. T., Karalunas, S. L., Feczko, E., & Fair, D. A. (2020a). Toward a revised nosology for Attention-Deficit/Hyperactivity Disorder heterogeneity. *Biological Psychiatry-Cognitive Neuroscience and Neuroimaging, 5*(8), 726–737. https://doi.org/10.1016/j.bpsc.2020.02.005

Nigg, J. T., Sibley, M. H., Thapar, A., & Karalunas, S. L. (2020b). Development of ADHD: Etiology, heterogeneity, and early life course. *Annual Review of Developmental Psychology, 2*(1), 559–583. https://doi.org/10.1146/annurev-devpsych-060320-093413

Noordermeer, S. D. S., Luman, M., Buitelaar, J. K., Hartman, C. A., Hoekstra, P. J., Franke, B., et al. (2020). Neurocognitive deficits in Attention-Deficit/Hyperactivity Disorder with and without comorbid Oppositional Defiant Disorder. *Journal of Attention Disorders, 24*(9), 1317–1329. https://doi.org/10.1177/1087054715606216

Norman, G. R., Sloan, J. A., & Wyrwich, K. W. (2003). Interpretation of changes in health-related quality of life - The remarkable universality of half a standard deviation. *Medical Care, 41*(5), 582–592. https://doi.org/10.1097/00005650-200305000-00004

Norman, L. J., Sudre, G., Bouyssi-Kobar, M., Sharp, W., & Shaw, P. (2021). An examination of the relationships between attention/deficit hyperactivity disorder symptoms and functional connectivity over time. *Neuropsychopharmacology: Official publication of the American College of Neuropsychopharmacology, 47*, 704–710. https://doi.org/10.1038/s41386-021-00958-y

Norman, L. J., Sudre, G., Price, J., Shastri, G. G., & Shaw, P. (2023). Evidence from "big data" for the default-mode hypothesis of ADHD: A mega-analysis of multiple large samples. *Neuropsychopharmacology, 48*(2), 281–289. https://doi.org/10.1038/s41386-022-01408-z

Nourredine, M., Gering, A., Fourneret, P., Rolland, B., Falissard, B., Cucherat, M., et al. (2021). Association of Attention-Deficit/Hyperactivity Disorder in childhood and adolescence with the risk of subsequent psychotic disorder A systematic review and meta-analysis. *Jama Psychiatry, 78*(5), 519–529. https://doi.org/10.1001/jamapsychiatry.2020.4799

O'Neill, J., Levitt, J. G., & Alger, J. R. (2013). Magnetic resonance spectroscopy studies of attention deficit hyperactivity disorder. In S. Blüml & A. Panigrahy (Eds.), *MR spectroscopy of pediatric brain disorders* (pp. 229–276). Springer.

O'Connor, L. J., & Price, A. L. (2018). Distinguishing genetic correlation from causation across 52 diseases and complex traits. *Nature Genetics, 50*(12), 1728. https://doi.org/10.1038/s41588-018-0255-0

O'Connor, T. G., Heron, J., Golding, J., Beveridge, M., & Glover, V. (2002). Maternal antenatal anxiety and children's behavioural/emotional problems at 4 years - Report from the Avon Longitudinal Study of Parents and Children. *British Journal of Psychiatry, 180*, 502–508. https://doi.org/10.1192/bjp.180.6.502

Oosterlaan, J., Logan, G. D., & Sergeant, J. A. (1998). Response inhibition in AD/HD, CD, comorbid AD/HD+CD, anxious, and control children: A meta-analysis of studies with the stop task. *Journal of Child Psychology and Psychiatry, 39*(3), 411–425. https://doi.org/10.1111/1469-7610.00336

Østergaard, S. D., Trabjerg, B. B., Als, T. D., Climent, C. A., Prive, F., Vilhjalmsson, B. J., et al. (2020). Polygenic risk score, psychosocial environment and the risk of attention-deficit/hyperactivity disorder. *Translational Psychiatry, 10*(1). https://doi.org/10.1038/s41398-020-01019-6

Otten, K., Keller, L., Puiu, A. A., Herpertz-Dahlmann, B., Seitz, J., Kohn, N., et al. (2022). Pre- and postnatal antibiotic exposure and risk of developing attention deficit hyperactivity disorder-A systematic review and meta-analysis combining evidence from human and animal studies. *Neuroscience and Biobehavioral Reviews, 140*, 104776. https://doi.org/10.1016/j.neubiorev.2022.104776

Overgaard, K. R., Aase, H., Torgersen, S., & Zeiner, P. (2016). Co-Occurrence of ADHD and anxiety in preschool Children. *Journal of Attention Disorders, 20*(7), 573–580. https://doi.org/10.1177/1087054712463063

Partty, A., Kalliomaki, M., Wacklin, P., Salminen, S., & Isolauri, E. (2015). A possible link between early probiotic intervention and the risk of neuropsychiatric disorders later in childhood: A randomized trial. *Pediatric Research, 77*(6), 823–828. https://doi.org/10.1038/pr.2015.51

Patros, C. H. G., Alderson, R. M., Kasper, L. J., Tarle, S. J., Lea, S. E., & Hudec, K. L. (2016). Choice-impulsivity in children and adolescents with attention-deficit/hyperactivity disorder (ADHD): A meta-analytic review. *Clinical Psychology Review, 43*, 162–174. https://doi.org/10.1016/j.cpr.2015.11.001

Pauli-Pott, U., & Becker, K. (2011). Neuropsychological basic deficits in preschoolers at risk for ADHD: A meta-analysis. *Clinical Psychology Review, 31*(4), 626–637. https://doi.org/10.1016/j.cpr.2011.02.005

Pennington, B. F., & Ozonoff, S. (1996). Executive functions and developmental psychopathology. *Journal of Child Psychology and Psychiatry, 37*(1), 51–87. https://doi.org/10.1111/j.1469-7610.1996.tb01380.x

Pereira-Sanchez, V., & Castellanos, F. X. (2021). Neuroimaging in attention-deficit/hyperactivity disorder. *Current Opinion in Psychiatry, 34*(2), 105–111. https://doi.org/10.1097/yco.0000000000000669

Perlov, E., Philipsen, A., Matthies, S., Drieling, T., Maier, S., Bubl, E., et al. (2009). Spectroscopic findings in attention-deficit/hyperactivity disorder: Review and meta-analysis. *World Journal of Biological Psychiatry, 10*(4), 355–365. https://doi.org/10.1080/15622970802176032

Peterson, B. S., Bansal, R., Sawardekar, S., Nati, C., Elgabalawy, E. R., Hoepner, L. A., et al. (2022). Prenatal exposure to air pollution is associated with altered brain structure, function, and metabolism in childhood. *Journal of Child Psychology and Psychiatry, 63*(11), 1316–1331. https://doi.org/10.1111/jcpp.13578

Pike, A., Iervolino, A. C., Eley, T. C., Price, T. S., & Plomin, R. (2006). Environmental risk and young children's cognitive and behavioral development. *International Journal of Behavioral Development, 30*(1), 55–66. https://doi.org/10.1177/0165025406062124

Pinto, R., Asherson, P., Ilott, N., Cheung, C. H. M., & Kuntsi, J. (2016). Testing for the mediating role of endophenotypes using molecular genetic data in a twin study of ADHD traits. *American Journal of Medical Genetics Part B-Neuropsychiatric Genetics, 171*(7), 982–992. https://doi.org/10.1002/ajmg.b.32463

Polanczyk, G., de Lima, M. S., Horta, B. L., Biederman, J., & Rohde, L. A. (2007). The worldwide prevalence of ADHD: A systematic review and metaregression analysis. *American Journal of Psychiatry, 164*(6), 942–948. https://doi.org/10.1176/appi.ajp.164.6.942

Polanczyk, G. V., Salum, G. A., Sugaya, L. S., Caye, A., & Rohde, L. A. (2015). Annual Research Review: A meta-analysis of the worldwide prevalence of mental disorders in children and adolescents. *Journal of Child Psychology and Psychiatry, 56*(3), 345–365. https://doi.org/10.1111/jcpp.12381

Posner, J., Polanczyk, G. V., & Sonuga-Barke, E. (2020). Attention-deficit hyperactivity disorder. *Lancet, 395*(10222), 450–462. https://doi.org/10.1016/s0140-6736(19)33004-1

Postema, M. C., Hoogman, M., Ambrosino, S., Asherson, P., Banaschewski, T., Bandeira, C. E., et al. (2021). Analysis of structural brain asymmetries in attention-deficit/hyperactivity disorder in 39 datasets. *Journal of Child Psychology and Psychiatry*. https://doi.org/10.1111/jcpp.13396

Price, T. S., Simonoff, E., & Waldman, I. (2001). Hyperactivity in preschool children is highly heritable. *Journal of the American Academy of Child and Adolescent Psychiatry, 40*(12), 1362–1364. https://doi.org/10.1097/00004583-200112000-00002

Ribasés, M., Mitjans, M., Hartman, C. A., Soler Artigas, M., Demontis, D., Larsson, H., et al. (2023). Genetic architecture of ADHD and overlap with other psychiatric disorders and cognition-related phenotypes. *Neuroscience & Biobehavioral Reviews*, 105313. https://doi.org/10.1016/j.neubiorev.2023.105313

Riddle, M. A., Yershova, K., Lazzaretto, D., Paykina, N., Yenokyan, G., Greenhill, L., et al. (2013). The Preschool Attention-Deficit/Hyperactivity Disorder Treatment Study (PATS) 6-year follow-up. *Journal of the American Academy of Child and Adolescent Psychiatry, 52*(3), 264–278. https://doi.org/10.1016/j.jaac.2012.12.007

Rivollier, F., Krebs, M. O., & Kebir, O. (2019). Perinatal exposure to environmental endocrine disruptors in the emergence of neurodevelopmental psychiatric diseases: A systematic review. *International Journal of Environmental Research and Public Health, 16*(8). https://doi.org/10.3390/ijerph16081318

Ronald, A., de Bode, N., & Polderman, T. J. C. (2021). Systematic review: How the Attention-Deficit/ Hyperactivity Disorder polygenic risk score adds to our understanding of ADHD and associated traits. *Journal of the American Academy of Child and Adolescent Psychiatry, 60*(10), 1234–1277. https://doi.org/10.1016/j.jaac.2021.01.019

Rosenau, P. T., Openneer, T. J. C., Matthijssen, A. F. M., Van de Loo-Neus, G. H. H., Buitelaar, J. K., van den Hoofdakker, B. J., et al. (2021). Effects of methylphenidate on executive functioning in children and adolescents with ADHD after long-term use: A randomized, placebo-controlled discontinuation study. *Journal of Child Psychology and Psychiatry, 62*(12), 1444–1452. https://doi.org/10.1111/jcpp.13419

Rubia, K. (2011). "Cool" inferior frontostriatal dysfunction in Attention-Deficit/Hyperactivity Disorder versus "Hot" ventromedial orbitofrontal-limbic dysfunction in conduct disorder: A review. *Developmental Psychology, 69*(12), E69–E87. https://doi.org/10.1016/j.biopsych.2010.09.023

Rucklidge, J. J., Eggleston, M. J. F., Johnstone, J. M., Darling, K., & Frampton, C. M. (2018). Vitamin-mineral treatment improves aggression and emotional regulation in children with ADHD: A fully blinded, randomized, placebo-controlled trial. *Journal of Child Psychology and Psychiatry, 59*(3), 232–246. https://doi.org/10.1111/jcpp.12817

Russell, A. E., Ford, T., Williams, R., & Russell, G. (2016). The association between socioeconomic disadvantage and Attention Deficit/Hyperactivity Disorder (ADHD): A systematic review. *Child Psychiatry & Human Development, 47*(3), 440–458. https://doi.org/10.1007/s10578-015-0578-3

Rydell, M., Lundstrom, S., Gillberg, C., Lichtenstein, P., & Larsson, H. (2018). Has the attention deficit hyperactivity disorder phenotype become more common in children between 2004 and 2014? Trends over 10 years from a Swedish general population sample. *Journal of Child Psychology and Psychiatry, 59*(8), 863–871. https://doi.org/10.1111/jcpp.12882

Samea, F., Soluki, S., Nejati, V., Zarei, M., Cortese, S., Eickhoff, S. B., et al. (2019). Brain alterations in children/adolescents with ADHD revisited: A neuroimaging meta-analysis of 96 structural and functional studies. *Neuroscience and Biobehavioral Reviews, 100*, 1–8. https://doi.org/10.1016/j.neubiorev.2019.02.011

Sandgren, A. M., & Brummer, R. J. M. (2018). ADHD-originating in the gut? The emergence of a new explanatory model. *Medical Hypotheses, 120*, 135–145. https://doi.org/10.1016/j.mehy.2018.08.022

Santosh, P. J., Taylor, E., Swanson, J., Wigal, T., Chuang, S., Davies, M., et al. (2005). Refining the diagnoses of inattention and overactivity syndromes: A reanalysis of the Multimodal Treatment study of attention deficit hyperactivity disorder (ADHD) based on ICD-10 criteria for hyperkinetic disorder. *Clinical Neuroscience Research, 5*(5-6), 307–314. https://doi.org/10.1016/j.cnr.2005.09.010

Saylor, K. E., & Amann, B. H. (2016). Impulsive aggression as a comorbidity of Attention-Deficit/Hyperactivity Disorder in children and adolescents. *Journal of Child and Adolescent Psychopharmacology, 26*(1), 19–25. https://doi.org/10.1089/cap.2015.0126

Schork, A. J., Brown, T. T., Hagler, D. J., Thompson, W. K., Chen, C. H., Dale, A. M., et al. (2019). Polygenic risk for psychiatric disorders correlates with executive function in typical development. *Genes Brain and Behavior, 18*(4). https://doi.org/10.1111/gbb.12480

Sergeant, J. A., Geurts, H., & Oosterlaan, J. (2002). How specific is a deficit of executive functioning for Attention-Deficit/Hyperactivity Disorder? *Behavioural Brain Research, 130*(1-2), 3–28. https://doi.org/10.1016/s0166-4328(01)00430-2

Shaffer, D., Gould, M. S., Brasic, J., Ambrosini, P., Fisher, P., Bird, H., & Aluwahlia, S. (1983). A Childrens Global Assessment Scale. *Archives of General Psychiatry, 40*(11), 1228–1231. https://doi.org/10.1001/archpsyc.1983.01790100074010

Shaw, P., Stringaris, A., Nigg, J., & Leibenluft, E. (2014). Emotion dysregulation in Attention Deficit Hyperactivity Disorder. *American Journal of Psychiatry, 171*(3), 276–293. https://doi.org/10.1176/appi.ajp.2013.13070966

Sibley, M. H., Bruton, A. M., Zhao, X., Johnstone, J. M., Mitchell, J., Hatsu, I., et al. (2023). Non-pharmacological interventions for attention-deficit hyperactivity disorder in children and adolescents. *The Lancet Child & Adolescent Health.* https://doi.org/10.1016/S2352-4642(22)00381-9

Siu, M. T., Goodman, S. J., Yellan, I., Butcher, D. T., Jangjoo, M., Grafodatskaya, D., et al. (2021). DNA methylation of the oxytocin receptor across neurodevelopmental disorders. *Journal Autism and Developmental Disorders, 51*, 3610–3623. https://doi.org/10.1007/s10803-020-04792-x

Sjowall, D., Roth, L., Lindqvist, S., & Thorell, L. B. (2013). Multiple deficits in ADHD: Executive dysfunction, delay aversion, reaction time variability, and emotional deficits. *Journal of Child Psychology and Psychiatry, 54*(6), 619–627. https://doi.org/10.1111/jcpp.12006

Skogheim, T. S., Weyde, K. V. F., Engel, S. M., Aase, H., Suren, P., Oie, M. G., et al. (2021). Metal and essential element concentrations during pregnancy and associations with autism spectrum disorder and attention-deficit/hyperactivity disorder in children. *Environment international, 152*, 106468–106468. https://doi.org/10.1016/j.envint.2021.106468

Smith, E., Meyer, B. J., Koerting, J., Laver-Bradbury, C., Lee, L., Jefferson, H., et al. (2017). Preschool hyperactivity specifically elevates long-term mental health risks more strongly in males than females: A prospective longitudinal study through to young adulthood. *European Child and Adolescent Psychiatry, 26*(1), 123–136. https://doi.org/10.1007/s00787-016-0876-8

Solanto, M. V., Abikoff, H., Sonuga-Barke, E. J. S., Schachar, R., Logan, G. D., Wigal, T., et al. (2001). The ecological validity of delay aversion and response inhibition as measures of impulsivity in AD/HD: A supplement to the NIMH multimodal treatment study of AD/HD. *Journal of Abnormal Child Psychology, 29*(3), 215–228. https://doi.org/10.1023/a:1010329714819

Solberg, B. S., Hegvik, T. A., Halmoy, A., Skjaerven, R., Engeland, A., Haavik, J., & Klungsoyr, K. (2021). Sex differences in parent-offspring recurrence of attention-deficit/hyperactivity disorder. *Journal of Child Psychology and Psychiatry, 62*(8), 1010–1018. https://doi.org/10.1111/jcpp.13368

Song, P. G., Zha, M. M., Yang, Q. W., Zhang, Y., Li, X., Rudan, I., & Global Health Epidemiology, R. (2021). The prevalence of adult attention-deficit hyperactivity disorder: A global systematic review and meta-analysis. *Journal of Global Health, 11*, 04009. https://doi.org/10.7189/jogh.11.04009

Sonuga-Barke, E. J. S., Dalen, L., & Remington, B. (2003). Do executive deficits and delay aversion make independent contributions to preschool attention-deficit/hyperactivity disorder symptoms? *Journal of the American Academy of Child and Adolescent Psychiatry, 42*(11), 1335–1342. https://doi.org/10.1097/01.chi.0000087564.34977.21

Sonuga-Barke, E. J. S., Auerbach, J., Campbell, S. B., Daley, D., & Thompson, M. (2005). Varieties of preschool hyperactivity: Multiple pathways from risk to disorder. *Developmental Science, 8*(2), 141–150. https://doi.org/10.1111/j.1467-7687.2005.00401.x

Sonuga-Barke, E. J. S., Brandeis, D., Cortese, S., Daley, D., Ferrin, M., Holtmann, M., et al. (2013). Nonpharmacological interventions for ADHD: Systematic review and meta-analyses of randomized controlled trials of dietary and psychological treatments. *American Journal of Psychiatry, 170*(3), 275–289. https://doi.org/10.1176/appi.ajp.2012.12070991

Sonuga-Barke, E. J. S., Kennedy, M., Kumsta, R., Knights, N., Golm, D., Rutter, M., et al. (2017). Child-to-adult neurodevelopmental and mental health trajectories after early life deprivation: The young adult follow-up of the longitudinal English and Romanian Adoptees study. *Lancet, 389*(10078), 1539–1548. https://doi.org/10.1016/s0140-6736(17)30045-4

Spencer, A. E., Uchida, M., Kenworthy, T., Keary, C. J., & Biederman, J. (2014). Glutamatergic dysregulation in pediatric psychiatric disorders: A systematic review of the magnetic resonance spectroscopy literature. *Journal of Clinical Psychiatry, 75*(11), 1226-+. https://doi.org/10.4088/JCP.13r08767

Spencer, N. J., Ludvigsson, J., Bai, G., Gauvin, L., Clifford, S. A., Abu Awad, Y., et al. (2022). Social gradients in ADHD by household income and maternal education exposure during early childhood: Findings from birth cohort studies across six countries. *Plos One, 17*(3), e0264709. https://doi.org/10.1371/journal.pone.0264709

Speyer, L. G., Eisner, M., Ribeaud, D., Luciano, M., Auyeung, B., & Murray, A. L. (2022). A symptom level perspective on reactive and proactive aggressive behaviours and ADHD symptoms in childhood. *Journal of Child Psychology and Psychiatry, 63*(9), 1017–1026. https://doi.org/10.1111/jcpp.13556

Sprich, S., Biederman, J., Crawford, M. H., Mundy, E., & Faraone, S. V. (2000). Adoptive and biological families of children and adolescents with ADHD. *Journal of the American Academy of Child and Adolescent Psychiatry, 39*(11), 1432–1437. https://doi.org/10.1097/00004583-200011000-00018

Steinberg, E. A., & Drabick, D. A. G. (2015). A developmental psychopathology perspective on ADHD and comorbid conditions: The role of emotion regulation. *Child Psychiatry & Human Development, 46*(6), 951–966. https://doi.org/10.1007/s10578-015-0534-2

Stern, A., Agnew-Blais, J., Danese, A., Fisher, H. L., Jaffee, S. R., Matthews, T., et al. (2018). Associations between abuse/neglect and ADHD from childhood to young adulthood: A prospective nationally-representative twin study. *Child Abuse and Neglect, 81*, 274–285. https://doi.org/10.1016/j.chiabu.2018.04.025

Stern, A., Agnew-Blais, J. C., Danese, A., Fisher, H. L., Matthews, T., Polanczyk, G. V., et al. (2020). Associations between ADHD and emotional problems from childhood to young adulthood: a longitudinal genetically sensitive study. *Journal of Child Psychology and Psychiatry, 61*(11), 1234–1242. https://doi.org/10.1111/jcpp.13217

Stevens, A. J., Purcell, R. V., Darling, K. A., Eggleston, M. J. F., Kennedy, M. A., & Rucklidge, J. J. (2019). Human gut microbiome changes during a 10 week Randomised Control Trial for micronutrient supplementation in children with attention deficit hyperactivity disorder. *Scientific Reports, 9*, 10128. https://doi.org/10.1038/s41598-019-461463

Stevenson, J. (2022). Editorial: Accumulating evidence for the benefit of micronutrients for children with attention-deficit/hyperactivity disorder. *Journal of the American Academy of Child and Adolescent Psychiatry, 61*(5), 599–600. https://doi.org/10.1016/j.jaac.2021.08.008

Stevenson, J., & Cate, I. P. (2004). The nature of hyperactivity in children and adolescents with hydrocephalus: A test of the dual pathway model. *Neural Plasticity, 11*(1-2), 13–21. https://doi.org/10.1155/np.2004.13

Stevenson, J., Buitelaar, J., Cortese, S., Ferrin, M., Konofal, E., Lecendreux, M., et al. (2014). Research Review: The role of diet in the treatment of attention-deficit/hyperactivity disorder - an appraisal of the evidence on efficacy and recommendations on the design of future studies. *Journal of Child Psychology and Psychiatry, 55*(5), 416–427. https://doi.org/10.1111/jcpp.12215

Sudre, G., Frederick, J., Sharp, W., Ishii-Takahashi, A., Mangalmurti, A., Choudhury, S., & Shaw, P. (2020). Mapping associations between polygenic risks for childhood neuropsychiatric disorders, symptoms of attention deficit hyperactivity disorder, cognition, and the brain. *Molecular Psychiatry, 25*(10), 2482–2492. https://doi.org/10.1038/s41380-019-0350-3

Sudre, G., Sharp, W., Kundzicz, P., Bouyssi-Kobar, M., Norman, L., Choudhury, S., & Shaw, P. (2021). Predicting the course of ADHD symptoms through the integration of childhood genomic, neural, and cognitive features. *Molecular Psychiatry, 26*(8), 4046–4054. https://doi.org/10.1038/s41380-020-00941-x

Sugaya, L. S., Salum, G. A., Gurgel, W. D., de Morais, E. M., Del Prette, G., Pilatti, C. D., et al. (2022). Efficacy and safety of methylphenidate and behavioural parent training for children aged 3-5 years with attentiondeficit hyperactivity disorder: A randomised, double-blind, placebo-controlled, and sham behavioural parent training-controlled trial. *Lancet Child & Adolescent Health, 6*(12), 845–856. https://doi.org/10.1016/s2352-4642(22)00279-6

Sugaya, L. S., Farhat, L. C., Califano, P., & Polanczyk, G. V. (2023). Efficacy of stimulants for preschool attention-deficit/hyperactivity disorder: A systematic review and meta-analysis. *JCPP Advances, e12146*. https://doi.org/10.1002/jcv2.12146

Sutcubasi, B., Metin, B., Kurban, M. K., Metin, Z. E., Beser, B., & Sonuga-Barke, E. (2020). Resting-state network dysconnectivity in ADHD: A system-neuroscience-based meta-analysis. *World Journal of Biological Psychiatry, 21*(9), 662–672. https://doi.org/10.1080/15622975.2020.1775889

Swanson, J. M., Sergeant, J. A., Taylor, E., Sonuga-Barke, E. J. S., Jensen, P. S., & Cantwell, D. P. (1998). Attention-deficit hyperactivity disorder and hyperkinetic disorder. *Lancet, 351*(9100), 429–433. https://doi.org/10.1016/s0140-6736(97)11450-7

Swanson, J. M., Schuck, S., Porter, M. M., Carlson, C., Hartman, C. A., Sergeant, J. A., et al. (2012). Categorical and dimensional definitions and evaluations of symptoms of ADHD: History of the SNAP and the SWAN rating scales. *The International Journal of Educational and Psychological Assessment, 10*(1), 51–70. PMID: 26504617.

Talebi, S., Miraghajani, M., Ghavami, A., & Mohammadi, H. (2022). The effect of zinc supplementation in children with attention deficit hyperactivity disorder: A systematic review and dose-response meta-analysis of randomized clinical trials. *Critical Reviews in Food Science and Nutrition, 62*(32), 9093–9102. https://doi.org/10.1080/10408398.2021.1940833

Tamm, L., Narad, M. E., Antonini, T. N., O'Brien, K. M., Hawk, L. W., & Epstein, J. N. (2012). Reaction time variability in ADHD: A review. *Neurotherapeutics, 9*(3), 500–508. https://doi.org/10.1007/s13311-012-0138-5

Taylor, E. (1998). Clinical foundations of hyperactivity research. *Behavioural Brain Research, 94*(1), 11–24. https://doi.org/10.1016/s0166-4328(97)00165-4

Taylor, E. (2017). Attention deficit hyperactivity disorder: Overdiagnosed or diagnoses missed? *Archives of Disease in Childhood, 102*(4), 376–379. https://doi.org/10.1136/archdischild-2016-310487

Taylor, M. J., Martin, J., Butwicka, A., Lichtenstein, P., D'Onofrio, B., Lundström, S., et al. (2023). A twin study of genetic and environmental contributions to attention-deficit/hyperactivity disorder over time. *Journal of Child Psychology and Psychiatry*. https://doi.org/10.1111/jcpp.13854

Thapar, A., Cooper, M., & Rutter, M. (2017). Neurodevelopmental disorders. *Lancet Psychiatry, 4*(4), 339–246. https://doi.org/10.1016/s2215-0366(16)30376-5

Thomas, R., Sanders, S., Doust, J., Beller, E., & Glasziou, P. (2015). Prevalence of Attention-Deficit/Hyperactivity Disorder: A systematic review and meta-analysis. *Pediatrics, 135*(4), E994–E1001. https://doi.org/10.1542/peds.2014-3482

Thompson, P. M., Jahanshad, N., Ching, C. R. K., Salminen, L. E., Thomopoulos, S. I., Bright, J., et al. (2020). ENIGMA and global neuroscience: A decade of large-scale studies of the brain in health and disease across more than 40 countries. *Translational Psychiatry, 10*(1). https://doi.org/10.1038/s41398-020-0705-1

Toplak, M. E., West, R. F., & Stanovich, K. E. (2013). Practitioner Review: Do performance-based measures and ratings of executive function assess the same construct? *Journal of Child Psychology and Psychiatry, 54*(2), 131–143. https://doi.org/10.1111/jcpp.12001

Tsang, T. W., Lucas, B. R., Olson, H. C., Pinto, R. Z., & Elliott, E. J. (2016). Prenatal alcohol exposure, FASD, and child behavior: A meta-analysis. *Pediatrics, 137*(3). https://doi.org/10.1542/peds.2015-2542

Tseng, P. T., Cheng, Y. S., Yen, C. F., Chen, Y. W., Stubbs, B., Whiteley, P., et al. (2018). Peripheral iron levels in children with attention-deficit hyperactivity disorder: A systematic review and meta-analysis. *Scientific Reports, 8*. https://doi.org/10.1038/s41598-017-19096-x

Uebel, H., Albrecht, B., Asherson, P., Boerger, N. A., Butler, L., Chen, W., et al. (2010). Performance variability, impulsivity errors and the impact of incentives as gender-independent endophenotypes for ADHD. *Journal of Child Psychology and Psychiatry, 51*(2), 210–218. https://doi.org/10.1111/j.1469-7610.2009.02139.x

Vainieri, I., Martin, J., Rommel, A.-S., Asherson, P., Banaschewski, T., Buitelaar, J., et al. (2021). Polygenic association between attention-deficit/hyperactivity disorder liability and cognitive impairments. *Psychological Medicine*, 1–9. https://doi.org/10.1017/s0033291720005218

Valera, E. M., Faraone, S. V., Murray, K. E., & Seidman, L. J. (2007). Meta-analysis of structural imaging findings in attention-deficit/hyperactivity disorder. *Developmental Psychology, 61*(12), 1361–1369. https://doi.org/10.1016/j.biopsych.2006.06.011

Van Liefferinge, D., Sonuga-Barke, E. J. S., Danckaerts, M., Van Broeck, N., & van der Oord, S. (2021). Do childhood emotional lability and ADHD symptoms have shared neuropsychological roots? *Journal of Psychopathology and Behavioral Assessment.* https://doi.org/10.1007/s10862-020-09859-8

Vidor, M. V., Panzenhagen, A. C., Martins, A. R., Cupertino, R. B., Bandeira, C. E., Picon, F. A., et al. (2022). Emerging findings of glutamate-glutamine imbalance in the medial prefrontal cortex in attention deficit/hyperactivity disorder: Systematic review and meta-analysis of spectroscopy studies. *European Archives of Psychiatry and Clinical Neuroscience, 272*(8), 1395–1411. https://doi.org/10.1007/s00406-022-01397-6

Viering, T., Hoekstra, P. J., Philipsen, A., Naaijen, J., Dietrich, A., Hartman, C. A., et al. (2021). Emotion dysregulation and integration of emotion-related brain networks affect intraindividual change in ADHD severity throughout late adolescence. *Neuroimage, 245*. https://doi.org/10.1016/j.neuroimage.2021.118729

Vink, J. M., Treur, J. L., Pasman, J. A., & Schellekens, A. (2021). Investigating genetic correlation and causality between nicotine dependence and ADHD in a broader psychiatric context. *American Journal of Medical Genetics Part B-Neuropsychiatric Genetics, 186B*, 423–429. https://doi.org/10.1002/ajmg.b.32822

Vos, M., Rommelse, N. N. J., Franke, B., Oosterlaan, J., Heslenfeld, D. J., Hoekstra, P. J., et al. (2021). Characterizing the heterogeneous course of inattention and hyperactivity-impulsivity from childhood to young adulthood. *European Child and Adolescent Psychiatry.* https://doi.org/10.1007/s00787-021-01764-z

Wang, Y., Huang, L., Zhang, L., Qu, Y., & Mu, D. Z. (2017). Iron status in Attention-Deficit/Hyperactivity Disorder: A systematic review and meta-analysis. *Plos One, 12*(1). https://doi.org/10.1371/journal.pone.0169145

Wetherill, L., Foroud, T., & Goodlett, C. (2018). Meta-analyses of externalizing disorders: Genetics or prenatal alcohol exposure? *Alcoholism-Clinical and Experimental Research, 42*(1), 162–172. https://doi.org/10.1111/acer.13535

Whitfield-Gabrieli, S., & Ford, J. M. (2012). Default mode network activity and connectivity in psychopathology. In S. Nolen-Hoeksema (Ed.), *Annual Review of Clinical Psychology, Vol 8* (Vol. 8, pp. 49–+).

Wilens, T. E., Biederman, J., Brown, S., Monuteaux, M., Prince, J., & Spencer, T. J. (2002). Patterns of psychopathology and dysfunction in clinically referred preschoolers. *Journal of Developmental and Behavioral Pediatrics, 23*(1), S31–S36. https://doi.org/10.1097/00004703-200202001-00006

Willcutt, E. G., Doyle, A. E., Nigg, J. T., Faraone, S. V., & Pennington, B. F. (2005). Validity of the executive function theory of attention-deficit/hyperactivity disorder: A meta-analytic review. *Developmental Psychology, 57*(11), 1336–1346. https://doi.org/10.1016/j.biopsych.2005.02.006

Willcutt, E. G., Nigg, J. T., Pennington, B. F., Solanto, M. V., Rohde, L. A., Tannock, R., et al. (2012). Validity of DSM-IV Attention Deficit/Hyperactivity Disorder symptom dimensions and subtypes. *Journal of Abnormal Psychology, 121*(4), 991–1010. https://doi.org/10.1037/a0027347

Willems, Y. E., Boesen, N., Li, J., Finkenauer, C., & Bartels, M. (2019). The heritability of self-control: A meta-analysis. *Neuroscience and Biobehavioral Reviews, 100*, 324–334. https://doi.org/10.1016/j.neubiorev.2019.02.012

Wood, A. C., Asherson, P., van der Meere, J. J., & Kuntsi, J. (2010). Separation of genetic influences on attention deficit hyperactivity disorder symptoms and reaction time performance from those on IQ. *Psychological Medicine, 40*(6), 1027–1037. https://doi.org/10.1017/s003329170999119x

Wootton, R. E., Riglin, L., Blakey, R., Agnew-Blais, J., Caye, A., Cadman, T., et al. (2022). Decline in attention-deficit hyperactivity disorder traits over the life course in the general population: trajectories across five population birth cohorts spanning ages 3 to 45 years. *International Journal of Epidemiology, 51*(3), 919–930. https://doi.org/10.1093/ije/dyac049

Chapter 10
Neurodevelopmental Aspects of Behavioural Differences II. Autism Spectrum Disorder (ASD)

There have been major revisions to the way autism has been conceptualised and studied in recent decades. Currently, the behaviours characterising autism spectrum disorder (ASD) in the DSM-5 are:

1. Persistent deficits in social communication and social interaction across multiple contexts including deficits in social-emotional reciprocity, deficits in nonverbal communicative behaviours used for social interaction, deficits in developing, maintaining, and understanding relationships.
2. Restricted, repetitive patterns of behaviour, interests, or activities, including: stereotyped or repetitive motor movements, use of objects, or speech, insistence on sameness, inflexible adherence to routines, or ritualised patterns of verbal or nonverbal behaviour, hyper-, or hyporeactivity to sensory input or unusual interest in sensory aspects of the environment.

These behaviours should show an onset at an early age, cause impairment of function and should not simply be associated with intellectual disability.

In reviewing the way the conceptualisation of autism has changed in the preceding 30 years, Happé and Frith (2020a) identify seven major changes. These are:

> (1) from a narrow definition to wide diagnostic criteria; (2) from a rare to a relatively common condition, although probably still under-recognised in women; (3) from something affecting children, to a lifelong condition; (4) from something discreet and distinct, to a dimensional view; (5) from one thing to many 'autisms', and a compound or 'fractionable' condition; (6) from a focus on 'pure' autism, to recognition that complexity and comorbidity is the norm; and finally, (7) from conceptualising autism purely as a 'developmental disorder', to recognising a neurodiversity perspective, operationalised in participatory research models. (Happé & Frith, 2020a, p. 218)

In discussing the question as to whether autism can be considered a categorical disorder, Happé and Frith (2020a) suggest that it is necessary to distinguish three levels of explanation – the biological, cognitive, and behavioural. This framework, and a personal account of the history of autism, was given in a paper by Frith (2012).

J. Stevenson, *Developmental Psychopathology*,
https://doi.org/10.1007/978-3-031-45787-6_10

In terms of the biological level, there is no evidence of a qualitative difference along the dimension in either genetics (Bralten et al., 2018) or pathophysiology (Kern et al., 2015). The same holds at the behavioural level. However, it may be that at the cognitive level, sub-groups of autism may represent qualitatively distinct categories whose abilities do not simply lie at the extreme of a continuum. Happé and Frith (2020b) suggest that as a consequence, children at the extreme of the ASD dimension process and experience the world in a distinct manner.

Rosen et al. (2021) reviewed the history of the diagnosis of ASD since its original formation by Kanner (1943). They concluded that the supposed alternative conceptualisation of ASD, as either dimensional or categorical, is false. Instead, they suggest that

> it may be helpful conceptualize ASD as a single diagnostic condition consisting of various categories of symptoms that can be evaluated in terms of dimensional severity (Pickles & Angold, 2003), where we choose to emphasize the dimensionality for some purposes (e.g., research and understanding mechanisms) and the category for others (e.g., practical issues related to service allocation or planning). (Rosen et al., 2021, p. 4258)

The global epidemiology and prevalence of autism was examined in an extensive systematic review (Baxter et al., 2015). They estimated the rate of ASD to be 76 per 10,000 and suggested that there was little between country variation in the rate. They also concluded that there had not been changes in the incidence of autism between 1990 and 2010. Their review was based on prevalence data from a range of sources that used comprehensive case-finding strategies. Consequently, their estimates were not biased by changes in diagnostic practice and levels of service referrals.

Rutter (2005) had previously concluded the incidence of ASD to be slightly lower 30–60 per 10,000. He pointed out the dramatic increase compared to the 4 per 10,000 in the first survey on the condition (Lotter, 1966). This is supported by the findings of a marked increase in the diagnosis of ASD in the UK over the period from 1998 to 2018 (Russell et al., 2022). This increase was most marked for females and for adults. Why the increase? Rutter (2005) suggests that:

> …it is largely a consequence of improved ascertainment and a considerable broadening of the diagnostic concept. (Rutter, 2005, p. 2)

This notion of a broadening of the diagnosis of ASD is supported by a meta-analysis by Rødgaard et al. (2019). They used the indirect, but subtle, device of examining the differences between participants with ASD and TD children in meta-analyses of neurocognitive functioning based on studies published from the mid-1960s onwards. The findings indicate that differences between individuals with autism and those without the diagnosis have been become less marked. They say this may be due to changes in the definition of autism from a:

> …narrowly defined and homogenous population toward an inclusive and heterogeneous population…. (Rødgaard et al., 2019, p. 1124)

However, there may also have been a true increase in the risk of ASD due to some as yet unknown environmental factor. Rutter (2005) is clear that there is no evidence for this being the measles–mumps–rubella vaccine or vaccines containing mercury from the preservative thimerosal, as had been suggested by Wakefield et al. (1998) and Bernard et al. (2001), respectively. Other environmental toxins have been suggested as contributing to this rise. Sulaiman et al. (2020) undertook a meta-analysis of studies on the levels of aluminium, cadmium, and mercury in hair, urine, blood, or teeth in those with ASD and controls. There were inconsistent results between studies. When aggregated in the meta-analysis, some significant associations were found but not always in the same direction. For example, the levels of aluminium in hair and urine were elevated in those with ASD but were lower in blood. An earlier meta-analysis by the same group on the association between ASD and inorganic arsenic and lead, showed consistent evidence supporting a positive association between early life inorganic arsenic exposure and ASD but inconsistent evidence for lead exposure and ASD risk (Wang et al., 2019). At present, it seems that with the exception of inorganic arsenic, little can be said of the risk for ASD from these environmental toxins or of the extent to which increases in these exposures may have contributed to the rise in the prevalence of ASD.

There is guidance that the sex ratio of children with ASD is 4:1 with an excess of boys (APA, 2013). In adults, it has been shown that the excess of males in limited to those with ASD and no or mild intellectual disability; the excess of males was not significant in those with moderate to profound disability (Brugha et al., 2016) However, it has been recognised that females have been underdiagnosed with ASD (Russell et al., 2011). A systematic review and meta-analysis of studies on the sex ratio for ASD has shown that if more reliance is placed studies with active case identification, i.e. not based on diagnoses by services, that the gender ratio is lower (Loomes et al., 2017). They suggest the ratio closer to 3:1 and that:

> there appears to be a diagnostic gender bias, meaning that girls who meet criteria for ASD are at disproportionate risk of not receiving a clinical diagnosis. (Loomes et al., 2017, p. 466)

10.1 Behavioural Aspects of ASD

Core Features Mandy and Skuse (2008) reviewed studies on the behavioural characteristics of children with ASD and argued that two elements of the disorder – social-communication impairment and the repetitive interests, behaviours, and activities (RIBAs) – are at best only modestly correlated. Consequently, these aspects need to be studied in their own right and may well have independent underlying causes. Happé and Ronald (2008) take this argument further to suggest that the three elements of the autism triad – namely, impairment in social interaction, impairment in communication and restricted, repetitive behaviours, and interests – are fractionable, i.e.they are influenced by largely independent causes. The three elements of the triad have been found to be influenced by largely independent genes and cognitive processes (Happé et al., 2006a, b). This fractionation can be seen at the biological (i.e., genetic) (Ronald et al., 2006a, b), cognitive (Brunsdon & Happé,

2014) and behavioural levels (Ronald et al., 2006a, b). These impairments do co-occur but, e.g., are seen to be only modestly correlated in a population-based study of 3000 twin pairs, both in terms of individual differences across the normal range (Ronald et al., 2006a, b) and at the extreme high end (Ronald et al., 2006a, b).

Associated Behaviour and Emotional Problems
Anxiety. There is good evidence that ASD is associated with internalising difficulties (Matson & Nebel-Schwalm, 2007). White et al. (2009) reviewed studies on the co-occurrence of ASD and anxiety and found that in those studies using diagnostic methods, about 50% of those with ASD also received an anxiety disorder diagnosis. A meta-analysis by van Steensel et al. (2011) of studies using questionnaires or diagnostic interviews found that 40% of those under 18 years with ASD had at least one comorbid anxiety disorder.

Hallett et al. (2012) used parent-reported data on 7311 twin pairs at age 7–8 years. They were interested in determining the patterns of overlap between the triad of autistic-like traits, i.e. social difficulties, communication problems, and repetitive/restricted behaviours, and four subtypes of internalising traits, namely, social anxiety, fears, generalized anxiety, and negative affect. Communication impairments and repetitive/restricted behaviours correlated most strongly with generalized anxiety and negative affect, both phenotypically and genetically. However, these correlations were small.

IQ and associated psychopathology. The role of IQ in the risk of developing anxiety in the those with ASD was studied in a meta-analysis by Mingins et al. (2021). They found that there was a significant, but modest, correlation between intelligence quotient and anxiety in ASD $r = 0.18$ (CI_{95} 0.11–0.25). It has been suggested that the mechanisms linking IQ and anxiety in those with ASD may change with age (Ronald & Hoekstra, 2011). In childhood, the association may arise due to environmental influences or an interaction between the two sets of behaviours. In contrast, in adolescence, a common genetic liability may be responsible.

There is a question as to whether the high level of comorbid behavioural problems seen in those with ASD arises, perhaps, as a consequence of the intellectual disability often found in that group. In a study of a large general population sample, Totsika et al. (2011) found that ASD and intellectual disability were independent risk factors for both behavioural and emotional problems. Brereton et al. (2006) compared two groups of 4–18-year-olds, one group with ASD and the other with intellectual disability but no ASD. They found that those with ASD showed significantly higher levels of psychopathology than young people with intellectual disability alone. This indicates that it is ASD per se that is responsible for the high psychiatric comorbidity seen in this group. Hofvander et al. (2009) investigated the mental health of adults with ASD but with IQs in the normal range. They found that mood and anxiety disorders were common, but ADHD and psychotic disorders were also present. This again supports the notion that it is ASD per se, rather than intellectual disability, that is associated with comorbid conditions.

Effects of Type of Schooling The question of whether children with ASD attending mainstream schools have high levels of emotional and behavioural problems was addressed by Hastings et al. (2022). This is an important issue as an increasing proportion of those with ASD are being taught in mainstream schools, and this setting presents particular challenges for such children. In a sample of 160 ASD children aged between 4 and 17 years in mainstream schools, Hastings et al. (2022) found that ASD children had higher scores on all the SDQ scales compared to UK norms. The risk of a high score within the ASD group was increased by male sex, living in a household with additional children, more severe autism symptoms, fewer adaptive skills, and lower socioeconomic status.

A study using the SDQ with children with ASD in special schools aged 4–19 years was reported by Salomone et al. (2014). The means scores on the SDQ in the ASD sample in mainstream schools by Hastings et al. (2022) and those in special schools by Salomone et al. (2014) are both elevated compared to the UK norm and approximately to the same extent. This suggests that whatever the type of school attended by children with ASD, there are a significant proportion of them with associated behavioural and emotional problems that would benefit from mental health support.

Continuity in Comorbid Psychopathology The continuities between psychopathology symptoms at ages 4–9 years and 13–17 years in children with an ASD diagnosis were studied by Leno et al. (2022). They found strong homotypic continuity in emotional, behavioural, and ADHD symptoms. The only significant heterotypic continuity was between childhood emotional symptoms and ADHD in adolescence. They found that those with ASD and an IQ below 70 showed greater homotypic continuity.

The role of cognitive factors in the association between ASD and emotional and behavioural problems was investigated by Ozsivadjian et al. (2020). They studied a number of cognitive mechanisms – cognitive inflexibility, intolerance of uncertainty, and alexithymia. Alexithymia is defined as difficulties in recognising, labelling, and processing one's own emotions, differentiating emotions from bodily sensations, and focusing on inner, rather than external experiences. They found that cognitive inflexibility may be a crucial factor in the development of externalising difficulties in ASD. It may also have an influence on intolerance of uncertainty, which in turn may play a role in the development of Internalising problems.

Pathological Demand Avoidance There is a debate about whether pathological demand avoidance should be considered as a central feature of ASD or whether it represents a comorbidity that can, in some circumstances, exist independently of ASD (Green et al., 2018a, b; O'Nions et al. 2018a, b). The term "pathological demand avoidance" was proposed by Newson et al. (2003) to describe children on the spectrum of pervasive developmental disorders who obsessively resist everyday demands and use "socially manipulative" behaviour to avoid complying. In addition, these children may show extreme mood variability and obsessive behaviour that is often focussed on other people. Newson et al. (2003) argued that this represents a distinctive pervasive developmental disorder separate from ASD. However, Green et al. (2018a, b) argued that the evidence does not support the validity of pathological demand avoidance as an independent syndrome. However, it does reflect important aspects of a range of co-occurring difficulties for many children with ASD that can substantially affect families.

Physical Health There is evidence that those with ASD are more likely to have a range of physical health conditions in addition to psychiatric comorbidities. In a review of 24 meta-analyses and systematic reviews addressing this issue, Rydzewska et al. (2021) found that comorbid physical conditions are common in ASD, and some are more prevalent than in the general population, e.g. sleep problems, epilepsy, sensory impairments, atopy, autoimmune disorders, and obesity.

10.2 Cognitive Aspects of ASD

Language Ability Difficulties in language development are a core component of ASD. However, there is wide variability in the extent and manner in which these difficulties are manifest. Some children may become fluent, others have delayed language, and some fail to develop useful or consistent use of words. One feature of the language of some children with ASD is language regression, where after a period of normal development, language skills are lost or fails to progress. It has been suggested that this pattern of regression in language and communication ability during the first years of life is common in ASD (Ozonoff & Iosif, 2019).

The significance for later development of this pattern was examined by Pickles et al. (2022). In this longitudinal study of 421 children with an autism diagnosis, 22% were found to show language regression. These children continued to show delays in expressive language development but not in language comprehension. The practical importance of this delay was thought to be progressively less significant as the child became older, as the average level of communication skills increases. A general feature in this study was the marked variability in the trajectory of communication development in children with ASD, both with and without regression.

Theory of Mind Two of the most influential cognitive theories of ASD have been the theory of mind (ToM) deficit and Weak Central Coherence (WCC). ToM was postulated as an explanation for the difficulties in social integration and reciprocal communication experienced by those with ASD (Baron-Cohen et al., 1985; Frith et al., 1991). This explanation suggests that children with ASD will not understand that people can have beliefs, feelings and attitudes that are different to their own. In the absence of this understanding it will be difficult to form and maintain social relationships. It will also create difficulties in a range of learning situations (Happé, 2015).

One measure of ToM is the Sally-Anne Test (Baron-Cohen et al., 1985). It assesses the attribution of a false belief. Here, the participant has to understand that another person (Sally in this test) will have a belief about the world that is different from the participant's own belief (see Fig. 10.1). Using both TD and IQ-matched Down Syndrome comparison groups the following striking result was obtained:

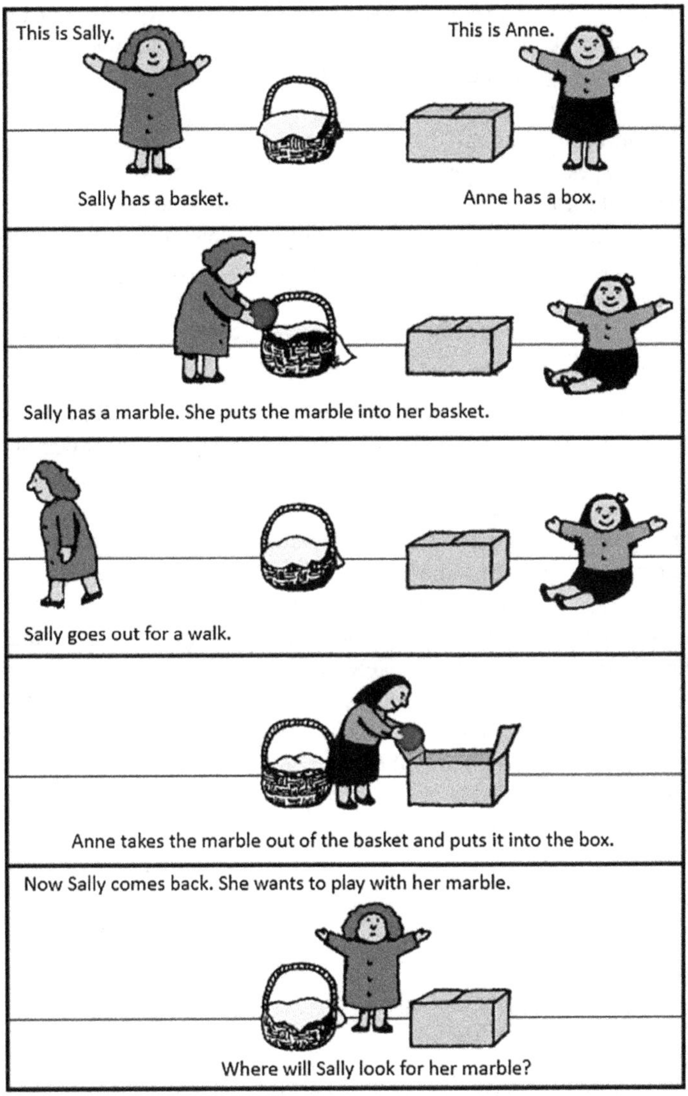

Fig. 10.1 The Sally–Anne test of the ability to attribute a false belief. (Reproduced with the permission of Axel Scheffler from Frith, U. (1989). *Autism: Explaining the Enigma.* Oxford: Blackwell)

> The critical question was, 'Where will Sally look?' after she returns. Here a group difference appeared: Autistic children answered this question in a distinctly different way from the others. The Down's Syndrome and normal preschool children answered by pointing to where the marble was put in the first place. Thus they must have appreciated that their own knowledge of where the marble actually was and the knowledge that could be attributed to the doll were different. That is, they predicted the doll's behaviour on the basis of the doll's belief. The autistic group, on the other hand, answered by pointing consistently to where the marble really was. They did not merely point to a 'wrong' location, but rather to the actual location of the marble. (Baron-Cohen et al., 1985, p. 42–43)

Perner and Lang (1999) examined the evidence that theory of mind (ToM) and executive function (EF) were closely associated during normal development at around the age of 4 years but could not identify which of a number of plausible mechanisms was responsible for the association. Marcovitch et al. (2015) went on to show that in a longitudinal study of a general population sample of over 200 children, EF at ages 3 and 4 years predicted ToM performance one year later. The reverse was not these case; ToM did not predict later EF. Wade et al. (2018) reviewed the evidence for EF and ToM having underlying brain mechanisms in common from a range of brain studies of normal and abnormal development. They concluded that it appears that ToM and EF share some overlapping neural structures, while also recruiting regions that are specially designed for mental representation and executive control, respectively.

Weak Central Coherence The Weak Central Coherence notion, developed by Frith, suggests that those with ASD combine a strength in local processing with a possible global processing deficit. The local processing strength was confirmed in a review of 50 studies by Happé and Frith (2006). This local processing strength resulted in a pattern of detailed focussed processing in those with ASD, meaning they concentrate on the trees rather than the wood. It has subsequently been shown that there is also a deficit in global processing alongside this relative strength in local processing (Booth & Happé, 2018). One measure of global processing was the fragmented-picture completion task. Here, the participants are required to identify a figure as it is gradually revealed in successive picture frames (see Fig. 10.2). Those with ASD they were significantly slower to integrate picture fragments than age- and IQ-matched controls to identify the pictures. This is indicative of reduced global integration.

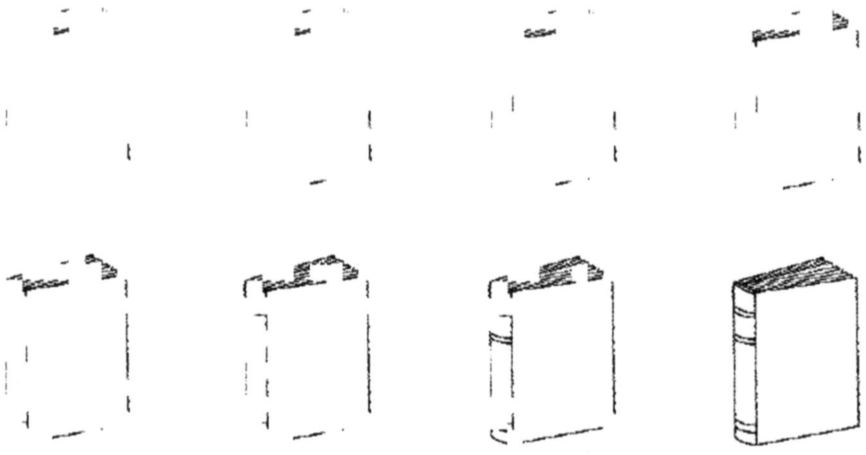

Fig. 10.2 Fragmented-picture completion task to measure global processing. (Reproduced with the permission of Springer Nature from Fig. 1 Booth and Happé (2018). *Journal of Autism and Developmental Disorders, 48*(4), 1397–1408; permission conveyed through Copyright Clearance Center, Inc.)

The fragmented-picture completion task was applied in a study of ASD traits in twins (Neufeld et al., 2020). They found that in accordance with the Weak Central Coherence theory, those with an ASD diagnosis or higher autistic traits needed more visual fragments to identify the figure on this task, which is taken to indicate a reduced global visual processing efficiency. The pattern of results of within MZ pair differences indicates that non-shared environmental influences are acting to produce the global processing deficit.

10.3 Biological Aspects of ASD

Gender There is an excess of males in those with ASD – the ratio of males to females is around 3:1. This has led to a number of investigations of the biological processes that may be linked to sex differences in ASD (Ferri et al., 2018). Baron-Cohen et al. (2001) produced an Autism-Spectrum Quotient (ASQ), which was designed to provide a dimensional measure of individual differences in ASD-rated traits in the general population. They showed marked differences on the ASQ between those with ASD and neurotypical controls. They also found that males scored higher than females. In a subsequent meta-analysis of the results from 73 publications, the effect size difference between males and females was SMD= 0.40 (Ruzich et al., 2015). It was suggested earlier by Baron-Cohen (2002) that autism can be considered as an extreme form of the male brain This was based on a generalisation that males are better at systematising than empathising, while for females, the opposite is true. These two dimensions of mentalising were defined as follows:

> 'Empathising' is the drive to identify another person's emotions and thoughts, and to respond to these with an appropriate emotion. Empathising allows you to predict a person's behaviour, and to care about how others feel.
>
> 'Systemising' is the drive to analyse the variables in a system, to derive the underlying rules that govern the behaviour of a system. Systemising also refers to the drive to construct systems. Systemising allows you to predict the behaviour of a system, and to control it. (Baron-Cohen, 2002, p. 248)

Ridley (2019) noted that, in the Ruzich et al. (2015) meta-analysis, neurotypical females had an ASQ of about 15 and males of 18. In contrast, females and males with ASD had mean scores of 39 and 36, respectively. She pertinently concluded that

> A female with autism therefore does not resemble a neurotypical man, she resembles an autistic man. That's because she has autism, not because she has a 'male brain', 'extreme' or otherwise. (Ridley, 2019, p. 23)

There is a clear gender bias in clinical referrals resulting in fewer girls receiving an ASD diagnosis. However, it is also the case that boys are more vulnerable to ASD than girls (Loomes et al., 2017). There is no consensus on what might constitute the basis of the excess of males in the ASD population. Ferri et al. (2018) concluded that a combination of factors that lead to possible protective effects in females and vulnerability effects in males are likely to be involved, and indeed, that there will complex interactions between these biological processes, both genetic and epigenetic, and environmental risks.

Minor Physical Anomalies There is evidence that the rate of minor physical anomalies (MPAs) may be elevated in those with ASD (Bolton, 2009; Ozgen et al., 2010). These anomalies are found in the morphology of the head, eyes, ears, mouth, hands, and feet. They are markers of first-trimester ectodermal developmental abnormalities and could be an indirect index for CNS maldevelopment during the same period (Hata et al., 2003). Bolton (2009) suggests that they may be particularly associated with ASD arising from de novo copy number variants and possibly other non-familial risk factors. The link with ASD was shown in a twin study of neurodevelopmental disorders (Myers et al., 2017). A specific association with ASD was found; MPAs were not related to ADHD. There was a stronger correlation between the MPAs within MZ than DZ pairs, which confirms the importance of genetic risks for MPAs.

Genetics

The genetics of autism is complex. Twin and family studies suggest that heritability is substantial. This was first shown in a classic twin study by Folstein and Rutter (1977a, b). They found that the concordance rate for both autism and related cognitive abnormalities for MZ twin pairs was substantially higher than that for DZ pairs in twin pairs where at least one member showed autism.

Ronald and Hoekstra (2011) reviewed over 30 twin studies on ASD and showed that they replicated the findings from the early twin studies of a marked discrepancy in the concordances for MZ and DZ twin pairs, with the former being over 75% and the latter below 30%. The twin studies have shown that both genetic and environmental factors influence autistic traits across development, both measured in the general population and in the extremes of the population. Multivariate genetic analysis based on measures of the triad of components of ASD (social impairment, communication impairments, and restrictive repetitive interests) suggests that there are at least partially independent genetic and environmental influences on each element of the triad. Ronald and Hoekstra (2011) suggest that the evidence from twin studies indicates that there may be a difference in the genetic factors influencing the risk of ASD in those with intellectual impairment and those with an IQ towards the normal range.

A meta-analysis of twin studies by Tick et al. (2016a, b) indicated that heritability of ASD was in the range of 0.64–0.91. It also suggested that the size of heritability does not change across the autistic spectrum. The notion of autism as the extreme on a dimension of ASD based on quantitative genetic analysis (Colvert et al., 2015) has been extended to examine the underlying biological processes shared between autism and autistic traits (Massrali et al., 2019).

However, some autistic individuals carry rare genetic mutations that add to the polygenic risks in influencing the development of autism (Sebat et al., 2007). Just which genes might be involved in this process is contentious (Myers et al., 2020). A Swedish study provided a synthesis of the various genetic and environmental contributions to the risk of developing ASD (Gaugler et al., 2014). They concluded that the single largest contribution came from common inherited genetic variants (49%) with an additional 3% for rare inherited variants. Genetic mutations arising in the individual contributed a further 3%. Non-additive genetic effects arising from interactions between genes produce an additional 4%. The remaining 41% are non-genetic influences. This analysis suggests that the common genetic variants are by far the largest contributors to the genetic causes of autism.

Subsequent studies have indicated that, for certain types of families, genetic de novo mutations may play a more substantial role. Yoon et al. (2021) estimated that for those from low-risk families, i.e. with few if any ASD relatives, copy-number variants (CNVs) (see Sect. 3.2) may contribute to over 50% of ASD cases. By contrast, in multiplex families, i.e. with 2 or more children with ASD, a combination of polygenic risk and de novo variants explained 50% and 15–20% of the genetic risk, respectively (Cirnigliaro et al., 2023). In these families, the ASD PRS is associated with both social dysfunction and language delay. The authors conclude that the findings on the genetics of ASD from their study suggest that language delay should be considered a core feature of the ASD diagnosis.

An important development was the recognition that families of children with ASD show a range of language-related cognitive deficits, social impairments, and stereotypic behaviours, but not mental retardation per se – what was called the broader autistic phenotype (BAP). Bolton et al. (1994) found that the BAP was much more common in the first degree relatives of children with ASD than in the relatives of a comparison group of children with Down syndrome. A systematic review of 41 subsequent studies replicated this finding but the rate of BAP in parents of children with ASD varied greatly depending on how it was measured but it is consistently found to be more prevalent in fathers than mothers (Rubenstein & Chawla, 2018).

Brain structure and Function To obtain a clear picture of the possible brain alterations in structure and function seen in those with ASD has proven difficult (Di Martino et al., 2014), with differences being found between studies and even between systematic reviews (Pua et al., 2017). However, mega-analyses (see Sect. 2.7) of studies comparing those with ASD to TD children have found smaller volumes for the putamen, amygdala, nucleus accumbens, and pallidum, increased frontal cortical thickness, and decreased temporal cortical thickness (van Rooij et al., 2018). The key findings on ASD from the Enhancing NeuroImaging Genetics through MetaAnalysis Consortium ASD Working Group, based on 1774 participants with ASD, were that there were altered morphometry in the cognitive and affective parts of the striatum, frontal cortex, and temporal cortex in ASD (Thompson et al., 2020).

An important study of brain growth in children at high familial risk and low risk of ASD was able to monitor changes in brain volume during the first year of life (Hazlett et al., 2017). They found that brain volume overgrowth was linked to the later emergence and severity of autistic social deficits. Within the high-risk sample, a machine learning algorithm was able to predict the diagnosis of autism at 24 months with reasonable accuracy based on MRI measures in the first year of life.

The mechanism whereby genetic factors influence the development of neuropathology underlying autism has been reviewed by de la Torres-Ubieta et al. (2016). They conclude that ASD is not a single disease but is a number of aetiologically distinct conditions with diverse pathophysiological mechanisms but which lead to similar behavioural characteristics.

The literature on neurosubtypes of ASD was reviewed by Hong et al. (2020). At the time of the review, only 12 studies had been published, and these suggested that indeed subtypes could be found on the basis of structural or functional MRI and EEG studies. The studies disagree on the number of possible neurosubtypes, which may be between 2 and 4. They make the point that the presence of such subtypes makes the use of case–control studies problematic to interpret given the heterogeneity in the cases (see Sect. 10.8). There is evidence that identifying neurotypes using fMRI data in conjunction with behavioural measures may be particularly productive in giving insights into brain–behaviour relationships in ASD (Easson et al., 2019; Horien et al., 2022).

The default mode network (DMN) is a distributed network of brain regions which are, somewhat paradoxically, more active when the brain is seemingly doing nothing (Whitfield-Gabrieli & Ford, 2012). It is suggested that DMN functioning is associated with the mind when it is in a free-wandering state, and its malfunction relates to the problems experienced by those with schizophrenia. Padmanabhan et al. (2017) reviewed the evidence on the characteristics of the default mode network (DMN) in those with ASD. These studies included those using resting-state functional magnetic resonance imaging (R-fMRI) methods. They found that there are structural and functional disruptions associated with ASD, and these contribute to atypical integration of information about the self in relation to "other" as well as to impairments in the ability to flexibly attend to socially relevant stimuli. A structure linked with the DMN is the cingulum bundle, which interconnects frontal, parietal, and medial temporal sites while also linking subcortical nuclei to the cingulate gyrus. The cingulum bundle is involved in executive, social, and emotional processes. A review of studies on the cingulum bundle has shown that there are structural changes associated with ASD (Bubb et al., 2018).

The salience network (SN) is a brain system that includes the insular cortex and dysfunctions of the SN can lead to a failure to recognise important features of stimuli as being salient or relevant to the individual. Such a deficit is characteristic of ASD, and it has become clear that both the activation levels and the functional connectivity patterns of the insular cortex are distinctive in those with ASD (Uddin, 2015; Chen et al., 2016a, b). These features of the insular cortex may play an important role in aspects of the ASD profile, including sensory overresponsivity (Green et al., 2016).

Alterations in the DMN and SN have been found to be related to dimensional scores on ASD (Neufeld et al., 2018). This study used a twin design that was able to control for genetic influences and provides evidence that environmental influences must play a role in the development of individual differences in the functional connectivity of both the DMN and the SN.

There is good evidence that there are abnormalities in gene expression in the brains of those with ASD, and that these underlie mechanisms of neuronal dysfunction in ASD (Voineagu et al., 2011). The genes that have been found to be associated with ASD are often expressed early in brain development. These risk genes have roles in regulation of gene expression or neuronal communication and thereby result in neurodevelopmental and neurophysiological changes (Satterstrom et al., 2020). It is known that many of the genetic variants that influence brain dysfunction or pathology are shared with other disorders such as schizophrenia and bipolar disorder (Gandal et al., 2018).

Brain Chemistry There is evidence that there are lower brain gamma-aminobutyric acid (GABA) levels in children with ASD (Schür et al., 2016). GABA is an inhibitory neurotransmitter. There is evidence from a meta-analysis that an excitatory neurotransmitter (glutamate) is higher in the blood of those with ASD compared to TD individuals (Zheng et al., 2016). It is known that blood and brain glutamate levels are highly correlated in those with ASD (Hassan et al., 2013). This pattern of high excitatory glutamate and low GABA has led to the development of a framework for understanding influences on ASD arising from an excitation-inhibition imbalance (Sohal & Rubenstein, 2019). The low levels of GABA and the high levels of glutamate may contribute to this imbalance in ASD (Robertson et al., 2016). There is evidence that the GABA/glutamate ratio in the striatum is related to the severity of social impairments in adults with ASD (Horder et al., 2018). However, there is uncertainty over whether levels of glutamate or GABA drive this imbalance in those with ASD.

In a detailed study of two families, Bonnet-Brilhault et al. (2016) have shown that a double hit of gene mutations influencing/inhibitory synapses in glutamate/GABA neurotransmission was related to ASD, but not learning disability, in these families. The complexity of these relationships was shown by Hollestein et al. (2023) in a study that examined the relationships between genetic variance, brain structure, and autism symptomatology in a sample of 359 children and adults with ASD and neurotypical comparison participants. They found that:

> ...glutamate genes are associated with core behavioral autism characteristics and GABA genes may be associated with sensory processing, and that increased expression of glutamate and GABA genes are associated with larger differences in cortical thickness between autistics and neurotypical controls in adolescents and adults but not in children. (Hollestein et al., 2023, p. 7)

These studies of GABA and glutamate have led to initial investigations of the possibility of pharmacological intervention to correct the imbalance. Huang et al. (2022) have shown that targeting GABA receptors can modify atypical visual sensory responses in adults with ASD by the use of arbaclofen, which is an agonist to $GABA_B$ receptors. There is some evidence that arbaclofen might improve symptoms in some children with ASD (Veenstra-Vander Weele et al., 2017). Glutamate has also been the target of a drug study in those with ASD. Riluzole inhibits glutamate production and was shown to modify the excitation–inhibition imbalance in adults with ASD (Ajram et al., 2017).

A field of investigation is developing on what has become known as the "microbiota–gut–brain axis" (Cryan et al., 2019). One of the actions of gut microbes is to produce or induce the production of glutamate and GABA (Needham et al., 2020), and this is being increasingly investigated as influences on neurodevelopmental conditions. The studies on gut microbiota in children with ASD were reviewed in a meta-analysis by Iglesias-Vazquez et al. (2020). They report that the abundance of gut microbes in children with ASD was found to be higher than in TD children. Sharon et al. (2019) have shown that gut microbiota from those with ASD can induce changes in mice of repetitive and social behaviour analogous to features of ASD. This study of mice has also illustrated some of the of the pathways linking the microbiome to genes and has shown that the ASD-like behaviours in mice can be modified by the administration of microbial neuroactive metabolites. There is evidence that treatments to improve the balance of gut microorganisms can change the behaviour of children with ASD (Grimaldi et al., 2018). The following conclusion gives a sense of the opportunities that may be opened up by these studies on the microbiota–gut–brain axis:

> ….development of microbiota-based interventions such as probiotics, fecal microbiota transplantation, or metabolites may offer a timely and tractable approach to addressing the lifelong challenges of ASD. (Sharon et al., 2019, p. 1612)

These studies on the relationship between brain chemistry, structure, and function are at a preliminary stage but hold promise for the development of possible treatments directly influencing core features of ASD.

Animal Brain Models An intriguing development is the use of animal brain models to inform studies on ASD and ADHD (Zhan et al., 2021). This study used R-fMRI to examine the connectivity in frontal and temporal cortices of monkey brains. The monkeys included transgenic monkeys who over expressed the MECP2 gene. The patterns in these data were then applied to a large brain imaging dataset on those with ADHD and ASD. It was found that for the ASD sample, but not the ADHD sample, that the monkey brain connectivity data could predict symptom severity scores, specifically communication ability scores.

Although providing an example of the potential value of the use of animal models to investigate the genetics of the neurobiology of human behaviours, the significance of these findings for the understanding of the development of ASD must be in doubt (van den Heuvel, 2021). A core feature of the logic leading to the Zhan et al. (2021) study was the suggestion that mutations in the MECP2 genes contribute to neurodevelopmental disorders, including autism. The condition most clearly related to MECP2 mutations is Rett syndrome. However, the full range of characteristic autistic behaviours are not observed in all individuals with Rett Syndrome, and a number of problems shown in Rett Syndrome are rarely seen in those with ASD (Mount et al., 2003). Furthermore, an early molecular genetic study found MECP2 mutations are infrequent, if not absent, in those with ASD (Vourc'h et al., 2001). In summary, the results of the Zhan et al. (2021) are intriguing, but their relevance to an understanding of the biological basis of ASD is moot.

Advanced Parental Reproductive Age A well-replicated risk factor for ASD is advanced paternal or maternal reproductive age (Lyall et al., 2017). This could be a reflection of a biological risk such as a germline mutation. However, it is also possible that parents who delay conceptions may show a mild form of ASD, and therefore, the effect is a result of shared common genetic variants (Lai et al., 2014). A meta -analysis of 27 studies found that the risk of ASD increased by 18% and 21% with a 10-year increase in maternal and paternal age, respectively (Wu et al., 2017). The relationship between reproductive age and ASD is made more complex by evidence that younger mothers may also represent a group with an increased risk of a child with ASD (Sari et al., 2022).

10.4 Environmental Risk Factors for ASD

In an extensive overview of previous systematic reviews and meta-analyses of environmental risk factors for autism, Modabbernia et al. (2017) conclude that some putative risk factors are unrelated causally to ASD. These include vaccination, maternal smoking, thimerosal exposure, and assisted reproductive technology. Some perinatal factors, such as hypoxia, are strongly related to ASD, but other pregnancy-related factors, such as maternal obesity, diabetes, and Caesarean section, are less so. See also Sect. 4.4 for a discussion of the studies on epidural anaesthesia and the risk of ASD. The evidence related to some of these environmental risk factors will now be summarised.

Psychogenic Hypothesis The formulation of ASD by Kanner (1943) included the observation that the 11 of the children being described came from families where there were:

> …very few really warm hearted fathers and mothers. (Kanner, 1943, p. 2)

This raised the question of the extent to which these parental characteristics may have contributed to the development of ASD. At the same time, Kanner recognised that the very early onset of the ASD behaviours was more consistent with a biological-based origin for the condition. The notion that autism might have its origins in the experience of being raised by cold and disengaged parents was taken further by Bettelheim (1967). For an account of the impact of this idea on parents and families, see Donvan and Zucker (2017).

This psychogenic hypothesis about the origins of autism was considered by Rutter (1968). He identified a number of objections to accepting that ASD might have its origins in experiences within the family. The first was that it seemed improbable that parenting could have such a severe disturbing effect so early in development. The second is that the direction of causality may run in the opposite direction. It may be that the atypical behaviour shown by the child with ASD may have a detrimental effect on the parents' ability to engage with the child. The third is that where a distinction had been made between ASD with and without a known a biological origin, there are no differences between the groups in parental characteristics. Rutter (1968) concludes that the psychogenic hypothesis is not supported by the evidence, but at the time he was writing, there were no decisive findings for or against. Thirty years later, Rutter (1999) was able to conclude that research had provided sufficient evidence that the notion of ASD as a psychogenic disorder had been superseded and was clearly a disorder based on organic brain dysfunction. The history of autism, its formulation and treatment, was reviewed by Wolff (2004).

Maternal Autoimmune Disease and Inflammation A meta-analysis found that antenatal exposure of children to maternal auto-immune conditions, such as psoriasis, systemic lupus erythematosus (SLE), and autoimmune thyroid disease, increased the risk of ASD in the children by 34% (Chen et al., 2016a, b). Maternal infections during pregnancy, such as rubella, were also linked to an increased risk of ASD, as was shown in a landmark paper by Chess (1971). These are examples of prenatal exposures to maternal immunological activation that is associated with ASD. The potential mechanisms linking of these exposures and post-natal aspects of immunological dysfunction to ASD have been reviewed (Estes & McAllister, 2015; Meltzer & Van de Water, 2017). In a prospective study of a total population sample of Norwegian children, a strong association was found between biomarkers of immune dysregulation in mothers blood as early as 17–21-week gestation and in cord blood of neonates later diagnosed with ASD (Che et al., 2022). The history of studies on the origins and nature ASD has been concisely summarised by Lipkin et al. (2023). They particularly emphasise the role of prospective birth cohort studies in elucidating the possible risk factors, including immune dysregulation for the development of ASD and the need to consider genetic vulnerabilities and environmental triggers as acting to produce ASD. They include a helpful time-line of major developments in research studies into ASD.

Environmental Toxins Modabbernai et al. (2017) concluded that studies on nutritional factors and on toxins have failed to provide consistent evidence of an association with ASD. However, there is some evidence that ADHD and ASD may share a common exposure to metals and elements antenatally. In a population database of cases of ADHD and ASD, the following were found to be elevated in maternal blood samples at 17-week gestation: arsenic, cadmium, copper, mercury, manganese, magnesium, and lead (Skogheim et al., 2021). The similarities among the metals and elements in their impact on ASD and ADHD led the authors to suggest that these two disorders share some neurochemical and neurodevelopmental pathways.

Vitamin D Deficiency There have been sporadic reports that vitamin D levels were reduced in those with ASD compared to TD children. This evidence from association studies was deemed to be inconsistent and imprecise by Modabbernia et al. (2017). A later meta-analysis of six studies on vitamin D supplementation for ASD yielded equivocal results (Zhang et al., 2023). The only significant changes were in stereotypical behaviours, and none in other core symptoms of ASD. At present there is no strong support for the notion that vitamin D deficiency is a cause of ASD in some children.

Air Pollution There have been suggestions that air pollutant exposure may contribute to the risk of ASD (Chun et al., 2020; Flores-Pajot et al., 2016; Lam et al., 2016). The effects, however, were slight and inconsistent between studies as to which aspect of pollution were implicated. A systematic review suggested that there is insufficient evidence to determine whether other factors, such as sex, socioeconomic status, or genotype, can modify the impact of air pollutants on the risk of ASD (Yu et al., 2022).

Demographic Characteristics It has been long recognised that referrals to specialist services for children with ASD are subject to a strong social class bias. Wing (1980) wed that in an epidemiological sample, there were no significant differences in social class between those with ASD and the general population. By contrast a sample of children referred to specialist services were of higher social class than the epidemiologically ascertained sample and the general population. It has also been suggested by Elsabbagh et al. (2012) that there are no marked cross-cultural differences in the prevalence of ASD. However, they note that there has been little research on ASD in low-income countries. Durkin et al. (2015) elaborate on this issue of under-resourcing of research and clinical provision for ASD in low-income countries. They suggest a range of possibilities to facilitate research collaboration and training globally.

There are divergences in the association between socioeconomic status (SES) and the diagnosis of ASD. In the USA, low SES is linked with a lower prevalence of ASD, while in Scandinavia, the reverse is the case, with ASD diagnosis more common in lower SES families (Lyall et al., 2017). There is evidence that the pattern in the USA may be changing (Winter et al., 2020). This study of ASD diagnoses in California between 1992 and 2018 found that this social gradient in ASD, for a higher level of diagnoses with higher SES, reversed for children of White and Asian mothers. The situation was complex in that this reversal did not happen for children of Black and Hispanic mothers. Over this time period, in this part of the USA, diagnoses of ASD were increasing but who was being diagnosed was changing.

The possible range of social, racial, and ethnicity factors influencing the rate of ASD diagnoses in the UK was studied by Roman-Urrestarazu et al. (2021). The database used was a census of just over 7,000,000 individuals under 21 years old in state-funded education in England. They found a prevalence of ASD of 1.76% ($CI_{.95}$ 1.75–1.77) with a male-to-female ratio of 4.32:1. In terms of race/ethnicity, Black children had the highest prevalence of 2.11% ($CI_{.95}$ 2.06–2.16) compared to 1.05% ($CI_{.95}$ 1.82–1.85) and 1.06 (1.04–1.09) in White and Asian children, respectively. Those with ASD were more likely to experience social disadvantage and this mediated the effects of ethnicity on ASD. There was also marked variation in the prevalence rate of ASD by geographical area and local authority districts. These prevalence figures are for ASD as identified in the English school system. The social differences in the prevalence could be due to a number of factors, including diagnostic biases, possible differences in detection and referral, or differential prevalence of the clinical diagnosis.

The association between ASD and immigration status was the subject of a systematic review by Crafa and Warfa (2015). They summarised the results from ten large-scale population studies. Across these studies, there was a higher rate of ASD in children of migrant mothers (2.69%) compared to those of non-migrant mothers (0.91%). They proposed that stress arising from pregnancy during migration and poor social economic circumstances may induce epigenetic changes during pregnancy and delivery that lead to ASD. The complexity of the relationship between race/ethnicity, social disadvantage, and immigration as risk factor for ASD has been clearly laid out by Lord (2013).

10.5 Outcome of ASD

Functioning in Adulthood Magiati et al. (2014) conducted a systematic review of studies that had examined the outcomes after age 16 years for children who had been identified with ASD. There were wide variations between the results from these studies but some patterns were discernible. In some studies, social functioning, cognitive ability, and language skills remained relatively stable but others reported a later deterioration. Adaptive functioning tended to improve with age in most studies. The severity of autism-related behavioural symptoms was often improved though the criteria for an ASD diagnosis were still met. The best predictors of a better outcome were childhood IQ and early language ability.

Simonoff et al. (2020) followed 158 participants with ASD in a longitudinal study from age 12 to 23 years. They found cognitive improvements for many, but the ASD symptoms themselves tended not to change. Howlin and Magiati (2017) reviewed studies on the functioning of adults with ASD. They showed that in this group there was very limited social integration, poor job prospects and high rates of mental health problems. A meta-analysis of 18 studies, with quantitative data on outcomes after age 18 years for those with ASD, showed that a good outcome was found for 20% of those with ASD, 27% had a fair outcome, and 49% a poor outcome (Mason et al., 2021). The main predictor of a poor outcome was IQ in adulthood. This latter finding holds across cultures, e.g. in Japan (Iwasa et al., 2022).

Using trait measures of ADHD and ASD in the longitudinally studied ALSPAC sample, Riglin et al. (2021) suggest that in young adults, ADHD and ASD symptoms have similar characteristics as they do in childhood. One difference identified was that the sex difference in ASD and ADHD trait scores was not as great in young adulthood as it was in childhood.

The possibility of those with ASD showing an improvement in their daily functioning has been widely recognised but little investigated. Livingston and Happé (2017) formulated an approach to this question and defined "compensation":

> ..as the processes contributing to improved behavioural presentation of a neurodevelopmental disorder, despite persisting core deficit(s) at cognitive and/or neurobiological levels. (Livingston & Happé, 2017, p. 739)

They suggest that this compensation process of improvement in behaviour with continuing underlying deficits may be seen in the following circumstances: good outcome, at risk individuals transitioning away from the autism phenotype, late diagnosis, and female autism presentation. The processes involved in these changes are poorly understood. Livingston et al. (2019) present some preliminary findings on compensatory strategies. They empathise that an understanding of compensation might aid clinicians identify those with underlying ASD deficits who compensate and thereby fail to receive beneficial mental health support.

There has been a recent commitment in a number of studies to shift the focus on the outcome of ASD away from dysfunction to a more balanced appraisal including identifying those with ASD who are "doing well" (McCauley et al., 2020). This rebalancing has come about in part by the advocacy of parents, the neurodiversty movement, and by those experiencing ASD themselves (see Kapp et al., 2013). There is a need to identify factors that are associated with "doing well" in adulthood. Szatmari et al. (2021) explored this issue adopting a framework suggested by Taylor (2017) that "doing well" could be indicated either by attaining a threshold of proficiency or by showing growth from an initial level of competence. They found that 80% of those with ASD could be considered to be "doing well" by one or other of these measures in one domain, from communication, activities of daily living, and socialisation. A number of factors were associated with "doing well" including child characteristics such as language ability and social context factors such as household income.

Circumscribed Exceptional Abilities There is a long history of studies examining those with ASD who have circumscribed exceptional abilities (O'Connor & Hermelin, 1991). Howlin et al. (2009) estimated that nearly a third of those with ASD showed an exceptional cognitive ability in one area. A similar proportion was identified in a study by Itzchak et al. (2013) who found that memory skills were the most frequently reported special ability, followed by musical, visuospatial, and reading skills. A number of components contribute to the development of exceptional talents in some with ASD including excellent attention to detail and the ability to recognise repeating patterns (Baron-Cohen et al., 2009). There is therefore a longstanding recognition that, for a sub-set of the those with ASD, high achievement can be obtained in circumscribed abilities.

Adverse Mental Health Outcomes Kirsch et al. (2020) used a population-based birth cohort to longitudinally assess the risk of multiple psychiatric comorbidities, specifically, clinically diagnosed depression, anxiety, and bipolar disorder, among individuals with ASD into middle adulthood. Their results suggested that individuals with ASD may be at increased risk for bipolar disorder (hazard ratio (HR) = 9.34), depression (HR = 2.81), and anxiety (HR = 3.45) compared to those without ASD. These estimates are all in broad agreement with prior studies.

A meta-analysis by Lai et al. (2019) of 96 studies produced the following estimated rates of co-occurring psychiatric conditions in autism: overall pooled prevalence estimates of 28% ($CI_{.95}$ 25–32) for attention-deficit hyperactivity disorder; 20% ($CI_{.95}$ 17–23) for anxiety disorders; 13% ($CI_{.95}$ 9–17) for sleep–wake disorders;

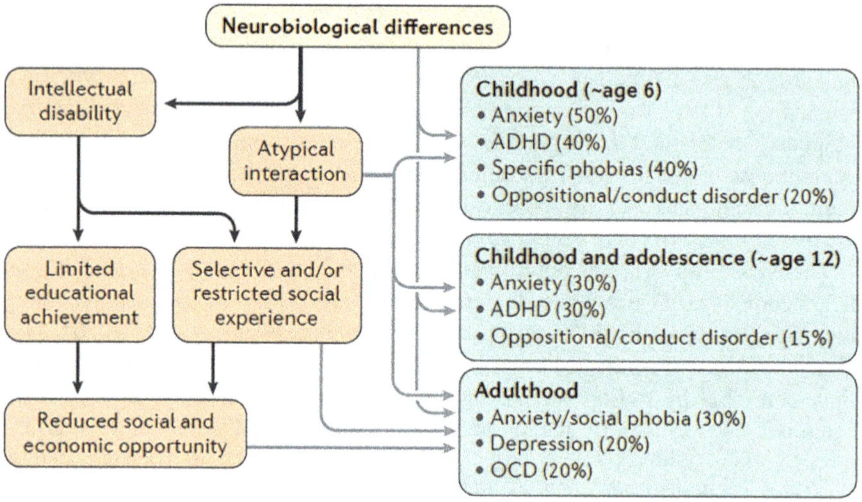

Fig. 10.3 Disorders co-occurring with ASD [OCD (obsessive-compulsive disorder)]. (Reproduced with the permission of Springer Nature from Fig. 5 Lord et al. (2020). *Nature Reviews Disease Primers*, *6*(1). doi:10.1038/s41572-019-0138-4; permission conveyed through Copyright Clearance Center, Inc.)

12% ($CI_{.95}$ 10–15) for disruptive, impulse-control, and conduct disorders; 11% ($CI_{.95}$ 9–13) for depressive disorders; 9% ($CI_{.95}$ 7–10) for obsessive-compulsive disorder; 5% ($CI_{.95}$ 3–6) for bipolar disorders; and 4% ($CI_{.95}$ 3–5) for schizophrenia spectrum disorders.

The changing developmental course of the problems co-occurring with ASD has been summaries by Lord et al. (2020) (see Fig. 10.3). These problems include primary and secondary disorders and disadvantages that can accrue in those with ASD. Lord et al. (2020) explain that the prevalence estimates of these associated disorders given in Fig. 10.3 are uncertain since they are largely based on studies of clinical populations and are not based on epidemiologically ascertained samples. There are three routes to these problems: via intellectual disability, via atypical interaction, and as a direct consequence of neurobiological differences.

A detailed study of the comorbidity between ASD and other psychiatric disorders was undertaken by Salazar et al. (2015). In a sample of 101 British children with ASD aged between 4 and 10 years of age, they found that most children met diagnostic criteria for additional psychopathology. The most common comorbidities were with generalised anxiety disorder (66%), specific phobias (53%), and ADHD (59%). Similar results were found in a sample of children with ASD from the USA (Joshi et al., 2010). In that study, the rate of comorbidity was even higher with 95% showing 3 or more comorbid psychiatric disorders. In a third country (Finland), a sample of high functioning children with ASD children also showed a high level of comorbidity (Mattila et al., 2010). They found comorbid psychiatric disorders in 74% of the ASD sample and often there multiple comorbidities.

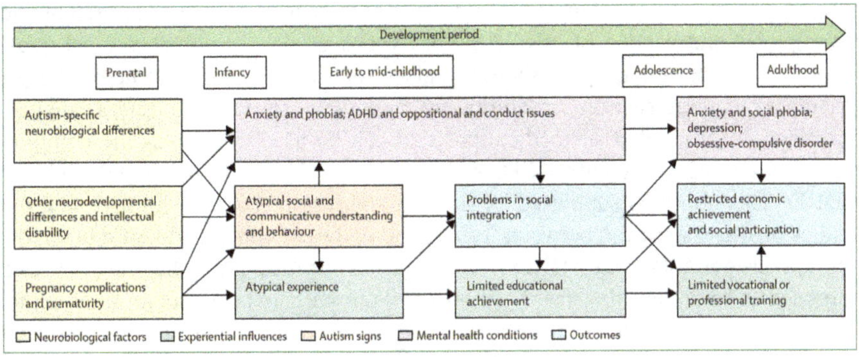

Fig. 10.4 Neurobiological and experiential influences on signs of autism, mental health, and life outcomes across development. (Reproduced with the permission of Elsevier from Fig. 2 Lord et al. (2022). *Lancet, 399*(10321), 271–334; permission conveyed through Copyright Clearance Center, Inc.)

Behavioural disorders were shown in 44%, anxiety disorders in 42%, and tic disorders in 26%. There is evidence that the degree of comorbidity in those with ASD declines with age (Lever & Geurts, 2016).

In ASD, there is a wide range of comorbidities with health related conditions which extends beyond psychiatric disorders (Kohane et al., 2012; Levy et al., 2010). The risk of dying prematurely is increased in both children with ADHD and ASD (Catalá-López et al., 2022). Across 27 studies, the relative risk of death was 2.13 for those with ADHD and 2.37 for those with ASD compared to the general population. Figures were not available for those with both ASD and ADHD.

An integrated summary of the biological and social influences on ASD across the life-span was provided by Lord et al. (2022). This is given in diagrammatic form in Fig. 10.4. This shows how neurobiological factors influence early behaviours, including those specific to ASD. These lead to mental health problems and cognitive, social, and communication difficulties during early childhood. They will also produce atypical experiences, for example, in the response from others to the behaviour of the child with ASD. Later, in childhood and adolescence, these aspects of behaviour and communication increase the risk of problems in integration and in poor education attainment. In adulthood, there may be consequent limitations on social participation and job opportunities alongside continuing mental health difficulties.

10.6 Treatment of ASD

Pharmacological Treatment Lord et al. (2018) have provided an overview of the current status of understanding about the origin and treatment for ASD. They emphasise that despite improvements in outcomes for those with ASD, many will still not gain full-time employment or independent living. Extensive research on the neurological and genetic basis of ASD has yet to result in pharmacological treatment for ASD per se, although there is a place for the use of drugs to help improve associated features such as irritability and agitation. Howes et al. (2018) suggest that there are a number of medications that can be used to address the common disorders co-occurring with ASD, such as methylphenidate and guanfacine for ADHD. This notion is supported by Antshel and Russo (2019), who reviewed the studies on the association between ADHD and ASD and concluded that it is important to consider comorbid ADHD if interventions for ASD are to be effective. One approach to treatment that has been attractive to parents is oxytocin nasal spray. Despite many clinical trials having been undertaken, a meta-analysis has produced non-significant effects (Ooi et al., 2017) and a large sample RCT also failed to show a significant benefit (Sikich et al., 2021).

Dietary Treatment A meta-analysis of 27 double-blind, randomized clinical trials of dietary treatments for ASD did not provide evidence of efficacy of this treatment approach (Fraguas et al., 2019). Despite the meta-analysis not supporting a general recommendation of dietary interventions in ASD, Fraguas et al. (2019) suggest that some dietary interventions could potentially have a benefit in managing some core and associated symptoms in those with ASD. As was discussed in Sect. 10.3, there is preliminary evidence that probiotic dietary treatments can improve the balance of gut microorganisms and can change the behaviour of children with ASD (Grimaldi et al., 2018).

Nonpharmacological Interventions Sandbank et al. (2020) undertook a comprehensive systematic review and meta-analysis of nonpharmacological early intervention studies for children with ASD. The interventions were classified as behavioural, developmental, naturalistic developmental behavioural intervention (NDBI), TEACCH (developed by Eric Schopler), sensory-based, animal-assisted, and technology-based. The meta-analysis included data on 6240 participants aged 0–8 years. The initial analysis suggested significant benefits from behavioural, developmental, and NDBI interventions but no effects for the other approaches. However, as more stringent design requirements on studies were made, i.e. an RCT design and no risk of detection bias (unblinded assessment), none of the interventions showed significant effects on any outcome. It is an unfortunate state of affairs that they have to conclude that currently:

> More high quality randomized-controlled trials that feature independently administered assessments are needed to unquestionably establish the efficacy of any intervention type. (Sandbank et al., 2020, p. 21)

Status of Research on Treatment Green and Garg (2018) reviewed the studies evaluating interventions for children with ASD. They concluded that many treatments in common use have no supporting evidence of efficacy. Some psychosocial interventions can improve the children's social interactions, but these effects are short-term. Evidence for more sustained benefits is largely lacking (Charman, 2021). Biologically based interventions are under development but as yet have not been subject to larger scale trials of effectiveness. Similar conclusions were reached by Baribeau et al. (2022).

The conclusions from Sandbank et al. (2020) concerning the lack of adequately conducted RCTs for treatment children with ASD were endorsed by Fuentes et al. (2021) in the European guidelines for the treatment of autism. It is also echoed by Charman (2019), who, commenting on the failure to replicate the initial promising findings on the Early Start Denver Model (see Rogers et al., 2019), suggests that:

> Developing a mature science of clinical trials in the early autism field will take time. (Charman, 2019, p. 847)

Nevertheless, there is reason for optimism for the possibility of effective interventions to change the course and outcome of ASD. Lord et al. (2022) produced an authoritative and wide ranging review of the state of knowledge about the needs and care of those with ASD. They suggest that:

> Autism was initially believed to be an intractable neurodevelopmental disorder with few effective treatment options, but a more optimistic view is emerging. Systematic reviews and meta-analyses of intervention studies for young children with autism published over the past 10 years have identified evidence-based psychosocial interventions that, when done in high-quality, university-led trials in HICs, resulted in change that could mitigate the influence of autism on development for some people. Furthermore, longitudinal research suggests that some individuals can compensate for difficulties associated with autism in ways that lead to very positive outcomes. Although not all people will change to the same degree, people with profound autism can have lives with social contacts, meaningful activity, and independence in some skills. Consequently, the question is no longer whether change and improvement are possible for people with autism, but rather what factors enable people with autism to live positive, fulfilling lives, what are the key elements of effective interventions, and what are the micro-environmental and macro-environmental barriers to change for autistic individuals. (Lord et al., 2022, p. 277)

This important paper from "The Lancet Commission on the future of care and clinical research in autism" should be required reading for anyone involved in the care of these children and their families.

Psychoanalysis In the welter of therapeutic approaches for children with ASD, there is one that has resisted evaluation. In France, psychoanalysis is frequently used as a therapeutic approach for children with ASD (Houzel, 2018). This approach has been subject to a stringent critique by Bishop and Swendsen (2021). In the context of its application to the treatment of those with ASD, they make the following powerful and damming conclusions:

> …psychoanalysis is qualitatively different from other forms of therapy. It is not only bereft of any evidence of effectiveness, but it is so ill-defined that it is unclear what such evidence would look like. It is only legitimised because it is promoted by authority figures and maintained by circles of power and influence. Moreover, in its more extreme forms, it has potential to cause damage to parents, especially mothers, who are demonised both for being too involved with and too remote from their children, and to children themselves, who are regarded as seducers rather than victims when involved in sexual relationships with adults. (Bishop & Swendsen, 2021, p. 90)

Prevention Given the difficulties in achieving effective long-term benefits from the treatment of children with ASD, an approach that focusses on interventions in the very early stages of ASD may be more fruitful. A number of such preventive interventions have been attempted, but only recently has one shown promising signs of efficacy. It is described as a pre-emptive intervention and this RCT was introduced to infants aged 9–14 months (Whitehouse et al., 2021). The infants were showing early signs of ASD. The intervention involved 10 sessions of a positive parenting programme. Caregiver–infant interactions were videotaped during each session, forming the basis for video feedback discussions. They found reduced ASD symptom severity across early childhood and reduced the odds of an ASD diagnosis at age 3 years in the treated group compared to a "care as usual" control group. There is some suggestion that the effect size, as reported in this paper, has been inflated by a statistical artefact (Ware, 2022). Nevertheless, follow-up studies of this sample will be awaited with interest.

10.7 Co-occurrence of ASD and ADHD

Extent of the Association Between ASD and ADHD The first study to investigate the co-occurrence of ASD with other psychiatric disorders using standardised assessments in a population-representative sample was conducted by Simonoff et al. (2008). They found a prevalence of 71% for any other psychiatric disorder, and 28% of this sample of children with ASD were also diagnosed with ADHD. Rong et al. (2021) produced a meta-analysis of 63 publications on the occurrence of ADHD in those with ASD. They found that the current and lifetime prevalence rates of ADHD in those with ASD were 38.5% ($CI_{.95}$ 34.0–43.2) and 40.2% ($CI_{.95}$ 34.9–45.7), respectively. Similarly, studies have found rates of ASD to be elevated in those with ADHD. A meta-analysis found that the rate of ASD in children and adolescents with ADHD was 21% and that the mean ASD trait scores for those with ADHD were significantly greater than for those without ADHD (SMD = 1.23) (Hollingdale et al., 2020).

Data from a national sample of 3–17-year-olds (N = 88,051) in the USA were used to estimate the prevalence of the co-occurrence of ADHD and ASD (Casseus, 2022). The overall prevalence was 1.2%, with boys over twice as likely to exhibit the combined condition than girls. The prevalence also varied by race/ethnicity, with the highest rate being for White/Non-Hispanic children. This same sample was used to estimate the rates of mental, behavioural, and developmental disorders in children with co-occurring ADHD and ASD (Casseus et al., 2023). They found that children with ADHD+ASD had higher rates of these co-occurring disorders than either those with ADHD or ASD alone.

The relationships between behaviours that characterise ADHD and ASD were examined by Krakowski et al. (2022). They used the Strengths and Weaknesses of ADHD and Normal Behavior (SWAN) (Swanson et al., 2012) and the Social Communication Questionnaire (SCQ) (for details of the SCQ, see Chesnut et al.,

2017) with 1497 children who had received either an ADHD or an ASD diagnosis. Combining the behaviour assessment from the two questionnaires, they applied both an EFA and CFA (see Sect. 2.4) to the data. They found that a four-factor structure fitted the data well. This model had two latent ADHD factors (inattention and hyperactivity/impulsivity) and two ASD factors (social communication and restrictive, repetitive behaviour and interests). This factor structure held across gender, age, and ADHD or ASD diagnosis. They suggest that this means that scores on these four latent factors can be compared in clinical sub-groups.

In a meta-analysis of 44 studies, children with ADHD, but no ASD diagnosis, performed significantly less well than TD children (SMD = 0.37) on measures of social cognition related to ASD (Bora & Pantells, 2016). These results support a dimensional approach when assessing children with suspected autism or ADHD. The focus should be on the degree to which the child shows ASD or ADHD traits rather than making a judgement as to whether the child meets the criteria for a diagnosis or not.

Antenatal Risk Factors for ASD and ADHD Co-occurrence There is evidence that both ADHD and ASD may arise in part from birth by Caesarean section delivery (Curran et al., 2015). In this meta-analysis, the putative effect of Caesarean section on ASD [OR = 1.23 ($CI_{.95}$ 1.07–1.40)] was somewhat larger than on ADHD [OR = 1.07 ($CI_{.95}$ 0.86–1.33)]. The estimate for ADHD was based on only two studies, and as the $CI_{.95}$ indicates, the OR was not significant. A subsequent study of 1.18 million births in Sweden suggested that the association between Caesarean section and neurodevelopmental disorders is most likely explained by confounding from familial, especially maternal, factors (Zhang et al., 2021).

A set of meta-analyses reviewed by Han et al. (2021) suggested that maternal inflammatory states are associated with ASD. These include obesity, gestational diabetes mellitus, pre-eclampsia, pollution, stress, depression, autoimmune diseases, and infection. As was commented in Sect. 9.4, these associations could arise from confounds such as gene–environment correlations. However, some of these inflammatory states are the same as those linked to ADHD, and the possibility that they represent a common causal factor needs to be considered.

The possible role of antipsychotic medication during pregnancy in increasing the risk of ADHD and ASD was examined by Wang et al. (2021). The study was based on a population cohort born in Hong Kong between 2001 and 2015. As this was an observational study, there was a need to take potential confounds into account. The study used a propensity score method (see Sect. 4.7) and sibling-matched controls to account for unmeasured environmental and genetic factors plus an additional negative control analysis (see Sect. 4.9). The findings did not suggest that exposure to prenatal antipsychotics increased the risk of ADHD or ASD.

Developmental Pathways Shephard et al. (2019) examined the behavioural development of high-risk and low-risk infants over the first two years of life. The high-risk group had an older sibling with ASD, and the low-risk did not. At age 7 years, the children were assessed on measures of ASD and ADHD symptoms. They found features of early-life that were uniquely correlated with later ADHD symptoms, but these did not correlate with ASD symptoms. This, therefore, suggested that these disorders may have distinct developmental origins and are unlikely to reflect a common condition.

However, Shephard et al. (2019) also examined anxiety at age 7 years, and the early developmental pathways suggested that anxiety and ASD may have shared developmental origins. The latter was also found in a twin study by Tick et al. (2016a, b) where co-occurrence of emotional symptoms in ASD is completely explained by common genetic effects with a genetic correlation between of 0.42. In that study, there were no shared genetic influences on conduct problems and ASD. The results for hyperactivity suggested that this early behaviour increased the likelihood that ASD traits would be identified rather than playing a direct causal role. This close connection between ADHD behaviours and ASD was found by Miller et al. (2020). They caution against the idea that ADHD and ASD are a single disorder but rather suggest that there is a mixture of overlapping and distinct early indicators of ASD- and ADHD-like profiles that can be difficult to disentangle early in life.

The co-development of ADHD and ASD behaviours between the ages of 4 and 25 years was studied in the ALSPAC sample by Shakeshaft et al. (2023). They identified three trajectories for the co-development of hyperactive-inattentive and social communication difficulties. One with low-stable ADHD-autistic traits, reflecting the typically developing majority (87%), and two smaller subgroups both with 6% prevalence, one with child/adolescent-declining ADHD-autistic traits, and the other with late-emerging ADHD-autistic traits. The general pattern was that ASD and ADHD traits were reciprocal, i.e. they decline, increase or persist in concert. Using a number of PRS, they found distinct profiles of scores for the three trajectory groups and also for a number of other associated characteristics. These findings suggest distinctive influences on the trajectory groups, which may have implications for clinical practice.

ASD Comorbidities These complex relationships between the causal factors underlying ADHD (and other comorbid conditions) and ASD were analysed by Hawks and Constantino (2020). They suggest three ways in which ADHD comorbidity with ASD could occur. The first is by shared genetic risk. The second is where ADHD arises as a secondary consequence of ASD. The third is a link arising by chance between a liability to ASD and an independent liability for ADHD which amplifies the risk for ASD. This latter process could occur in utero or postnatally. They suggest that the co-occurrence of ASD and ADHD can arise through either via shared genetic risk or this third mechanism of a chance conjunction of independent liabilities.

Genetics The genetic basis of the association between ASD and ADHD was examined in family studies by Jokiranta-Olkoniemi et al. (2016) and Ghirardi et al. (2018). Jokiranta-Olkoniemi et al. (2016) analysed a large dataset of siblings from a population-based cohort to identify whether ASD and ADHD might have common risk factors. The siblings for those with ASD showed a significant relative risk (RR) for ASD adjusted RR = 11.8 ($CI_{.95}$ 9.4–14.7) and for ADHD adjusted RR = 3.7 ($CI_{.95}$

2.9–4.7). These findings suggest that ADHD and ASD may have common risk factors. Ghirardi et al. (2018) studied individuals with ASD and their relatives and found an increased risk of ADHD. The findings from such family studies supports the following evidence of a genetic correlation between ASD and ADHD in twin studies and molecular genetic studies.

Using a large population cohort of 2906 MZ twin pairs and 3689 (same sex) DZ twin pairs, Pettersson et al. (2013) applied structural equation modelling to test whether common genetic and environmental influences could be detected for ADHD, ASD, and other neurodevelopmental problems. They found that a general genetic factor accounted for a large proportion of the phenotypic covariance between the measures of neurodevelopmental problems. In addition, specific genetic factors were found to influence "impulsivity", "learning problems", and "tics and autism". Three unique (non-shared) environmental factors were identified as influencing "autism", "hyperactivity and impulsivity", and "inattention and learning problems". There was no significant contribution to the phenotypic covariation from shared environmental factors. This quantitative genetic study provided an important precursor for subsequent molecular genetic studies on the overlap between ADHD and ASD.

The shared genetic basis of ADHD and ASD has been identified in twins (Pinto et al., 2016) and in molecular genetic studies (Grove et al., 2019). These contrasting methodologies suggest a genetic correlation between ASD and ADHD of around $r_G = 0.40$. This estimate is replicated in Lee et al. (2019) who found a single nucleotide polymorphism (SNP) based genetic correlation between ASD and ADHD of 0.37. There is also evidence of genetic contribution to their association from studies on ADHD and ASD traits. For example, in a study of child twins, Taylor et al. (2015) identified a genetic correlation of about 0.50 between ASD communication difficulties and traits of ADHD. Similarly, in a study of adults twins, the inattentive and hyperactivity/impulsivity components of ADHD showed genetic correlations with ASD social interaction communication abilities of 0.42 and 0.33 (Ghirardi et al., 2019). There appears to be genetic mediation between developmental changes in the ADHD/ASD relationship with early ADHD traits influencing later communication difficulties (Taylor et al., 2013). Stergiakouli et al. (2017) have shown that in the general population, genetic origins of variation on the dimensions of social-communication difficulties and ADHD symptoms are linked throughout childhood and adolescence.

Polygenic risk scores (PRS) for ASD and ADHD were calculated for 15,205 children from the Norwegian mother, father, and child cohort study (Askeland et al., 2022). In a longitudinal follow-up to 8 years of age, significant associations were found between these scores and dimensional measures of ASD and ADHD behaviours. The size of these associations was small – none of the standardised regression weights were greater than $\beta = 0.05$. However, they do indicate that risk based on genetics can be identified at an early age. It is of interest to note that the correlation between the PRS for ADHD and for ASD was $r = 0.20$ ($CI_{.95}$ 0.18–0.22). This suggests that genetic factors contribute to the association between ASD and ADHD, at least for dimensional measures in the general population.

A GWAS was undertaken on a large sample diagnosed with ADHD and/or ASD, including a total of 34,462 cases and 41,201 controls (Mattheisen et al., 2022). There were 7 loci that were shared between ADHD and ASD plus 5 loci that were associated with just one of the conditions. Those with both ADHD and ASD were found to carry the genetic risk factors for each of the conditions. This landmark study provides the basis for developing a better understanding as to the biological origins of ADHD and ASD.

The association between ASD and a range of neurodevelopmental and psychiatric conditions has been shown to be substantially influenced by genetic factors by an analysis of familial resemblance in a total population sample of over two million Swedish children (Ghirardi et al., 2021). They reported the following genetic correlations between ASD and other conditions: neurodevelopmental disorders $r_G = 0.73$ ($CI_{.95} = 0.66–0.79$), anxiety disorders $r_G = 0.47$ ($CI_{.95} = 0.33–0.61$), depression $r_G = 0.52$ ($CI_{.95} = 0.37–0.66$), and intentional self-harm $r_G = 0.54$ ($CI_{.95} = 0.36–0.71$). A direct test of the possible shared genetic influences on ASD and ADHD was undertaken by Peyre et al. (2021) in the analysis of two GWAS datasets. They found common genetic variants and genes shared by ASD and ADHD and also some specific to each disorder. Approximately, a quarter of the common genetic variants associated with one disorder were also linked to the other disorder.

An extensive meta-analysis of genetic and environmental influences on neurodevelopmental disorders (NDDs) was produced by Gidziela et al. (2023). This synthesised findings based on studies of family resemblance, such as twin studies, that provide estimates of h^2 and molecular genetic studies that provided estimates of h^2_{SNP}. The values of these heritabilities and estimates of shared and non-shared environmental influences were computed for NDDs (including ADHD and ASD). The family based and SNP based genetic correlations between these NDDs and between NDDs and disruptive, impulse control and conduct disorders (DICCs) were also calculated. They found that all NDDs to be substantially heritable (family-based heritability, 0.66; SNP heritability, 0.19). These estimates of heritability and of environmental effects are displayed in Fig. 10.5 for each of the NDDs. The genetic correlations between NDDs were moderate – family-based genetic correlation = 0.36 and SNP-based genetic correlation = 0.39 but differed substantially between pairs of disorders. The family-based genetic correlation between ASD and ADHD was 0.67 and the SNP-based genetic correlation was 0.39 The genetic overlap between NDDs and DICCs was strong – family-based genetic correlation = 0.62.

Network Approaches The association between ADHD and ASD dimensions was examined using a network analysis approach (Farhat et al., 2022). The children were aged between 6 and 17 years and were a general population sample living in an urban area of Brazil. Two questionnaires were used, one to measure ADHD symptoms (SNAP-IV, Bussing et al., 2008) and one to measure ASD symptoms (CAST)(Scott et al., 2002). There were strong connections in the network between symptoms within the ADHD and within the ASD groupings but only weak connectivity between these groupings. This suggests that in the general population ASD and ADHD symptoms do not have a causal impact across the diagnostic groupings.

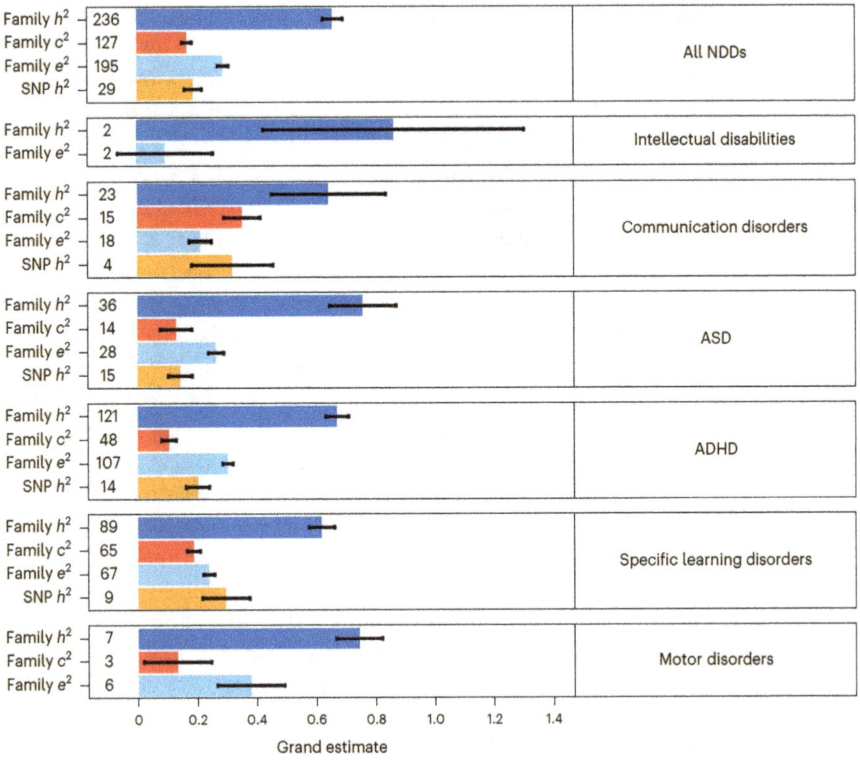

Fig. 10.5 Genetic and environmental sources of variation in NDDs. Meta-analytic family and SNP-based heritability (h2) of NDDs and shared environmental influences (c2) and non-shared environmental influences (e2) on variation in NDDs. The number preceding each bar on the y axis denotes the number of studies identified that provided estimates for specific NDDs. The error bars signify standard errors of the grand estimates of heritability and environmental influences. (Reproduced with the permission of Nature Research from Fig. 3 Gidziela et al. (2023). *Nature Human Behaviour, 7*(4), 642–656; permission conveyed through Copyright Clearance Center, Inc.)

This study was the first to use a network approach with these sets of symptoms in a general population sample.

An analysis of the pattern of associations between the behavioural features of ASD and ADHD was undertaken by Sokolova et al. (2017). They used a novel causal discovery procedure to identify a possible network of direct and indirect links between behaviours and to identify possible latent common causes. The novelty of the method and the exploratory nature of the method mean that the results must be treated as preliminary and, as the authors recognise, require replication in further data sets and by other methods. Their findings suggest that there are three routes by which ADHD and ASD can co-occur. The first is a pathway where impulsivity leads to social ineptness. A second pathway develops from hyperactivity to stereotyped behaviour. The third is a common cause leading to the association between inattention, social ineptness, and low verbal IQ.

Common Cognitive Factors The co-occurrence of ASD and ADHD raises the question of whether some of the underlying cognitive features of these conditions share a common basis. Rommelse et al. (2011) reviewed studies on factors that might be associated with both ASD and ADHD and where there was good evidence of heritability. The cognitive factors they identified as being common to both were pragmatics (appropriate use of language in social contexts), executive functions, error and feedback processing, facial emotion recognition, arousal and reward in response to social stimuli, sustained attention, and reaction time (RT) variability. They suggest that delay aversion, theory of mind and central coherence only relate to one of the conditions. Emotion regulation, defined as monitoring, evaluating, and modifying emotional responses and experiences, was found to be a feature common to ASD and ADHD in narrative review (England-Mason, 2020). She concluded that deficits in emotion regulation were a mechanism underlying the co-occurrence of these two neurodevelopmental conditions. This is suggestion is supported by the results of a co-twin control study (Astenvald et al., 2022), which found a strong association between ADHD, ASD, and deficits in emotional regulation. This study also showed that emotional regulation deficits persisted in those with ADHD, even after controlling for ASD symptoms. The pattern of results is consistent with a genetic basis for the association between ADHD and emotional dysregulation.

Visser et al. (2016) surveyed studies that examined the association between ASD and ADHD in early childhood. They concluded that co-occurrence of ASD and ADHD increases with age, severity of symptoms and lower IQ. Attention problems provide a key link between early ASD and ADHD. Both ASD and ADHD show high levels of negative affect, but possibly the factors leading to negative affect are different in the two. They also both have problems with aspects of EF. A comparison of EF in ADHD and ASD concluded that there were less severe and persistent EF deficits in ASD than in ADHD (Happé et al. 2006a, b). There is a suggestion that EF may carry a specific genetic risk for ASD. Torske et al. (2020) used scores on the BRIEF (see Sect. 9.2) to examine whether polygenic scores for ASD, ADHD, and IQ were associated with EF ratings within a clinical sample with ASD symptoms. They found that only the polygenic score for ASD was significantly related to the EF measure.

The cognitive impairments in ASD and ADHD were examined in a study of children aged 7 to 15 with ADHD ($n = 509$), ASD no ADHD ($n = 32$), ASD plus ADHD (58) and TD children ($n = 301$) (Karalunas et al., 2018). Children with ASD plus ADHD were impaired on attention/arousal, processing speed, working memory, and response inhibition, but did not differ from TD children on measures of delayed reward discounting, set-shifting, or interference control. Children with ASD are conservative in the pattern of responses in a RT task opting for accuracy over speed. Karalunas et al. (2018) argue that this response style may be a unique marker of ASD pathology that helps partially differentiate the two disorders at the cognitive level.

Brain Structure, Function, and Chemistry Children with ASD and those with ADHD have been found to show both differences and similarities in brain structure and functional connectivity compared to neurotypical children (Bethlehem et al.,

2017). Using diffusion tensor imaging (DTI), Aoki et al. (2017) found that a dimensional or trait approach was more sensitive in detecting brain–behaviour relationships with ASD traits and ADHD traits than the categorical approach. They suggest that their study indicates that the co-occurrence of ASD and ADHD arises from shared underlying neural mechanisms.

A large collaborative study is examining whether there are shared characteristics between ASD and ADHD in terms of brain organisation. They have found that subcortical volumes are similarly affected in ASD and ADHD, albeit with small effect sizes (Boedhoe et al., 2020; Hoogman et al., 2020). However, analysis of the cortex identified unique differences in each disorder, but also considerable overlap between the two, specifically in cortical thickness. A direct comparison of the gray matter volumes in children with ADHD, with ASD and TD children was undertaken by Sáenz et al. (2020). They found ADHD had a disorder-specific larger grey matter volume in the left precuneus and decreased grey matter volume in the right thalamus. An analysis to examine the correlation between genetics and structural MRI measures of selective brain region vulnerability found no significant shared associations between ASD and ADHD (Radonjic et al., 2021).

A review by Padmanabhan et al. (2017) indicated that there were robust findings of atypical functional connectivity in the DMN in those with ASD. This raises the possibility that the DMN might link ASD and ADHD. Studies on R-fMRI in children with ASD and ADHD were reviewed by Harikumar et al. (2021). There were contrasting findings with studies on ASD showing both over- and under-connectivity and those on ADHD showing overconnectivity. They concluded that there have been too few studies on the DMN in those with both ADHD and ASD to provide any guidance on its possible role in the co-occurrence of ADHD and ASD.

One possible common influence on the risk for ASD and ADHD is branched-chain amino acids (BCAAs). These BCAAs, i.e. leucine, isoleucine, and valine, are essential amino acids and have an important cellular signalling role in brain functioning. They have been found to be elevated in cord blood in mothers of children with ADHD (Anand et al., 2021) and elevated in the plasma of obese/diabetic mothers with a child with ASD (Panjwani et al., 2019). They may then be a candidate mechanism that leads to the association between ADHD and ASD.

Glutamatergic system changes associated with ADHD and ASD were reviewed by Naaijen et al. (2015). They conclude that there was a possible increase in glutamate, glutamine, and GABA in the striatum across ADHD, OCD, and ASD. A similar increase is seen in the anterior cingulate cortex of children with ADHD but a lower values occur in adults with ADHD. As was discussed in Sect. 10.3, a meta-analysis by Schür et al. (2016) provided evidence for lower brain GABA levels in children with ASD. A subsequent investigation found that there are genetic associations that may be involved in both the excitatory and inhibitory transmitter systems in ADHD and in the development of ASD symptom severity in those with ADHD (Naaijen et al., 2017). There are also an initial suggestions that the balance between glutamatergic and GABAergic neurotransmitter systems may differentiate between ADHD and ASD (Lee et al., 2022). This study used a measure of synaptic activity in the retina to monitor abnormal glutamate and GABA neurotransmission. These retinal responses were in the opposite direction in those with ADHD and those with ASD.

Age-Related Changes in the Association Between ASD and ADHD Hartman et al. (2016) addressed the question of age related changes in the association between ASD and ADHD, particularly from a life-span perspective. They reviewed previously published studies and presented their own findings from an analysis of ASD and ADHD symptom ratings from 17,173 participants aged 0 to 84 years. Within toddlerhood, the correlation between ADHD and ASD was estimated as 0.06, within preschool as 0.24, within childhood as 0.51, within adolescence as 0.60, within young adulthood as 0.50, within middle adulthood as 0.50, and finally, within late adulthood as 0.39. This indicates that the ASD/ADHD association peaks during adolescence and they concluded that this overlap is maximal at this age due to the increased demands for social adaptation and use of executive functioning skills.

Extreme Early Deprivation It is well-established that maltreatment in childhood can have an adverse long-term impact on mental health (Gilbert et al., 2009). A study of children who spend their first months or years of life in Romanian orphanages have also demonstrated the severity of the long-term harm to these children's well-being and mental health (the ERA study). A number of deprivation-specific patterns have been identified in the ERA study (Rutter et al., 2012). On the basis of their clinical presentation, these patterns were termed quasi-autism, disinhibited social engagement disorder, cognitive impairment (including IQ below 80 and deficits in inhibitory control, planning, working memory, and verbal fluency), and inattention/overactivity, which shows many features of ADHD (Kumsta et al., 2015).

The ERA study has also shown that a time-limited period of early severe deprivation can have influences on patterns of behaviour into adulthood (Golm et al., 2020; Rodriguez-Perez et al., 2023; Sonuga-Barke et al., 2017). Patterns enduring into adulthood include ASD spectrum behaviours, disinhibited social engagement, and inattention and overactivity. This suggests that in some extreme conditions, early severe deprivation may lead to the co-occurrence of ADHD and ASD behaviours. However, in this sample, the cognitive impairments seen in childhood remitted by the early adult years. The authors make the following striking conclusion:

> extended early deprivation was associated with long-term deleterious effects on wellbeing that seem insusceptible to years of nurturance and support in adoptive families. (Sonuga-Barke et al., 2017, p. 1359)

10.8 Heterogeneity in ASD and ADHD

The question of whether there are distinct sub-types of neurodevelopmental disorders exist has become a major focus of research. The issues concerning the study of such heterogeneity are similar for ADHD and ASD and are therefore being discussed together in this section.

Heterogeneity within those with ASD or ADHD can arise for a variety of reasons – some systematic, others less so. A variety of circumstances under which heterogeneity is seen is presented in Fig. 10.6. The situation where there is a clear

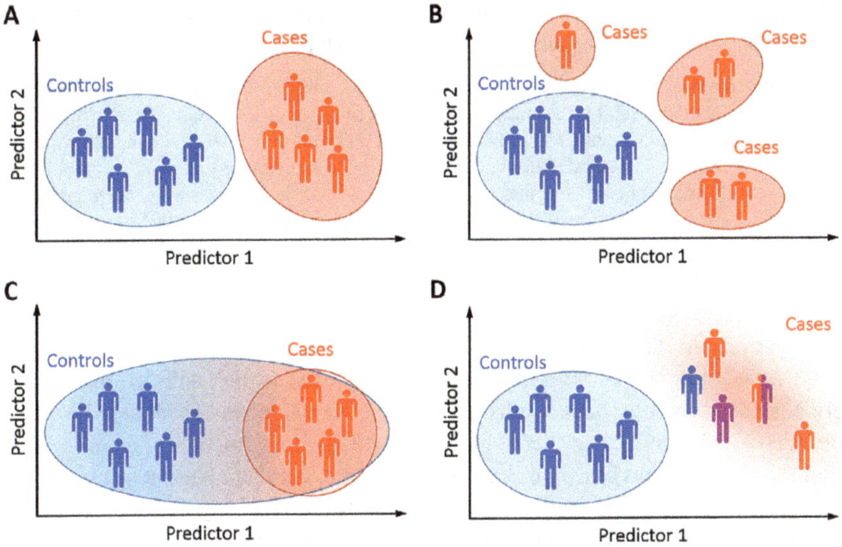

Fig. 10.6 Types of heterogeneity. (Reproduced from Fig. 1 Marquand et al. (2016). *Biological Psychiatry, 80*(7), 552–561. doi:10.1016/j.biopsych.2015.12.023; CC-BY-4.0 (https://creativecommons.org/licenses/by/4.0/))

separation between cases (those with ASD or ADHD) and TD controls is shown in Fig. 10.6a. Sharp differences between cases and controls can be found but that may be rare. For example, in the Sally-Anne Test referred to in Sect. 10.2, there is a striking difference in performance of the ASD and TD comparison group but even here 20% of the ASD group passed the test (Baron-Cohen et al., 1985). Heterogeneity might arise because the cases are comprised of different sub-groups with distinct aetiology (Fig. 10.6b). As seems to be the case with both ASD and ADHD children in these groups are at the extreme of normal variation (Fig. 10.6c). Beyond these systematic effects, there may be residual individual differences – for example, in brain development (Foulkes & Blakemore, 2018). These will overlay any systemic group differences that may be present and may arise from a number of influences including random events (Frith, 2019; Mitchell, 2007). This pattern is shown in Fig 10.6D.

Feczko et al. (2019) suggest that the identification of sub-types of psychopathology and their structure is made more complex by the "heterogeneity problem". This concerns two issues. The first is equifinality where the same condition can arise from a variety of underlying mechanisms. The second is the variety of sub-groups within a condition whose characteristics may vary depending on the feature being examined e.g. brain structure or environmental influences. Heterogeneity in presentation is a feature of many conditions, and the issues related to heterogeneity have become more complex as dimensional rather than categorical frameworks have been adopted (Grzadzinski et al., 2013). This is the case for both ADHD (Karaluna et al., 2019) and ASD (Constantino & Charman, 2016).

These issues are summarised in the opening paragraph of the Constantino and Charman paper on ASD (similar issues hold for ADHD):

> Until little more than a decade ago, autism was considered to be rare and usually accompanied by intellectual disability; standardised methods to calibrate the nature and severity of symptoms were not available, and only rarely could the syndrome be traced to a biological cause. All of that has changed. Although clinician diagnosis maintains its tentative hold as the current standard for case designation, the diagnostic process is increasingly informed by scientific discoveries that have challenged traditional perspectives on the appropriate threshold for assigning a clinical diagnosis and on how diagnosis should relate to the specific cause of an autism spectrum disorder (ASD) in an individual patient. (Constantino & Charman, 2016, p. 279)

Heterogeneity in ASD An extensive review of attempts to identify homogenous sub-types in ASD was produce by Rabot et al. (2023) who concluded that as yet there has not been consistent results. A similar conclusion was reached by Wolfers et al. (2019) who suggested that some replicated findings on sub-types have been found for classification based on cognitive measures, but there have as yet been few such analyses based on biological differences in ASD. Wolfers et al. (2019) identified two broad types of approach to the study of heterogeneity: pattern classification and stratification. The main distinction between these two approaches is that in pattern classification, the groups being characterised are known, whereas stratification generates its own groups based on the inherent structure in the data.

Pattern Classification Pattern classification is a supervised machine learning approach that optimizes the discrimination between classes – in this case, between those with ASD and TD comparison participants. The approach is based on a statistical method developed by Ronald Fisher – discriminant function analysis (DFA) (Stevenson, 1993). This attempts to identify a discriminant score, a linear weighted combination of measures, that maximises the differences in the score between two or more classes. Duffy and Als (2019) provided an example of the application of DFA in a study on ASD. They used cluster analysis of EEG data to identify two distinct sub-groups within a prospectively studied sample of children with ASD. They then used DFA to test how well these clusters could be distinguished from each other and from a comparison group of typically developing children. With two being predicted by DFA there is a single equation (function) but with three groups, as is the case here, two equations are needed to adequately separate the groups. The results of this DFA are shown in Fig. 10.7. The variables obtained from the EEG recording can be aggregated into two functions that can distinguish the two ASD clusters and the controls. Duffy and Als (2019) suggest that EEG data can aid the discovery of clinically relevant autism sub-populations and may come to provide valuable additional information in the diagnosis of ASD.

Stratification Stratification is a set of unsupervised analyses that attempts to identify relative homogeneous classes within the data. There are a number of methods of types of stratification that have been applied to heterogeneity issue in ASD – cluster analysis, finite mixture models, machine learning, and normative modelling.

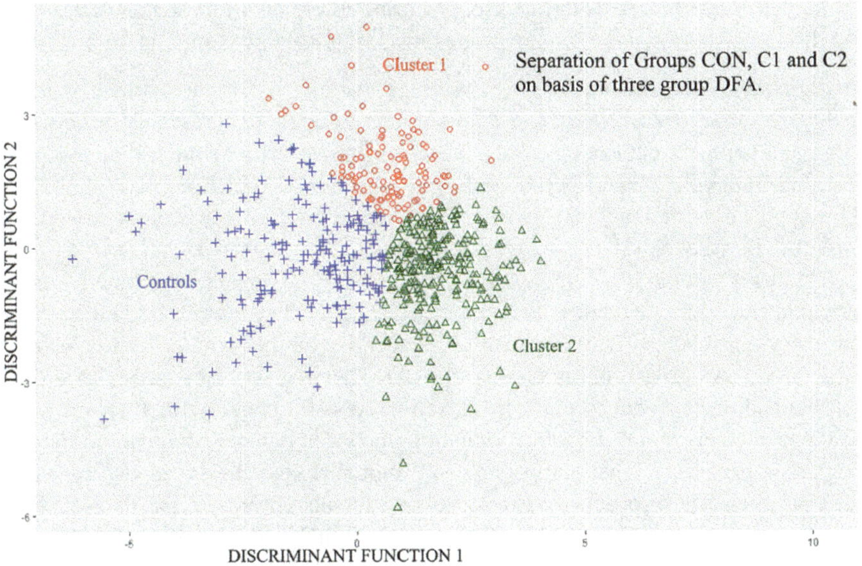

Fig. 10.7 Discriminant function analysis showing clear separation of groups identified from EEG recordings of children with ASD and controls. (Reproduced from Fig. 6 Duffy and Als (2019) *BMC Neurology, 19*(1), 27. doi:10.1186/s12883-019-1254-1; CC-BY-4.0 (https://creativecommons.org/licenses/by/4.0/))

Stratification – Cluster Analysis Cluster analysis has been described in Sect. 2.3. Using items from the Autism Diagnostic Interview-Revised (Lord et al., 1994), a cluster analysis was produced by Hu and Steinberg (2009). They identified four clusters: the first showing severe language deficits, the second had milder symptoms across the domains, the third cluster showed a higher frequency of savant skills, and the fourth group intermediate severity across all domains. They were able to use this sub-grouping to show that heterogeneity in those with ASD was related to differential gene expression with some expressed genes unique to a cluster and some genes shared across all clusters (Hu et al., 2009).

Stratification – Finite Mixture Modelling Finite mixture modelling is a form of latent variable analysis (see Sect. 2.4), which identifies a categorical latent variable that groups the participants into a discrete number of relatively homogenous classes. Each individual in the dataset can be assigned a probabilistic class membership, which indicates the degree to which they fit within a latent class. See Prince and Fidler (2021) for an introduction to finite mixture modelling and for illustrations of its application to ASD and other neurodevelopmental conditions.

An example of finite mixture modelling applied to ASD is a study by Eagle et al. (2010). They analysed a wide variety of measures of behaviour, cognitive ability, and direct observations of behaviour in a sample of 43 children aged between 3 and 12 years with diagnosed ASD. Using finite mixture modelling, they were able to identify two broad groups. These groups differed markedly on language, IQ, and social behaviour scores, with one group scoring lower on all these measures, with the difference between the groups producing SMDs ranging from 1.88 to 2.76.

Stratification – Machine Learning Machine learning is a group of mathematical techniques that exploit the power of the modern computer to identify patterns in large and complex dataset (see Sect. 2.8). For an overview of the use of machine learning in developmental psychopathology, see Dwyer and Koutsouleris (2022). The application of machine learning in studies on ASD has been reviewed by Parlett-Pelleriti et al. (2022), and two examples will be discussed.

The first example is a demonstration of the potential value of machine learning to guide treatment decisions (Stevens et al., 2019). They used a combination of unsupervised machine learning analyses to identify the behavioural sub-types in a large group ($N = 2400$) of children with ASD. They had available an archival data set that had been produced to record the children's ability and to monitor progress in eight developmental domains, including social, language, adaptive, academic, cognitive, executive functioning, play, and motor skills. They used two machine learning methods to produce a structure for the subs-groups in the dataset. This structure comprised 16 sub-groups nested within two broader behavioural phenotypes.

A distinctive feature of the study was that they were able to relate sub-group membership to treatment response. The children were receiving forms of Applied Behaviour Analysis (ABA) treatments. These treatments are based on the notion that changes to the environment will modify behaviour and employs intensive interventions from an early age. The range of related treatment approaches to ASD that has emerged from ABA has been reviewed and have been labelled 'Naturalistic Developmental Behavioral Interventions (NDBI) (Schreibman et al., 2015). Stevens et al. (2019) were able to show that treatment response varied between the sub-groups. The results are seen as preliminary and need replicating but they do point to a way in which addressing heterogeneity in ASD could lead to tailoring treatments to individuals for optimal impact.

The second example of machine learning applied to children with ASD is by Feczko et al., (2018). They aimed to identify subtypes of children with ASD and typically developing children based on their cognitive profiles. They tested whether the sub-types could be differentiated in terms of R-fMRI. Random forest methods use machine learning to estimate the similarity between participants on, in this case, their measures of cognition. To identify sub-groups, a community detection algorithm was applied. This algorithm identifies sub-groups that are similar to one another and that are distant from other sub-groups.

They identified three sub-groups in the ASD sample and four sub-groups in the TD sample based on scores on seven information processing tasks. These sub-groups were found to differ in functional connectivity in R-fMRI but did not differ in ASD symptom severity. This suggests that heterogeneity in the cognitive profiles of children with ASD arises from differences in brain processes. The authors emphasised that the study must be treated as preliminary, as the sample sizes were modest (ASD N = 47 and TD N = 58), and the sub-groups identified are only putative and require replication in larger samples.

Stratification – Normative Modelling A fourth unsupervised approach, normative modelling, has a different aim in that it has a focus on identifying how individuals are placed in the range of normative functioning on multiple measures. It is being increasingly adopted to map variation between cognitive, clinical, or demographic variables and relating these to quantitative measures obtained from neuroimaging (Marquand et al., 2019). For an introduction to normative modelling and an illustration of its application to ADHD, see Marquand et al. (2016), and for its application to ASD, see Zabihi et al. (2019).

The recognition that ASD is characterised by differences that are seen as deviations from a normal pattern of functioning has led to the suggestion that case–control comparisons, such as in pattern classification, are less appropriate (Marquand et al., 2016). For both ASD and ADHD, the frameworks that have been developed, which see the disorders as being on a continuum and blending into variation in the general population, suggest that the pattern seen Fig. 10.6c might apply. In the normative modelling approach, the variation seen in a large sample of the general population is studied, and individuals at the extreme of the range are identified. Marquand et al. (2016) suggest that

> Normative modeling provides a natural framework to study disorders at the individual participant level without dichotomizing the cohort. Instead, disease can be considered as an extreme of the normal range or as—possibly idiosyncratic—deviation from normal functioning. It also enables inferences over the degree to which behavioral variables, including diagnostic labels, map onto biology. (Marquand et al., 2016, p. 552)

Zabihi et al. (2019) used the normative modelling to investigate deviations from a typical pattern of neuroanatomical development in those with ASD and concluded that "individuals with ASD show distinct, highly individualised trajectories of brain development" (p. 567).

The approaches to heterogeneity in ASD discussed so far have been based on parsing multivariate data using a variety of mathematical techniques. An alternative route to identifying heterogeneity has been developed based on genetics.

"Genetics First" Rather addressing heterogeneity from groupings of cognitive abilities or variation in behavioural or brain development, an alternative approach to heterogeneity in ASD based on biological differences is that of "genetics-first". This approach starts with the known heterogeneity in genetic variants such copy number variants (CNV) associated with ASD (see Sect. 10.3). Chawner et al. (2021) used these differences to examine whether there was heterogeneity in ASD presentation that was related to these CNVs. Based on a number of international consortia, participants were identified as being in one of 4 CNV groups. These CNV groups differed in the rate of associated ASD ranging between 23% (22q11.2 deletion) and 58% (16p11.2 duplication). There were group differences between the CNVs in several aspects of the autism phenotype, including autism symptom severity, symptom domain profile, and cognitive profile, but only 1%–21% of the variance is explained by genetic variant group, depending on the autism trait. These results suggest that there is no simple one-to-one relationship between the type of genetic variant and the ASD phenotype. Rather, the ASD profiles are distinct but overlapping. Chawner et al. (2021) draw attention to the issue of those with the genetic variants that do not show the full ASD profile but may still have clinically significant symptoms. These individuals are unlikely to receive suitable support.

There are a number of outstanding questions, including which genetic and environmental factors account for phenotypic variation within the genetic variant groups. There are also the unresolved issues of how the same CNV can lead to different neurodevelopmental disorders and the same neurodevelopmental disorder can be influenced by different CNVs (Silva et al., 2022). There is some evidence that delays in expressive language and gross motor development might be indicators of the distinctive developmental trajectories of different genetic variants leading to ASD (Wickstrom et al., 2021).

Heterogeneity in ADHD The complexities in dealing with the heterogeneity of possible causal factors and patterns of deficits in ADHD have been laid out by Nigg et al. (2020). The *first* approach to these problems is to identify distinct sub-groups of children with ADHD. The same methods for identifying subgroups in ASD have been employed in studies of ADHD.

Pattern Classification Arnett et al. (2013) used DFA to address the question of whether there were features of development and behaviour in the first years of life that could predict high levels of ADHD symptoms at 8–9 years of age in a sample of 1106 from the general population. They found that such a prediction from a DFA could be made based on cognitive and behavioural measures obtained before the age of 2 years. However, the accuracy of the prediction was not sufficient to warrant routine screening for early risks with the measurers currently available.

Stratification – Latent Class Analysis Latent class analysis was used by Lambek et al. (2018) to investigate a dual route model of ADHD. This proposes that ADHD can arise from delay aversion and from executive function deficits, and a battery of measures testing these routes was subjected to a latent profile analysis (a form of latent class analysis). They found that the measures could be accounted for by three factors in a CFA – two reflecting EF (working memory/inhibition and shifting) and a delay aversion factor. As would be expected, the two EF factors were correlated ($r = 0.65$). However, the delay aversion factor was also correlated with the EF factors ($r = 0.55$ and $r = 0.43$). Despite this at least partial dissociation, they were unable to identify distinct sub-groups based on a latent profile analysis of the EF and delay aversion scores, suggesting that there are not distinct sub-groups of children with ADHD based on the dual route model.

Stratification – Network Analysis A community detection algorithm can be used to identify clusters within a network (see Sect. 2.6), in this case a network of individuals (not symptoms). The algorithm identifies sub-groups that are similar to one another and that are distant from other sub-groups. Fair et al. (2012) provide an illustration of community detection applied to neuropsychological function in children with ADHD and to TD children. The study was undertaken as proof of principle to demonstrate the potential of the methods to uncover details of the heterogeneity of ADHD. The sub-groups had the following characteristics. One had suggestions of altered visual processing mechanisms and another altered attention mechanism. There was also evidence of a sub-group that showed atypicality in both systems. These findings need to be treated with caution and require replication in a larger sample. A partial replication was obtained in a study that identified three subgroups – poor inhibitory control, poor set-shifting/speed, and intact task performance (Roberts et al., 2017).

Stratification – Cluster Analysis Roberts et al. (2017) used cluster analysis to group children with ADHD into three clusters based on EF test performance. The groups were characterised by poor set-shifting/speed, poor inhibitory control, and relatively intact task performance. Importantly, they were able to validate the distinction between the clusters with reference to other disruptive behaviour and anxiety/mood symptoms, as well as intelligence and academic achievement.

Morris et al. (2023) used a similar cluster analysis approach but with based on measures of parasympathetic and sympathetic functioning. These divisions of the autonomic nervous system are characterised as follows:

> The parasympathetic nervous system (PNS) is one of the two functionally distinct and continuously active divisions of the autonomic nervous system (ANS). It is in opposition to the other, the sympathetic nervous system (SNS). The parasympathetic nervous system predominates in quiet "rest and digest" conditions while the sympathetic nervous system drives the "fight or flight" response in stressful situations. The main purpose of the PNS is to conserve energy to be used later and to regulate bodily functions like digestion and urination. (Tindle & Tadi, 2023, p. 1)

Morris et al. (2023) proposed the functioning of these aspects of the autonomic nervous system as a source of heterogeneity in ADHD based on the temperament model proposed by Nigg (2006). Measures were taken whilst the child completed an emotion-based task. Respiratory sinus arrhythmia was used as an index of parasympathetic activity (emotion regulation), and electrodermal activity (skin conductance) indicated sympathetic activity (arousal). A k-means cluster analysis (see Sect. 2.3) identified three biological profiles differing in regulation and arousal levels among the children with ADHD. These profile were: Profile 1 – underregulated, hyperaroused (negative contexts only), Profile 2 – typically regulated, underaroused, and Profile 3 – overregulated (positive contexts only).

Morris et al. (2023) speculated that those with ADHD in each of these prolife groups may vary in their response to behavioural and pharmacological treatments. For example, those in Profile 2 may benefit more from methylphenidate treatment as this has been shown to increase autonomic nervous system activity, and those in Profile 3 may benefit more from reward-based behavioural interventions.

Stratification – Normative Modelling Marquand et al. (2016) used normative modelling to study the brain activity in a general population sample of young adults. They mapped the range of normal variation in functional MRI reward-related brain responses to a gambling task. They were able to identify participants with the extreme of normal variation in brain activity that merges with the general population. The extent of this deviance was then related to ADHD symptoms. However, in addition, there were individuals more idiosyncratic in their brain responses. An additional feature of these results was that the normative brain activity model related well to individual differences in hyperactivity but not to variation in inattention. Marquand et al. (2016) summarised their findings as follows:

> We identified two distinct mechanisms through which participants have high hyperactivity: participants either fit the normative model well, suggesting they are at the extreme of a normal axis of variation, or showed patterns of abnormality that were highly individualized but still meaningfully related to symptoms. These reflect a convergence of different biological mechanisms on the same symptoms. In other words, the extreme clinical phenotype is characterized by mechanistic heterogeneity, which is a key feature of many psychiatric disorders, including ADHD. We also showed domain specificity because the degree of abnormality correlated with hyperactivity but not inattention. (Marquand et al., 2016, p. 559)

A subsequent study by this same group (Wolfers et al., 2020) showed that when the brain volumes of a sample of young adults with persistent ADHD were compared to a healthy sample in terms of mean values, there were significantly reduced grey matter in the cerebellum and hippocampus in those with ADHD. However, when normative modelling was applied, there was substantial inter-individual variation in brain volumes in the group with ADHD. They conclude that studies based on case–control comparison alone will fail to capture the important biological features of individuals, which may be key to the development of precision medicine for those with ADHD.

Precision Medicine Precision medicine is the notion that treatment can be tailored to the specific underlying cause of the condition in the patient (Posner, 2018). There are some initial steps in this direction in the treatment of ADHD. Although methylphenidate is a successful treatment for ADHD (Cortese et al., 2018), there may be 35% of patients that do not respond to methylphenidate treatment, and their characteristics are poorly understood, and non-response is difficult to predict (Hodgkins et al., 2012). It may be possible to use brain imaging to predict treatment response. Norman et al. (2021) found that better treatment responses were associated with a stable level of resting-sate connectivity shown in fMRI between nodes of the cingulo-opercular network during childhood and adolescence, whereas worse responses were associated with increased connectivity with increasing age.

A *second* approach to identity heterogeneity in ADHD is to identify distinct neurobiological pathways underlying the ADHD phenotype.

This approach was adopted in a set of studies on a large sample of children with ADHD and their siblings, and a control sample of sibling pairs without ADHD (e.g. Cheung et al., 2016; Kuntsi et al., 2010; Michelini et al., 2021). These studies applied measures of ADHD symptomology, neuropsychological tests and neurophysiological measures (electroencephalography and event-related potentials). The study design provides the possibility of estimating familial influences but it cannot separate the effects of genetic factors from that of the shared environment. Kuntsi et al. (2010) identified two familial factors. One reflected mean reaction time and reaction time variability, these being influenced by sub-cortical dysfunction and are the prime familial influence on ADHD behaviours. The second reflected executive control, which is influenced by prefrontal cortex functions.

The role of these factors (response variability and executive functions) in influencing the course of ADHD was tested by Cheung et al. (2016). They found that response variability was a marker of remission of ADHD, that low IQ was a potential moderator of ADHD outcome, and that executive function processes were not significantly associated with ADHD outcome in adolescence. Michelini et al. (2021) studied older sibling pairs aged 11–27 years. In these older participants they found three partially separable etiological pathways leading to cognitive-neurophysiological impairments in pubertal and adult ADHD.

> The familial processes underlying both slower and more variable RTs and lower IQ in adolescents and young adults with ADHD may be partially distinct from familial influences on memory dysfunction and on impairments in sustained attention and brain activity of inhibitory/error-detection processes. These partially distinct etiological pathways may underlie dysfunctional brain networks, which are, in turn, associated with impaired cognition and behaviour in the disorder. (Michelini et al., 2021, p. 100)

The research on heterogeneity in ADHD has been summarised by Nigg et al. (2020). They suggest that progress has been made towards identifying a temperament profile of emotional dysregulation as a sub-type of ADHD and that sub-grouping based on cognitive profiles may prove useful in planning treatment. Findings such as these led Nigg et al. (2020) to be optimistic that the problems of heterogeneity in ADHD can be solved:

> Overall, the future is bright. The problem of creating neurobiologically and clinically superior nosology to reduce ADHD heterogeneity is becoming tractable. (Nigg et al., 2020, p. 734)

10.9 State of Play in the Study of Developmental Psychopathology

In 1974, developmental psychopathology was described as "…a field that hardly exists yet" (Achenbach, 1974,p. 3). Ten years later, it was designated an "emergent" discipline by Sroufe and Rutter in their landmark 1984 paper (p. 18). In reviewing the progress made in the subsequent 30 years, Rutter clarified that in his view developmental psychopathology

> ... is not a theory and it is not a discipline. It is not a theory because it does not propose an overall explanatory account. It is not a discipline because it does not refer to a definable body of knowledge, and it does not involve a single profession. Rather, it constitutes a conceptualization that leads to crucial questions on continuities and discontinuities and which is dedicated to the discovery of mediating mechanisms. (Rutter, 2013, p. 1210)

In a companion paper, Sroufe (2013) concludes that

> We have learned much about brain development, gene expression and its relation to experience, and the role of early experience. (Sroufe, 2013, p. 1222)

Indeed, these areas have features centrally in the studies reported in this book – brain development, genes as a biological basis for development, the role of experiences, and environmental exposures, but perhaps most crucially the interplay between genetic differences and the environment in influencing behavioural variation.

There are now attempts to provide integrated models of the development of this interplay. For example, building on the theoretical insights relating to gene–environment correlation and interaction (Plomin et al., 1977) and the notion of the "nature of nurture" (Plomin & Bergeman, 1991), a gene–environment cascade theory of developmental psychopathology has been proposed by Elam et al. (2023). They suggest that:

> …genetic predisposition for psychopathology, as well as stable traits and behaviors, can lead to negative environments via gene-environment correlations that can be exacerbated or buffered by an individual's social information processing. Moreover, these "environments" range from dyadic social relationships to broader sociocultural contexts. Over time, these processes exacerbate one another as part of developmental cascades, resulting in accumulating risk for psychopathology. (Elam et al., 2023, p. 287)

Elam et al. (2023) proposed that through developmental periods, the succession of passive r_{GE}, evocative r_{GE}, and active r_{GE} leads to differentiation into the experience of negative environments ranging from the narrow (e.g. social relationships) to the broad (e.g. cultural processes). An example of these cultural processes is the way temperament styles are evaluated differently in various cultures (Super et al., 2008).

A second example of an integrated model of gene–environment interplay is that of Nigg (2023). He places an emphasis on the role of epigenetics (defined broadly to refer to any biological mechanism that modifies the expression of genes) as providing one common pathway via which a range of gene and environmental converge to influence a range of psychopathologies.

There has been a step-change in the use of information on genetic risk in the analysis of the interplay between genes and the environment to study developmental psychopathology. This has come about as a result of enhanced data analysis methods (Evans et al., 2021), theoretical insights into routes whereby genes can have their effects (e.g. genetic nurture, Kong et al. (2018)), the incorporation of causal modelling concepts into the analysis of intergenerational transmission data (Frach et al., 2023), the development of microarrays that can genotype thousands of genes to provide polygenetic risk scores (e.g. Allegrini et al., 2022) and by the application of structural equation modelling to molecular genetic data (e.g. Genomic SEM (Grotzinger et al., 2019)).

A key component has been the application of PRS derived from GWAS to study gene–environment interplay. These have been widely employed in studies in developmental psychopathology, but there are caveats over their application. Barker et al. (2022) identify three aspects of the science that are problematic. The first is that PRS are usually based on gene–behaviour relationships derived from GWAS on samples of adults. It is known that the genetic influences on phenotypes can change with age and that the PRS derived from adults may be less accurate predictors of behaviour in children and adolescents. The second is that the discovery GWAS, on which the gene–behaviour relationships are estimated, require very large samples and are often based on pooling data from disparate samples from different countries. The measurement of behaviour for these samples may vary, and the pooling of data across studies may result in an aggregated index of behaviour of uncertain validity and reliability. The third is that when measures of the environment are employed, these may be under considerable genetic influence. When then applied in models with PRS estimates, spurious gene–environment associations may thereby be created. The fourth limitation of PRS is that they are estimated on the overall risk of genetic differences being related to an outcome (e.g. ADHD). In studies of gene–environment interaction, these PRS may not capture the vulnerability to environmental exposures. To achieve, this requires GWAS to have more extensive and refined measures of these environmental exposures.

A further limitation of PRS studies is that they are based on samples of unrelated individuals; this is necessary to avoid confounds from shared environmental influences. They are also based on a model of additive effects of common genetic variants. This leads to gaps in knowledge such as missing heritability and in understanding the mechanisms of the transmission of genetic effects. Cheesman et al. (2023) have shown how these problems can at least be partially overcome by integrating DNA based indicators, such as PRS, with the quantitative genetic analysis of data form related individuals in families.

The state of play in genetic research has been summarised as follows:

> A substantial and growing body of genetic research has begun to elucidate the underlying structure of psychopathology. Before the modern era of genomic research, family and twin studies demonstrated that all major psychiatric disorders aggregate in families and are heritable. Over the past decade, the success of large-scale genomic studies has confirmed several key principles: (1) psychiatric disorders are highly polygenic, reflecting the contribution of hundreds to thousands of common variants of small effect and rare (often de novo) SNVs and CNVs (2) genetic influences on psychopathology commonly transcend the diagnostic boundaries of our clinical DSM nosology. At the level of genetic etiology, there are no sharp boundaries between diagnostic categories or between disorder and normal variation. In the coming years, ever-larger studies incorporating DNA sequencing, environmental exposures, and phenome-wide analyses will facilitate a more granular understanding of the genetic etiology and phenotypic spectrum of mental illness. (Smoller et al., 2019, p. 417)

However, a systematic review of research on biomarkers for neurodevelopmental disorders came to the sobering conclusions that *none* of those markers (including gene variants) investigated in the 780 studies, that met their inclusion criteria, showed adequate sensitivity and specificity for use as diagnostic indicators for ASD or ADHD (Cortese et al., 2023). There has also been little advance in our understanding of just which genes and their combined action influences behavioural variation. Indeed, the complexity of investigating the way genes may influence the expression of other genes has barely been broached. This includes the question of epistasis or gene–gene interaction. For example, to date, studies developing PRS largely have been based on the assumption that the effects of genes are additive, not interactive (Brandes et al., 2022). The importance of adopting an emergent systems approach to address this question was emphasised by Flint et al. (2020):

> Single genes do not specify a behaviour, but in combination with each other and with the environment they may.

> ...it may be more appropriate to examine genes in networks and assign function to combination of genes, rather than to individual entities. (Flint et al., 2020, p. 280)

The same emergent systems orientation is needed in the examination of environmental influences in the exposome – this term has been defined as follows:

> the cumulative measure of environmental influences and associated biological responses throughout the lifespan, including exposures from the environment, diet, behavior, and endogenous processes. (Miller & Jones, 2014, p. 2)

The exposome measure attempts to capture the totality of exposures in a lifetime from conception onward. It aims to provide an environmental complement to the measurement of genetic risk (Guloksuz et al., 2018).

The next step is to integrate an understanding of these networks of genetic and environmental influences. An indication of how such a research programme might develop is given by the findings presented by Choi et al. (2022). They suggest that

> In this study, we applied advanced statistical genetics methods in a longitudinal cohort of preadolescent youth to address fundamental questions about the role of 'nature and nurture' in developmental psychopathology. Because of our ability to explicitly model joint genomic and exposomic effects as well as their potential interactions, this represents to our knowledge the most comprehensive decomposition to date of genetic and environmental influences on mental health in youth using molecular genetic data. Choi et al. (2022) p. 5.

The situation has now been reached where aggregates can be used to estimate the risk of behaviour and emotional problems based on genetic influences, brain structure variants, and environmental factors (e.g. ACEs). This is valuable for prediction and general frameworks for understanding the interactions of influences. These aggregate risk indicators can identify individuals that might benefit from preventive interventions but do not, as yet, give insight into specific mechanisms that might provide a basis for developing effective treatments (Derks et al., 2022).

> While a translational science of child psychiatric genetics may be currently no more than a distant dream, it is essential that practitioners remain informed about progress in this vital field. Maughan and Sonuga-Barke (2014)

The "distant dream" identified in the above quote might still be distant some 10 years later. However, what has emerged over the past decade is the realisation that by combining findings from molecular genetic studies, for example PRS, with quantitative genetic designs such as twin and family studies, insights can be gained into the causal role of social experiences and environmental exposures in influencing individual differences in behaviour. So, somewhat paradoxically, the progress made in genetics has resulted in advances in our understanding of the place of the environment in gene–environment interplay as an influence on developmental psychopathology.

References

Achenbach, T. M. (1974). *Developmental psychopathology*. Ronald Press.

Ajram, L. A., Horder, J., Mendez, M. A., Galanopoulos, A., Brennan, L. P., Wichers, R. H., et al. (2017). Shifting brain inhibitory balance and connectivity of the prefrontal cortex of adults with autism spectrum disorder. *Translational Psychiatry, 7*, e1137. https://doi.org/10.1038/tp.2017.104

Allegrini, A. G., Baldwin, J. R., Barkhuizen, W., & Pingault, J.-B. (2022). Research review: A guide to computing and implementing polygenic scores in developmental research. *Journal of Child Psychology and Psychiatry, 63*, 1111–1124. https://doi.org/10.1111/jcpp.13611

Anand, N. S., Ji, Y. L., Wang, G. Y., Hong, X. M., van der Rijn, M., Riley, A., et al. (2021). Maternal and cord plasma branched-chain amino acids and child risk of attention-deficit hyperactivity disorder: a prospective birth cohort study. *Journal of Child Psychology and Psychiatry, 62*(7), 868–875. https://doi.org/10.1111/jcpp.13332

Antshel, K. M., & Russo, N. (2019). Autism spectrum disorders and ADHD: Overlapping phenomenology, diagnostic issues, and treatment considerations. *Current Psychiatry Reports, 21*(5), Article 34. https://doi.org/10.1007/s11920-019-1020-5

Aoki, Y., Yoncheva, Y. N., Chen, B., Nath, T., Sharp, D., Lazar, M., et al. (2017). Association of white matter structure with autism spectrum disorder and attention-deficit/hyperactivity disorder. *Jama Psychiatry, 74*(11), 1120–1128. https://doi.org/10.1001/jamapsychiatry.2017.2573

APA. (2013). *Diagnostic and statistical manual* (5th ed.). American Psychiatric Association.

Arnett, A. B., MacDonald, B., & Pennington, B. F. (2013). Cognitive and behavioral indicators of ADHD symptoms prior to school age. *Journal of Child Psychology and Psychiatry, 54*(12), 1284–1294. https://doi.org/10.1111/jcpp.12104

Askeland, R. B., Hannigan, L. J., Ask, H., Ayorech, Z., Tesli, M., Corfield, E., et al. (2022). Early manifestations of genetic risk for neurodevelopmental disorders. *Journal of Child Psychology and Psychiatry, 63*(7), 810–819. https://doi.org/10.1111/jcpp.13528

Astenvald, R., Frick, M. A., Neufeld, J., Bolte, S., & Isaksson, J. (2022). Emotion dysregulation in ADHD and other neurodevelopmental conditions: a co-twin control study. *Child and Adolescent Psychiatry and Mental Health, 16*(1). https://doi.org/10.1186/s13034-022-00528-0

Baribeau, D., Vorstman, J., & Anagnostou, E. (2022). Novel treatments in autism spectrum disorder. *Current Opinion in Psychiatry, 35*(2), 101–110. https://doi.org/10.1097/yco.0000000000000775

Barker, E. D., Maughan, B., Allegrini, A., Pingault, J. B., & Sonuga-Barke, E. (2022). Editorial: Does the polygenic revolution herald a watershed in the study of GE interplay in developmental psychopathology? Some considerations for the Special Issue reader. *Journal of Child Psychology and Psychiatry, 63*(10), 1107–1110. https://doi.org/10.1111/jcpp.13692

Baron-Cohen, S. (2002). The extreme male brain theory of autism. *Trends in Cognitive Sciences, 6*(6), 248–254. https://doi.org/10.1016/s1364-6613(02)01904-6

Baron-Cohen, S., Leslie, A. M., & Frith, U. (1985). Does the autistic-child have a theory of mind. *Cognition, 21*(1), 37–46. https://doi.org/10.1016/0010-0277(85)90022-8

Baron-Cohen, S., Wheelwright, S., Skinner, R., Martin, J., & Clubley, E. (2001). The Autism-Spectrum Quotient (AQ): Evidence from Asperger syndrome/high-functioning autism, males and females, scientists and mathematicians. *Journal of Autism and Developmental Disorders, 31*(1), 5–17. https://doi.org/10.1023/a:1005653411471

Baron-Cohen, S., Ashwin, E., Ashwin, C., Tavassoli, T., & Chakrabarti, B. (2009). Talent in autism: Hyper-systemizing, hyper-attention to detail and sensory hypersensitivity. *Philosophical Transactions of the Royal Society B-Biological Sciences, 364*(1522), 1377–1383. https://doi.org/10.1098/rstb.2008.0337

Baxter, A. J., Brugha, T. S., Erskine, H. E., Scheurer, R. W., Vos, T., & Scott, J. G. (2015). The epidemiology and global burden of autism spectrum disorders. *Psychological Medicine, 45*(3), 601–613. https://doi.org/10.1017/s003329171400172x

Bernard, S., Enayati, A., Redwood, L., Roger, H., & Binstock, T. (2001). Autism: A novel form of mercury poisoning. *Medical Hypotheses, 56*(4), 462–471. https://doi.org/10.1054/mehy.2000.1281

Bethlehem, R. A. I., Romero-Garcia, R., Mak, E., Bullmore, E. T., & Baron-Cohen, S. (2017). Structural covariance networks in children with autism or ADHD. *Cerebral Cortex, 27*(8), 4267–4276. https://doi.org/10.1093/cercor/bhx135

Bettelheim, B. (1967). *The empty fortress: Infantile autism and the birth of self.* The Free Press.

Bishop, D. V. M., & Swendsen, J. (2021). Psychoanalysis in the treatment of autism: Why is France a cultural outlier? *Bjpsych Bulletin, 45*(2), 89–93. https://doi.org/10.1192/bjb.2020.138

Boedhoe, P. S. W., van Rooij, D., Hoogman, M., Twisk, J. W. R., Schmaal, L., Abe, Y., et al. (2020). Subcortical brain volume, regional cortical thickness, and cortical surface area across disorders: Findings from the ENIGMA ADHD, ASD, and OCD Working Groups. *American Journal of Psychiatry, 177*(9), 834–843. https://doi.org/10.1176/appi.ajp.2020.19030331

Bolton, P. F. (2009). Medical conditions in autism spectrum disorders. *Journal of Neurodevelopmental Disorders, 1*(2), 102–113. https://doi.org/10.1007/s11689-009-9021-z

Bolton, P., Macdonald, H., Pickles, A., Rios, P., Goode, S., Crowson, M., et al. (1994). A case – control family history study of autism. *Journal of Child Psychology and Psychiatry, 35*(5), 877–900. https://doi.org/10.1111/j.1469-7610.1994.tb02300.x

Bonnet-Brilhault, F., Alirol, S., Blanc, R., Bazaud, S., Marouillat, S., Thepault, R. A., et al. (2016). GABA/Glutamate synaptic pathways targeted by integrative genomic and electrophysiological explorations distinguish autism from intellectual disability. *Molecular Psychiatry, 21*(3), 411–418. https://doi.org/10.1038/mp.2015.75

Booth, R. D. L., & Happé, F. G. E. (2018). Evidence of reduced global processing in Autism Spectrum Disorder. *Journal of Autism and Developmental Disorders, 48*(4), 1397–1408. https://doi.org/10.1007/s10803-016-2724-6

Bora, E., & Pantelis, C. (2016). Meta-analysis of social cognition in attention-deficit/hyperactivity disorder (ADHD): comparison with healthy controls and autistic spectrum disorder. *Psychological Medicine, 46*(4), 699–716. https://doi.org/10.1017/s0033291715002573

Bralten, J., van Hulzen, K. J., Martens, M. B., Galesloot, T. E., Vasquez, A. A., Kiemeney, L. A., et al. (2018). Autism spectrum disorders and autistic traits share genetics and biology. *Molecular Psychiatry, 23*(5), 1205–1212. https://doi.org/10.1038/mp.2017.98

Brandes, N., Weissbrod, O., & Linial, M. (2022). Open problems in human trait genetics. *Genome Biology, 23*(1). https://doi.org/10.1186/s13059-022-02697-9

Brereton, A. V., Tonge, B. J., & Einfeld, S. L. (2006). Psychopathology in children and adolescents with autism compared to young people with intellectual disability. *Journal of Autism and Developmental Disorders, 36*(7), 863–870. https://doi.org/10.1007/s10803-006-0125-y

Brugha, T. S., Spiers, N., Bankart, J., Cooper, S. A., McManus, S., Scott, F. J., et al. (2016). Epidemiology of autism in adults across age groups and ability levels. *British Journal of Psychiatry, 209*(6), 498–503. https://doi.org/10.1192/bjp.bp.115.174649

Brunsdon, V. E. A., & Happé, F. (2014). Exploring the 'fractionation' of autism at the cognitive level. *Autism, 18*(1), 17–30. https://doi.org/10.1177/1362361313499456

Bubb, E. J., Metzler-Baddeley, C., & Aggleton, J. P. (2018). The cingulum bundle: Anatomy, function, and dysfunction. *Neuroscience and Biobehavioral Reviews, 92*, 104–127. https://doi.org/10.1016/j.neubiorev.2018.05.008

Bussing, R., Fernandez, M., Harwood, M., Hou, W., Garvan, C. W., Eyberg, S. M., & Swanson, J. M. (2008). Parent and teacher SNAP-IV ratings of attention deficit hyperactivity disorder symptoms – Psychometric properties and normative ratings from a school district sample. *Assessment, 15*(3), 317–328. https://doi.org/10.1177/1073191107313888

Casseus, M. (2022). Prevalence of co-occurring autism spectrum disorder and attention deficit/hyperactivity disorder among children in the United States. *Autism, 26*(6), 1591–1597. https://doi.org/10.1177/13623613221083279

Casseus, M., Kim, W. J., & Horton, D. B. B. (2023). Prevalence and treatment of mental, behavioral, and developmental disorders in children with co-occurring autism spectrum disorder and

attention-deficit/hyperactivity disorder: A population-based study. *Autism Research.* https://doi.org/10.1002/aur.2894
Catalá-López, F., Hutton, B., Page, M. J., Driver, J. A., Ridao, M., Alonso-Arroyo, A., et al. (2022). Mortality in persons with Autism Spectrum Disorder or Attention-Deficit/Hyperactivity Disorder – A systematic review and meta-analysis. *JAMA Pediatrics, 176*(4). https://doi.org/10.1001/jamapediatrics.2021.6401
Charman, T. (2019). Editorial: Trials and tribulations in early autism intervention research. *Journal of the American Academy of Child and Adolescent Psychiatry, 58*(9), 846–848. https://doi.org/10.1016/j.jaac.2019.03.004
Charman, T. (2021). Editorial: One good thing (sometimes) leads to another: Demonstrating mechanistic connections between parent and child outcomes in a community implementation autism trial. *Journal of the American Academy of Child and Adolescent Psychiatry, 60*(3), 338–339. https://doi.org/10.1016/j.jaac.2020.12.005
Chawner, S., Doherty, J. L., Anney, R. J. L., Antshel, K. M., Bearden, C. E., Bernier, R., et al. (2021). A genetics-first approach to dissecting the heterogeneity of autism: Phenotypic comparison of autism risk copy number variants. *American Journal of Psychiatry, 178*(1), 77–86. https://doi.org/10.1176/appi.ajp.2020.20010015
Che, X. Y., Hornig, M., Bresnahan, M., Stoltenberg, C., Magnus, P., Suren, P., et al. (2022). Maternal mid-gestational and child cord blood immune signatures are strongly associated with offspring risk of ASD. *Molecular psychiatry, 27*(3), 1527–1541. https://doi.org/10.1038/s41380-021-01415-4
Cheesman, R., Ayorech, Z., Eilertsen, E. M., & Ystrom, E. (2023). Why we need families in genomic research on developmental psychopathology. *JCPP Advances, 3*(1), e12138. https://doi.org/10.1002/jcv2.12138
Chen, H., Duan, X., Liu, F., Lu, F., Ma, X., Zhang, Y., et al. (2016a). Multivariate classification of autism spectrum disorder using frequency-specific resting-state functional connectivity-A multi-center study. *Progress in Neuro-Psychopharmacology & Biological Psychiatry, 64*, 1–9. https://doi.org/10.1016/j.pnpbp.2015.06.014
Chen, S. W., Zhong, X. S., Jiang, L. N., Zheng, X. Y., Xiong, Y. Q., Ma, S. J., et al. (2016b). Maternal autoimmune diseases and the risk of autism spectrum disorders in offspring: A systematic review and meta-analysis. *Behavioural Brain Research, 296*, 61–69. https://doi.org/10.1016/j.bbr.2015.08.035
Chesnut, S. R., Wei, T. L., Barnard-Brak, L., & Richman, D. M. (2017). A meta-analysis of the social communication questionnaire: Screening for autism spectrum disorder. *Autism, 21*(8), 920–928. https://doi.org/10.1177/1362361316660065
Chess, S. (1971). Autism in children with congenital rubella. *Journal of Autism and Childhood Schizophrenia, 1*(1), 33–47. https://doi.org/10.1007/bf01537741
Cheung, C. H. M., Rijsdijk, F., McLoughlin, G., Brandeis, D., Banaschewski, T., Asherson, P., & Kuntsi, J. (2016). Cognitive and neurophysiological markers of ADHD persistence and remission. *British Journal of Psychiatry, 208*(6), 548. https://doi.org/10.1192/bjp.bp.114.145185
Choi, K. W., Wilson, M., Ge, T., Kandola, A., Patel, C. J., Lee, S. H., & Smoller, J. W. (2022). Integrative analysis of genomic and exposomic inlfuences on youth mental health. *Journal of Child Psychology and Psychiatry, 63*(10), 1196–1205. https://doi.org/10.1111/jcpp.13664
Chun, H., Leung, C., Wen, S. W., McDonald, J., & Shin, H. H. (2020). Maternal exposure to air pollution and risk of autism in children: A systematic review and meta-analysis. *Environmental Pollution, 256*. https://doi.org/10.1016/j.envpol.2019.113307
Cirnigliaro, M., Chang, T. S., Arteaga, S. A., Perez-Cano, L., Ruzzo, E. K., Gordon, A., et al. (2023). The contributions of rare inherited and polygenic risk to ASD in multiplex families. *Proceedings of the National Academy of Sciences of the United States of America, 120*(31), e2215632120. https://doi.org/10.1073/pnas.2215632120
Colvert, E., Tick, B., McEwen, F., Stewart, C., Curran, S. R., Woodhouse, E., et al. (2015). Heritability of autism spectrum disorder in a UK population-based twin sample. *Jama Psychiatry, 72*(5), 415–423. https://doi.org/10.1001/jamapsychiatry.2014.3028

Constantino, J. N., & Charman, T. (2016). Diagnosis of autism spectrum disorder: Reconciling the syndrome, its diverse origins, and variation in expression. *Lancet Neurology, 15*(3), 279–291. https://doi.org/10.1016/s1474-4422(15)00151-9

Cortese, S., Adamo, N., Del Giovane, C., Mohr-Jensen, C., Hayes, A. J., Carucci, S., et al. (2018). Comparative efficacy and tolerability of medications for attention-deficit hyperactivity disorder in children, adolescents, and adults: A systematic review and network meta-analysis. *Lancet Psychiatry, 5*(9), 727–738. https://doi.org/10.1016/s2215-0366(18)30269-4

Cortese, S., Solmi, M., Michelini, G., Bellato, A., Blanner, C., Canozzi, A., et al. (2023). Candidate diagnostic biomarkers for neurodevelopmental disorders in children and adolescents: A systematic review. *World Psychiatry: Official Journal of the World Psychiatric Association (WPA), 22*(1), 129–149. https://doi.org/10.1002/wps.21037

Crafa, D., & Warfa, N. (2015). Maternal migration and autism risk: Systematic analysis. *International Review of Psychiatry, 27*(1), 64–71. https://doi.org/10.3109/09540261.2014.995601

Cryan, J. F., O'Riordan, K. J., Cowan, C. S. M., Sandhu, K. V., Bastiaanssen, T. F. S., Boehme, M., et al. (2019). The microbiota-gut-brain-axis. *Physiological Reviews, 99*(4), 1877–2013. https://doi.org/10.1152/physrev.00018.2018

Curran, E. A., O'Neill, S. M., Cryan, J. F., Kenny, L. C., Dinan, T. G., Khashan, A. S., & Kearney, P. M. (2015). Research Review: Birth by caesarean section and development of autism spectrum disorder and attention-deficit/hyperactivity disorder: A systematic review and meta-analysis. *Journal of Child Psychology and Psychiatry, 56*(5), 500–508. https://doi.org/10.1111/jcpp.12351

de la Torre-Ubieta, L., Won, H. J., Stein, J. L., & Geschwind, D. H. (2016). Advancing the understanding of autism disease mechanisms through genetics. *Nature Medicine, 22*(4), 345–361. https://doi.org/10.1038/nm.4071

Derks, E. M., Thorp, J. G., & Gerring, Z. F. (2022). Ten challenges for clinical translation in psychiatric genetics. *Nature Genetics, 54*(10), 1457–1465. https://doi.org/10.1038/s41588-02201174-0

Di Martino, A., Yan, C. G., Li, Q., Denio, E., Castellanos, F. X., Alaerts, K., et al. (2014). The autism brain imaging data exchange: Towards a large-scale evaluation of the intrinsic brain architecture in autism. *Molecular Psychiatry, 19*(6), 659–667. https://doi.org/10.1038/mp.2013.78

Donvan, J., & Zucker, C. (2017). *In a different key: the story of autism.* Penguin. ISBN: 9780241958179.

Duffy, F. H., & Als, H. (2019). Autism, spectrum or clusters? An EEG coherence study. *BMC Neurology, 19*(1), 27. https://doi.org/10.1186/s12883-019-1254-1

Durkin, M. S., Elsabbagh, M., Barbaro, J., Gladstone, M., Happe, F., Hoekstra, R. A., et al. (2015). Autism screening and diagnosis in low resource settings: Challenges and opportunities to enhance research and services worldwide. *Autism Research, 8*(5), 473–476. https://doi.org/10.1002/aur.1575

Dwyer, D., & Koutsouleris, N. (2022). Annual research review: Translational machine learning for child and adolescent psychiatry. *Journal of Child Psychology and Psychiatry, 63*(4), 421–443. https://doi.org/10.1111/jcpp.13545

Eagle, R. F., Romanczyk, R. G., & Lenzenweger, M. F. (2010). Classification of children with autism spectrum disorders: A finite mixture modeling approach to heterogeneity. *Research in Autism Spectrum Disorders, 4*(4), 772–781. https://doi.org/10.1016/j.rasd.2010.02.001

Easson, A. K., Fatima, Z., & McIntosh, A. R. (2019). Functional connectivity-based subtypes of individuals with and without autism spectrum disorder. *Network Neuroscience, 3*(2), 344–362. https://doi.org/10.1162/netn_a_00067

Elam, K. K., Lemery-Chalfant, K., & Chassin, L. (2023). A Gene-Environment cascade theoretical framework of developmental psychopathology. *Journal of Psychopathology and Clinical Science, 132*(3), 287–296. https://doi.org/10.1037/abn0000546

Elsabbagh, M., Divan, G., Koh, Y. J., Kim, Y. S., Kauchali, S., Marcin, C., et al. (2012). Global prevalence of autism and other pervasive developmental disorders. *Autism Research, 5*(3), 160–179. https://doi.org/10.1002/aur.239

England-Mason, G. (2020). Emotion regulation as a transdiagnostic feature in children with neurodevelopmental disorders. *Current Developmental Disorders Reports, 7*(3), 130–138. https://doi.org/10.1007/s40474-020-00200-2

Estes, M. L., & McAllister, A. K. (2015). Immune mediators in the brain and peripheral tissues in autism spectrum disorder. *Nature Reviews Neuroscience, 16*(8), 469–486. https://doi.org/10.1038/nrn3978

Evans, D. M., Medland, S. E., & Prom-Wormley, E. (2021). Introduction to the Special Issue on statistical genetic methods for human complex traits. *Behavior Genetics, 51*(3), 165–169. https://doi.org/10.1007/s10519-021-10057-9

Fair, D. A., Bathula, D., Nikolas, M. A., & Nigg, J. T. (2012). Distinct neuropsychological subgroups in typically developing youth inform heterogeneity in children with ADHD. *Proceedings of the National Academy of Sciences of the United States of America, 109*(17), 6769–6774. https://doi.org/10.1073/pnas.1115365109

Farhat, L. C., Brentani, H., de Toledo, V. H. C., Shephard, E., Mattos, P., Baron-Cohen, S., et al. (2022). ADHD and autism symptoms in youth: A network analysis. *Journal of Child Psychology and Psychiatry, 63*(2), 143–151. https://doi.org/10.1111/jcpp.13436

Feczko, E., Balba, N. M., Miranda-Dominguez, O., Cordova, M., Karalunas, S. L., Irwin, L., et al. (2018). Subtyping cognitive profiles in autism spectrum disorder using a functional random forest algorithm. *Neuroimage, 172*, 674–688. https://doi.org/10.1016/j.neuroimage.2017.12.044

Feczko, E., Miranda-Dominguez, O., Marr, M., Graham, A. M., Nigg, J. T., & Fair, D. A. (2019). The heterogeneity problem: Approaches to identify psychiatric subtypes. *Trends in Cognitive Sciences, 23*(7), 584–601. https://doi.org/10.1016/j.tics.2019.03.009

Ferri, S. L., Abel, T., & Brodkin, E. S. (2018). Sex differences in autism spectrum disorder: A review. *Current Psychiatry Reports, 20*(2). https://doi.org/10.1007/s11920-018-0874-2

Flint, J., Greenspan, R. J., & Kendler, K. S. (2020). *How genes influence behaviour* (2nd ed.). Oxford University Press.

Flores-Pajot, M. C., Ofner, M., Do, M. T., Lavigne, E., & Villeneuve, P. J. (2016). Childhood autism spectrum disorders and exposure to nitrogen dioxide, and particulate matter air pollution: A review and meta-analysis. *Environmental Research, 151*, 763–776. https://doi.org/10.1016/j.envres.2016.07.030

Folstein, S., & Rutter, M. (1977a). Genetic influences and infantile-autism. *Nature, 265*(5596), 726–728. https://doi.org/10.1038/265726a0

Folstein, S., & Rutter, M. (1977b). Infantile autism – Genetic study of 21 twin pairs. *Journal of Child Psychology and Psychiatry, 18*(4), 297–321. https://doi.org/10.1111/j.1469-7610.1977.tb00443.x

Foulkes, L., & Blakemore, S. J. (2018). Studying individual differences in human adolescent brain development. *Nature Neuroscience, 21*(3), 315–323. https://doi.org/10.1038/s41593-018-0078-4

Frach, L., Jami, E. S., McAdams, T. A., Dudbridge, F., & Pingault, J. B. (2023). Causal inference methods for intergenerational research using observational data. *Psychological Review*. https://doi.org/10.1037/rev0000419

Fraguas, D., Diaz-Caneja, C. M., Pina-Camacho, L., Moreno, C., Duran-Cutilla, M., Ayora, M., et al. (2019). Dietary interventions for Autism spectrum disorder: A meta-analysis. *Pediatrics, 144*(5). https://doi.org/10.1542/peds.2018-3218

Frith, U. (1989). *Autism: Explaining the enigma*. Blackwell.

Frith, U. (2012). The 38th Sir Frederick Bartlett Lecture why we need cognitive explanations of autism. *Quarterly Journal of Experimental Psychology, 65*(11), 2073–2092. https://doi.org/10.1080/17470218.2012.697178

Frith, U. (2019). Flux of life. *Developmental Cognitive Neuroscience, 38*. https://doi.org/10.1016/j.dcn.2019.100669

Frith, U., Morton, J., & Leslie, A. M. (1991). The cognitive basis of a biological disorder – Autism. *Trends in Neurosciences, 14*(10), 433–438. https://doi.org/10.1016/0166-2236(91)90041-r

Fuentes, J., Hervas, A., Howlin, P., & Party, E. A. W. (2021). ESCAP practice guidance for autism: A summary of evidence-based recommendations for diagnosis and treatment. *European Child and Adolescent Psychiatry, 30*(6), 961–984. https://doi.org/10.1007/s00787-020-01587-4

Gandal, M. J., Haney, J. R., Parikshak, N. N., Leppa, V., Ramaswami, G., Hartl, C., et al. (2018). Shared molecular neuropathology across major psychiatric disorders parallels polygenic overlap. *Science, 359*(6376), 693–697. https://doi.org/10.1126/science.aad6469

Gaugler, T., Klei, L., Sanders, S. J., Bodea, C. A., Goldberg, A. P., Lee, A. B., et al. (2014). Most genetic risk for autism resides with common variation. *Nature Genetics, 46*(8), 881–885. https://doi.org/10.1038/ng.3039

Ghirardi, L., Brikell, I., Kuja-Halkola, R., Freitag, C. M., Franke, B., Asherson, P., et al. (2018). The familial co-aggregation of ASD and ADHD: A register-based cohort study. *Molecular Psychiatry, 23*(2), 257–262. https://doi.org/10.1038/mp.2017.17

Ghirardi, L., Pettersson, E., Taylor, M. J., Freitag, C. M., Franke, B., Asherson, P., et al. (2019). Genetic and environmental contribution to the overlap between ADHD and ASD trait dimensions in young adults: A twin study. *Psychological Medicine, 49*(10), 1713–1721. https://doi.org/10.1017/s003329171800243x

Ghirardi, L., Kuja-Halkola, R., Butwicka, A., Martin, J., Larsson, H., D'Onofrio, B. M., et al. (2021). Familial and genetic associations between autism spectrum disorder and other neurodevelopmental and psychiatric disorders. *Journal of Child Psychology and Psychiatry, 62*(11), 1274–1284. https://doi.org/10.1111/jcpp.13508

Gidziela, A., Ahmadzadeh, Y. I., Michelini, G., Allegrini, A. G., Agnew-Blais, J., Lau, L. Y., et al. (2023). A meta-analysis of genetic effects associated with neurodevelopmental disorders and co-occurring conditions. *Nature Human Behaviour, 7*(4), 642–656. https://doi.org/10.1038/s41562-023-01530-y

Gilbert, R., Widom, C. S., Browne, K., Fergusson, D., Webb, E., & Janson, S. (2009). Child Maltreatment 1 Burden and consequences of child maltreatment in high-income countries. *Lancet, 373*(9657), 68–81. https://doi.org/10.1016/s0140-6736(08)61706-7

Golm, D., Maughan, B., Barker, E. D., Hill, J., Kennedy, M., Knights, N., et al. (2020). Why does early childhood deprivation increase the risk for depression and anxiety in adulthood? A developmental cascade model. *Journal of Child Psychology and Psychiatry, 61*(9), 1043–1053. https://doi.org/10.1111/jcpp.13205

Green, J., & Garg, S. (2018). Annual research review: The state of autism intervention science: Progress, target psychological and biological mechanisms and future prospects. *Journal of Child Psychology and Psychiatry, 59*(4), 424–443. https://doi.org/10.1111/jcpp.12892

Green, S. A., Hernandez, L., Bookheimer, S. Y., & Dapretto, M. (2016). Salience network connectivity in autism Is related to brain and behavioral markers of sensory overresponsivity. *Journal of the American Academy of Child and Adolescent Psychiatry, 55*(7), 618–626. https://doi.org/10.1016/j.jaac.2016.04.013

Green, J., Absoud, M., Grahame, V., Malik, O., Simonoff, E., Le Couteur, A., & Baird, G. (2018a). Pathological demand avoidance: symptoms but not a syndrome. *Lancet Child & Adolescent Health, 2*(6), 455–464. https://doi.org/10.1016/s2352-4642(18)30044-0

Green, J., Absoud, M., Grahame, V., Malik, O., Simonoff, E., Le Couteur, A., & Baird, G. (2018b). Demand avoidance is not necessarily defiance. *Lancet Child & Adolescent Health, 2*(9), E21–E21. https://doi.org/10.1016/s2352-4642(18)30221-9

Grimaldi, R., Gibson, G. R., Vulevic, J., Giallourou, N., Castro-Mejía, J. L., Hansen, L. H., et al. (2018). A prebiotic intervention study in children with autism spectrum disorders (ASDs). *Microbiome, 6*(1), 133. https://doi.org/10.1186/s40168-018-0523-3

Grotzinger, A. D., Rhemtulla, M., de Vlaming, R., Ritchie, S. J., Mallard, T. T., Hill, W. D., et al. (2019). Genomic structural equation modelling provides insights into the multivariate genetic architecture of complex traits. *Nature Human Behaviour, 3*(5), 513–525. https://doi.org/10.1038/s41562-019-0566-x

Grove, J., Ripke, S., Als, T. D., Mattheisen, M., Walters, R. K., Won, H., et al. (2019). Identification of common genetic risk variants for autism spectrum disorder. *Nature Genetics, 51*(3), 431. https://doi.org/10.1038/s41588-019-0344-8

Grzadzinski, R., Huerta, M., & Lord, C. (2013). DSM-5 and autism spectrum disorders (ASDs): an opportunity for identifying ASD subtypes. *Molecular Autism, 4*. https://doi.org/10.1186/2040-2392-4-12

Guloksuz, S., van Os, J., & Rutten, B. P. F. (2018). The exposome paradigm and the complexities of environmental research in psychiatry. *JAMA Psychiatry, 75*, 985–986.

Hallett, V., Ronald, A., Rijsdijk, F., & Happe, F. (2012). Disentangling the associations between autistic-Llke and internalizing traits: A community based twin study. *Journal of Abnormal Child Psychology, 40*(5), 815–827. https://doi.org/10.1007/s10802-011-9596-1

Han, V. X., Patel, S., Jones, H. F., Nielsen, T. C., Mohammad, S. S., Hofer, M. J., et al. (2021). Maternal acute and chronic inflammation in pregnancy is associated with common neurodevelopmental disorders: A systematic review. *Translational Psychiatry, 11*(1). https://doi.org/10.1038/s41398-021-01198-w

Happe, F. (2015). Autism as a neurodevelopmental disorder of mind-reading. *Journal of the British Academy, 3*, 197–209.

Happe, F., & Frith, U. (2006). The weak coherence account: Detail-focused cognitive style in autism spectrum disorders. *Journal of Autism and Developmental Disorders, 36*(1), 5–25. https://doi.org/10.1007/s10803-005-0039-0

Happe, F., & Frith, U. (2020a). Annual research review: Looking back to look forward – Changes in the concept of autism and implications for future research. *Journal of Child Psychology and Psychiatry, 61*(3), 218–232. https://doi.org/10.1111/jcpp.13176

Happe, F., & Frith, U. (2020b). Dimensional or categorical approaches to Autism? Both are needed. A reply to Nick Chown and Julia Leatherland. *Journal of Autism and Developmental Disorders*. https://doi.org/10.1007/s10803-020-04728-5

Happe, F., & Ronald, A. (2008). The 'Fractionable Autism Triad': A review of evidence from behavioural, genetic, cognitive and neural research. *Neuropsychology Review, 18*(4), 287–304. https://doi.org/10.1007/s11065-008-9076-8

Happe, F., Booth, R., Charlton, R., & Hughes, C. (2006a). Executive function deficits in autism spectrum disorders and attention-deficit/hyperactivity disorder: Examining profiles across domains and ages. *Brain and Cognition, 61*(1), 25–39. https://doi.org/10.1016/j.bandc.2006.03.004

Happe, F., Ronald, A., & Plomin, R. (2006b). Time to give up on a single explanation for autism. *Nature Neuroscience, 9*(10), 1218–1220. https://doi.org/10.1038/nn1770

Harikumar, A., Evans, D. W., Dougherty, C. C., Carpenter, K. L. H., & Michael, A. (2021). A review of the default mode network in autism spectrum disorders and Attention Deficit Hyperactivity Disorder. *Brain Connectivity*. https://doi.org/10.1089/brain.2020.0865

Hartman, C. A., Geurts, H. M., Franke, B., Buitelaar, J. K., & Rommelse, N. N. J. (2016). Changing ASD-ADHD symptom co-occurrence across the lifespan with adolescence as crucial time window: Illustrating the need to go beyond childhood. *Neuroscience and Biobehavioral Reviews, 71*, 529–541. https://doi.org/10.1016/j.neubiorev.2016.09.003

Hassan, T. H., Abdelrahman, H. M., Fattah, N. R. A., El-Masry, N. M., Hashim, H. M., El-Gerby, K. M., & Fattah, N. R. A. (2013). Blood and brain glutamate levels in children with autistic disorder. *Research in Autism Spectrum Disorders, 7*(4), 541–548. https://doi.org/10.1016/j.rasd.2012.12.005

Hastings, S. E., Hastings, R. A., Swales, M. A., & Hughes, J. C. (2022). Emotional and behavioural problems of children with autism spectrum disorder attending mainstream schools. *International Journal of Developmental Disabilities, 68*(5), 633–640. https://doi.org/10.1080/20473869.2020.1869414

Hata, K., Iida, J., Iwasaka, H., Negoro, H. I., Ueda, F., & Kishimoto, T. (2003). Minor physical anomalies in childhood and adolescent onset schizophrenia. *Psychiatry and Clinical Neurosciences, 57*(1), 17–21. https://doi.org/10.1046/j.1440-1819.2003.01074.x

Hawks, Z. W., & Constantino, J. N. (2020). Neuropsychiatric "comorbidity" as causal influence in autism. *Journal of the American Academy of Child and Adolescent Psychiatry, 59*(2), 229–235. https://doi.org/10.1016/j.jaac.2019.07.008

Hazlett, H. C., Gu, H. B., Munsell, B. C., Kim, S. H., Styner, M., Wolff, J. J., et al. (2017). Early brain development in infants at high risk for autism spectrum disorder. *Nature, 542*(7641), 348. https://doi.org/10.1038/nature21369

Hodgkins, P., Shaw, M., Coghill, D., & Hechtman, L. (2012). Amfetamine and methylphenidate medications for attention-deficit/hyperactivity disorder: complementary treatment options. *European Child and Adolescent Psychiatry, 21*(9), 477–492. https://doi.org/10.1007/s00787-012-0286-5

Hofvander, B., Delorme, R., Chaste, P., Nyden, A., Wentz, E., Stahlberg, O., et al. (2009). Psychiatric and psychosocial problems in adults with normal-intelligence autism spectrum disorders. *BMC Psychiatry, 9*. https://doi.org/10.1186/1471-244x-9-35

Hollestein, V., Poelmans, G., Forde, N. J., Beckmann, C. F., Ecker, C., Mann, C., et al. (2023). Excitatory/inhibitory imbalance in autism: the role of glutamate and GABA gene-sets in symptoms and cortical brain structure. *Translational Psychiatry, 13*(1). https://doi.org/10.1038/s41398-023-02317-5

Hollingdale, J., Woodhouse, E., Young, S., Fridman, A., & Mandy, W. (2020). Autistic spectrum disorder symptoms in children and adolescents with attention-deficit/hyperactivity disorder: A meta-analytical review. *Psychological Medicine, 50*(13), 2240–2253. https://doi.org/10.1017/s0033291719002368

Hong, S. J., Vogelstein, J. T., Gozzi, A., Bernhardt, B. C., Yeo, B. T., Milham, M. P., & Di Martino, A. (2020). Toward neurosubtypes in autism. *Biological Psychiatry, 88*(1), 111–128. https://doi.org/10.1016/j.biopsych.2020.03.022

Hoogman, M., van Rooij, D., Klein, M., Boedhoe, P., Ilioska, I., Li, T., et al. (2020). Consortium neuroscience of attention deficit/hyperactivity disorder and autism spectrum disorder: The ENIGMA adventure. *Human Brain Mapping, 43*(1), 37–55. https://doi.org/10.1002/hbm.25029

Horder, J., Petrinovic, M. M., Mendez, M. A., Bruns, A., Takumi, T., Spooren, W., et al. (2018). Glutamate and GABA in autism spectrum disorder-a translational magnetic resonance spectroscopy study in man and rodent models. *Translational Psychiatry, 8*, Article 106. https://doi.org/10.1038/s41398-018-0155-1

Horien, C., Floris, D. L., Greene, A. S., Noble, S., Rolison, M., Tejavibulya, L., et al. (2022). Functional connectome-based predictive modeling in autism. *Biological Psychiatry, 92*(8), 626–642. https://doi.org/10.1016/j.biopsych.2022.04.008

Houzel, D. (2018). Autism and psychoanalysis in the French context. *International Journal of Psychoanalysis, 99*(3), 725–745. https://doi.org/10.1080/00207578.2018.1468220

Howes, O. D., Rogdaki, M., Findon, J. L., Wichers, R. H., Charman, T., King, B. H., et al. (2018). Autism spectrum disorder: Consensus guidelines on assessment, treatment and research from the British Association for Psychopharmacology. *Journal of Psychopharmacology, 32*(1), 3–29. https://doi.org/10.1177/0269881117741766

Howlin, P., & Magiati, I. (2017). Autism spectrum disorder: outcomes in adulthood. *Current Opinion in Psychiatry, 30*(2), 69–76. https://doi.org/10.1097/yco.0000000000000308

Howlin, P., Goode, S., Hutton, J., & Rutter, M. (2009). Savant skills in autism: psychometric approaches and parental reports. *Philosophical Transactions of the Royal Society B-Biological Sciences, 364*(1522), 1359–1367. https://doi.org/10.1098/rstb.2008.0328

Hu, V. W., & Steinberg, M. E. (2009). Novel clustering of items from the Autism Diagnostic Interview-Revised to define phenotypes within Autism Spectrum Disorders. *Autism Research, 2*(2), 67–77. https://doi.org/10.1002/aur.72

Hu, V. W., Sarachana, T., Kim, K. S., Nguyen, A., Kulkarni, S., Steinberg, M. E., et al. (2009). Gene expression profiling differentiates autism case-controls and phenotypic variants of autism spectrum disorders: Evidence for circadian rhythm dysfunction in severe autism. *Autism Research, 2*(2), 78–97. https://doi.org/10.1002/aur.73

Huang, Q. Y., Pereira, A. C., Velthuis, H., Wong, N. M. L., Ellis, C. L., Ponteduro, F. M., et al. (2022). GABA(B) receptor modulation of visual sensory processing in adults with and without autism spectrum disorder. *Science Translational Medicine, 14*(626). https://doi.org/10.1126/scitranslmed.abg7859

Iglesias-Vazquez, L., Van Ginkel Riba, G., Arija, V., & Canals, J. (2020). Composition of gut microbiota in children with Autism Spectrum Disorder: A systematic review and meta-analysis. *Nutrients, 12*(3), 792. https://doi.org/10.3390/nu12030792

Itzchak, E.-B., Aviva, B., & Zachor, D. A. (2013). Are special abilities in autism spectrum disorder associated with a distinct clinical presentation? *Research in Autism Spectrum Disorders, 7*(9), 1122–1128. https://doi.org/10.1016/j.rasd.2013.05.003

Iwasa, M., Shimizu, Y., Sasayama, D., Imai, M., Ohzono, H., Ueda, M., et al. (2022). Twenty-year longitudinal birth cohort study of individuals diagnosed with autism spectrum disorder before seven years of age. *Journal of Child Psychology and Psychiatry, 63*(12), 1563–1573. https://doi.org/10.1111/jcpp.13614

Jokiranta-Olkoniemi, E., Cheslack-Postava, K., Sucksdorff, D., Suominen, A., Gyllenberg, D., Chudal, R., et al. (2016). Risk of psychiatric and neurodevelopmental disorders among siblings of probands with autism spectrum disorders. *Jama Psychiatry, 73*(6), 622–629. https://doi.org/10.1001/jamapsychiatry.2016.0495

Joshi, G., Petty, C., Wozniak, J., Henin, A., Fried, R., Galdo, M., et al. (2010). The heavy burden of psychiatric comorbidity in youth with Autism Spectrum Disorders: A large comparative study of a psychiatrically referred population. *Journal of Autism and Developmental Disorders, 40*(11), 1361–1370. https://doi.org/10.1007/s10803-010-0996-9

Kanner, L. (1943). Autistic disturbances of affective contact. *Nervous Child, 2*(3), 217–250.

Kapp, S. K., Gillespie-Lynch, K., Sherman, L. E., & Hutman, T. (2013). Deficit, difference, or both? Autism and neurodiversity. *Developmental Psychology, 49*(1), 59–71. https://doi.org/10.1037/a0028353

Karalunas, S. L., Hawkey, E., Gustafsson, H., Miller, M., Langhorst, M., Cordova, M., et al. (2018). Overlapping and distinct cognitive impairments in Attention-Deficit/Hyperactivity and autism spectrum disorder without intellectual disability. *Journal of Abnormal Child Psychology, 46*(8), 1705–1716. https://doi.org/10.1007/s10802-017-0394-2

Karalunas, S. L., Gustafsson, H. C., Fair, D., Musser, E. D., & Nigg, J. T. (2019). Do we need an irritable subtype of ADHD? Replication and extension of a promising temperament profile approach to ADHD subtyping. *Psychological Assessment, 31*(2), 236–247. https://doi.org/10.1037/pas0000664

Kern, J., Geier, D., Sykes, L., Geier, M., & Detha, R. (2015). Are ASD and ADHD a continuum? A comparison of pathophysiological similarities between the disorders. *Journal of Attention Disorders, 19*, 805–827. https://doi.org/10.1177/1087054712459886

Kirsch, A. C., Huebner, A. R. S., Mehta, S. Q., Howie, F. R., Weaver, A. L., Myers, S. M., et al. (2020). Association of comorbid mood and anxiety disorders with autism spectrum disorder. *JAMA Pediatrics, 174*(1), 63–70. https://doi.org/10.1001/jamapediatrics.2019.4368

Kohane, I. S., McMurry, A., Weber, G., MacFadden, D., Rappaport, L., Kunkel, L., et al. (2012). The co-morbidity burden of children and young adults with Autism Spectrum Disorders. *Plos One, 7*(4), e33224. https://doi.org/10.1371/journal.pone.0033224

Kong, A., Thorleifsson, G., Frigge, M. L., Vilhjalmsson, B. J., Young, A. I., Thorgeirsson, T. E., et al. (2018). The nature of nurture: Effects of parental genotypes. *Science, 359*(6374), 424–428. https://doi.org/10.1126/science.aan6877

Krakowski, A. D., Cost, K. T., Szatmari, P., Anagnostou, E., Crosbie, J., Schachar, R., et al. (2022). Characterizing the ASD-ADHD phenotype: Measurement structure and invariance in a clinical sample. *Journal of Child Psychology and Psychiatry, 63*(12), 1534–1543. https://doi.org/10.1111/jcpp.13609

Kumsta, R., Kreppner, J., Kennedy, M., Knights, N., Rutter, M., & Sonuga-Barke, E. (2015). Psychological consequences of early global deprivation An overview of findings from the English & Romanian Adoptees Study. *European Psychologist, 20*(2), 138–151. https://doi.org/10.1027/1016-9040/a000227

Kuntsi, J., Wood, A. C., Rijsdijk, F., Johnson, K. A., Andreou, P., Albrecht, B., et al. (2010). Separation of cognitive impairments in Attention-Deficit/Hyperactivity Disorder Into 2 familial factors. *Archives of General Psychiatry, 67*(11), 1159–1167. https://doi.org/10.1001/archgenpsychiatry.2010.139

Lai, M. C., Lombardo, M. V., & Baron-Cohen, S. (2014). Autism. *Lancet, 383*(9920), 896–910. https://doi.org/10.1016/s0140-6736(13)61539-1

Lai, M. C., Kassee, C., Besney, R., Bonato, S., Hull, L., Mandy, W., et al. (2019). Prevalence of co-occurring mental health diagnoses in the autism population: A systematic review and meta-analysis. *Lancet Psychiatry, 6*(10), 819–829. https://doi.org/10.1016/s2215-0366(19)30289-5

Lam, J., Sutton, P., Kalkbrenner, A., Windham, G., Halladay, A., Koustas, E., et al. (2016). A systematic review and meta-analysis of multiple airborne pollutants and Autism Spectrum Disorder. *Plos One, 11*(9), e0161851. https://doi.org/10.1371/journal.pone.0161851

Lambek, R., Sonuga-Barke, E., Tannock, R., Sorensen, A. V., Damm, D., & Thomsen, P. H. (2018). Are there distinct cognitive and motivational sub-groups of children with ADHD? *Psychological Medicine, 48*(10), 1722–1730. https://doi.org/10.1017/s0033291717003245

Lee, P. H., Anttila, V., Won, H., Feng, Y.-C. A., Rosenthal, J., Zhu, Z., et al. (2019). Genomic relationships, novel Loci, and pleiotropic mechanisms across eight psychiatric disorders. *Cell, 179*(7), 1469. https://doi.org/10.1016/j.cell.2019.11.020

Lee, I. O., Skuse, D. H., Constable, P. A., Marmolejo-Ramos, F., Olsen, L. R., & Thompson, D. A. (2022). The electroretinogram b-wave amplitude: A differential physiological measure for Attention Deficit Hyperactivity Disorder and Autism Spectrum Disorder. *Journal of Neurodevelopmental Disorders, 14*(1), Article: 30. https://doi.org/10.1186/s11689-022-09440-2

Leno, V. C., Hollocks, M. J., Chandler, S., White, P., Yorke, I., Charman, T., et al. (2022). Homotypic and heterotypic continuity in psychiatric symptoms from childhood to adolescence in autistic youth. *Journal of the American Academy of Child and Adolescent Psychiatry, 61*(12), 1445–1454. https://doi.org/10.1016/j.jaac.2022.05.010

Lever, A. G., & Geurts, H. M. (2016). Psychiatric co-occurring symptoms and disorders in young, middle-aged, and older adults with Autism Spectrum Disorder. *Journal of Autism and Developmental Disorders, 46*(6), 1916–1930. https://doi.org/10.1007/s10803-016-2722-8

Levy, S. E., Giarelli, E., Lee, L. C., Schieve, L. A., Kirby, R. S., Cunniff, C., et al. (2010). Autism Spectrum Disorder and co-occurring developmental, psychiatric, and medical conditions among children in multiple populations of the United States. *Journal of Developmental and Behavioral Pediatrics, 31*(4), 267–275. https://doi.org/10.1097/DBP.0b013e3181d5d03b

Lipkin, W. I., Bresnahan, M., & Susser, E. (2023). Cohort-guided insights into gene-environment interactions in autism spectrum disorders. *Nature Reviews Neurology, 19*(2), 118–125. https://doi.org/10.1038/s41582-022-00764-0

Livingston, L. A., & Happe, F. (2017). Conceptualising compensation in neurodevelopmental disorders: Reflections from autism spectrum disorder. *Neuroscience and Biobehavioral Reviews, 80*, 729–742. https://doi.org/10.1016/j.neubiorev.2017.06.005

Livingston, L. A., Shah, P., & Happé, F. (2019). Compensatory strategies below the behavioural surface in autism: a qualitative study. *Lancet Psychiatry, 6*(9), 766–777. https://doi.org/10.1016/s2215-0366(19)30224-x

Loomes, R., Hull, L., & Mandy, W. P. L. (2017). What Is the male-to-female ratio in autism spectrum disorder? A systematic review and meta-analysis. *Journal of the American Academy of Child and Adolescent Psychiatry, 56*(6), 466–474. https://doi.org/10.1016/j.jaac.2017.03.013

Lord, C. (2013). Fetal and sociocultural environments and autism. *American Journal of Psychiatry, 170*(4), 355–358. https://doi.org/10.1176/appi.ajp.2013.13010078

Lord, C., Rutter, M., & Lecouteur, A. (1994). Autism diagnostic interview-revised – A revised version of a diagnostic interview for caregivers of individuals with possible pervasive developmental disorders. *Journal of Autism and Developmental Disorders, 24*(5), 659–685. https://doi.org/10.1007/bf02172145

Lord, C., Elsabbagh, M., Baird, G., & Veenstra-Vanderweele, J. (2018). Autism spectrum disorder. *Lancet, 392*(10146), 508–520. https://doi.org/10.1016/s0140-6736(18)31129-2

Lord, C., Brugha, T. S., Charman, T., Cusack, J., Dumas, G., Frazier, T., et al. (2020). Autism spectrum disorder. *Nature Reviews Disease Primers, 6*(1), Article 5. https://doi.org/10.1038/s41572-019-0138-4

Lord, C., Charman, T., Havdahl, A., Carbone, P., Anagnostou, E., Boyd, B., et al. (2022). The Lancet Commission on the future of care and clinical research in autism. *Lancet, 399*(10321), 271–334. https://doi.org/10.1016/s0140-6736(21)01541-5

Lotter, V. (1966). Epidemiology of autistic conditions in young children: 1. Prevalence. *Social Psychiatry, 1*, 124–137.

Lyall, K., Croen, L., Daniels, J., Fallin, M. D., Ladd-Acosta, C., Lee, B. K., et al. (2017). In J. E. Fielding (Ed.), *The changing epidemiology of Autism Spectrum Disorders* (Vol. 38, pp. 81–102). Annual Review of Public Health. https://doi.org/10.1146/annurev-publhealth-031816-044318

Magiati, I., Tay, X. W., & Howlin, P. (2014). Cognitive, language, social and behavioural outcomes in adults with autism spectrum disorders: A systematic review of longitudinal follow-up studies in adulthood. *Clinical Psychology Review, 34*(1), 73–86. https://doi.org/10.1016/j.cpr.2013.11.002

Mandy, W. P. L., & Skuse, D. H. (2008). Research review: What is the association between the social-communication element of autism and repetitive interests, behaviours and activities? *Journal of Child Psychology and Psychiatry, 49*(8), 795–808. https://doi.org/10.1111/j.1469-7610.2008.01911.x

Marcovitch, S., O'Brien, M., Calkins, S. D., Leerkes, E. M., Weaver, J. M., & Levine, D. W. (2015). A longitudinal assessment of the relation between executive function and theory of mind at 3, 4, and 5 years. *Cognitive Development, 33*, 40–55. https://doi.org/10.1016/j.cogdev.2014.07.001

Marquand, A. F., Rezek, I., Buitelaar, J., & Beckmann, C. F. (2016). Understanding heterogeneity in clinical cohorts using normative models: Beyond case-control studies. *Biological Psychiatry, 80*(7), 552–561. https://doi.org/10.1016/j.biopsych.2015.12.023

Marquand, A. F., Kia, S. M., Zabihi, M., Wolfers, T., Buitelaar, J. K., & Beckmann, C. F. (2019). Conceptualizing mental disorders as deviations from normative functioning. *Molecular Psychiatry, 24*(10), 1415–1424. https://doi.org/10.1038/s41380-019-0441-1

Mason, D., Capp, S. J., Stewart, G. R., Kempton, M. J., Glaser, K., Howlin, P., & Happe, F. (2021). A meta-analysis of outcome studies of autistic adults: Quantifying effect size, quality, and meta-regression. *Journal of Autism and Developmental Disorders, 51*, 3165–3179. https://doi.org/10.1007/s10803-020-04763-2

Massrali, A., Brunel, H., Hannon, E., Wong, C., Baron-Cohen, S., Warrier, V., & i, P.-M. E. G. (2019). Integrated genetic and methylomic analyses identify shared biology between autism and autistic traits. *Molecular Autism, 10*. https://doi.org/10.1186/s13229-019-0279-z

Matson, J. L., & Nebel-Schwalm, M. S. (2007). Comorbid psychopathology with autism spectrum disorder in children: An overview. *Research in Developmental Disabilities, 28*(4), 341–352. https://doi.org/10.1016/j.ridd.2005.12.004

Mattheisen, M., Grove, J., Als, T. D., Martin, J., Voloudakis, G., Meier, S., et al. (2022). Identification of shared and differentiating genetic architecture for autism spectrum disorder, attention-deficit hyperactivity disorder and case subgroups. *Nature Genetics, 54*(10), 1470. https://doi.org/10.1038/s41588-022-01171-3

Mattila, M. L., Hurtig, T., Haapsamo, H., Jussila, K., Kuusikko-Gauffin, S., Kielinen, M., et al. (2010). Comorbid psychiatric disorders associated with Asperger Syndrome/High-functioning Autism: A community- and clinic-based study. *Journal of Autism and Developmental Disorders, 40*(9), 1080–1093. https://doi.org/10.1007/s10803-010-0958-2

Maughan, B., & Sonuga-Barke, E. J. S. (2014). Editorial: Translational genetics of child psychopathology: A distant dream? *Journal of Child Psychology and Psychiatry, 55*(10), 1065–1067. https://doi.org/10.1111/jcpp.12323

McCauley, J. B., Pickles, A., Huerta, M., & Lord, C. (2020). Defining positive outcomes in more and less cognitively able autistic adults. *Autism Research, 13*(9), 1548–1560. https://doi.org/10.1002/aur.2359

Meltzer, A., & Van de Water, J. (2017). The role of the immune system in Autism Spectrum Disorder. *Neuropsychopharmacology, 42*(1), 284–298. https://doi.org/10.1038/npp.2016.158

Michelini, G., Cheung, C. H. M., Kitsune, V., Brandeis, D., Banaschewski, T., McLoughlin, G., et al. (2021). The etiological structure of cognitive-neurophysiological impairments in ADHD in adolescence and young adulthood. *Journal of Attention Disorders, 25*(1), 91–104. https://doi.org/10.1177/1087054718771191

Miller, G. W., & Jones, D. P. (2014). The nature of nurture: Refining the definition of the exposome. *Toxicological Sciences, 137*(1), 1. https://doi.org/10.1093/toxsci/kft251

Miller, M., Austin, S., Iosif, A. M., de la Paz, L., Chuang, A. N., Hatch, B., & Ozonoff, S. (2020). Shared and distinct developmental pathways to ASD and ADHD phenotypes among infants at familial risk. *Developmental Psychopathology, 32*(4), 1323–1334. https://doi.org/10.1017/s0954579420000735

Mingins, J. E., Tarver, J., Waite, J., Jones, C., & Surtees, A. D. R. (2021). Anxiety and intellectual functioning in autistic children: A systematic review and meta-analysis. *Autism, 25*(1), 18–32. https://doi.org/10.1177/1362361320953253

Mitchell, K. J. (2007). The genetics of brain wiring: From molecule to mind. *Plos Biology, 5*(4), 690–692. https://doi.org/10.1371/journal.pbio.0050113

Modabbernia, A., Velthorst, E., & Reichenberg, A. (2017). Environmental risk factors for autism: an evidence-based review of systematic reviews and meta-analyses. *Molecular Autism, 8*, Article 13. https://doi.org/10.1186/s13229-017-0121-4

Morris, S. S. J., Timmons, A., & Musser, E. D. (2023). An individualized, data-driven biological approach to Attention-Deficit/Hyperactivity Disorder (ADHD) heterogeneity. *Research on Child and Adolescent Psychopathology*. https://doi.org/10.1007/s10802-023-01104-6

Mount, R. H., Charman, T., Hastings, R. P., Reilly, S., & Cass, H. (2003). Features of autism in Rett syndrome and severe mental retardation. *Journal of Autism and Developmental Disorders, 33*(4), 435–442. https://doi.org/10.1023/a:1025066913283

Myers, L., Anderlid, B. M., Nordgren, A., Willfors, C., Kuja-Halkola, R., Tammimies, K., & Bolte, S. (2017). Minor physical anomalies in neurodevelopmental disorders: a twin study. *Child and Adolescent Psychiatry and Mental Health, 11*, Article 57. https://doi.org/10.1186/s13034-017-0195-y

Myers, S. M., Challman, T. D., Bernier, R., Bourgeron, T., Chung, W. K., Constantino, J. N., et al. (2020). Insufficient evidence for "autism-specific" genes. *American Journal of Human Genetics, 106*(5), 587–595. https://doi.org/10.1016/j.ajhg.2020.04.004

Naaijen, J., Lythgoe, D. J., Amiri, H., Buitelaar, J. K., & Glennon, J. C. (2015). Fronto-striatal glutamatergic compounds in compulsive and impulsive syndromes: A review of magnetic resonance spectroscopy studies. *Neuroscience and Biobehavioral Reviews, 52*, 74–88. https://doi.org/10.1016/j.neubiorev.2015.02.009

Naaijen, J., Bralten, J., Poelmans, G., Glennon, J. C., Franke, B., Buitelaar, J. K., & Consortium, I. (2017). Glutamatergic and GABAergic gene sets in attention-deficit/hyperactivity disorder: association to overlapping traits in ADHD and autism. *Translational Psychiatry, 7*, e999. https://doi.org/10.1038/tp.2016.273

Needham, B. D., Kaddurah-Daouk, R., & Mazmanian, S. K. (2020). Gut microbial molecules in behavioural and neurodegenerative conditions. *Nature Reviews Neuroscience, 21*(12), 717–731. https://doi.org/10.1038/s41583-020-00381-0

Neufeld, J., Kuja-Halkola, R., Mevel, K., Cauvet, E., Fransson, P., & Bolte, S. (2018). Alterations in resting state connectivity along the autism trait continuum: A twin study. *Molecular Psychiatry, 23*(7), 1659–1665. https://doi.org/10.1038/mp.2017.160

Neufeld, J., Hagstrom, A., Van't Westeinde, A., Lundin, K., Cauvet, E., Willfors, C., et al. (2020). Global and local visual processing in autism – A co-twin-control study. *Journal of Child Psychology and Psychiatry, 61*(4), 470–479. https://doi.org/10.1111/jcpp.13120

Newson, E., Le Marechal, K., & David, C. (2003). Pathological demand avoidance syndrome: a necessary distinction within the pervasive developmental disorders. *Archives of Disease in Childhood, 88*(7), 595–600. https://doi.org/10.1136/adc.88.7.595

Nigg, J. T. (2006). Temperament and developmental psychopathology. *Journal of Child Psychology and Psychiatry, 47*(3–4), 395–422. https://doi.org/10.1111/j.1469-7610.2006.01612.x

Nigg, J. T. (2023). Considerations toward an epigenetic and common pathways theory of mental disorder. *Journal of Psychopathology and Clinical Science, 132*(3), 297–313. https://doi.org/10.1037/abn0000748

Nigg, J. T., Karalunas, S. L., Feczko, E., & Fair, D. A. (2020). Toward a revised nosology for Attention-Deficit/Hyperactivity Disorder heterogeneity. *Biological Psychiatry-Cognitive Neuroscience and Neuroimaging, 5*(8), 726–737. https://doi.org/10.1016/j.bpsc.2020.02.005

Norman, L. J., Sudre, G., Bouyssi-Kobar, M., Sharp, W., & Shaw, P. (2021). A longitudinal study of resting-state connectivity and response to psychostimulant treatment in ADHD. *American Journal of Psychiatry, 178*(8), 744–751. https://doi.org/10.1176/appi.ajp.2021.20091342

O'Connor, N., & Hermelin, B. (1991). Talents and preoccupations in idiots-savants. *Psychological Medicine, 21*(4), 959–964. https://doi.org/10.1017/s0033291700029949

O'Nions, E., Happe, F., Viding, E., Gould, J., & Noens, I. (2018a). Demand avoidance is not necessarily defiance. *Lancet Child & Adolescent Health, 2*(7), E14–E14. https://doi.org/10.1016/s2352-4642(18)30171-8

O'Nions, E., Viding, E., Floyd, C., Quinlan, E., Pidgeon, C., Gould, J., & Happe, F. (2018b). Dimensions of difficulty in children reported to have an autism spectrum diagnosis and features of extreme/'pathological' demand avoidance. *Child and Adolescent Mental Health, 23*(3), 220–227. https://doi.org/10.1111/camh.12242

Ooi, Y. P., Weng, S.-J., Kossowsky, J., Gerger, H., & Sung, M. (2017). Oxytocin and Autism Spectrum Disorders: A systematic review and meta-analysis of randomized controlled trials. *Pharmacopsychiatry, 50*(1), 5–13. https://doi.org/10.1055/s-0042-109400

Ozgen, H. M., Hop, J. W., Hox, J. J., Beemer, F. A., & van Engeland, H. (2010). Minor physical anomalies in autism: A meta-analysis. *Molecular psychiatry, 15*(3), 300–307. https://doi.org/10.1038/mp.2008.75

Ozonoff, S., & Iosif, A. M. (2019). Changing conceptualizations of regression: What prospective studies reveal about the onset of autism spectrum disorder. *Neuroscience and Biobehavioral Reviews, 100*, 296–304. https://doi.org/10.1016/j.neubiorev.2019.03.012

Ozsivadjian, A., Hollocks, M. J., Magiati, I., Happe, F., Baird, G., & Absoud, M. (2020). Is cognitive inflexibility a missing link? The role of cognitive inflexibility, alexithymia and intolerance of uncertainty in externalising and internalising behaviours in young people with autism spectrum disorder. *Journal of Child Psychology and Psychiatry, 62*(6), 715–724. https://doi.org/10.1111/jcpp.13295

Padmanabhan, A., Lynch, C. J., Schaer, M., & Menon, V. (2017). The default mode network in autism. *Biological Psychiatry-Cognitive Neuroscience and Neuroimaging, 2*(6), 476–486. https://doi.org/10.1016/j.bpsc.2017.04.004

Panjwani, A. A., Ji, Y., Fahey, J. W., Palmer, A., Wang, G., Hong, X., et al. (2019). Maternal obesity/diabetes, plasma branched-chain amino acids, and Autism Spectrum Disorder risk in urban low-income children: Evidence of sex difference. *Autism Research, 12*(10), 1562–1573. https://doi.org/10.1002/aur.2177

Parlett-Pelleriti, C. M., Stevens, E., Dixon, D., & Linstead, E. J. (2022). Applications of unsupervised machine learning in Autism Spectrum Disorder research: A review. *Review Journal of Autism and Developmental Disorders.* https://doi.org/10.1007/s40489-021-00299-y

Perner, J., & Lang, B. (1999). Development of theory of mind and executive control. *Trends in Cognitive Sciences, 3*(9), 337–344. https://doi.org/10.1016/s1364-6613(99)01362-5

Pettersson, E., Anckarsater, H., Gillberg, C., & Lichtenstein, P. (2013). Different neurodevelopmental symptoms have a common genetic etiology. *Journal of Child Psychology and Psychiatry, 54*(12), 1356–1365. https://doi.org/10.1111/jcpp.12113

Peyre, H., Schoeler, T., Liu, C. Y., Williams, C. M., Hoertel, N., Havdahl, A., & Pingault, J. B. (2021). Combining multivariate genomic approaches to elucidate the comorbidity between autism spectrum disorder and attention deficit hyperactivity disorder. *Journal of Child Psychology and Psychiatry, 62*(11), 1285–1296. https://doi.org/10.1111/jcpp.13479

Pickles, A., & Angold, A. (2003). Natural categories or fundamental dimensions: On carving nature at the joints and the rearticulation of psychopathology. *Developmental Psychopathology, 15*(3), 529–551. https://doi.org/10.1017/s0954579403000282

Pickles, A., Wright, N., Bedford, R., Steiman, M., Duku, E., Bennett, T., et al. (2022). Predictors of language regression and its association with subsequent communication development in children with autism. *Journal of Child Psychology and Psychiatry, 63*(11), 1243–1252. https://doi.org/10.1111/jcpp.13565

Pinto, R., Rijsdijk, F., Ronald, A., Asherson, P., & Kuntsi, J. (2016). The genetic overlap of Attention-Deficit/Hyperactivity Disorder and autistic-like traits: An investigation of individual symptom scales and cognitive markers. *Journal of Abnormal Child Psychology, 44*(2), 335–345. https://doi.org/10.1007/s10802-015-0037-4

Plomin, R., & Bergeman, C. S. (1991). The nature of nurture – genetic influences on environmental measures. *Behavioral and Brain Sciences, 14*(3), 373–385. https://doi.org/10.1017/s0140525x00070278

Plomin, R., DeFries, J. C., & Loehlin, J. C. (1977). Genotype-environment interaction and correlation in analysis of human-behavior. *Psychological Bulletin, 84*(2), 309–322. https://doi.org/10.1037/0033-2909.84.2.309

Posner, J. (2018). The role of precision medicine in child psychiatry: What can we expect and when? *Journal of the American Academy of Child and Adolescent Psychiatry, 57*(11), 813–817. https://doi.org/10.1016/j.jaac.2018.07.874

Prince, M. A., & Fidler, D. J. (2021). Chapter Two – Analytic approaches to heterogeneity in neurogenetic syndrome research. In R. M. Hodapp & D. J. Fidler (Eds.), *International review of research in developmental disabilities* (Vol. 60, pp. 55–73). Academic Press.

Pua, E. P. K., Bowden, S. C., & Seal, M. L. (2017). Autism spectrum disorders: Neuroimaging findings from systematic reviews. *Research in Autism Spectrum Disorders, 34*, 28–33. https://doi.org/10.1016/j.rasd.2016.11.005

Rabot, J., Rodgaard, E. M., Joober, R., Dumas, G., Bzdok, D., Bernhardt, B., et al. (2023). Genesis, modelling and methodological remedies to autism heterogeneity. *Neuroscience and Biobehavioral Reviews, 150*. https://doi.org/10.1016/j.neubiorev.2023.105201

Radonjic, N. V., Hess, J. L., Rovira, P., Andreassen, O., Buitelaar, J. K., Ching, C. R. K., et al. (2021). Structural brain imaging studies offer clues about the effects of the shared genetic etiology among neuropsychiatric disorders. *Molecular Psychiatry, 26*, 2101–2110. https://doi.org/10.1038/s41380-020-01002-z

Ridley, R. (2019). Some difficulties behind the concept of the 'Extreme male brain' in autism research. A theoretical review. *Research in Autism Spectrum Disorders, 57*, 19–27. https://doi.org/10.1016/j.rasd.2018.09.007

Riglin, L., Leppert, B., Langley, K., Thapar, A. K., O'Donovan, M. C., Smith, G. D., et al. (2021). Investigating attention-deficit hyperactivity disorder and autism spectrum disorder traits in the general population: What happens in adult life? *Journal of Child Psychology and Psychiatry, 62*(4), 449–457. https://doi.org/10.1111/jcpp.13297

Roberts, B. A., Martel, M. M., & Nigg, J. T. (2017). Are there executive dysfunction subtypes within ADHD? *Journal of Attention Disorders, 21*(4), 284–293. https://doi.org/10.1177/1087054713510349

Robertson, C. E., Ratai, E. M., & Kanwisher, N. (2016). Reduced GABAergic action in the autistic brain. *Current Biology, 26*(1), 80–85. https://doi.org/10.1016/j.cub.2015.11.019

Rødgaard, E. M., Jensen, K., Vergnes, J. N., Soulieres, I., & Mottron, L. (2019). Temporal changes in effect sizes of studies comparing individuals with and without autism – A meta-analysis. *Jama Psychiatry, 76*(11), 1124–1132. https://doi.org/10.1001/jamapsychiatry.2019.1956

Rodriguez-Perez, M., Kennedy, M., Barker, E. D., Kreppner, J., Solerdelcoll, M., & Sonuga-Barke, E. J. S. (2023). The adult outcome of childhood quasi-autism arising following extreme institutional deprivation. *Journal of Child Psychology and Psychiatry, 64*(9), 1292–1302. https://doi.org/10.1111/jcpp.13767

Rogers, S. J., Estes, A., Lord, C., Munson, J., Rocha, M., Winter, J., et al. (2019). A multisite randomized controlled two-phase trial of the early start Denver model compared to treatment as usual. *Journal of the American Academy of Child and Adolescent Psychiatry, 58*(9), 853–865. https://doi.org/10.1016/j.jaac.2019.01.004

Roman-Urrestarazu, A., van Kessel, R., Allison, C., Matthews, F. E., Brayne, C., & Baron-Cohen, S. (2021). Association of race/ethnicity and social disadvantage with autism prevalence in 7 million school children in England. *JAMA Pediatrics, 175*(6), e210054. https://doi.org/10.1001/jamapediatrics.2021.0054

Rommelse, N. N. J., Geurts, H. M., Franke, B., Buitelaar, J. K., & Hartman, C. A. (2011). A review on cognitive and brain endophenotypes that may be common in autism spectrum disorder and attention-deficit/hyperactivity disorder and facilitate the search for pleiotropic genes. *Neuroscience and Biobehavioral Reviews, 35*(6), 1363–1396. https://doi.org/10.1016/j.neubiorev.2011.02.015

Ronald, A., & Hoekstra, R. A. (2011). Autism Spectrum Disorders and autistic traits: A decade of new twin studies. *American Journal of Medical Genetics Part B-Neuropsychiatric Genetics, 156B*(3), 255–274. https://doi.org/10.1002/ajmg.b.31159

Ronald, A., Happé, F., Bolton, P., Butcher, L. M., Price, T. S., Wheelwright, S., et al. (2006a). Genetic heterogeneity between the three components of the autism spectrum: A twin study. *Journal of the American Academy of Child and Adolescent Psychiatry, 45*(6), 691–699. https://doi.org/10.1097/01.chi.0000215325.13058.9d

Ronald, A., Happé, F., Price, T. S., Baron-Cohen, S., & Plomin, R. (2006b). Phenotypic and genetic overlap between autistic traits at the extremes of the general population. *Journal of the American Academy of Child and Adolescent Psychiatry, 45*(10), 1206–1214. https://doi.org/10.1097/01.chi.0000230165.54117.41

Rong, Y., Yang, C. J., Jin, Y., & Wang, Y. (2021). Prevalence of attention-deficit/hyperactivity disorder in individuals with autism spectrum disorder: A meta-analysis. *Research in Autism Spectrum Disorders, 83*, 101759. https://doi.org/10.1016/j.rasd.2021.101759

Rosen, N. E., Lord, C., & Volkmar, F. R. (2021). The diagnosis of autism: From Kanner to DSM-III to DSM-5 and beyond. *Journal of Autism and Developmental Disorders, 51*, 4253–4270. https://doi.org/10.1007/s10803-021-04904-1

Rubenstein, E., & Chawla, D. (2018). Broader autism phenotype in parents of children with autism: A systematic review of percentage estimates. *Journal of Child and Family Studies, 27*(6), 1705–1720. https://doi.org/10.1007/s10826-018-1026-3

Russell, G., Steer, C., & Golding, J. (2011). Social and demographic factors that influence the diagnosis of autistic spectrum disorders. *Social Psychiatry and Psychiatric Epidemiology, 46*(12), 1283–1293. https://doi.org/10.1007/s00127-010-0294-z

Russell, G., Stapley, S., Newlove-Delgado, T., Salmon, A., White, R., Warren, F., et al. (2022). Time trends in autism diagnosis over 20 years: a UK population-based cohort study. *Journal of Child Psychology and Psychiatry, 63*(6), 674–682. https://doi.org/10.1111/jcpp.13505

Rutter, M. (1968). Concepts of autism – A review of research. *Journal of Child Psychology and Psychiatry, 9*(1), 1–25. https://doi.org/10.1111/j.1469-7610.1968.tb02204.x

Rutter, M. (1999). The Emanuel Miller Memorial Lecture 1998 – Autism: Two-way interplay between research and clinical work. *Journal of Child Psychology and Psychiatry, 40*(2), 169–188. https://doi.org/10.1111/1469-7610.00431

Rutter, M. (2005). Incidence of autism spectrum disorders: Changes over time and their meaning. *Acta Paediatrica, 94*(1), 2–15. https://doi.org/10.1080/08035250410023124

Rutter, M. (2013). Developmental psychopathology: A paradigm shift or just a relabeling? *Developmental Psychopathology, 25*(4), 1201–1213. https://doi.org/10.1017/s0954579413000564

Rutter, M., Kumsta, R., Schlotz, W., & Sonuga-Barke, E. J. S. (2012). Longitudinal studies using a 'Natural Experiment' design: The case of adoptees from Romanian institutions. *Journal of the American Academy of Child and Adolescent Psychiatry, 51*(8), 762–770. https://doi.org/10.1016/j.jaac.2012.05.011

Ruzich, E., Allison, C., Smith, P., Watson, P., Auyeung, B., Ring, H., & Baron-Cohen, S. (2015). Measuring autistic traits in the general population: A systematic review of the Autism-Spectrum Quotient (AQ) in a nonclinical population sample of 6900 typical adult males and females. *Molecular Autism, 6*, Article 2. https://doi.org/10.1186/2040-2392-6-2

Rydzewska, E., Dunn, K., & Cooper, S. A. (2021). Umbrella systematic review of systematic reviews and meta-analyses on comorbid physical conditions in people with autism spectrum disorder. *British Journal of Psychiatry, 218*(1), 10–19. https://doi.org/10.1192/bjp.2020.167

Sáenz, A. A., Van Schuerbeek, P., Baijot, S., Septier, M., Deconinck, N., Defresne, P., et al. (2020). Disorder-specific brain volumetric abnormalities in attention-deficit/hyperactivity disorder relative to Autism spectrum disorder. *Plos One, 15*(11), e0241856. https://doi.org/10.1371/journal.pone.0241856

Salazar, F., Baird, G., Chandler, S., Tseng, E., O'Sullivan, T., Howlin, P., et al. (2015). Co-occurring psychiatric disorders in preschool and elementary school-aged children with autism spectrum disorder. *Journal of Autism and Developmental Disorders, 45*(8), 2283–2294. https://doi.org/10.1007/s10803-015-2361-5

Salomone, E., Kutlu, B., Derbyshire, K., McCloy, C., Hastings, R. P., Howlin, P., & Charman, T. (2014). Emotional and behavioural problems in children and young people with autism spectrum disorder in specialist autism schools. *Research in Autism Spectrum Disorders, 8*(6), 661–668. https://doi.org/10.1016/j.rasd.2014.03.004

Sandbank, M., Bottema-Beutel, K., Crowley, S., Cassidy, M., Dunham, K., Feldman, J. I., et al. (2020). Project AIM: Autism intervention meta-analysis for studies of young children. *Psychological Bulletin, 146*(1), 1–29. https://doi.org/10.1037/bul0000215

Sari, N. P., Jansen, P. W., Blanken, L. M. E., Ruigrok, A. N. V., Prinzie, P., Tiemeier, H., et al. (2022). Maternal age, autistic-like traits and mentalizing as predictors of child autistic-like traits in a population-based cohort. *Molecular Autism, 13*(1), Article 26. https://doi.org/10.1186/s13229-022-00507-4

Satterstrom, F. K., Kosmicki, J. A., Wang, J. B., Breen, M. S., De Rubeis, S., An, J. Y., et al. (2020). Large-scale exome sequencing study implicates both developmental and functional changes in the neurobiology of autism. *Cell, 180*(3), 568. https://doi.org/10.1016/j.cell.2019.12.036

Schreibman, L., Dawson, G., Stahmer, A. C., Landa, R., Rogers, S. J., McGee, G. G., et al. (2015). Naturalistic developmental behavioral interventions: Empirically validated treatments for Autism Spectrum Disorder. *Journal of Autism and Developmental Disorders, 45*(8), 2411–2428. https://doi.org/10.1007/s10803-015-2407-8

Schür, R. R., Draisma, L. W. R., Wijnen, J. P., Boks, M. P., Koevoets, M. G. J. C., Joels, M., et al. (2016). Brain GABA levels across psychiatric disorders: A systematic literature review and meta-analysis of H-1-MRS studies. *Human Brain Mapping, 37*(9), 3337–3352. https://doi.org/10.1002/hbm.23244

Scott, F. J., Baron-Cohen, S., Bolton, P., & Brayne, C. (2002). The CAST (Childhood Asperger Syndrome Test) – Preliminary development of a UK screen for mainstream primary-school-age children. *Autism, 6*(1), 9–31. https://doi.org/10.1177/1362361302006001003

Sebat, J., Lakshmi, B., Malhotra, D., Troge, J., Lese-Martin, C., Walsh, T., et al. (2007). Strong association of de novo copy number mutations with autism. *Science, 316*(5823), 445–449. https://doi.org/10.1126/science.1138659

Shakeshaft, A., Heron, J., Blakey, R., Riglin, L., Smith, G. D., Stergiakouli, E., et al. (2023). Co-development of attention deficit hyperactivity disorder and autistic trait trajectories from childhood to early adulthood. *Journal of Child Psychology and Psychiatry.* https://doi.org/10.1111/jcpp.13851

Sharon, G., Cruz, N. J., Kang, D. W., Gandal, M. J., Wang, B., Kim, Y. M., et al. (2019). Human gut microbiota from Autism Spectrum Disorder promote behavioral symptoms in mice. *Cell, 177*(6), 1600. https://doi.org/10.1016/j.cell.2019.05.004

Shephard, E., Bedford, R., Milosavljevic, B., Gliga, T., Jones, E. J. H., Pickles, A., et al. (2019). Early developmental pathways to childhood symptoms of attention-deficit hyperactivity disorder, anxiety and autism spectrum disorder. *Journal of Child Psychology and Psychiatry, 60*(9), 963–974. https://doi.org/10.1111/jcpp.12947

Sikich, L., Kolevzon, A., King, B. H., McDougle, C. J., Sanders, K. B., Kim, S. J., et al. (2021). Intranasal oxytocin in children and adolescents with Autism Spectrum Disorder. *New England Journal of Medicine, 385*(16), 1462–1473. https://doi.org/10.1056/NEJMoa2103583

Silva, A. I., Ehrhart, F., Ulfarsson, M. O., Stefansson, H., Stefansson, K., Wilkinson, L. S., et al. (2022). Neuroimaging findings in neurodevelopmental copy number variants: Identifying molecular pathways to convergent phenotypes. *Biological Psychiatry, 92*(5), 341–361. https://doi.org/10.1016/j.biopsych.2022.03.018

Simonoff, E., Pickles, A., Charman, T., Chandler, S., Loucas, T., & Baird, G. (2008). Psychiatric disorders in children with autism spectrum disorders: Prevalence, comorbidity, and associated factors in a population-derived sample. *Journal of the American Academy of Child and Adolescent Psychiatry, 47*(8), 921–929. https://doi.org/10.1097/CHI.0b013e318179964f

Simonoff, E., Kent, R., Stringer, D., Lord, C., Briskman, J., Lukito, S., et al. (2020). Trajectories in symptoms of autism and cognitive ability in autism from childhood to adult life: Findings from a longitudinal epidemiological cohort. *Journal of the American Academy of Child and Adolescent Psychiatry, 59*(12), 1342–1352. https://doi.org/10.1016/j.jaac.2019.11.020

Skogheim, T. S., Weyde, K. V. F., Engel, S. M., Aase, H., Suren, P., Oie, M. G., et al. (2021). Metal and essential element concentrations during pregnancy and associations with autism spectrum disorder and attention-deficit/hyperactivity disorder in children. *Environment international, 152*, 106468–106468. https://doi.org/10.1016/j.envint.2021.106468

Smoller, J. W., Andreassen, O. A., Edenberg, H. J., Faraone, S. V., Glatt, S. J., & Kendler, K. S. (2019). Psychiatric genetics and the structure of psychopathology. *Molecular psychiatry, 24*(3), 409–420. https://doi.org/10.1038/s41380-017-0010-4

Sohal, V. S., & Rubenstein, J. L. R. (2019). Excitation-inhibition balance as a framework for investigating mechanisms in neuropsychiatric disorders. *Molecular psychiatry, 24*(9), 1248–1257. https://doi.org/10.1038/s41380-019-0426-0

Sokolova, E., Oerlemans, A. M., Rommelse, N. N., Groot, P., Hartman, C. A., Glennon, J. C., et al. (2017). A causal and mediation analysis of the comorbidity between Attention Deficit Hyperactivity Disorder (ADHD) and Autism Spectrum Disorder (ASD). *Journal of Autism and Developmental Disorders, 47*(6), 1595–1604. https://doi.org/10.1007/s10803-017-3083-7

Sonuga-Barke, E. J. S., Kennedy, M., Kumsta, R., Knights, N., Golm, D., Rutter, M., et al. (2017). Child-to-adult neurodevelopmental and mental health trajectories after early life deprivation: The young adult follow-up of the longitudinal English and Romanian Adoptees study. *Lancet, 389*(10078), 1539–1548. https://doi.org/10.1016/s0140-6736(17)30045-4

Sroufe, L. A. (2013). The promise of developmental psychopathology: Past and present. *Developmental Psychopathology, 25*(4), 1215–1224. https://doi.org/10.1017/s0954579413000576

Sroufe, L. A., & Rutter, M. (1984). The domain of developmental psychopathology. *Child Development, 55*(1), 17–29. https://doi.org/10.2307/1129832

Stergiakouli, E., Smith, G. D., Martin, J., Skuse, D. H., Viechtbauer, W., Ring, S. M., et al. (2017). Shared genetic influences between dimensional ASD and ADHD symptoms during child and adolescent development. *Molecular Autism, 8*, Article 18. https://doi.org/10.1186/s13229-017-0131-2

Stevens, E., Dixon, D. R., Novack, M. N., Granpeesheh, D., Smith, T., & Linstead, E. (2019). Identification and analysis of behavioral phenotypes in autism spectrum disorder via unsupervised machine learning. *International Journal of Medical Informatics, 129*, 29–36. https://doi.org/10.1016/j.ijmedinf.2019.05.006

Stevenson, J. (1993). Multivariate-statistics. 6. The place of discriminant function-analysis in psychiatric research. *Nordic Journal of Psychiatry, 47*(2), 109–122. https://doi.org/10.3109/08039489309095021

Sulaiman, R., Wang, M., & Ren, X. F. (2020). Exposure to aluminum, cadmium, and mercury and autism spectrum disorder in children: A systematic review and meta-analysis. *Chemical Research in Toxicology, 33*(11), 2699–2718. https://doi.org/10.1021/acs.chemrestox.0c00167

Super, C. M., Axia, G., Harkness, S., Welles-Nystrom, B., Zylicz, P. O., Parmar, P., et al. (2008). Culture, temperament, and the "Difficult Child": A study in seven Western cultures. *International Journal of Developmental Science, 2*, 136–157. https://doi.org/10.3233/DEV-2008-21209

Swanson, J. M., Schuck, S., Porter, M. M., Carlson, C., Hartman, C. A., Sergeant, J. A., et al. (2012). Categorical and dimensional definitions and evaluations of symptoms of ADHD: history of the SNAP and the SWAN rating scales. *The International Journal of Educational and Psychological Assessment, 10*(1), 51–70.

Szatmari, P., Cost, K. T., Duku, E., Bennett, T., Elsabbagh, M., Georgiades, S., et al. (2021). Association of child and family attributes with outcomes in children with autism. *Jama Network Open, 4*(3), e212530. https://doi.org/10.1001/jamanetworkopen.2021.2530

Taylor, J. L. (2017). When is a good outcome actually good? *Autism, 21*(8), 918–919. https://doi.org/10.1177/1362361317728821

Taylor, M. J., Charman, T., Robinson, E. B., Plomin, R., Happe, F., Asherson, P., & Ronald, A. (2013). Developmental associations between traits of autism spectrum disorder and attention deficit hyperactivity disorder: A genetically informative, longitudinal twin study. *Psychological Medicine, 43*(8), 1735–1746. https://doi.org/10.1017/s003329171200253x

Taylor, M. J., Charman, T., & Ronald, A. (2015). Where are the strongest associations between autistic traits and traits of ADHD? evidence from a community-based twin study. *European Child and Adolescent Psychiatry, 24*(9), 1129–1138. https://doi.org/10.1007/s00787-014-0666-0

Thompson, P. M., Jahanshad, N., Ching, C. R. K., Salminen, L. E., Thomopoulos, S. I., Bright, J., et al. (2020). ENIGMA and global neuroscience: A decade of large-scale studies of the brain in health and disease across more than 40 countries. *Translational Psychiatry, 10*(1), 100. https://doi.org/10.1038/s41398-020-0705-1

Tick, B., Bolton, P., Happe, F., Rutter, M., & Rijsdijk, F. (2016a). Heritability of autism spectrum disorders: A meta-analysis of twin studies. *Journal of Child Psychology and Psychiatry, 57*(5), 585–595. https://doi.org/10.1111/jcpp.12499

Tick, B., Colvert, E., McEwen, F., Stewart, C., Woodhouse, E., Gillan, N., et al. (2016b). Autism Spectrum Disorders and other mental health problems: Exploring etiological overlaps and phenotypic causal associations. *Journal of the American Academy of Child and Adolescent Psychiatry, 55*(2), 106–113. https://doi.org/10.1016/j.jaac.2015.11.013

Tindle, J., & Tadi, P. (2023). Neuroanatomy, parasympathetic nervous system. [Updated 2022 Oct 31]. In *StatPearls [Internet]. Treasure Island (FL)*. StatPearls Publishing. https://www.ncbi.nlm.nih.gov/books/NBK553141/

Torske, T., Naerland, T., Bettella, F., Bjella, T., Malt, E., Hoyland, A. L., et al. (2020). Autism spectrum disorder polygenic scores are associated with every day executive function in children admitted for clinical assessment. *Autism Research, 13*(2), 207–220. https://doi.org/10.1002/aur.2207

Totsika, V., Hastings, R. P., Emerson, E., Lancaster, G. A., & Berridge, D. M. (2011). A population-based investigation of behavioural and emotional problems and maternal mental health: Associations with autism spectrum disorder and intellectual disability. *Journal of Child Psychology and Psychiatry, 52*(1), 91–99. https://doi.org/10.1111/j.1469-7610.2010.02295.x

Uddin, L. Q. (2015). Salience processing and insular cortical function and dysfunction. *Nature Reviews Neuroscience, 16*(1), 55–61. https://doi.org/10.1038/nrn3857

van den Heuvel, O. A. (2021). Can transgenic monkeys help us innovate transdiagnostic therapies? *American Journal of Psychiatry, 178*(1), 8–10. https://doi.org/10.1176/appi.ajp.2020.20111590

van Rooij, D., Anagnostou, E., Arango, C., Auzias, G., Behrmann, M., Busatto, G. F., et al. (2018). Cortical and subcortical brain morphometry differences between patients With Autism Spectrum Disorder and healthy individuals across the lifespan: Results from the ENIGMA ASD Working Group. *American Journal of Psychiatry, 175*(4), 359–369. https://doi.org/10.1176/appi.ajp.2017.17010100

van Steensel, F. J. A., Bogels, S. M., & Perrin, S. (2011). Anxiety disorders in children and adolescents with Autistic Spectrum Disorders: A meta-analysis. *Clinical Child and Family Psychology Review, 14*(3), 302–317. https://doi.org/10.1007/s10567-011-0097-0

Veenstra-Vander Weele, J., Cook, E. H., King, B. H., Zarevics, P., Cherubini, M., Walton-Bowen, K., et al. (2017). Arbaclofen in children and adolescents with Autism Spectrum Disorder: A randomized, controlled, Phase 2 trial. *Neuropsychopharmacology, 42*(7), 1390–1398. https://doi.org/10.1038/npp.2016.237

Visser, J. C., Rommelse, N. N., Greven, C. U., & Buitelaar, J. K. (2016). Autism spectrum disorder and attention-deficit/hyperactivity disorder in early childhood: A review of unique and shared characteristics and developmental antecedents. *Neuroscience and Biobehavioral Reviews, 65*, 229–263. https://doi.org/10.1016/j.neubiorev.2016.03.019

Voineagu, I., Wang, X. C., Johnston, P., Lowe, J. K., Tian, Y., Horvath, S., et al. (2011). Transcriptomic analysis of autistic brain reveals convergent molecular pathology. *Nature, 474*(7351), 380. https://doi.org/10.1038/nature10110

Vourc'h, P., Bienvenu, T., Beldjord, C., Chelly, J., Barthelemy, C., Muh, J. P., & Andres, C. (2001). No mutations in the coding region of the Rett syndrome gene MECP2 in 59 autistic patients. *European Journal of Human Genetics, 9*(7), 556–558. https://doi.org/10.1038/sj.ejhg.5200660

Wade, M., Prime, H., Jenkins, J. M., Yeates, K. O., Williams, T., & Lee, K. (2018). On the relation between theory of mind and executive functioning: A developmental cognitive neuroscience perspective. *Psychonomic Bulletin & Review, 25*(6), 2119–2140. https://doi.org/10.3758/s13423-018-1459-0

Wakefield, A. J., Murch, S. H., Anthony, A., Linnell, J., Casson, D. M., Malik, M., et al. (1998). RETRACTED: Ileal-lymphoid-nodular hyperplasia, non-specific colitis, and pervasive developmental disorder in children (Retracted article. See vol 375, pg 445, 2010). *Lancet, 351*(9103), 637–641. https://doi.org/10.1016/s0140-6736(97)11096-0

Wang, M., Hossain, F., Sulaiman, R., & Ren, X. F. (2019). Exposure to inorganic arsenic and lead and Autism Spectrum Disorder in children: A systematic review and meta-analysis. *Chemical Research in Toxicology, 32*(10), 1904–1919. https://doi.org/10.1021/acs.chemrestox.9b00134

Wang, Z. X., Chan, A. Y. L., Coghill, D., Ip, P., Lau, W. C. Y., Simonoff, E., et al. (2021). Association between prenatal exposure to antipsychotics and Attention-Deficit/Hyperactivity Disorder, Autism Spectrum Disorder, preterm birth, and small for gestational age. *Jama Internal Medicine, 181*(10), 1332–1340. https://doi.org/10.1001/jamainternmed.2021.4571

Ware, R. S. (2022). Reporting both unadjusted and adjusted estimates Is essential to the interpretation of randomized clinical trial results. *JAMA Pediatrics, 176*(3), 325. https://doi.org/10.1001/jamapediatrics.2021.5544

White, S. W., Oswald, D., Ollendick, T., & Scahill, L. (2009). Anxiety in children and adolescents with autism spectrum disorders. *Clinical Psychology Review, 29*(3), 216–229. https://doi.org/10.1016/j.cpr.2009.01.003

Whitehouse, A. J. O., Varcin, K. J., Pillar, S., Billingham, W., Alvares, G. A., Barbaro, J., et al. (2021). Effect of preemptive intervention on developmental outcomes among infants showing early signs of autism A randomized clinical trial of outcomes to diagnosis. *JAMA Pediatrics, 175*(11). https://doi.org/10.1001/jamapediatrics.2021.3298

Whitfield-Gabrieli, S., & Ford, J. M. (2012). In S. Nolen-Hoeksema (Ed.), *Default Mode Network activity and connectivity in psychopathology* (Vol. 8, p. 49). Annual Review of Clinical Psychology.

Wickstrom, J., Farmer, C., Snyder, L. G., Mitz, A. R., Sanders, S. J., Bishop, S., & Thurm, A. (2021). Patterns of delay in early gross motor and expressive language milestone attainment in probands with genetic conditions versus idiopathic ASD from SFARI registries. *Journal of Child Psychology and Psychiatry, 62*(11), 1297–1307. https://doi.org/10.1111/jcpp.13492

Wing, L. (1980). Childhood autism and social class - a question of selection. *British Journal of Psychiatry, 137*(NOV), 410–417. https://doi.org/10.1192/bjp.137.5.410

Winter, A. S., Fountain, C., Cheslack-Postava, K., & Bearman, P. S. (2020). The social patterning of autism diagnoses reversed in California between 1992 and 2018. *Proceedings of the National Academy of Sciences of the United States of America, 117*(48), 30295–30302. https://doi.org/10.1073/pnas.2015762117

Wolfers, T., Floris, D. L., Dinga, R., van Rooij, D., Isakoglou, C., Kia, S. M., et al. (2019). From pattern classification to stratification: Towards conceptualizing the heterogeneity of Autism Spectrum Disorder. *Neuroscience and Biobehavioral Reviews, 104*, 240–254. https://doi.org/10.1016/j.neubiorev.2019.07.010

Wolfers, T., Beckmann, C. F., Hoogman, M., Buitelaar, J. K., Franke, B., & Marquand, A. F. (2020). Individual differences v. the average patient: Mapping the heterogeneity in ADHD using normative models. *Psychological Medicine, 50*(2), 314–323. https://doi.org/10.1017/s0033291719000084

Wolff, S. (2004). The history of autism. *European Child and Adolescent Psychiatry, 13*(4), 201–208. https://doi.org/10.1007/s00787-004-0363-5

Wu, S., Wu, F., Ding, Y., Hou, J., Bi, J., & Zhang, Z. (2017). Advanced parental age and autism risk in children: A systematic review and meta-analysis. *Acta Psychiatrica Scandinavica, 135*(1), 29–41. https://doi.org/10.1111/acps.12666

Yoon, S., Munoz, A., Yamrom, B., Lee, Y. H., Andrews, P., Marks, S., et al. (2021). Rates of contributory de novo mutation in high and low-risk autism families. *Communications Biology, 4*(1), Article 1026. https://doi.org/10.1038/s42003-021-02533-z

Yu, X., Rahman, M. M., Wang, Z. Y., Carter, S. A., Schwartz, J., Chen, Z. H., et al. (2022). Evidence of susceptibility to autism risks associated with early life ambient air pollution: A systematic review. *Environmental Research, 208*, Article 112590. https://doi.org/10.1016/j.envres.2021.112590

Zabihi, M., Oldehinkel, M., Wolfers, T., Frouin, V., Goyard, D., Loth, E., et al. (2019). Dissecting the heterogeneous cortical anatomy of Autism Spectrum Disorder using normative models. *Biological Psychiatry-Cognitive Neuroscience and Neuroimaging, 4*(6), 567–578. https://doi.org/10.1016/j.bpsc.2018.11.013

Zhan, Y., Wei, J., Liang, J., Xu, X., He, R., Robbins, T. W., & Wang, Z. (2021). Diagnostic classification for human autism and obsessive-compulsive disorder based on machine learning from a primate genetic model. *American Journal of Psychiatry, 178*(1), 65–76. https://doi.org/10.1176/appi.ajp.2020.19101091

Zhang, T., Brander, G., Mantel, A., Kuja-Halkola, R., Stephansson, O., Chang, Z., et al. (2021). Assessment of cesarean delivery and neurodevelopmental and psychiatric disorders in the children of a population-based Swedish birth cohort. *Jama Network Open, 4*(3), e210837. https://doi.org/10.1001/jamanetworkopen.2021.0837

Zhang, M., Wu, Y. R., Lu, Z. X., Song, M. Y., Huang, X. L., Mi, L. L., et al. (2023). Effects of Vitamin D supplementation on children with Autism Spectrum Disorder: A systematic review and meta-analysis. *Clinical Psychopharmacology and Neuroscience, 21*(2), 240–251. https://doi.org/10.9758/cpn.2023.21.2.240

Zheng, Z., Zhu, T. T., Qu, Y., & Mu, D. Z. (2016). Blood glutamate levels in Autism Spectrum Disorder: A systematic review and meta-analysis. *Plos One, 11*(7), e0158688. https://doi.org/10.1371/journal.pone.0158688

Index

J. Stevenson, *Developmental Psychopathology*, https://doi.org/10.1007/978-3-031-45787-6